# SURGERY OF THE EAR

### THIRD EDITION

## GEORGE E. SHAMBAUGH, Jr., M.D.

Emeritus Professor of Otolaryngology
Northwestern University
Chicago, Illinois

## MICHAEL E. GLASSCOCK, III, M.D.

Clinical Associate Professor of Surgery
    and of Hearing and Speech
Vanderbilt University
Nashville, Tennessee

W. B. SAUNDERS COMPANY
Philadelphia  London  Toronto

W. B. Saunders Company:   West Washington Square
Philadelphia, PA   19105

1 St. Anne's Road
Eastbourne, East Sussex BN21 3UN, England

1 Goldthorne Avenue
Toronto, Ontario M8Z 5T9, Canada

**Library of Congress Cataloging in Publication Data**

Shambaugh, George Elmer, 1903–

Surgery of the ear.

1. Ear — Surgery.      I. Glasscock, Michael E., 1933–
   joint author.     II. Title. [DNLM: 1. Ear — Surgery.
   WV200 S528s]

RF126.S5 1980        617.8′059        79–92613

ISBN 0–7216–8142–5

Surgery of the Ear                                              ISBN   0-7216-8142-5

Last digit is the print number:    9    8    7    6    5    4    3    2

*To the Memory of*

# GUNNAR HOLMGREN

Father of Microsurgery of the Ear

*this book is dedicated*

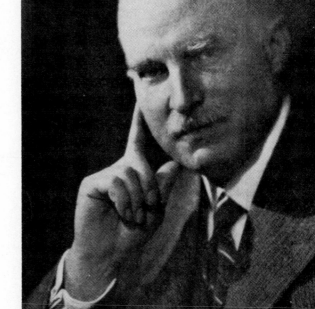

*Gunnar Holmgren*

BORN 1875
DIED 1954

Pioneer in fenestration surgery, the first to use the binocular operating microscope, founder of the *Acta oto-laryngologica*.

Author of the First and Second Editions of *Surgery of the Ear* and Senior Co-author of the Third Edition. Emeritus Professor of Otolaryngology, Northwestern University. Recipient of Honorary Doctorate, University of Freiburg, 1967, and University of Bordeaux, 1980. Founder of the Shambaugh Ear Institute.

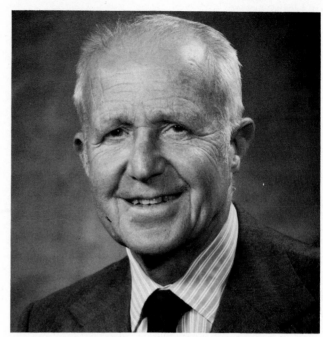

*George E. Shambaugh, Jr.*

Founder of *The American Journal of Otology* and student of William F. House. Special interest in teaching anatomy of the temporal bone and in neurotology.

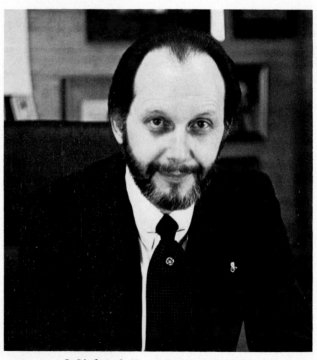

*Michael E. Glasscock, III*

# Preface

Thirteen years have elapsed since preparation of the Second Edition of *Surgery of the Ear*. Most of the principles and techniques described in the Second Edition remain valid today and have been retained with few changes. Added to this Third Edition are intact canal wall techniques and osteoplastic epitympanotomy for chronic ear surgery, with improved tympanoplasty methods that are yielding better hearing results. New are middle fossa surgery pioneered by William House and skull base operations pioneered by Ugo Fisch that contribute to the new sub-specialty of Neurotology.

Co-author of this Third Edition is Michael Glasscock who has rewritten parts of some chapters, most of a few chapters.

The authors wish to thank all those who have assisted in the monumental task of revising an entire text. Particular gratitude is due to Galdino Valvassori who within two decades has become recognized as the world's foremost authority in radiologic diagnosis of ear disease. Mrs. Lorayn Disosway has worked faithfully and well to complete the innumerable details in preparing and correcting the manuscript.

The senior author acknowledges once again the support and encouragement of his wife, Gene, and son, David, without whom the task would still remain unfinished.

Last, but by no means least, the authors wish to thank Richard J. Wiet for his well-done *Surgical Anatomy of the Temporal Bone Through Dissection* that is a companion to *Surgery of the Ear*, Third Edition, and that replaces the dissection instructions in the Second Edition.

George E. Shambaugh, Jr.
Shambaugh Ear Institute
40 South Clay Street
Hinsdale, Illinois 60521

Michael E. Glasscock, III
The Otology Group
1811 State Street
Nashville, Tennessee 37203

# Contents

*Part one   Introduction to Surgery of the Ear*

*Chapter 1*
DEVELOPMENTAL ANATOMY OF THE EAR........................................................ 5

*Chapter 2*
SURGICAL ANATOMY OF THE TEMPORAL BONE.................................... 31

*Chapter 3*
DIAGNOSIS OF EAR DISEASE........................................................ 53

*Chapter 4*
CONVENTIONAL RADIOLOGIC EXAMINATION OF THE TEMPORAL BONE................ 84
    *by W. E. Compere, Jr.*

*Chapter 5*
TOMOGRAPHY OF THE TEMPORAL BONE........................................ 112
    *by Galdino E. Valvassori*

*Chapter 6*
PRINCIPLES OF TEMPORAL BONE SURGERY ............................... 155

*Part two   Surgery of Infections of the Ear*

*Chapter 7*
PATHOLOGY AND CLINICAL COURSE OF INFLAMMATORY DISEASES OF
THE MIDDLE EAR........................................................ 186

*Chapter 8*
OPERATIONS ON THE AURICLE, EXTERNAL MEATUS AND TYMPANIC
MEMBRANE ........................................................ 221

*Chapter 9*
THE SIMPLE MASTOID OPERATION ............................... 251

*Chapter 10*
THE RADICAL AND BONDY MODIFIED RADICAL MASTOID OPERATIONS.................. 267

*Chapter 11*
MENINGEAL COMPLICATIONS OF OTITIS MEDIA.............................. 289

*Chapter 12*
NON-MENINGEAL COMPLICATIONS OF OTITIS MEDIA ....................... 317

*Part three   Surgery of Deafness*

*Chapter 13*
MECHANICS OF HEARING ........................................... 351

*Chapter 14*
SURGICAL CORRECTION OF CONGENITAL MALFORMATIONS OF THE
SOUND-CONDUCTING MECHANISM ..................................... 380

*Chapter 15*
CLOSURE OF TYMPANIC MEMBRANE PERFORATIONS......................... 408

*Chapter 16*
TYMPANOPLASTY .................................................. 425

*Chapter 17*
DIAGNOSIS, INDICATIONS FOR SURGERY AND MEDICAL THERAPY OF
OTOSPONGIOSIS (OTOSCLEROSIS)..................................... 455

*Chapter 18*
STAPES OPERATIONS FOR OTOSPONGIOSIS (OTOSCLEROSIS)................ 477

*Chapter 19*
FENESTRATION OPERATION FOR OTOSPONGIOSIS (OTOSCLEROSIS) ......... 501

*Part four   Surgery of the Facial Nerve, Endolymphatic
              Hydrops and Tumors of the Ear*

*Chapter 20*
FACIAL NERVE DECOMPRESSION AND REPAIR............................. 519

*Chapter 21*
SURGICAL TREATMENT OF ENDOLYMPHATIC HYDROPS...................... 559

*Chapter 22*
SURGERY OF TUMORS OF THE EAR .................................... 595

*Chapter 23*
ACOUSTIC NEUROMA AND TUMORS OF THE CEREBELLOPONTINE ANGLE................ 637

*Surgical Anatomy of the Temporal Bone Through Dissection* ............. 675

INDEX OF NAMES......................................................................... 727

INDEX OF SUBJECTS ...................................................................... 733

# Surgery of the Ear

*As to Diseases, make a habit of two things: to help or at least to do no harm.*

HIPPOCRATES

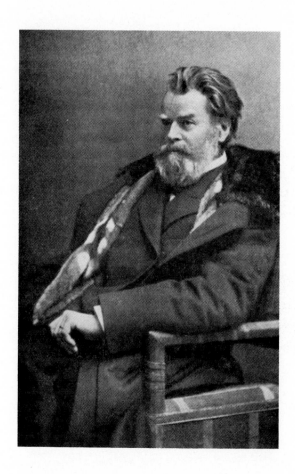

*Friedrich Bezold*

BORN 1842
DIED 1908

Clarified the differentiation by tuning fork tests of conductive and sensorineural hearing losses and the clinical diagnosis of otosclerosis (otospongiosis). His clear and concise Textbook of Otology served as a model for this Surgery of the Ear.

# Part One

*"You will easily recognize that there is hardly another part of the body which calls for higher qualifications on the part of the operator as to anatomical knowledge than the temporal bone. . . ."*

BEZOLD

# Introduction to Surgery of the Ear

## Theodore H. Bast

BORN 1890
DIED 1959

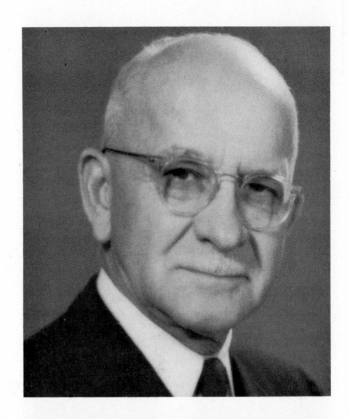

First described the utriculo-endolymphatic valve, and with Barry Anson restudied the developmental anatomy of the ear and temporal bone.

## Barry J. Anson

BORN 1894
DIED 1974

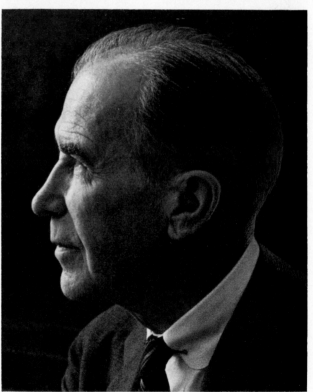

Student and investigator par excellence of the gross and developmental anatomy of the temporal bone.

# Chapter 1

# Developmental Anatomy of the Ear

This chapter is based on the original researches of
PROFESSOR BARRY ANSON
and PROFESSOR T. H. BAST.[1]

ORIGIN AND DEVELOPMENT OF THE ENDOLYMPHATIC
  (OTIC) LABYRINTH
DEVELOPMENT OF THE PERILYMPHATIC (PERIOTIC)
  LABYRINTH
DEVELOPMENT OF THE BONY LABYRINTH
DEVELOPMENT OF THE OUTER AND MIDDLE EAR
DEVELOPMENT OF THE PNEUMATIC CELLS OF THE
  TEMPORAL BONE
TEMPORAL BONE OF THE INFANT COMPARED TO THAT
  OF THE CHILD AND ADULT

An intimate knowledge of the **embryology** of the ear is necessary for the surgeon of the temporal bone, to help him to anticipate the anatomic variations that render operations within this crowded area difficult and hazardous, and to aid him in recognizing and surgically correcting congenital malformations of the sound-conducting system.

The developmental history of the ear is remarkable and without parallel in other organs of the human body in these respects:

The inner ear is the only organ that reaches full adult size and complete differentiation by midterm, even before the tiny fetus has become a viable premature infant.

The labyrinthine capsule and ossicles are the only parts of the osseous skeleton that retain primitive endochondral bone throughout the life span of the individual, and it is here that the unique disease of otospongiosis (otosclerosis) occurs. Everywhere else endochondral bone initially formed in cartilage is later removed and replaced by haversian periosteal bone.

The two functional parts of the hearing mechanism come from different and widely separated anlages. The sound-perceiving sensorineural apparatus of the inner ear comes from the ectodermal otocyst; the sound-conducting mechanism is derived from the branchial or gill structure of the embryo. In no other organ of the human body have our lowly phylogenetic ancestors left their trace more clearly.

## ORIGIN AND DEVELOPMENT OF THE ENDOLYMPHATIC (OTIC) LABYRINTH

The earliest beginning of the ear is seen in the 3 week old human embryo as a platelike thickening of ectoderm on either side of the head near the hindbrain. This **otic placode** invaginates in a few days to form the **otic pit** (Fig. 1–1), and in a few more days, by the fourth week of embryonic life, the mouth of the pit has narrowed and fused to form the **otocyst.** The ectodermal-lined, fluid-filled otocyst constitutes the primitive otic or endolymphatic labyrinth, and it proceeds to differentiate by a series of folds and elongations as follows:

At 4½ weeks the oval-shaped otocyst has elongated and begun to divide into an endolymphatic duct and sac portion and a utricular-saccular portion. In a few more days archlike outpocketings of the utricular portion of the otic vesicle appear, which by 7 weeks have formed the three **semicircular canals.** Meanwhile, at 6 weeks (Fig. 1–2) the last part of the otic labyrinth to appear begins as a short evagination of the saccule, the **cochlea.** By 8 weeks it has elongated and begun to coil, and by 11 weeks it has formed nearly all of its two and a half turns.

As these appendages of the otic vesicle appear and develop, a constriction occurs between the utricle and saccule to form the longer **utricular duct** and the shorter **saccular duct,** which join to form the common **endolymphatic duct.** The otic or endolymphatic labyrinth, at first quite small, steadily enlarges despite its encasement in cartilage until midterm, at which time the endolymphatic labyrinth has reached the complicated adult form from which it derives its name (Fig. 1–3). The cartilaginous otic capsule then ossifies, preventing any further growth.

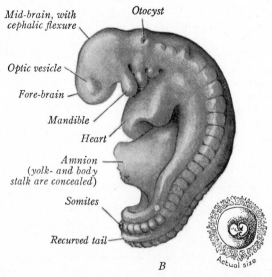

*Mid-brain, with cephalic flexure*

*Otocyst*

*Optic vesicle*

*Fore-brain*

*Mandible*

*Heart*

*Amnion (yolk- and body stalk are concealed)*

*Somites*

*Recurved tail*

*B*

*Actual size*

**Figure 1–1**  Human embryo of 26 days, showing first and second branchial grooves and the otic pit preliminary to formation of otocyst. (From Arey, L. B.: Developmental Anatomy, 7th ed., revised. Philadelphia, W. B. Saunders Co., 1974.)

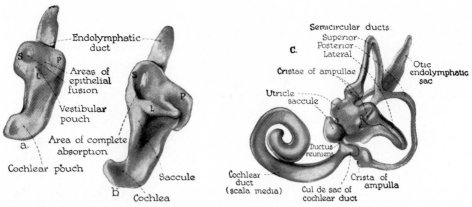

**Figure 1–2** Development in a 3 week period of the membranous labyrinth, shown by reconstructions. *a*, Five weeks (8 mm.), ×27. *b*, Six weeks (13 mm.), ×27. *c*, Eight weeks (30 mm.), ×14. (From Anson, B. J.: Morris' Human Anatomy, 12th ed. New York, McGraw-Hill Book Co., 1966.)

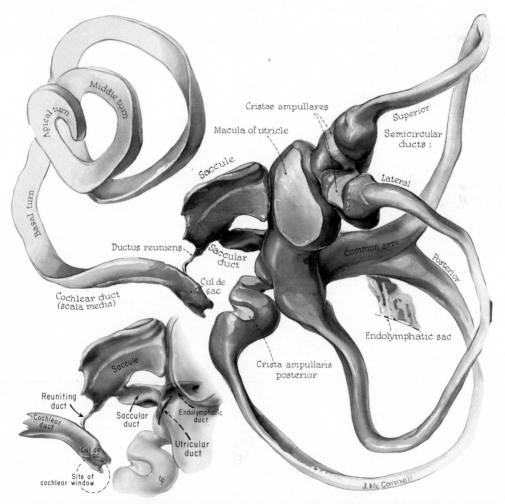

**Figure 1–3** Drawing of a reconstruction of the lumen of the membranous labyrinth. Anterolateral view. Mature form. Only the proximal part of the endolymphatic sac is included. Inset: Demonstrating the ducts that bring the utricle into communication with the saccule and the cochlear duct. (From Anson, B. J., Harper, D. G., and Winch, T. R.: The vestibular system. Anatomic considerations. Arch. Otol., 85:497–514, 1967.)

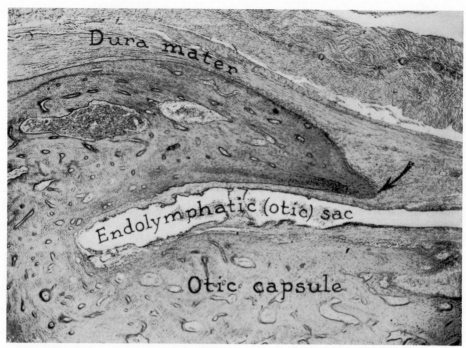

**Figure 1–4**   Photomicrograph of endolymphatic sac, infant of 10 weeks, showing osseous portion with rugose epithelium and dural portion with smooth epithelium. (From Anson, B. J., and Bast, T. H. *In* Coates, G. N., et al.: Otolaryngology. Hagerstown, Md., W. F. Prior Co., 1955.)

Noteworthy is the fact that the endolymphatic duct and sac are the earliest appendages of the otic vesicle to appear; and unlike the rest of the endolymphatic labyrinth that reaches adult shape and size by midterm, the duct and sac continue to change and enlarge throughout infancy and childhood until after puberty. The adult endolymphatic sac lies half within bone, where its epithelium is in many folds with a vascular subepithelial connective tissue, and half between two layers of the

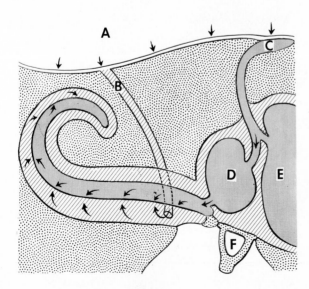

**Figure 1–5**   Increased cerebrospinal fluid pressure (*A*) causes cerebrospinal fluid to enter the perilymphatic system through the cochlear aqueduct (*B*). Pressure on the walls of the endolymphatic sac (*C*) forces endolymph into the labyrinth to equalize pressure on the walls of the endolymphatic labyrinth, including the cochlear partition. *D*, Saccule. *E*, Utricle. *F*, Stapes. (From Allen, G. W.: Endolymphatic sac and cochlear aqueduct. Arch. Otol., 79:322, 1964.)

dura mater, where its walls are smooth (Fig. 1–4). This morphology, and the fact that the sac appears so early in embryonic life and continues to enlarge until in the adult it is threefold larger than at birth, point toward definite and important functions. Resorption of endolymph is one probability; a hydrostatic equilibratory mechanism has been suggested more recently[2, 3] to equalize intracranial and intralabyrinthine pressure in the endolymphatic system (Fig. 1–5), as is accomplished by the perilymphatic duct (cochlear aqueduct) for the perilymphatic system. The rugose walls of the endolymphatic duct and proximal portion of the sac, its columnar epithelium with the nuclei lying in the outer portion of the cells, as in resorptive epithelium elsewhere, and the rich venous drainage from the surrounding loose connective tissue all provide a structure suited for fluid resorption.

Mention should be made of a flaplike fold at the opening of the utricular duct to the utricle (Fig. 1–6), a constant finding in man and all common laboratory animals.

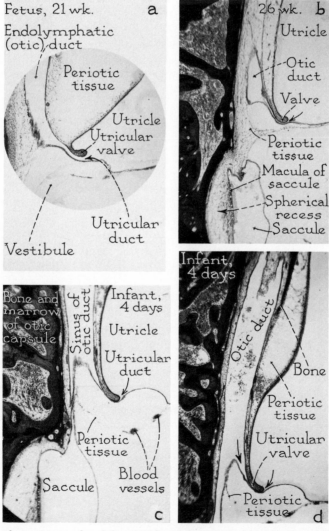

**Figure 1–6** Photomicrographs of the utriculoendolymphatic fold, or valve of Bast, in the 21 and 26 week fetus (a and b) and in the newborn (c and d). Observe that adult form and size are attained in the fetus. (Courtesy of Dr. Barry J. Anson.)

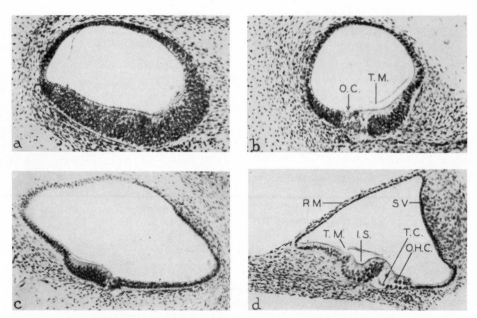

**Figure 1–7** Photomicrograph of development of the cochlear duct. *a*, Apical turn in 12 week fetus showing thickening of epithelium of sensory area. *b*, Middle turn at 12 weeks showing organ of Corti *(O.C.)* and tectorial membrane *(T.M.)*. *c*, Apical turn in 15 week fetus. *d*, Basal turn in 15 week fetus: *(R.M.)* Reissner's membrane, *(S.V.)* stria vascularis, *(I.S.)* internal sulcus, *(T.C.)* cortis tunnel, *(O.H.C.)* outer hair cells. (From Anson, B. J., and Bast, T. H. *In* Coates, G. N., et al.: Otolaryngology. Hagerstown, Md., W. F. Prior Co., 1955.)

Its shape suggests a valve function, as though to prevent utricular endolymph from returning to the endolymphatic duct. It is known as the utriculoendolymphatic valve of Bast, after its discoverer.

As the complicated convolutions of the endolymphatic labyrinth develop, its sensory end-organs begin to appear as localized thickenings of the epithelium. First in the utricle and saccule between weeks 7 and 8, then in the semicircular canals at 8 weeks, and lastly in the cochlea at 12 weeks, the epithelium in localized areas assumes a pseudostratified form and then begins to differentiate into two types of cells, the sensory cells with bristlelike hairs at their free margin and the supporting cells that secrete a gelatinous substance to form the cushionlike membrane into which the hairs penetrate (Fig. 1–7). Complete differentiation in the cochlea lags until after midterm. Thus the order of acquisition in phylogenetic evolution of the sensory end-organs of the labyrinth parallels their order of embryonic development. The more recently acquired cochlear end-organ not only is the last in the labyrinth to differentiate, but also is less stable and more subject to developmental malformation and acquired disease than the older vestibular end-organs.

## DEVELOPMENT OF THE PERILYMPHATIC (PERIOTIC) LABYRINTH

As the otocyst begins to differentiate, the mesenchyme surrounding it begins to condense at 6½ weeks, becoming precartilage at 7 weeks. At 8 weeks the precartilage surrounding the otic labyrinth changes to an outer zone of true cartilage to form the otic capsule, while the inner zone begins to loosen and vacuolize to form the periotic or perilymphatic space. Fluid-filled spaces appear first around the vestibule, then on either side of the endolymphatic cochlear duct to form the scala tympani and scala vestibuli, and last around the semicircular canals. These spaces fuse until there is a continuous fluid-filled perilymphatic labyrinth containing a delicate mesh of arachnoid-like connective tissue, except in the scala tympani and scala vestibuli where the connective tissue network is absent to permit a completely free to-and-fro vibratory movement of the perilymph between the oval and round windows. The scala tympani ends at the round window membrane in the basal coil of the cochlea, and its only connection with the rest of the perilymphatic system is through the helicotrema to the scala vestibuli around the blind end of the endolymphatic cochlear duct.

The perilymphatic space has three principal prolongations into the surrounding osseous otic capsule: the **perilymphatic** (periotic) **duct** (or cochlear aqueduct), the **fissula ante fenestram** and the **fossula post fenestram.**

The **perilymphatic duct** is not a true duct, since it is not lined by epithelium. Rather it is a narrow space filled with fluid and an arachnoid-type connective tissue, that extends from the scala tympani near the round window to the subarachnoid space near the emergence of the glossopharyngeal nerve. It varies considerably in size in the adult; it is usually flaring at its extremities and constricted in its midportion, where the fluid space may be extremely narrow. Cerebrospinal fluid is believed to filter through the perilymphatic duct into the scala tympani and from there to go via the helicotrema and scala vestibuli to the remainder of the perilymphatic spaces. However, such filtration, at least in man, must be extremely slow in view of the narrowness of the fluid spaces within the perilymphatic duct. This accounts for the clinical observation that when the perilymphatic space is opened surgically the perilymph does not escape in considerable quantities. The profuse flow of perilymph encountered occasionally upon perforating or removing the stapes footplate is probably due to an abnormally wide and patent perilymphatic duct (cochlear aqueduct). See Figure 1–8.

The **fissula ante fenestram** is of great clinical interest because of its relationship to otosclerosis. It consists of an irregular ribbon of connective tissue that extends through the bony otic capsule from the vestibule just anterior to the oval window ("ante fenestram") to the tympanic cavity near the processus cochleariformis (Fig. 1–9). The moderately vascular connective tissue in the fissula is continuous with the perilymphatic connective tissue mesh in the labyrinth at one end of the fissula and with the subepithelial connective tissue in the middle ear at its other end.

This constant structure is unique to man, although a rudimentary incomplete fissula was observed by the senior author in a rhesus monkey. It appears quite early in the human embryo, at 9 weeks, but does not extend all the way through the cartilaginous capsule from the middle ear to the vestibule until 10 or 12 weeks. It proceeds to grow in size from week 12 to 21, at which time the ossification of the otic capsule approaches completion. The fissula ante fenestram, once it is completely formed in midfetal life, remains remarkably constant until old age, but it shows considerable individual variations in size and shape. At first it is bordered by a rim of cartilage separating its connective tissue from the surrounding bone, but with advancing age this rim of cartilage is reduced and largely disappears. The constancy of the fissular tract in man suggests a function — perhaps, as suggested by Bast, that of supplementing the limited opportunities for perilymph resorption.

Two types of pathologic tissue are frequently found in the fissular region: a mass of newly formed cartilage (Fig. 1–10) or a mass of newly formed gnarly bone (Fig.

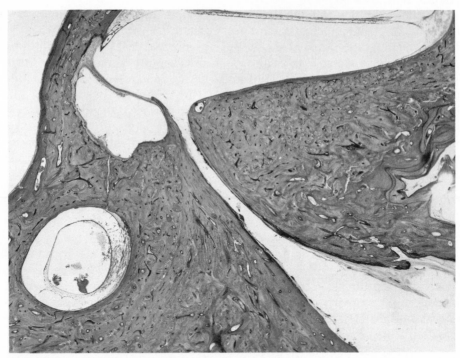

**Figure 1–8**  Large abnormally patent cochlear aqueduct, adult human. (Courtesy of Dr. H. F. Schuknecht.)

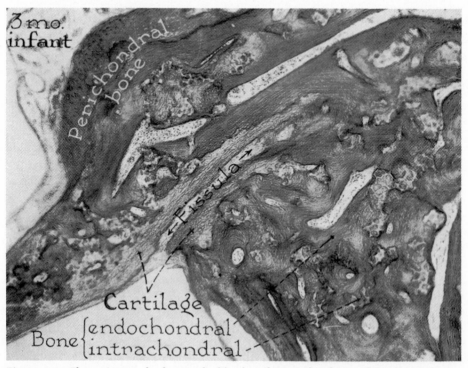

**Figure 1–9**  Photomicrograph of 3 month old infant showing fissula ante fenestram with vascular spaces of adjacent otic capsule nearly obliterated by endochondral bone. (From Anson, B. J., and Bast, T. H. *In* Coates, G. M., et al.: Otolaryngology. Hagerstown, Md., W. F. Prior Co., 1955.)

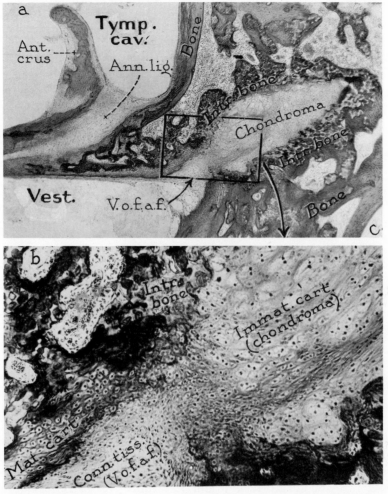

**Figure 1–10**  Photomicrographs of fissula ante fenestram in which the normal connective tissue was replaced by cartilage. *a*, The fissula and related structures. *b*, Detail of the area blocked in *a*. *Ann. lig.*, Annular ligament; *Ant. crus*, anterior crus; *C.*, cochlea; *Conn. tiss.*, connective tissue; *Immat. cart.*, immature cartilage; *Intr. bone*, intrachondral bone; *Mat. cart.*, mature cartilage; *Tymp. cav.*, tympanic cavity; *Vest.*, vestibule; *V.o.f.a.f.*, vestibular orifice of fissula ante fenestram. (From Anson, B. J., Cauldwell, E. W., and Bast, T. H.: The fissula ante fenestram of the human otic capsule. II. Aberrant form and contents. Ann. Otol. Rhin. & Laryng., 57:103, 1948.)

1–11). These occur in especially wide fissulas, as though to reduce the excessive amount of connective tissue. The new bone may remain confined to the fissula, or it may extend beyond into the adjacent endochondral layer of the capsule, replacing the solid avascular endochondral and intrachondral bone by a relatively spongy vascular bone with irregularly arranged lamellae and lacking the islands of ossified cartilage that characterize the normal endochondral layer of the capsule. Such a focus of new bone may remain inactive, or, according to Bast and Anson, it may undergo remodeling and slow expansion to become an active focus of otospongiosis, or so-called otosclerosis. Since this new bone at first is less dense than the endochondral capsule that it replaces, it should be termed otospongiosis instead of the popular misnomer otosclerosis. The nodule of otospongiosis may recalcify and become inactive, or it may slowly enlarge to approach or reach the cochlear

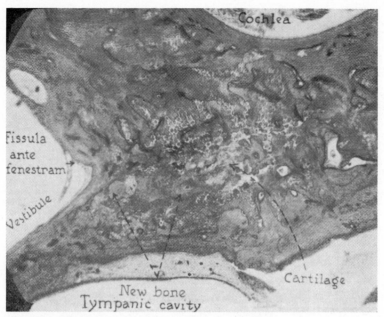

**Figure 1–11** Photomicrograph showing new bone formation in fissula ante fenestram, child age 10. This may represent the earliest stage of histologic otosclerosis.

endosteum or the oval window, causing a sensorineural loss in the former or a conductive loss due to stapes fixation in the latter situation (Fig. 1–12).

The **fossula post fenestram** is a connective tissue tract just behind the oval window, resembling the fissula ante fenestram but as a rule smaller and less constant. It is found in about two thirds of human ears, and in only 15 per cent of ears does it extend through the capsule to the tympanic cavity, being pouchlike and confined to the vestibule in most cases. Like the fissula ante fenestram, the fossula post fenestram may be the site for the later occurrence of a focus of gnarly new bone of otospongiosis.

## DEVELOPMENT OF THE BONY LABYRINTH

The ossification of the fetal cartilaginous otic capsule is unique in several respects. In other bones ossification begins soon after the first cartilage appears and proceeds as the cartilage is added to, whereas in the otic capsule the cartilage attains maximum growth and maturity before ossification begins. Ossification of its capsule is an important event in the development of the inner ear, for once it has occurred, further growth of the rigidly encased inner ear structure ceases. The other peculiarity of the otic capsule (and ossicles), already alluded to, is that the endochondral bone initially formed from cartilage is never removed and replaced by periosteal haversian bone, as occurs in all other bones of the skeleton, but remains throughout life as a primitive, relatively avascular type of bone of petrous hardness, poor in its osteogenic response, with scant bone remodeling activity, and subject to local replacement by pathologic otospongiotic bone in about 10 per cent of human ears.

The first ossification center appears around the cochlea when it reaches adult size in the 16th week of fetal life. The last center appears around the semicircular

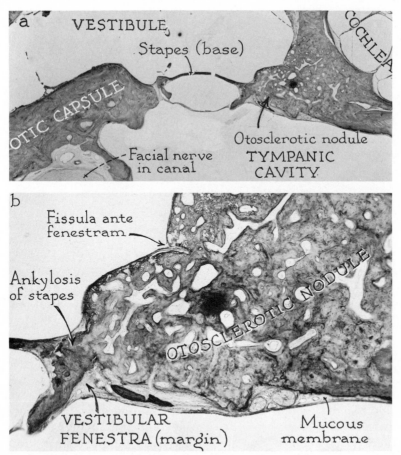

**Figure 1–12** Photomicrograph of an otosclerotic lesion in a female 50 years of age. The patient, diagnosed 15 years earlier, had a successful fenestration by the senior author of this text two years before her death. *a,* Showing the entire stapes and the adjacent areas of the temporal bone. *b,* Details of histologic structure. (Courtesy of Dr. Barry J. Anson.)

canals when they cease to grow in the 21st or 22nd week. There are 14 centers in all. Once it has begun, ossification occurs rapidly, until by the 23rd week it is complete except for an area over the horizontal semicircular canal, and a narrow rim of cartilage that remains around the oval window and the fissula ante fenestram.

The first step in the ossification of the fetal cartilaginous otic capsule begins with an enlargement of the cartilage cells in their lacunas and a simultaneous deposition of calcium in the cartilage matrix between them (Fig. 1–13). Several osteogenic cells from the periosteum now migrate into the lacuna of each enlarged cartilage cell and proceed to lay down **intrachondral bone** inside the lacuna. While this is occurring, capillary buds from the periosteum enter and excavate irregular areas of cartilage, but leave irregular islands of unexcavated cartilage, which is being ossified by the deposition of calcium in its matrix and of intrachondral bone in its lacunas (Fig. 1–14). As the final step osteoblasts line up around the island of ossified cartilage and proceed to lay down concentric layers of dense **endochondral bone**, gradually narrowing the wide vascular spaces until the original cartilaginous otic capsule has been replaced by an excessively hard, almost avascular endochondral bone containing irregular spicules of intrachondral bone. Meanwhile a thin uniform layer of **endosteal bone** is laid down against the endosteal membrane that lines the

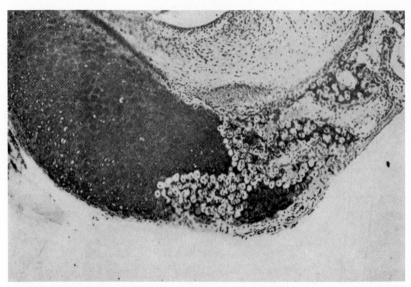

**Figure 1–13** Photomicrograph of 15 cm. pig embryo showing first step in ossification of the cartilaginous otic capsule, with excavation of cartilage by vascular loops from the perichondrium. (Figures 1–13, 1–14 and 1–15 from sections made by George Shambaugh, Sr., circa 1903.)

labyrinth, while outside the endochondral layer periosteal bone is laid down in parallel lamellae (Fig. 1–15).

Once they have formed in midfetal life, the thin inner endosteal layer and the thicker middle endochondral layer of the labyrinthine capsule remain relatively inert and unchanged throughout life, except for gradual conversion of the fetal cancellous endochondral layer into the petrous endochondral bone of the adult (Fig. 1–16). In response to infection or trauma to the endosteal membrane lining the

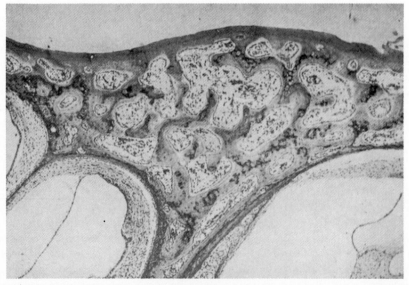

**Figure 1–14** Photomicrograph of 18 cm. pig embryo showing second step in ossification of the otic capsule. Islands of unexcavated cartilage show beginning ossification, with osteoblasts lining the numerous wide vascular spaces.

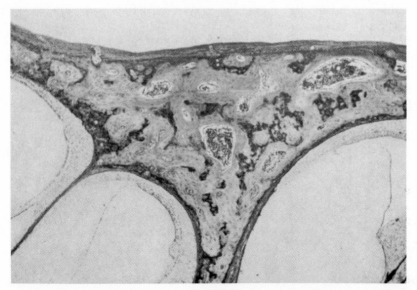

**Figure 1–15**  Photomicrograph of 25 cm. pig embryo showing last stage of ossification of the otic capsule. Whorls of bone are filling the vascular spaces between the islands of ossified cartilage to form the endochondral layer of the otic capsule. Parallel lamellae of periosteal bone are beginning to form around the endochondral layer. A thin layer of endosteal bone has formed between the endosteum and the endochondral layer.

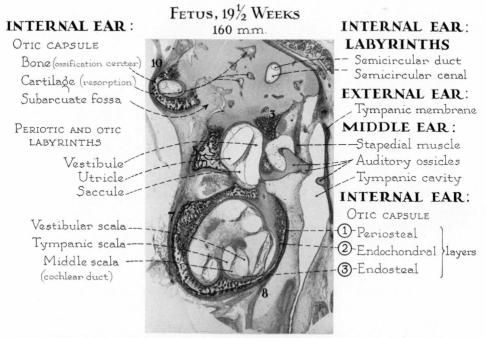

FETUS, 19½ WEEKS
160 mm.

INTERNAL EAR :

OTIC CAPSULE

  Bone (ossification center)   10

  Cartilage (resorption)

  Subarcuate fossa

PERIOTIC AND OTIC
LABYRINTHS

    Vestibule

    Utricle

    Saccule

Vestibular scala

Tympanic scala

Middle scala
(cochlear duct)

INTERNAL EAR :
LABYRINTHS

  Semicircular duct

  Semicircular canal

EXTERNAL EAR :

  Tympanic membrane

MIDDLE EAR :

  Stapedial muscle

  Auditory ossicles

  Tympanic cavity

INTERNAL EAR :

OTIC CAPSULE

  ① Periosteal

  ② Endochondral ⎱ layers

  ③ Endosteal

**Figure 1–16**  Stages in ossification of human cartilaginous labyrinthine capsule: Formation of foci of endochondral bone with thin endosteal layer of bone and thicker periosteal layer. (8 and 10 refer to ossification centers according to T. H. Bast's 1930 investigation.)

labyrinth, the endosteal layer of bone may proliferate, partially or completely obliterating the lumen of the labyrinth. The endochondral layer may also participate to a limited extent in osteogenic repair, but very poorly compared to periosteal bone, so that fractures through the labyrinth may remain unhealed except for fibrous union. The poor osteogenic response of endochondral bone makes possible the construction of a labyrinthine fenestra that remains permanently open in operations for stapedial otospongiosis. In some cases fracture of the stapes footplate (composed of endochondral bone) will fail to heal by new bone formation.

The periosteal bone of the labyrinthine capsule, at first a thin layer, rapidly thickens and continues to be added to during infancy and childhood until early adult life. Like periosteal bone elsewhere it is later removed and replaced by haversian bone containing marrow spaces, and eventually pneumatic cells invade most of the periosteal layer of the capsule along with much of the remainder of the temporal bone. Like all periosteal bone, that of the capsule undergoes remodeling and reacts readily to infection or trauma with osteogenesis.

## DEVELOPMENT OF THE OUTER AND MIDDLE EAR

The sound-conducting apparatus of the outer and middle ear is derived from the branchial or gill apparatus of the embryo (Fig. 1–17). The unique evolutionary process by which this occurred has clinical implications.

Water-borne sound vibrations pass easily through the skin of the head of aquatic forms to the fluid-filled otocyst, with but little loss of energy. However, owing to the differences in the physical properties of air and water, sound vibrations in air are largely reflected away from the surface of water, very little of the sound energy of air being transmitted to water. Actually 99.9 per cent of the energy of air-borne sound is reflected away, only 0.1 per cent entering the water. This very great **air-water sound barrier** may be observed by the underwater swimmer who hears very little of the sounds originating in the air above the water, but who hears very clearly sounds originating under water, such as two stones clicked together (Fig. 1–18).

As certain aquatic forms in the course of evolution began to emerge onto dry land, they required for survival a mechanism that would overcome the air-water sound barrier. Such a mechanism would convert air vibrations of large amplitude but small force into water vibrations of small amplitude but large force. As the lungs were developed for respiration, the abandoned gill apparatus became available for transformation into such an "impedance-matching" mechanism. As we shall see in Chapter 13, the sound-conducting apparatus of the middle ear effectively overcomes the air-water sound barrier.

The first primordium of the sound-conducting apparatus appears in the 4 week old human embryo when three protuberant branchial arches separated by two branchial grooves appear on either side of the embryonic head (Fig. 1–1). The third arch and the second branchial groove soon disappear except in rare cases when a cyst or cleft persists in the neck behind and below the external auditory meatus, sometimes extending inward as far as the tonsil (Fig. 1–19).

Meanwhile the first branchial groove deepens to become the primitive external auditory meatus, while the corresponding evagination from the pharynx, the first pharyngeal pouch, presses outward toward it. For a brief time the epithelium of the first branchial groove comes in contact with the entoderm of the first pharyngeal pouch, but soon mesoderm grows between and separates these two epithelial layers.

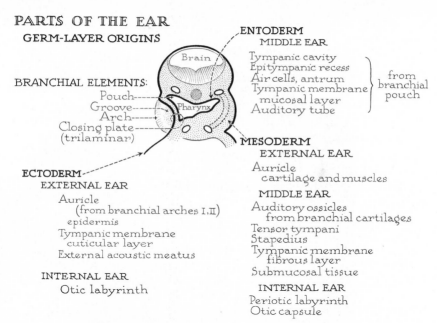

## PARTS OF THE EAR
### GERM-LAYER ORIGINS

Brain

Pharynx

**BRANCHIAL ELEMENTS:**
Pouch
Groove
Arch
Closing plate
(trilaminar)

**ENTODERM**
MIDDLE EAR
Tympanic cavity
Epitympanic recess
Air cells, antrum          } from
Tympanic membrane    } branchial
  mucosal layer          } pouch
Auditory tube

**MESODERM**
  EXTERNAL EAR
  Auricle
    cartilage and muscles
  MIDDLE EAR
  Auditory ossicles
    from branchial cartilages
  Tensor tympani
  Stapedius
  Tympanic membrane
    fibrous layer
  Submucosal tissue
  INTERNAL EAR
  Periotic labyrinth
  Otic capsule

**ECTODERM**
  EXTERNAL EAR
  Auricle
    (from branchial arches I, II)
    epidermis
  Tympanic membrane
    cuticular layer
  External acoustic meatus

  INTERNAL EAR
  Otic labyrinth

**Figure 1–17** Parts of the external, middle and internal divisions of the ear, listed on the basis of origin from the three germ layers of the embryonic body.

The primordium of the membranous (otic) labyrinth is the first element to appear, being derived from the ectodermal otocyst. The osseous (periotic) labyrinth, represented in the adult by the system of perilymphatic spaces, is formed around the membranous labyrinth through the resolution of mesenchymal tissue of mesodermal origin. From the same germ layer come the otic capsule and the auditory ossicles, the latter bones being made over, so to speak, from portions of the first and second branchial arches. The entoderm contributes the auditory tube and its continuities, namely, the epitympanic recess and antrum, the air cells of the mastoid and petrous parts of the temporal bone. Beginning as an extension of the first branchial pouch on the wall of the primitive pharynx, the constituent mucous membrane, in the course of its prolongation, invests the auditory ossicles and contributes the inner layer to the trilaminar tympanic membrane. (Courtesy of Dr. Barry J. Anson.)

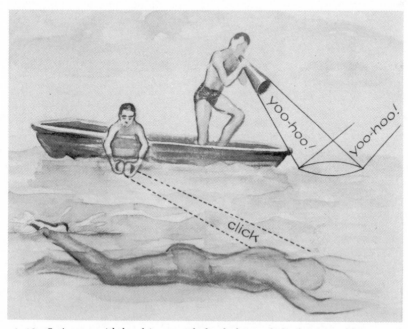

**Figure 1–18** Swimmer with head immersed clearly hears click of stones under water but not the voice above water.

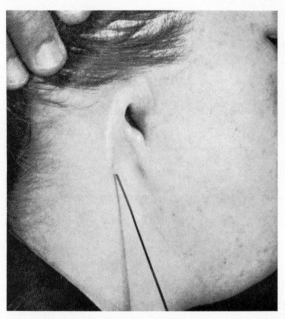

**Figure 1–19** Second branchial fistula (at end of pointer) in child with congenital absence of auricle and deformed meatus (first branchial groove).

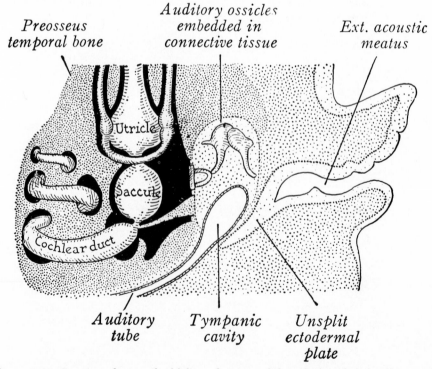

**Figure 1–20** Drawing of 3 month old fetus showing solid cord of epithelial cells extending toward the first pharyngeal pouch from the primitive meatus. (From Arey, L. B.: Developmental Anatomy, 7th ed., revised. Philadelphia, W. B. Saunders Co., 1974.)

Near the close of the second fetal month a solid core of epithelial cells grows inward from the primitive funnel-shaped meatus toward the epithelium of the pharyngeal pouch until only a thin seam of connective tissue intervenes, destined to become the circular and radiating fibers of the tense portion of the tympanic membrane (Fig. 1–20). The cord of epithelial cells remains solid until near the end of fetal life; meanwhile the connective tissue around the margin of the tympanic membrane ossifies to form the tympanic sulcus, beginning in the third month. Finally, in the seventh month of fetal life when all other structures of the outer, middle and inner ear are well differentiated, the solid core of epithelial cells splits, first in its deepest portion to form the outer surface of the tympanic membrane, and then extending outward to join the lumen of the primitive meatus. Thus it is that congenital atresia of the meatus may occur with a normally formed and functioning tympanic membrane and ossicular chain, as well as with various malformations of these structures, depending upon the age at which development was delayed or arrested.

The auricle develops around the first branchial groove from six knoblike outgrowths from the first and second branchial arches, which appear in the sixth week of embryonic life and then gradually fuse by the third month to form the auricle (Fig. 1–21). Earlier authors stated that the tragus and helix came from the first (mandibular) arch, and that the antihelix and antitragus were from the second

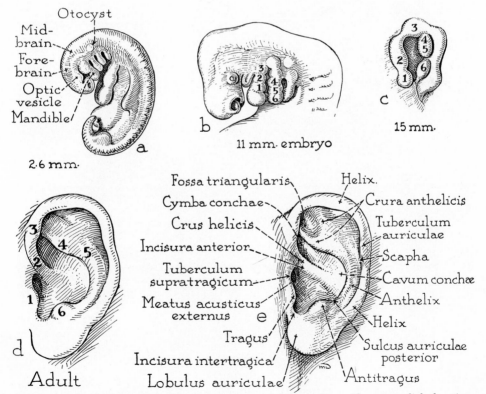

**Figure 1–21** Developmental and adult anatomy of the auricle. *a*, The primordial elevations on the first (mandibular) and second (hyoid) arches *(b)* which fuse *(c)* to form the adult auricle *(d)*, marked with numerals to indicate the derived parts. *e*, Adult form of the auricle with the parts identified. (From Anson, B. J.: Morris' Human Anatomy, 12th ed. New York, McGraw-Hill Book Co., 1966.)

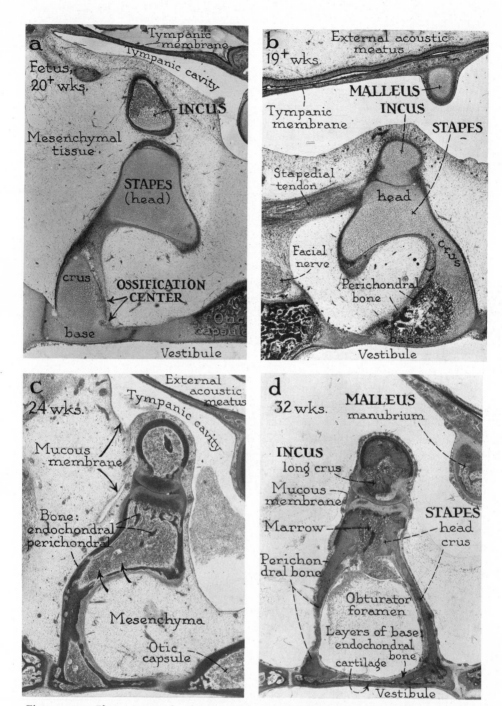

**Figure 1–22** Photomicrographs showing major steps in the development of the stapes. *a,* In the 5 month fetus the single ossification center has appeared at the crurobasal junction. *b,* In another specimen of approximately the same age, bone formation is further advanced, there being a thin layer of periosteal bone over the area of excavated cartilage. *c,* In the 6 month fetus the newly formed periosteal layer is being removed on the obturator aspect of the ossicle. *d,* At 8 months this process has been virtually completed; concurrently a thin layer of endosteal bone is deposited on the cartilage of the base (footplate) and of the head. (From Anson, B. J., and Bast, T. H., *In* Coates, G. M., et al.: Otolaryngology. Hagerstown, Md., W. F. Prior Co., 1955.)

(hyoid) arch, but more recent investigators conclude that all of the auricle save the tragus is from the second arch.

The first pharyngeal pouch becomes the eustachian tube and middle ear cavity; the cartilages of the first and second branchial arches proceed to form the ossicles, as follows:

In the 8 week fetus the tympanic cavity is present only in the lower part of the future middle ear, cellular mesenchyme occupying the upper half. Cartilaginous condensations within the mesenchyme of the first branchial arch begin to form most of the malleus and incus, and from the second branchial arch are formed the stapes, lenticular process of the incus and malleus handle. At first the malleus, incus and cartilaginous mandible are continuous as Meckel's cartilage of the first branchial arch, and the styloid process, hyoid, stapes, lenticular process of incus and malleus handle are continuous as Reichert's cartilage of the second branchial arch. Soon the ossicles separate from their parent cartilages and begin an independent growth. Their subsequent development is important to the surgeon because of the variations and not infrequent malformations encountered in operations.

The ossicles, like the otic capsule and labyrinth, grow only through the first half of uterine life, and then ossify. Each ossicle ossifies from a single center of ossification that appears in the incus at 16 weeks, in the malleus at 16½ weeks and in the stapes at 18 weeks. The ossicles are alike in that each is formed of endochondral bone that persists for the rest of the individual's life, just as does the endochondral layer of the labyrinthine capsule. The ossicles differ in that the incus and malleus remain solid and relatively constant in size and shape, whereas the stapes undergoes a curious process of erosion and thinning soon after it ossifies; the adult stapes is actually less bulky and considerably more delicate and fragile than in midfetal life (Fig. 1–22). With this diminution in bulk and weight there develop rather extraordinary variations in size, shape and strength of the adult crura and footplate, differences of critical importance in surgical attempts to mobilize the stapes in stapes fixation otospongiosis. The stapes footplate is formed by fusion of the primitive ring-shaped cartilage of the stapes with the wall of the cartilaginous otic capsule. The footplate partakes of the same variability in thickness and form as does the remainder of the stapes. Thus the normal footplate varies between a uniformly blue, thin, bony plate to a thicker plate with irregular ridges, or a plate that may be dehiscent in its central portion with the tympanic mucous membrane lying directly against the endosteum of the vestibule. The differentiation by the surgeon of a thick footplate due to a developmental anomaly from a footplate invaded by otospongiotic bone may be difficult, requiring careful inspection of the entire oval window area under the operating microscope.

As the ossicles differentiate and begin to ossify, the surrounding mesenchymal connective tissue becomes looser and less cellular until by 18 to 21 weeks the connective tissue filling the middle ear is very loose, somewhat vacuolated and mucoid in character. Then at 22 weeks this loosened mucoid connective tissue gives way to the expanding tympanic epithelium of the pharyngeal pouch. The latter encroaches upon and wraps around the ossicles and their tendons and ligaments until by the 30th week pneumatization of the tympanum proper is almost complete. Pneumatization of the antrum soon follows and progresses rapidly from the 34th to the 35th week, but in the epitympanum it lags and is not complete until the last month of fetal life.

In rare cases the surgeon will encounter in the adult a mass of gelatinous connective tissue filling the oval window niche, and more often he will find webs or

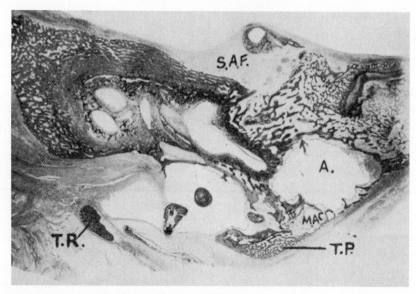

**Figure 1–23**  Photomicrograph of 34 week fetus showing beginning pneumatization of antral air cells (arrow). (T.R.) Tympanic ring, (T.P.) tympanic process of squamous temporal, (MAC) mastoid air cell, (A.) antrum, (S.A.F.) subarcuate fossa. (From Anson, B. J. and Bast, T. H. *In* Coates, G. M., et al.: Otolaryngology. Hagerstown, Md., W. F. Prior Co., 1955.)

strands of connective tissue across the oval or round window niche. Some of these strands may be residues of inflammatory middle ear infections, but more often they are remnants of the embryonic loose connective tissue that once filled the tympanic cavity.

The air-containing space of the tympanic cavity expands immediately after birth with the onset of respiration as air entering the middle ear permits the remaining loose subepithelial connective tissue to condense and thin until it becomes the extremely delicate tunica propria of the mucoperiosteal membrane of the normal middle ear cavity.

## DEVELOPMENT OF THE PNEUMATIC CELLS OF THE TEMPORAL BONE

The **air cells** of the temporal bone develop as outpouchings from the tympanum, epitympanum, antrum and eustachian tube. Epithelium-lined evaginations begin to appear from the antrum as early as 34 weeks in the fetus (Fig. 1–23). However, it is not until air enters the middle ear at birth, permitting the loose embryonic connective tissue to condense and thin, that pneumatization accelerates, continuing throughout infancy and early childhood. In the petrous apex, pneumatization may continue into early adult life.

Pneumatization of the mastoid process occurs partially by epithelium-lined projections into soft tissue between spicules of new bone that is just forming, and partly by a degeneration and dedifferentiation of bone marrow into a loose connective tissue, which is then invaded by pneumatic pockets. The surrounding bony trabeculae proceed to resorb to permit epithelial expansion and enlargement of the pneumatic cells. Thus air cells never press into bone marrow directly, but only after the latter has been converted into a loose mesenchymal tissue.

From the antrum grow air cells of the mastoid process and squama, but a tract of pneumatic cells also frequently grows directly from the posterior wall of the tympanic cavity lateral to the facial nerve, the facial recess, or medial to the facial nerve, the sinus tympani, into the tip of the mastoid process.

From the antrum and the epitympanum, cells grow into the root of the zygoma and into the base of the petrous pyramid around the semicircular canals, in some cases extending into the petrous apex.

From the floor of the tympanum, cells extend below the eustachian tube and sometimes between the cochlea and jugular bulb. From the anterior aspect of the tympanum, cells extend in front of, behind and above the carotid artery, and often in front of and above the cochlea, medially into the petrous apex.

Not infrequently some peritubal cells develop directly from the floor of the eustachian tube.

The extent and pattern of pneumatization vary greatly among individuals, but with a tendency toward symmetry between the two temporal bones of the same individual except as the result of middle ear disease. As a general rule, the most peripheral cell in any cell system is the largest.

Failure of pneumatization or partial arrest of pneumatization of a temporal bone is believed to be the result of middle ear infection occurring in infancy or early childhood. Wittmaack[4] believed that an otitis media occurring soon after birth either in the form of a sterile inflammation due to meconium in the eustachian tube or middle ear or in the form of a bacterial infection causes the loose embryonic subepithelial connective tissue to fibrose, preventing its normal condensation and thinning. Persistent thickening of this subepithelial connective tissue then inhibits or arrests the normal process of pneumatization. Heredity also plays a part in pneumatization.[5]

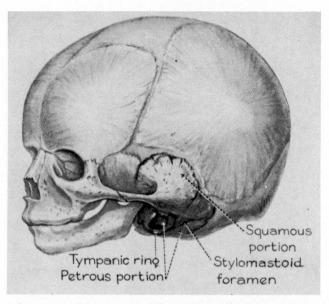

**Figure 1–24**  Infant temporal bone, quite different from adult bone in shape and position, occupies the latero-inferior surface of the skull rather than the lateral aspect as in the adult.

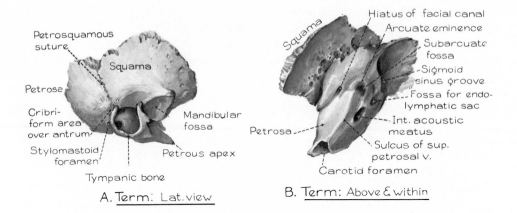

A. Term: Lat. view

B. Term: Above & within

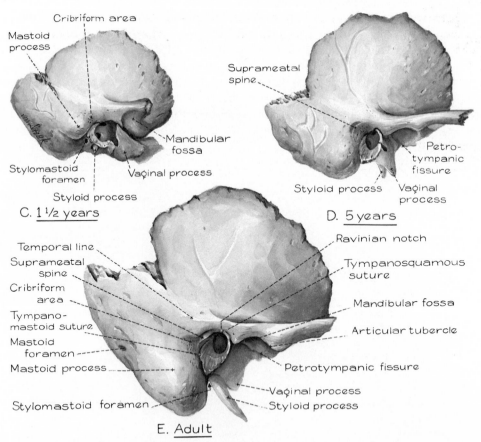

C. 1½ years

D. 5 years

E. Adult

**Figure 1–25** Stages of development of the temporal bone from birth to adulthood. *A* and *B*, At term. *C*, Child of 1½ years. *D*, Child of 5 years. *E*, Adult.

## TEMPORAL BONE OF THE INFANT COMPARED
## TO THAT OF THE CHILD AND ADULT

At birth the hearing mechanism is fully formed and of adult size save for the external auditory meatus, which is short owing to absence of its osseous portion. But the remainder of the temporal bone is small and quite different from the adult bone in shape and position, occupying the latero-inferior surface of the skull, rather than the lateral aspect as in the adult (Figs. 1–24 and 1–25).

Viewed from the side, the infant's temporal bone consists of a relatively large squamous portion, a tympanic portion that is confined to a thin incomplete sulcus just large enough to support the annulus tympanicus, and no mastoid process. Instead of the latter, the petrous portion is seen lying behind the tympanic sulcus and below the squamous portion. The middle ear cavity is enclosed by the tympanic portion laterally, the squamous portion superiorly and the petrous portion medially. The antrum is well formed at birth and is enclosed by the squamous portion laterally and in front and by the petrous portion medially and behind.

The bone of the squama lateral to the antrum is cribriform at birth and until several months of age, so that an otitis media readily produces a subperiosteal inflammation in this area.

Noteworthy is the fact that since there is no mastoid process in the infant, the facial nerve emerges from the stylomastoid foramen onto the lateral surface of the skull where it can be cut by the usual vertical postaural incision. Therefore the incision for a postaural subperiosteal abscess in an infant must be made in a more horizontal plane, rather than vertically as in the adult (Chapter 6, p. 168, and Fig. 6–7D).

The petrous portion of the temporal bone in the newborn has two striking features: on the middle fossa surface the facial canal is not yet bridged over by bone in the region of the geniculate ganglion, and on the posterior surface there is a large subarcuate fossa just beneath and behind the arch of the superior semicircular canal (Fig. 1–25B).

The mastoid process begins to develop during the second year of life by downward extensions of the squamous portion to partially conceal the petrous portion, and of the petrous portion to form the mastoid tip (Fig. 1–25C). These two parts of the mastoid process may fuse imperfectly leaving a more or less distinct petrosquamous suture line on the lateral surface (Fig. 1–26). Within the mastoid process pneumatic cells grow from the antrum vertically in the petrous portion of the mastoid tip, and laterally and radially in the squamous portion. A well marked septum known as Körner's septum may persist between these cell tracts. The mastoid surgeon may be misled by this septum and fail to discover the deeper system of cells in the petrous portion of the mastoid process (Fig. 1–27).

As the mastoid process develops, the thin incomplete sulcus of the infant's tympanic portion grows laterally and inferiorly to form the osseous external auditory meatus with two suture lines: a well marked deep tympanosquamous suture in the anterosuperior meatal wall and a shallower less distinct tympanomastoid suture in the posterior meatal wall (Fig. 1–25E). Connective tissue fibers enter these sutures from the skin of the osseous meatus and must be divided in elevating a meatal skin flap for endomeatal surgery.

The lateral growth of the tympanic portion and mastoid process causes the lateral surface of the temporal bone to assume a vertical position in the adult. At the same time, the stylomastoid foramen and facial nerve come to lie quite deeply to the

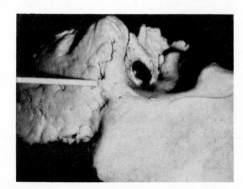

**Figure 1–26**  Petrosquamous suture line. (From Batson, O. V., *In* Coates, G. M., et al.: Otolaryngology. Hagerstown, Md., W. F. Prior Co., 1955.)

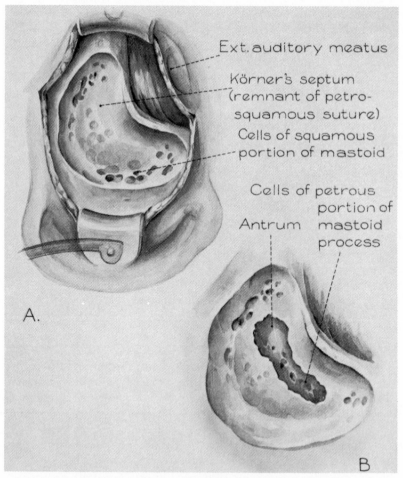

**Figure 1–27**  Körner's septum. *A*, Septum intact. *B*, Septum partially removed.

lateral surface of the mastoid process, well protected from the usual vertical postaural incision.

## REFERENCES

1. Bast, T. H., and Anson, B. J.: The Temporal Bone and the Ear. Charles C Thomas, Springfield, Ill.,
       1949.
2. Allen, G. W.: Endolymphatic sac and cochlear aqueduct. Arch. Otol., 79:322, 1964.
3. House, W. F.: Subarachnoid shunt for drainage of hydrops. Arch. Otol., 79:338, 1964.
4. Wittmaack, K.: Über die normale und die pathologische Pneumatisation des Schläfenbeines. Fischer,
       Jena, 1918.
5. Diamant, M.: Chronic Otitis, a Critical Analysis. S. Karger, New York, 1952.

*Antonio Maria Valsalva*

BORN 1666
DIED 1723

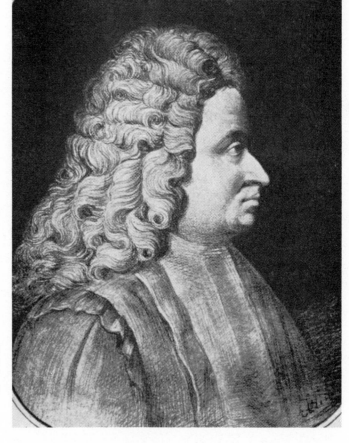

Described self-inflation of the eustachian tube and middle ear by the patient and in 1707 first observed fluid within the labyrinth.

# Chapter 2

# Surgical Anatomy of the Temporal Bone

APPLIED ANATOMY OF SOFT PARTS OVER THE
  TEMPORAL BONE
SURGICAL LANDMARKS OF THE LATERAL SURFACE OF
  THE TEMPORAL BONE
SURGICAL LANDMARKS OF THE SUPERIOR SURFACE OF
  THE TEMPORAL BONE
SURGICAL RELATIONSHIPS BETWEEN THE TEMPORAL
  BONE AND ADJACENT STRUCTURES
SURGICAL RELATIONSHIPS WITHIN THE TEMPORAL
  BONE

The surgical anatomy of the temporal bone is not easily learned, for many more important structures are crowded together in this small space than in any other area of comparable size in the human body. The problem for the surgeon is further complicated by the variability of certain of the anatomic relationships among structures concealed in bone. Add to this the functional importance of such parts as the facial nerve and organ of hearing, and the fragile construction and minute size of portions of the hearing mechanism that must be dealt with surgically, and it is easily understood that here **the dangers of an incompetent operator are particularly great.**

Contrariwise, modern surgery of the temporal bone, in the hands of the otologist who has made the effort to become thoroughly familiar with the surgical anatomy, and who observes the strict rules of surgical asepsis, has proved to be remarkably safe and relatively free from risk of serious complication, as well as deeply satisfying in the results that can be achieved.

Otologic surgical technique and the mastery of the difficult surgical anatomy of the ear cannot be learned from a book alone, nor solely in the operating room. It can be acquired only by time-consuming and painstaking cadaver dissections in the laboratory, until the intricacies of the temporal bone and its variations become as familiar to the surgeon as his own home. Not until the surgeon is comfortably "at home" within the temporal bone can he operate effectively and with complete safety to the patient.

The student of otologic surgery should utilize Wiet's *Surgical Anatomy of the Temporal Bone Through Dissection,* at the end of this *Surgery of the Ear.*

## APPLIED ANATOMY OF THE SOFT PARTS OVER THE TEMPORAL BONE

The external ear includes the auricle, the external meatus and the outer surface of the drum membrane.

### Cartilage

The shape of the auricle is determined by the thin, convoluted, continuous sheet of yellow elastic cartilage that curves forward to enclose the floor and anterior wall of the external cartilaginous meatus, but not the roof (Fig. 2–1). Superiorly the cartilage of the meatus is lacking, leaving a deep cleft, the **incisura terminalis,** utilized by the surgeon in making the extracartilaginous endaural incision for surgical exposure of the temporal bone (Chapter 6).

### Skin

The skin of the meatus and outer surface of the auricle is tightly bound down to the perichondrium, lacking the usual loose subcutaneous layer. Hemorrhage from trauma to the auricle therefore cannot easily diffuse and be absorbed but elevates the perichondrium and, unless evacuated, organizes to produce a "cauliflower ear." The skin of the osseous meatus is thin and closely adherent to the periosteum, and lacks

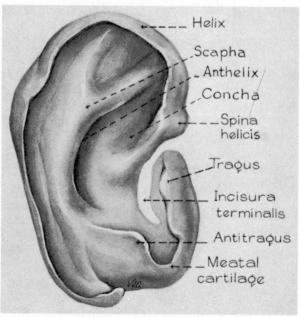

**Figure 2–1**   Auricular cartilage.

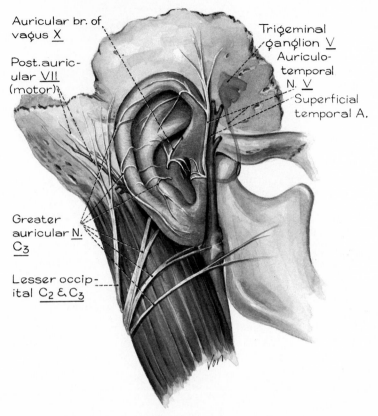

Auricular br. of vagus X

Post. auricular VII (motor)

Greater auricular N. C₃

Lesser occipital C₂ & C₃

Trigeminal ganglion V
Auriculotemporal N. V
Superficial temporal A.

**Figure 2–2** Innervation of external ear (front view).

hair follicles and glands, whereas that of the cartilaginous meatus is supplied with stiff hairs and ceruminous glands. Furuncles, therefore, occur only in the cartilaginous meatus and cause severe pain because of the close attachment of skin to perichondrium.

On its posterior surface the skin of the auricle is thin and delicate with a loose subcutaneous layer. It, with a border of adjacent skin over the mastoid process, is free from large hair follicles, but it is liberally supplied with sebaceous glands, making this a frequent site for sebaceous cysts.

### Attachment of Auricle

The meatal cartilage is firmly attached to the tympanic bone of the osseous meatus. Except for this, the auricle is only loosely attached to the side of the head by connective tissue and by six or seven poorly developed intrinsic muscles innervated by the **posterior auricular nerve,** a branch of the facial nerve (VII).

### Sensory Nerves

The sensory nerve supply of the auricle and meatus comes from the trigeminal, facial and vagus cranial nerves and the third cervical nerve (Figs. 2–2 and 2–3). The **great auricular nerve** (C₃) curves around the posterior border of the sternocleido-

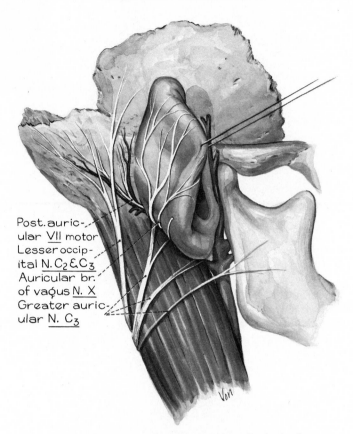

Post. auric-
ular <u>VII</u> motor
Lesser occip-
ital N. C<sub>2</sub> & C<sub>3</sub>
Auricular br.
of vagus <u>N. X</u>
Greater auric-
ular <u>N. C<sub>3</sub></u>

**Figure 2-3**   Innervation of external ear (back view).

mastoid muscle and ascends the side of the neck vertically to supply the skin of the mastoid process and both sides of the auricle. The **auriculotemporal nerve,** from the mandibular division of the trigeminal (V), reaches the mandibular fossa side of the cartilaginous meatus from deep within the mandibular fossa. It gives off two twigs that pass between the cartilaginous and bony anterior meatal walls to supply the skin of the meatus and the tympanic membrane. The auriculotemporal nerve then accompanies the superficial temporal artery upward just in front of the ear to supply the anterior part of the auricle and the skin of the temple.

The **auricular branch of the vagus** (X) passes from the fossa of the jugular bulb into the vertical portion of the bony canal of the facial nerve, where it lies alongside the facial nerve down to the stylomastoid foramen, whence it emerges and then curves laterally and upward on the anterior surface of the mastoid process to supply the floor of the external auditory meatus and a small part of the auricle (Fig. 2–2). Twigs from the facial nerve and chorda tympani supply the skin of the upper posterior aspect of the bony external auditory canal.

For operations on the ear under local anesthesia the great auricular nerve is blocked by infiltration of the anesthetic agent over the lateral surface of the mastoid process; the auricular branch of the vagus is blocked by infiltration of the periosteum and soft tissues on the anterior surface of the mastoid process and by a second injection into the skin and perichondrium of the outer portion of the floor of the meatus; the sensory twigs from the facial nerve to the osseous meatus are blocked by injecting the skin of the posterior wall; the branches of the auriculotemporal nerve to the tympanic membrane are blocked by an injection into the anterior wall of the external auditory meatus at the junction of the osseous and cartilaginous meatus, and with infiltration into the incisura terminalis of the auricle to block branches of the auriculotemporal nerve to the upper part of the auricle (Fig. 2–4). If 1 or 2 per cent Xylocaine is used for local infiltration, the same solution can be instilled into the tympanic cavity attic and antrum as these are opened surgically, to anesthetize the muscosa. Local infiltration anesthesia, which is very effective for operations on a noninfected ear, is less satisfactory when the skin and periosteum of the outer ear are inflamed, and when the mucoperiosteum of the middle ear is thickened and inflamed.

### Vessels

The blood supply of the outer ear is partly from the **posterior auricular artery,** one of the branches of the external carotid artery. It runs upward on the anterior surface of the mastoid process to supply the bone and skin of the mastoid and auricle, having first given off a stylomastoid branch that enters the facial canal. The **superficial temporal artery**, another branch of the external carotid, provides additional blood supply to the meatus and auricle from three or four twigs that run horizontally backward. Veins accompanying these arteries empty into the external jugular or common facial and thence into the internal jugular vein.

The postauricular incision usually cuts across the posterior auricular artery or its larger branches. The endaural incision generally avoids any large vessels but may cut across one or two small horizontal twigs of the superficial temporal artery and vein.

### Muscles

The attachment of the **sternocleidomastoid muscle** to the outer surface of the mastoid tip may be cut without disturbing its function. The **posterior belly of the**

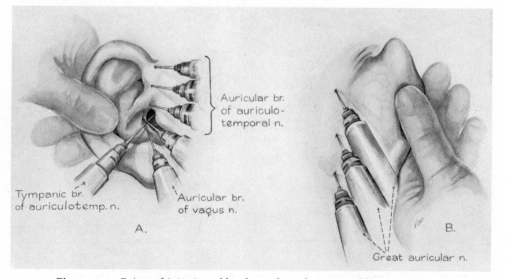

**Figure 2–4**   Points of injection of local anesthetic for temporal bone operations.

**digastric muscle** attaches to the **digastric groove** (incisura mastoidea) on the inner surface of the mastoid tip. This groove is the surgeon's infallible guide to the facial nerve at the point where it emerges from the stylomastoid foramen at the anterior end of the groove. The inferior edge of the **temporal muscle** is exposed and may be cut into by the postaural and the endaural incision. A piece of this muscle may conveniently be removed to place against an accidental tear of the dura, and a section of the temporalis fascia that covers this muscle may be used for repair or replacement of the tympanic membrane. Pedicle flaps consisting of portions of the temporalis or sternocleidomastoid muscles attached to mastoid periosteum may be used to obliterate an operative cavity in the mastoid process.

## SURGICAL LANDMARKS ON THE LATERAL SURFACE OF THE TEMPORAL BONE

When the lateral surface of the mastoid process is exposed by either the postaural or the endaural incision, the following landmarks come into view (Fig. 2–5). (See also Wiet's dissection manual at the end of this *Surgery of the Ear*.)

The upper posterior angle of the meatus is usually but not invariably marked by a small spine, the **suprameatal spine of Henle.** About 1 cm. posterior to it, where there is generally a shallow depression, the cortex is perforated by numerous blood vessels, especially in the infant and child. This is the **fossa mastoidea,** or cribriform area.

The suprameatal spine is commonly taken as a guide to the antrum, which generally lies directly inward from it. However, in a poorly pneumatized bone, or in certain anomalies, the middle fossa dura, the sigmoid sinus or the facial nerve may be encountered by the surgeon who proceeds directly inward from the spine to find the antrum. The safest approach to the antrum in such a bone is first to enter the attic by following the superior osseous meatal wall inward as described in Chapter 10 under the Atticotomy Approach.

The posterior root of the zygomatic process forms the outermost limit of the anterosuperior osseous meatal wall. Extending horizontally backward from it as a

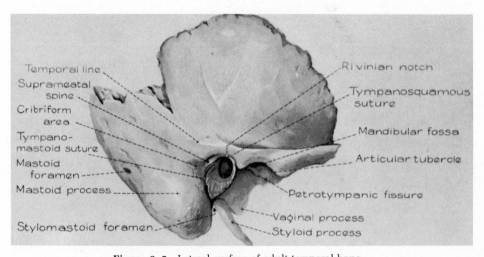

**Figure 2–5**  Lateral surface of adult temporal bone.

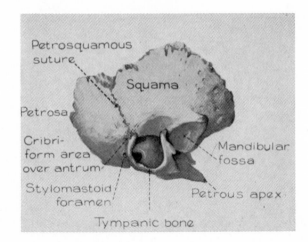

**Figure 2–6** Lateral view of infant's temporal bone.

slight ridge, the **temporal line** marks the inferior margin of the insertion of the temporal muscle. It is sometimes used as an approximate guide to the level of the middle fossa dura within, but it is only very roughly approximate.

Elevation of the periosteum far posteriorly will expose the mastoid foramen containing the **mastoid emissary vein** that passes from the scalp to the sigmoid sinus.

On the lateral surface of the mastoid process the remnant of the **petrosquamous suture** may or may not be discerned; within the mastoid cells this suture sometimes persists as a distinct partition extending upward to the antrum as Körner's septum (see Fig. 1–27).

Elevation of the periosteum from the superior and posterior osseous meatal walls reveals two fissures. In the anterosuperior angle of the meatus there is a well marked fissure, the **tympanosquamous suture,** with a band of connective tissue from the periosteum entering it. This is the suture that develops between the squama and the tympanic bone as the latter grows outward, leaving the gap superiorly corresponding to the notch of Rivinus. At about the middle of the posterior osseous meatal wall a similar but weaker band of connective tissue from the periosteum enters the **tympanomastoid suture** between the mastoid process and tympanic bone. The periosteum of the meatus elevates easily from the squamous portion of the temporal bone that forms the roof of the meatus between these sutures, but at the sutures the periosteum is bound down and needs to be freed by sharp dissection, especially at the tympanosquamous suture.

### Landmarks on the Infant's Temporal Bone

The surgeon must remember that the infant has no external osseous meatus and no mastoid process (Fig. 2–6). The facial nerve emerges from the stylomastoid foramen onto the lateral surface just behind the tympanic membrane, and may be severed by the usual postaural incision. The bone over the infant's antrum is cribriform, so that an otitis media is actually subperiosteal with early edema and redness. Not until the second year of life does the mastoid process begin to appear and the osseous meatus begin to develop by lateral growth of the early incomplete ring of the tympanic bone.

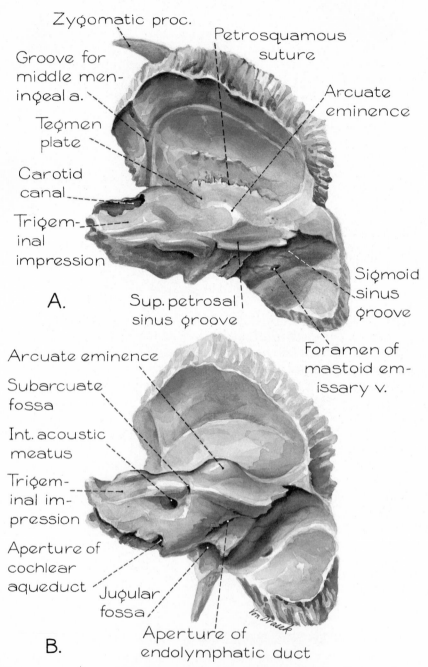

Figure 2–7   *A,* Temporal bone viewed from above. *B,* Temporal bone viewed posteriorly.

## SURGICAL LANDMARKS ON THE SUPERIOR
## SURFACE OF THE TEMPORAL BONE

The surgical landmarks of the superior surface of the temporal bone become important in middle fossa procedures (Fig. 2–7).[1] Once the craniectomy has been performed and the temporal lobe dura elevated, these following landmarks are noted. The most anterior limit of the exposure is determined by locating the **middle meningeal artery** as it enters the cranial vault through the **foramen spinosum.** Medial to the artery are the **greater and lesser superficial petrosal nerves,** which lead posteriorly to the **facial hiatus.** This is a bony foramen for the exit of the greater superficial petrosal nerve as it leaves the **geniculate ganglion.** Posterior to the hiatus one finds a bulge in the surface of the bone, the **arcuate eminence** (Fig. 2–7). This area corresponds to the location of the **superior semicircular canal.** Medial to all these landmarks is a groove running along the edge of the petrous bone that contains the **superior petrosal sinus.** See Wiet's dissection manual at the end of this *Surgery of the Ear* for further orientation.

## SURGICAL RELATIONSHIPS BETWEEN THE
## TEMPORAL BONE AND ADJACENT STRUCTURES

### Jaw Joint

The bone of the anterior meatal wall forms the posterior wall of the mandibular (glenoid) fossa, but the function of this joint is not endangered by resection of the anterior osseous meatal wall, since the posterior half of the fossa is filled with loose connective tissue and is nonarticular. The articular cartilage is confined to the anterior half of the mandibular fossa, extending forward to include the articular eminence. When the mouth is opened the condyloid process slides forward onto the articular eminence (Fig. 2–8), this being a sliding rather than a hinge joint. Dislocation occurs when the condyloid process slides forward beyond the articular eminence as a result of cavernous yawning or wide opening of the jaws under general anesthesia. Pressure downward on the mandible behind the molars replaces the joint.

The proximity of the mandibular joint to the meatus and tympanic membrane and their common innervation by the mandibular division of the trigeminal nerve account for the referred otalgia so common in disease of the molar teeth or of the joint.

### Meninges

A tomogram of the base of the skull (Fig. 2–9) reveals the tympanic cavity a full third of the distance from the outer surface of the head to the center of the skull. In a well pneumatized temporal bone, nearly all of its middle fossa surface from the squama to the petrous tip may be occupied by the middle ear spaces, including the attic, antrum and pneumatic cells, their mucoperiosteum being separated from the dura mater only by a very thin plate of bone. Two small areas not usually pneumatized are the arcuate eminence produced by the arch of the superior semicircular canal on the middle fossa surface, and the bone over the geniculate ganglion at the hiatus of the facial canal. The posterior surface of the petrous

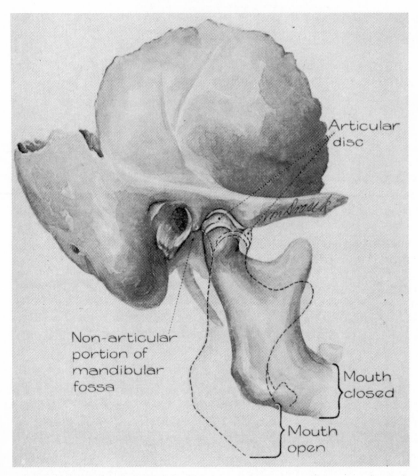

**Figure 2–8**  Mandibular joint closed and open in relation to osseous meatus. (Redrawn from Spalteholz.)

pyramid is partially occupied by the sigmoid sinus, jugular bulb, endolymphatic sac and internal auditory meatus; otherwise, pneumatic cells are close to the posterior fossa dura, too, from the sigmoid sinus to the petrous tip. It is not surprising that most cases of meningitis not due to the meningococcus, as well as the majority of brain abscesses, are of otitic origin.

Observe in the tomogram (Fig. 2–9) that the posterior surface of the petrous bone lies at a 45 degree angle to the median plane, and the internal and external auditory meatuses run nearly perpendicular to this plane. The surgeon thus runs sharply against the posterior fossa plate if he proceeds medially from the mastoid process and antrum.

In surgical procedures the middle fossa dura elevates quite easily from the squama and from the tegmen plate above the attic and antrum, and medially as far as the arcuate eminence where it is more tightly adherent. This portion of the dura may be exposed during operations without fear of serious consequences. Should it be torn accidentally, any depressed bone fragment holding the tear open must be removed and a piece of temporal muscle should be placed on the laceration. The cerebrospinal fluid leak soon repairs itself by proliferation of the adjacent arachnoid mesh.

The posterior fossa dura medial to the sigmoid sinus is more adherent to the bone and therefore more vulnerable to accidental tear when exposed. Because of the arachnoid-free lateral prolongation of the basal cistern to and beyond the internal auditory meatus, the resulting spinal fluid leak is more profuse and heals more slowly with greater danger of meningitis.

### Venous Sinuses

The veins of the head and neck rely upon gravity for the direction of flow, and are without valves except at the junction of the internal jugular with the subclavian vein and at the mouths of the diploic veins of the skull where they join the veins of the scalp. Thus the direction of flow in the veins of the head is easily reversed by change of position, edema or occluding thrombosis. This probably favors the spread of infection by retrograde thrombophlebitis from the mucoperiosteum of the middle ear spaces to the meninges and brain.

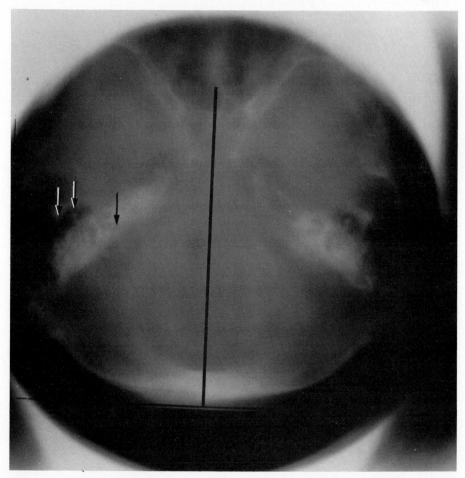

**Figure 2–9** Horizontal tomographic section through the external meatus and internal ear showing relationship of tympanic membrane and middle ear to lateral surface and center of skull. Arrows from left to right point to the tympanic membrane, middle ear, and internal auditory meatus. (Courtesy of Dr. G. E. Valvassori.)

The cranial venous sinuses are the great collecting veins for blood from the brain, dura, labyrinth, temporal bone, orbit and to some extent the diploë of the skull. These sinuses lie in a split of the dura, usually where the tentorium of the cerebellum or the falx of the cerebrum or cerebellum attaches. In contrast to veins elsewhere in soft tissue, they have a constant caliber because of their rigid walls, and this may predispose to stagnation and thrombosis in the presence of infection, and to propagation of a thrombus within the sinus.

The largest of the venous sinuses, carrying most of the intracranial venous blood to the neck, are the **lateral (transverse) sinuses.** These begin at the occipital protuberance, extend horizontally forward in the posterior attachment of the tentorium as far as the mastoid and then curve downward and medially in a deep groove on the inner wall of the mastoid process as the **sigmoid portion,** ending in the domelike **jugular bulb** just beneath the hypotympanum and cochlea. At this point the **internal jugular vein** begins its vertical descent.

The two lateral sinuses usually start as a confluence of the **superior longitudinal (sagittal) sinus** in the attachment of the cerebral falx to the middle of the skull, of the **straight (rectus) sinus** in the attachment of the falx to the tentorium and of the **occipital sinus** in the attachment of the cerebellar falx to the occipital bone. This confluence, known as the **torcular Herophili** (literally, the "wine-press of Herophilus"), is more often incomplete, the large superior longitudinal sinus flowing into a large right lateral sinus, and the smaller straight sinus flowing into a smaller left lateral sinus (Fig. 2–10).

The sigmoid portion at its junction with the horizontal portion of the lateral sinus receives the **superior petrosal sinus.** This lies in the attachment of the tentorium to the petrous ridge and carries blood from the **cavernous sinus,** from the temporal bone and from the mucosa of its air cells. The sigmoid sinus then receives the **mastoid emissary vein** from the scalp at about its midportion, and veins from the endolymphatic sac and duct; at the jugular bulb the sigmoid sinus receives the **inferior petrosal sinus,** containing blood from the cavernous sinus and petrous bone, running along the lower border of the posterior surface of the petrous pyramid. In addition there is the **inferior petro-occipital sinus of Englisch,** lying outside of the cranial cavity in a groove between the petrous and occipital bones on the lower surface of the skull. It carries blood to the jugular bulb from the cavernous sinus, petrous tip and bodies of the sphenoid and occipital bones.

In a well pneumatized temporal bone the sigmoid portion of the lateral sinus (or sigmoid sinus) is in close relation to mastoid air cells from its beginning to the jugular bulb, with only the very thin bone of the sinus plate separating the mucoperiosteum of the pneumatic cells from the dural wall of the sinus. Thrombophlebitis of the sigmoid sinus is understandably one of the common complications of acute and chronic suppurative otitis media with mastoiditis.

The thin outer dural wall of the sigmoid sinus may be exposed accidentally or purposely at surgery. If it is torn or incised, there is profuse venous bleeding, readily controlled by a Gelfoam pack placed against the sinus wall and held with neurosurgical cottonoid until the bleeding stops. The cottonoid may then be removed, the Gelfoam pack left in place and the operation resumed. Healing of a torn sinus wall generally occurs without infection or other complication provided there is not a depressed fragment of bone left projecting into the sinus.

The jugular bulb may be the seat of a primary thrombosis from a suppurative otitis media, but more often it is involved secondary to a sigmoid sinus thrombosis. The superior and inferior petrosal sinuses may become infected and carry infection to the cavernous and sigmoid sinuses. The cavernous sinus, in the dura that bridges

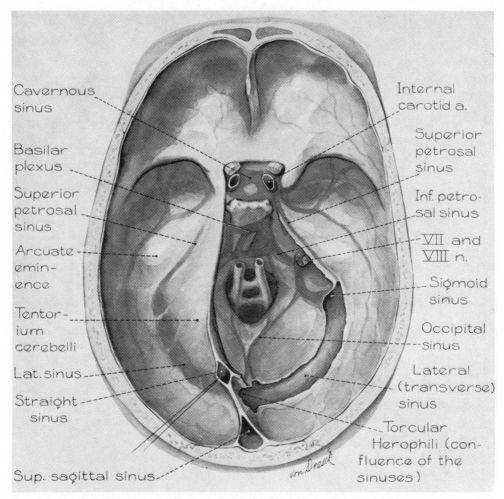

Cavernous sinus

Basilar plexus

Superior petrosal sinus

Arcuate eminence

Tentorium cerebelli

Lat. sinus

Straight sinus

Sup. sagittal sinus

Internal carotid a.

Superior petrosal sinus

Inf. petrosal sinus

VII and VIII n.

Sigmoid sinus

Occipital sinus

Lateral (transverse) sinus

Torcular Herophili (confluence of the sinuses)

von Drasek

**Figure 2–10** Cranial venous sinuses in relation to the temporal bone.

the suture between the petrous tip and sphenoid bone, is, like the superior longitudinal sinus, interlaced by connective tissue bands which may predispose to the lodging of septic emboli and the dread cavernous sinus thrombosis.

Occlusion of both lateral sinuses or ligation of both internal jugular veins may not always cause cerebral venous stasis with increased intracranial pressure and choked disc, because of anastomoses that include the mastoid emissary vein connecting the sigmoid sinus with the external jugular vein, and connections between the occipital sinus and the vertebral veins. These anastomoses also account for the unreliable results sometimes encountered in the Tobey-Ayer (Queckenstedt) test (Chapter 12, p. 304).

There is **no reliable surface landmark for the location of the sigmoid sinus.** The position of this large venous channel in relation to the mastoid cortex and the posterior osseous meatal wall is so extremely variable that the surgeon must be ever alert for an unusually far forward or superficially lying sinus. The position of the sigmoid sinus determines the pattern of pneumatization in the mastoid process. In an unusually well pneumatized mastoid, air cells may extend laterally and pos-

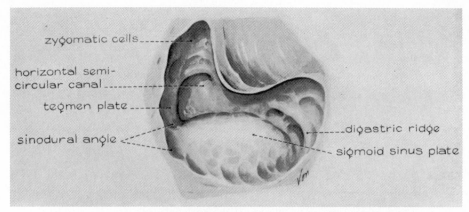

zygomatic cells

horizontal semi-
circular canal

tegmen plate

sinodural angle

digastric ridge

sigmoid sinus plate

**Figure 2–11**   Sigmoid sinus plate defined by simple complete mastoidectomy.

teriorly beyond the sigmoid sinus, but in the bone of average pneumatization the sinus wall usually marks the posterior limit of the mastoid cells. Thus the sigmoid sinus is a useful surgical guide for complete exenteration of mastoid cells (Fig. 2–11).

### Carotid Artery

Considering its long course within the temporal bone and its proximity to the eustachian tube, cochlea and petrous air cells, the internal carotid artery is of surprisingly slight clinical importance in otology. It may be the source of a pulsating tinnitus, audible to patient and examiner alike in the case of an aneurysm. Its chief interest to the otologic surgeon is as the best guide to the cells of the petrous apex when the surgeon is unable to find a surgically accessible cell tract leading to the apex (Chapter 12). To the knowledge of the senior author, there is only one recorded instance of an aberrant carotid producing an elevation in the medial wall of the tympanic cavity sufficient to prompt the operator to take a biopsy. The profuse bleeding, probably from the venous plexus around the carotid rather than from the artery itself, was controlled by firm packing.[2]

The internal carotid artery enters the temporal bone just in front of the jugular bulb and at first progresses vertically, forming a bulge covered by thin bone on the medial wall of the eustachian tube near its tympanic orifice. The artery then turns at right angles and runs horizontally medially in the anterior portion of the petrous apex. In its bony canal in the temporal bone the artery is surrounded by a rich venous plexus, probably as a cushion to prevent its pulsations from eroding the bony wall or being communicated to the hearing mechanism.

### Nerves

The nerves adjacent to or passing into or through the temporal bone have considerable clinical importance. The fifth, sixth, seventh, eighth, ninth, tenth and eleventh cranial nerves may become involved in ear disease.

The sixth (abducens) nerve, motor to the lateral rectus muscle of the eye, runs through a canal of the dura between the petrous tip and the sphenoid bone called

**Dorello's canal.** The trigeminal ganglion (fifth) lies in a shallow depression (impressio trigemini) on the petrous apex. Both may become involved from suppuration within the apex to produce **Gradenigo's syndrome:** pain behind the eye, diplopia and aural discharge.

The facial (seventh) and acoustic (eighth) nerves enter the internal acoustic meatus together. The acoustic is the first nerve to become involved by an acoustic neurinoma (neurilemmoma), and the sensory portion of the facial is the next involved.

The glossopharyngeal (ninth), vagus (tenth) and accessory (eleventh) nerves emerge from the skull through the jugular foramen alongside and just medial to the jugular bulb, and may become involved in a glomus jugularis tumor arising from the dome of the jugular bulb.

## SURGICAL RELATIONSHIPS WITHIN THE TEMPORAL BONE

The complicated and surgically important relationships within the temporal bone will be considered as they relate to the individual surgical procedures. At this point we will consider only the more general relationships and certain special terms.

In describing surgical relationships within or around the ear, "anteriorly" or "in front" means toward the face; "posteriorly" or "behind" is toward the occiput; "superiorly" or "above" is toward the vertex; "inferiorly" or "below" is toward the neck and feet; "deep" is medial, toward the center of the skull; and "superficial" is toward the lateral surface.

Study of Wiet's *Surgical Anatomy of the Temporal Bone Through Dissection* at the end of this *Surgery of the Ear* should accompany the remainder of this chapter.

### Middle Ear Spaces

The middle ear cavity, fully developed and of approximately adult size at birth, includes the **tympanum** just medial to the tympanic membrane, the **hypotympanum** below the lower edge of the sulcus tympanicus, the **epitympanum** or **attic** above the tympanic canal of the facial nerve and the **antrum** lying just behind the attic. The aditus ad antrum is the opening from the epitympanum to the antrum. The outpouchings from the various portions of the middle ear cavity that form the pneumatic cells carry a continuation of the mucoperiosteum of the middle ear cavity, and therefore are extensions of the middle ear spaces.

The antrum is a particularly important landmark because, except in an extremely rare congenital malformation usually associated with atresia, it is always present and lies just posterior to the attic and just above and behind the posterosuperior osseous meatal wall. Osteitis of the bone around the antrum causes edema of the skin of the adjacent meatal wall and the "sagging of the wall" seen clinically in surgical coalescent mastoiditis or large cholesteatomas.

The roof or **tegmen** of the attic and antrum lies in a horizontal plane except anterior to the incudomalleolar joint where the tegmen slopes sharply downward in a forward direction.

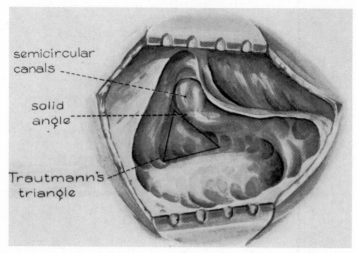

semicircular
canals

solid
angle

Trautmann's
triangle

**Figure 2–12**   Simple mastoidectomy showing Trautmann's triangle.

The roughly triangular area of posterior fossa plate behind the antrum, bounded by the sigmoid sinus, superior petrosal sinus and bony labyrinth, is called **Trautmann's triangle** (Fig. 2–12). The solid bone medial to the antrum in the angle formed by the three semicircular canals is known as the **solid angle.** The angle between the middle fossa above and the posterior fossa and sigmoid sinus behind the antrum is called the **sinodural angle** (Fig. 2–11).

### Facial Nerve

The surgical relationships of the facial nerve are of particular concern to the surgeon because of the ease with which it may be injured or severed accidentally in various operations on the temporal bone.

The facial nerve enters the internal acoustic meatus just above the acoustic nerve and at the medial end enters a bony canal of its own, the facial canal or Aqueduct of Fallopius. This canal with its enclosed nerve continues almost directly laterally, close to the middle fossa as far as the geniculate ganglion, with a short "jog" anteriorly just before it reaches the ganglion. In the newborn the ganglion is not yet covered by bone and lies against the middle fossa dura. In the adult it is usually covered by a thin bony plate except for the hiatus of the facial canal for the emergence of the greater superficial petrosal nerve and lesser superficial petrosal nerve onto the surface of the petrous apex. The first portion of the facial nerve, partly in the internal acoustic meatus and partly in its bony canal, is its petrous portion.

At the geniculate ganglion the facial nerve turns (knee) posteriorly to begin its tympanic course in the medial wall of the middle ear, where it stands out clearly in its bony canal just above the niche of the oval window. This portion of the facial nerve is called the tympanic portion. It is also sometimes called the horizontal portion, but inaccurately since it slopes downward at an angle of about 30 degrees from the horizontal as it proceeds backward.

In about 30 per cent of stapedectomy operations the senior author has observed a dehiscence of a portion of the bony tympanic facial canal, the nerve being covered only by the tympanic mucoperiosteum. In congenital malformation of the middle ear, usually with meatal atresia, the facial nerve may have quite an abnormal course.

In one case it crossed the tympanic cavity **below** rather than above the oval window, clothed only in mucoperiosteum. In another case it emerged from the deformed temporal bone into soft tissue at the posterior end of its tympanic course. **Fortunately these anomalies of the facial nerve are rare,** the tympanic portion in its bony canal being an important and dependably constant surgical landmark.

The anterior end of the tympanic facial canal is marked by the cochleariform process, and the pyramidal eminence for the stapedius tendon and muscle marks the posterior end (Fig. 2–13). The bony tympanic facial canal is fused with the bony horizontal semicircular canal, the nerve generally lying superficial to the perilymphatic space and membranous labyrinth at the ampulla, and deep to or level with the membranous labyrinth at the posterior end of its tympanic portion. However, this exact relationship varies considerably and cannot be relied upon.

A useful surgical guide to the approximate position of the tympanic portion of the facial nerve is the last "bridge" of superior osseous meatal wall to be removed in a radical mastoidectomy, the nerve lying directly inward from the bridge and separated from it by the neck of the malleus, long crus of the incus and chorda tympani nerve. As long as the posterior or short crus of the incus is in its normal position the surgeon need not worry about the facial nerve while taking down the "bridge," for the nerve always lies deep to the incus.

At the pyramidal eminence for the stapedius muscle the facial nerve makes its second turn, curving downward to begin its vertical or mastoid course to the stylomastoid foramen. This **pyramidal turn** is a more gentle curve than the "knee," and carries the nerve just posterior to the tympanic cavity at the posterior extremity of the sulcus tympanicus (Fig. 2–14).

The surgical landmarks for the **vertical or mastoid portion** of the facial nerve are especially important, for this is where the nerve is most often accidentally injured at surgery. The beginning of the vertical portion is approximately at the same depth from the lateral surface of the mastoid process as the bulge of the posterior half of the bony horizontal semicircular canal on the floor and medial wall of the antrum. The tympanomastoid suture in the posterior osseous meatal wall is the landmark to its

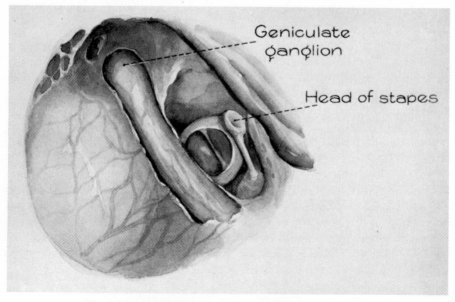

**Figure 2–13** Relations of tympanic portion of facial nerve.

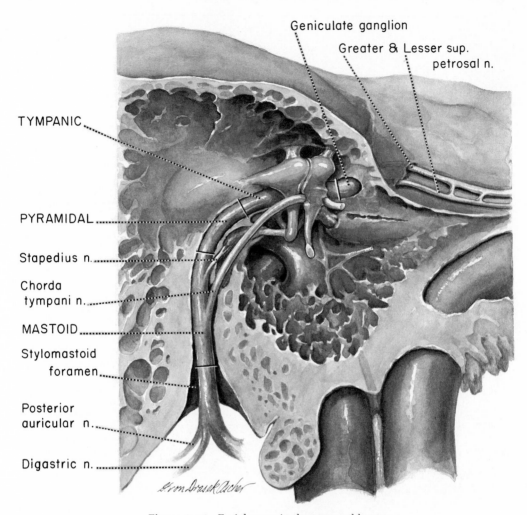

**Figure 2–14**   Facial nerve in the temporal bone.

vertical course, the nerve lying directly inward, sometimes a little posterior but never anterior to this plane. As stated earlier, the nerve emerges from the stylomastoid foramen at the anterior end of the digastric groove (Fig. 2–15). By locating the posterior end of the bony horizontal semicircular canal in the floor of the antrum, by following the digastric groove to the stylomastoid foramen and by noting the tympanomastoid suture in the posterior osseous meatal wall, the surgeon can determine the approximate position of the vertical mastoid portion of the facial nerve.

During intact canal wall procedures, the area referred to as the "facial recess"[3] is a triangle-shaped area bounded superiorly by the incudal fossa, inferiorly by the chorda tympani and medially by the facial nerve. In opening this recess, the surgeon gains access not only to the facial nerve itself but to the pyramidal process, stapes and round window. It is possible to expose the tympanic portion of the facial nerve in this manner without having to remove the incus.

Deliberate surgical exposure of the facial nerve to explore, decompress or repair it may begin in the internal auditory canal and proceed through its labyrinthine, tympanic and mastoid course (Chapter 20).

## Labyrinth

The osseous labyrinthine capsule almost completely blocks the surgeon from entering the apex of the petrous pyramid. Anteriorly the cochlea and carotid artery generally lie against the middle fossa plate; superiorly the geniculate ganglion, the petrous portion of the facial nerve and the arcuate eminence of the superior semicircular canal are usually in contact with the tegmen; posteriorly the posterior semicircular canal is frequently in contact with the posterior fossa plate; and inferiorly the cochlea is usually in contact with the bony wall of the jugular bulb. Nevertheless, some pneumatization of the petrous apex and of the basal peri-labyrinthine portion of the petrous pyramid does occur in about two thirds of adults, one or more cell tracts finding their way around the labyrinth or through the arch of the superior canal. These tracts may be discovered and sometimes followed into the apex, as described in Chapter 12.

The basal coil of the cochlea produces the **promontory** on the medial wall of the tympanic cavity, with the apical coil lying anteriorly. The vestibule of the labyrinth

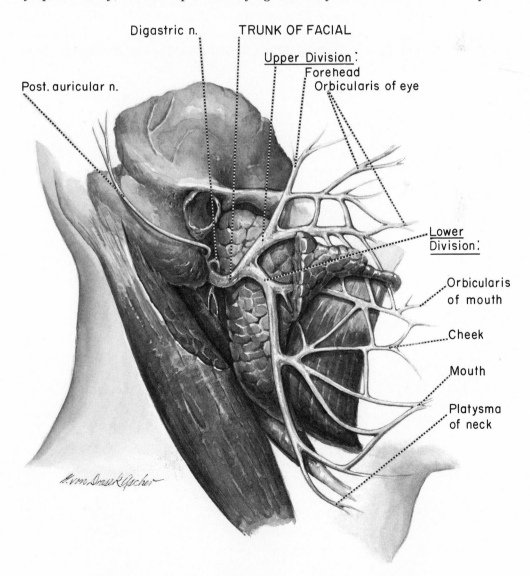

**Figure 2–15** Facial nerve peripheral from the stylomastoid foramen.

lies medial to the oval window, cochleariform process and tympanic portion of the facial nerve (Fig. 2–16). The semicircular canals lie in the medial wall of the attic and antrum (Fig. 2–17). Effective surgical drainage of the labyrinth, once considered a hazardous technical feat, is a relatively simple procedure by today's endaural approach with magnification (Chapter 12).

### Pneumatic Cells

The pneumatic cells of the temporal bone are distinctive features that offer surgical access to the structures within and adjacent to this bone, and have a considerable influence on the development and course of suppurative disease. As we saw in Chapter 1, these air cells begin to appear as epithelium-lined outpouchings from the antrum during the eighth month of fetal life. The major and most constant pneumatization of the mastoid process occurs by air cells that grow out from the antrum downward to the mastoid tip, backward lateral to the sigmoid sinus, posterosuperiorly into the sinodural angle and medially into the perilabyrinthine portion of the petrous portion. In a well pneumatized bone, cells extend from the attic laterally into the root of the zygoma and medially above the geniculate ganglion

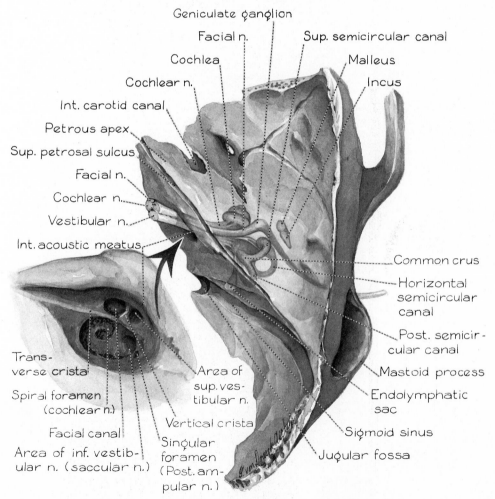

**Figure 2–16**  Internal acoustic meatus: anatomical relationships.

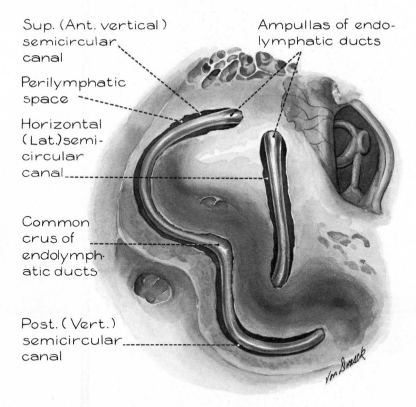

Sup. (Ant. vertical)
semicircular
canal

Perilymphatic
space

Horizontal
(Lat.)semi-
circular
canal

Common
crus of
endolymph-
atic ducts

Post. (Vert.)
semicircular
canal

Ampullas of endo-
lymphatic ducts

**Figure 2-17**   Semicircular canals opened from mastoid approach.

and ampullated end of the superior semicircular canal toward the petrous apex. A separate tract of cells may proceed through the arch of the superior semicircular canal into the apex.

In extensively pneumatized temporal bones, cells often develop directly from the tympanum posteriorly into the mastoid process, one tract extending medial to the vertical portion of the facial nerve into the mastoid tip, and a second tract lateral to the upper end of the vertical portion of the facial nerve via the facial recess into the mastoid process. From the hypotympanum, cells may extend medially between the jugular bulb and the cochlea into the petrous apex; another tract begins at the tympanic orifice of the eustachian tube and extends medially into the apex in the triangular area that lies between the cochlea behind, the tegmen tympani above and the carotid artery anteriorly.

The exact pattern and degree of pneumatization varies greatly among temporal bones, but with a tendency toward symmetry between the two sides of a particular individual. Inherited tendency toward greater or lesser degrees of pneumatization is a controlling factor, but otitis media, especially in infancy and early childhood, is believed to be the cause of arrested pneumatization, especially when there is a well pneumatized mastoid process on the opposite side.

## REFERENCES

1. Glasscock, M. E.: The middle fossa approach to the temporal bone: An otologic frontier. Arch. Otolaryngol., 90:41, 1969.
2. House, H.: Personal communication.
3. Sheehy, J. L., and Patterson, M. E.: Intact canal wall tympanoplasty with mastoidectomy. Laryngoscope, 77:1502, 1967.

## Heinrich Adolph Rinne

BORN 1819
DIED 1868

In 1855 described the tuning fork test, still the best method for diagnosis of conductive versus sensori-neural hearing loss. (From Heck, W. E.: Dr. A. Rinne. Laryngoscope, 72: 647, 1962.)

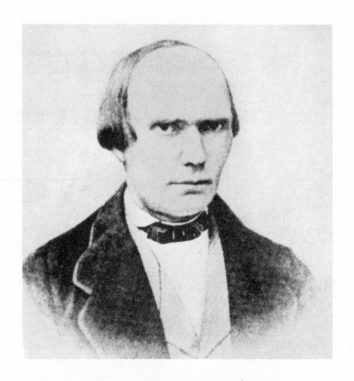

## Adam Politzer

BORN 1835
DIED 1920

Foremost teacher of otologic diagnosis and therapy of the Vienna school.

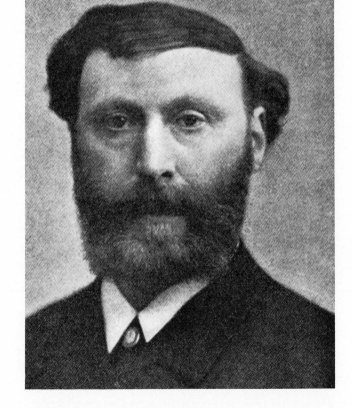

# Chapter 3

# Diagnosis of Ear Disease

OFFICE PROCEDURE
OFFICE EQUIPMENT
HISTORY
HEARING TESTS
VESTIBULAR TESTS
OTOSCOPIC INSPECTION
EXAMINATION OF THE EUSTACHIAN TUBE
DIFFERENTIAL DIAGNOSIS OF HEARING LOSSES
ETIOLOGIC TYPES OF SENSORINEURAL LOSS
ETIOLOGIC TYPES OF CONDUCTIVE LOSS

The otologist is first a Doctor of Medicine and second a surgical specialist in diseases of the ear. Surgical intervention should be based on an accurate and definitive diagnosis, and appropriate conservative treatment should be utilized before resorting to operative procedures.

Unlike the ophthalmologist, who can peer into the eye and see as far as the endings of the optic nerve, the otologist can see no farther into the ear than the tympanic membrane unless it is perforated. What lies beyond must be deduced from the history the patient gives, hearing tests, vestibular tests, examination of eustachian tube function and radiography. Since ear disease is rarely fatal to today's patient, the otologist must depend upon the pathologic findings disclosed by the operating microscope, and ultimately on temporal bone sectioning, to verify the accuracy of the clinical diagnosis.

It has been estimated that only a third of all patients who consult a general physician have a purely physical disease requiring only medical or surgical therapy; a third have organic findings but with superimposed emotional factors; and a third have symptoms with no definite bodily disease to account for them.[1] A good rule is that when the sum of the symptoms does not equal the sum of the organic findings, the difference represents a psychosomatic factor. The occurrence of nonorganic disease is far less in private patients consulting the otologist; nevertheless he must be alert to detect symptoms that have an emotional basis or psychogenic overlay, as is often the case with tinnitus, vertigo and psychogenic deafness.

This chapter on the diagnosis of organic ear disease will consider the diagnostic methods that are most useful and practical for everyday office practice of otology. A brief differential diagnosis of some common ear symptoms will include mention of nonsurgical as well as surgical methods of therapy, but for more detailed consideration of medical treatment of ear disease the reader is referred elsewhere. Radiogra-

**53**

phy of the ear, usually done outside the otologist's office, will be considered in the next two chapters.

## OFFICE PROCEDURE

Every office detail that the patient senses reflects the personality of the doctor himself. Courteous, considerate and kind receptionist and nurse, efficient and businesslike office routine, clean office linen and neatly attired personnel engender an atmosphere of quiet competence and meticulous regard for the best interests of the one patient under consideration. A thorough history and examination with time taken to explain the diagnosis and prognosis in language that the patient understands will create confidence and dispel unnecessary apprehension, for no fear is greater than that of the unknown. It pays to be completely frank and honest with the patient and his family, avoiding mysterious terminology, and neither exaggerating the probable benefits of the proposed medical or surgical therapy nor minimizing the possibilities of failure. Today's intelligent patient seeks the plain truth, not medical sorcery.

Seven simple rules are helpful for dealing with patients in the office:[2]

1.   Never consider the preliminary history and examination of casual importance, but establish and adhere to a routine so that you will not fail to take a complete history and make a complete otolaryngologic examination of every patient.

2.   Never convey to a patient the impression of haste. Avoid unnecessary interruptions. He must feel that his problem is important to you, and that your full attention and serious consideration are being concentrated upon it.

3.   Avoid inflicting pain, by gentle manipulation and the use of local anesthetics whenever necessary. If momentary pain is unavoidable, warn the patient first, especially a child, who will never forgive or forget if you hurt him after promising not to do so.

4.   Never jest with a patient concerning an ailment, nor attempt to belittle his complaints. If he did not regard them seriously he would not be in your office. But do not hesitate to reassure him that he does not have serious organic disease **after** your examination if such be your findings.

5.   Know normal findings and do not ascribe present symptoms to congenital anomalies or residues of no longer active disease.

6.   Make positive statements on the history and to the patient about normal findings; do not describe the results as "negative." Use the positive approach regarding hearing that is still present or can be restored rather than the negative emphasis on hearing that has been lost irretrievably. The best medicine for many patients with minimal or irreversible disease is sincere reassurance based on a careful history and thorough examination.

7.   Never deviate from the Golden Rule: Advise and do for the patient exactly what you would choose for yourself or your family, including adequate but not excessive charges for your services. Free advice is rarely followed, and the patient who receives free medical or surgical treatment often becomes the dissatisfied patient who imagines neglect or incompetent care and may consult an attorney.

## OFFICE EQUIPMENT

The equipment required for careful diagnosis and efficient office treatment of ear disease need not be very elaborate or excessively costly.

An examining chair for the patient, a light and head mirror for the doctor, a set of examining instruments, a 10 cc. hypodermic syringe for caloric tests, a set of magnesium alloy tuning forks with a device for narrow-band masking (Fig. 3–1), a calibrated audiometer for conducting pure tone air and bone conduction audiograms and speech tests, and an impedance bridge (Fig. 3–2 shows an impedance bridge in use) comprise the basic essentials.

The examining instruments will include nasal and ear speculums, a magnifying pneumatic ear speculum, eustachian catheter with auscultation tube and Politzer bag, blunt ear hook, thin metal cotton applicators, attic cannula, postnasal mirror and nasopharyngoscope. Suction and compressed air with a pressure gauge and regulating valve are useful conveniences. An office microscope is desirable.

A very desirable adjunct for the office practice of otology is training and equipment for the diagnosis and management of allergic diseases of the ear. The details concerning these are beyond the scope of this book, except to list the allergic ear conditions frequently encountered by the otologic surgeon, but rarely recognized or properly treated by him unless he has had training in allergy techniques. Common allergic diseases of the ear include:

A good proportion of cases of chronic external otitis.

A high percentage of cases of recurring or chronic secretory otitis media, both in children and in adults.

A considerable number of cases of chronic suppurative otitis media with persistent mucoid discharge from a central perforation.

A small percentage (about 10 per cent) of cases of endolymphatic hydrops.

Certain cases of recurring persistent otorrhea from a once healed radical mastoid or fenestration cavity.

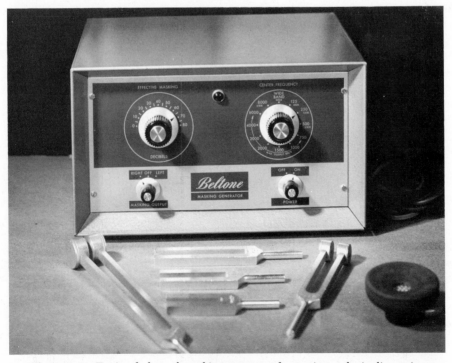

**Figure 3–1**  Tuning forks and masking apparatus for routine otologic diagnosis.

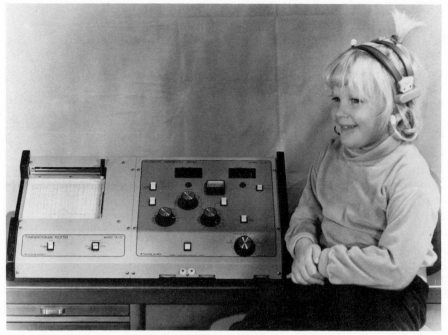

**Figure 3–2**   Impedance bridge in use.

## HISTORY

The **presenting complaint,** or what really brings the patient to the doctor, is of more than passing interest, for it provides the clue to fears that need to be allayed or emotional factors that need attention. For the first several minutes the patient should be encouraged to talk freely and tell his own story in his own words. Thereafter the physician by interjecting specific questions should guide the development of a clear, coherent, consecutive and concise history to be entered on the history sheet. Since certain patients, although not intending to be evasive, give vague, wandering and indefinite replies to specific questions, the physician will need to insist gently but firmly that they keep to the subject and give a definite reply to each question. Did the symptoms begin abruptly, gradually or following an illness or other incident? Have they gone on for days, months or years? Are they intermittent, recurrent or continuous, and what seems to influence them?

Questions to every ear patient should cover: history of draining ear, pain, vertigo, hearing loss, allergic symptoms (including sensitivity to any antibiotic or other drug) and previous medical or surgical therapy. As the story develops the experienced clinician learns to ask further pertinent questions, since practical necessity precludes asking every patient all possible questions. For example, if the complaint is dizziness, a typical attack should be described with respect to frequency of occurrence, duration of the attack, its relation to change of position, the presence of ataxia, nausea or vomiting, tinnitus, hearing loss, distortion of hearing and fullness or pressure in the ears. If the problem is one of impaired hearing, the specific questions should include the family history, age and mode of onset, progression, fluctuation or stability of the hearing level, influence of pregnancy, antecedent illness or history of an ototoxic drug, history of syphilis and of previous noise exposure and use of a hearing aid.

## HEARING TESTS

The minimal routine hearing tests needed for the office diagnosis of ear diseases are:

Pure tone air and bone conduction audiograms
Speech reception threshold and speech discrimination scores
Rinne, Schwabach, Weber, and a tuning fork test for diplacusis

In certain cases, the following tests may be appropriate:

Impedance measurements, including acoustic reflexes
Tone decay test
Performance-intensity function
Alternate binaural loudness balance test (ABLB)
Short increment sensitivity index (SISI)
Békésy audiometry
Central auditory tests
Evoked response audiometry (ERA)

### Pure Tone Audiometry

Audiometric pure tone testing should be conducted in a quiet room, preferably a prefabricated steel sound-treated room. If a prefabricated room is not available, a carpeted floor, acoustic tiles on the walls and ceiling, and a double or steel door can minimize noise levels in the test room. The audiometer should be electronically calibrated at least once a year, and a daily listening check should be conducted by the tester to monitor the calibration and to detect mechanical defects in the equipment.

Thresholds are determined at each frequency by the presentation of interrupted tones until the softest level to which the patient responds 50 per cent of the time is found. Narrow-band masking noise should be utilized in all bone conduction testing, and in air conduction testing when the threshold is 40 decibels or greater than the bone conduction threshold of the opposite ear.

*Interpretation of Thresholds.* Air conduction thresholds are a measure of the entire auditory system. Bone conduction thresholds are a measure of the perceptive mechanism of the ear (cochlea and auditory nerve), with some influence of the middle ear system.*

Air conduction thresholds alone cannot diagnose the type of hearing loss, that is, whether it is conductive or sensorineural. For example, a greater loss for low frequencies than for high frequencies occurs in the purely cochlear loss of endolymphatic hydrops as well as in many conductive losses (Fig. 3–3A). Conversely, a greater loss for high frequencies, so characteristic of many inner ear losses, occurs also in the pure conductive loss of secretory (serous) otitis media (Fig. 3–3B; also see Mechanics of Hearing, Chapter 13).

In normal hearing and in pure sensorineural hearing losses, air and bone conduction thresholds interweave. In conductive losses, bone conduction thresholds are essentially normal with a depression of the air conduction thresholds. In mixed hearing losses, there is a loss for both air and bone, but with the bone better than air.

---

*In stapes ankylosis a mechanical shift in the bone conduction thresholds, known as the Carhart notch, is observed in about half the cases (see Chapter 13).

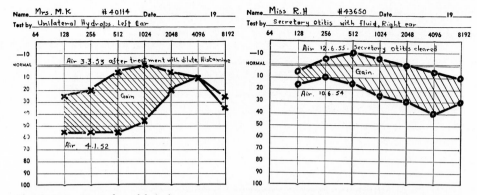

**Figure 3–3**  Examples of low frequency pure sensori-neural loss and high frequency pure conductive loss. *A,* Audiogram of patient with endolymphatic hydrops. Lower curve shows greater loss for low frequencies. Upper curve shows hearing gain after treatment with dilute histamine, with disappearance of symptoms. *B,* Audiogram of patient with secretory otitis with fluid in middle ear. Lower curve shows greater loss for high frequencies. Upper curve shows gain after treatment with repeated inflations, myringotomy and control of allergy with Hansel's dust.

An air–bone gap of 20 to 30 decibels indicates a mild or very early conductive loss. An air–bone gap of 30 to 45 decibels indicates a moderate conductive loss. An air–bone gap of 45 to 60 decibels indicates a maximum conductive loss, such as produced by interruption of the ossicular chain or by complete otosclerotic (otospongiotic) ankylosis of the stapes. Because of a possible 10 decibel variation inherent in air and bone conduction audiometry, an air–bone gap of less than 20 decibels may not indicate a conductive loss unless confirmed by an equal or negative Rinne test with the 256 tuning fork.

### Speech Audiometry

The old-fashioned spoken or whispered voice tests, with the result recorded in feet from the ear, are so variable among examiners, even when done at different times by the same examiner, as to be of limited diagnostic value. They have been replaced by the much more accurate and diagnostically dependable speech reception threshold and speech discrimination tests.

*Speech Reception Threshold.*  The speech reception threshold (SRT) is the minimum intensity required for a patient to just understand speech. Spondaic words (two syllable words with equal accent on each syllable, such as "baseball") are presented via monitored live voice or recorded materials. The lowest intensity level at which 50 per cent of the words are repeated correctly by the patient is the SRT. The SRT is usually equivalent to the three-frequency pure tone average (500–2000 Hz). An SRT that is better than the pure tone average by more than 10 decibels suggests a psychogenic hearing loss.

*Speech Discrimination Testing.*  Speech discrimination testing measures the patient's ability to distinguish phonetic elements of speech. The most common speech test materials used are single syllable words selected to represent the phonetic composition of the spoken English language. These word lists are presented via monitored live voice or recorded materials at 25 to 40 decibels above the SRT or pure tone average (sensation level), and the percentage repeated correctly by the patient is the speech discrimination score.

A discrimination score of 90 to 100 per cent indicates excellent speech discrimination ability, and is usually seen in persons with normal hearing, pure conductive losses and some cochlear losses. A score of less than 90 per cent is indicative of impaired ability to discriminate speech and is seen in some patients with cochlear or retrocochlear lesions.

### Tuning Fork Tests

Spurious conductive hearing losses can occur audiometrically due to ear canal collapse induced by the pressure of the earphone[3] or because of vibro-tactile response to the bone oscillator. Because of these possibilities, as well as daily variations in equipment, personnel, and patient response, serious diagnostic errors can be avoided only if the initial air and bone conduction audiogram for each patient is checked routinely by a careful but quick series of tuning fork tests. If a discrepancy exists between the audiogram and the results of the tuning fork tests, diagnostic information can be provided by additional impedance measurements or a bone-conducted speech reception threshold (SRT), with the spondaic words presented through the bone oscillator.

### *Rinne Test*

The **Rinne test** is made with the 256, 512 and 1024 tuning forks, **while the opposite ear is masked.** It is not good technique to use a stop watch to time the duration of audible vibration with continuous placement of the stem of the tuning fork on the mastoid and of the tines in front of the ear, because this introduces two sources of error: differences in the initial intensity of vibration, and adaptation (sometimes termed tone decay) when the ear is subjected to a continuous stimulus. A more accurate and at the same time quicker and easier method for performing the Rinne test is alternately to place the stem of the fork on the patient's mastoid at about the fossa mastoidea, and ½ inch away from his external meatus until he no longer hears it at one of these positions. The result is expressed as "Rinne positive" when heard longer by air, "Rinne equal" when heard the same by air and by bone and "Rinne negative" when heard longer by bone.

### *Schwabach Test*

The **Schwabach test** is made with the 256, 512, 1024 and 2048 tuning forks while the opposite ear is masked. Again an intermittent stimulus is applied by placing the stem of the vibrating tuning fork first on the mastoid of the patient and then on the examiner's, alternating until one or the other no longer hears it. The result is expressed as "Schwabach normal" if heard the same by both, "Schwabach prolonged" if heard longer by the patient and "Schwabach shortened" if heard longer by the examiner. The degree of shortening can be qualified as "slightly," "moderately," "much" or "not heard."

*Weber Test*

The **Weber test** is made by placing the vibrating tuning fork, usually the 256 or 512, on the vertex or the midline of the forehead just above the glabella and noting whether the sound is heard in the midline, expressed as "Weber negative," or whether it is definitely referred to one or the other ear, expressed as "Weber right" or "Weber left."

*64 Fork by Air Test*

The **64 fork by air** test also utilizes an intermittent stimulus, with the tines of the fork placed alternately ½ inch from the meatus of the patient and examiner. The result is "normal," "slightly shortened," "moderately shortened," "much shortened" or "not heard."

*Diplacusis Test*

**Diplacusis** is tested for by placing a vibrating tuning fork in front of each ear of the patient alternately, adjusting the distance until it is heard equally loudly in both ears, and then asking if the sound is exactly the same in both ears. If the tuning fork is higher pitched in one ear or if it has a rough, non-musical quality contrasted with the musical tone heard in the opposite ear, the test is positive. Since diplacusis may be present in only part of the tone range it should be tested for with forks of several pitches.

*Interpretation of Tuning Fork Tests.*   The experienced examiner should be able to predict the size of an air–bone gap to within 10 or 15 decibels by his tuning fork Rinne tests. For example, a Rinne test that is equal or negative for 256 but positive for 512 and 1024 indicates a mild conductive loss with an air–bone gap of 20 to 30 decibels* (Fig. 3–4A). A Rinne test that is negative for 256 and 512 but positive for 1024 indicates a moderate conductive loss with a 30 to 45 decibel air–bone gap (Fig. 3–4B). A negative Rinne test for all three forks tested indicates a maximum conductive loss and air–bone gap of 45 to 60 decibels (Fig. 3–4C).

Similarly the examiner should be able to predict the bone audiogram from his tuning fork Schwabach tests.

The Weber test is the least valuable and reliable of the common tuning fork tests, and frequently its results must be disregarded.

The 64 fork, when heard normally by the patient and when accompanied by a positive Rinne test for the 256 fork, rules out a significant conductive hearing loss. If the patient has a pure conductive loss and the 64 fork is not heard at its loudest intensity, the conductive loss is maximum with an air–bone gap of 45 to 60 decibels.

Diplacusis when definitely present indicates an end-organ cochlear lesion of the nature of a labyrinthine hydrops, serous labyrinthitis, labyrinthine hemorrhage or a mechanical disruption of the organ of Corti from concussion or explosive noise.[4] The absence of demonstrable diplacusis does not, however, exclude these conditions, since some persons are unable to distinguish pitch differences.

---

*Mention should be made of unilateral sensorineural losses of severe degree when a falsely negative Rinne test with the 256 fork usually occurs owing to the impossibility of completely masking the low pitch frequencies in the normal ear. The Rinne test with the 512 fork will be strongly positive in such cases when the normal ear is masked by narrow-band noise.

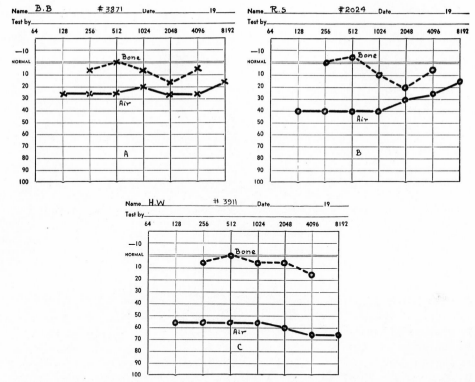

**Figure 3–4** Examples of mild, moderate and maximum conductive loss. *A*, Audiogram of early otosclerosis with air-bone gap of 20 to 30 decibels. Rinne test negative for 256 tuning fork, positive for 512 and 1024 tuning forks. *B*, Audiogram of otosclerosis with air-bone gap of 30 to 45 decibels. Rinne test negative for 256 and 512 tuning forks and positive for 1024 tuning fork. *C*, Audiogram of otosclerosis with air-bone gap of 45 to 60 decibels. Rinne negative for 256, 512 and 1024 tuning forks.

## Special Auditory Tests

A number of tests are available to differentiate conductive, cochlear, auditory nerve or central lesions and to objectively determine hearing levels. Because a clinical audiologist has the expertise to administer and interpret these tests, they will be described only briefly here. For additional information, refer to any recent audiology textbook.[5]

### Impedance Measurements

In impedance audiometry, the integrity of the middle ear system is assessed by means of two basic tests: (1) tympanometry and (2) acoustic reflex measurements. In tympanometry, variance in air pressure introduced into a sealed ear canal provides information regarding the amount of air pressure in the middle ear cavity, as well as the mobility (compliance) of the tympanic membrane and ossicular chain. The graphic recording of this information is called a tympanogram, and it is usually classified into one of five basic types, described in Figure 3–5.

In acoustic reflex measurements, observation is made of the changes in compliance caused by contraction of the middle ear muscles in response to auditory

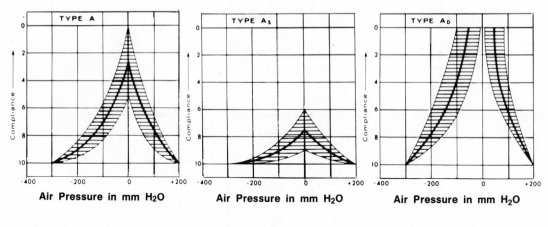

Type A - Normal pressure (±100 mm $H_2O$) and normal static compliance (.25 - 1.6 cc)

Type As - Normal pressure (±100 mm $H_2O$) and reduced static compliance (less than .25 cc)

Type Ad - Normal pressure (±100 mm $H_2O$) and high static compliance (greater than 1.6 cc)

*Static compliance is 0 mm $H_2O$ or peak compliance value minus +200 mm $H_2O$ compliance value.

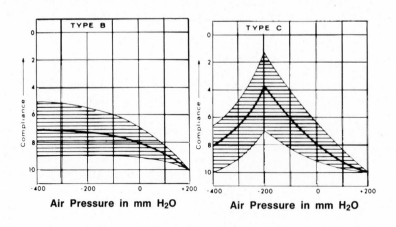

Type B - Extreme negative pressure (greater than −250 mm $H_2O$) and low static compliance (.10 - .25 cc)

Type C - Negative pressure (−100 to −250 mm $H_2O$) and normal compliance (.25 - 1.6 cc)

**Figure 3–5**  Five major types of tympanogram.

**TYPICAL PATTERNS of TYMPANOMETRY and ACCOUSTIC REFLEXES in VARIOUS DISORDERS**

| DISORDER | TYMPANOGRAM | ACOUSTIC REFLEXES | REFLEX DECAY |
|---|---|---|---|
| Normal | Type A | Present > 60 dB above threshold | Normal |
| Cochlear lesion - mild to severe | Type A | Present < 60 dB above threshold | Normal |
| Cochlear hearing loss - profound | Type A | Absent | — |
| Retrocochlear lesion | Type A | Absent or elevated | Abnormal |
| Early stapedial fixation | Type A or A$_S$ | Present with on-off effect | Normal |
| Late stapedial fixation | Type A or A$_S$ | Absent | — |
| Ossicular discontinuity peripheral to stapedial muscle | Type A$_D$ | Absent | — |
| Ossicular discontinuity medial to stapedial muscle | Type A$_D$ | Present | Normal |
| Flaccid tympanic membrane | Type A$_D$ | Present | Normal |
| Facial nerve lesion medial to stapedial muscle | Type A | Absent | — |
| Facial nerve lesion peripheral to stapedial muscle | Type A | Present | Normal |
| Malleus fixation | Type A$_S$ | Absent | — |
| Tympanosclerosis | Type A$_S$ | Present or absent | Normal |
| Otitis media | Type B | Absent | — |
| Occluded Eustachian tube | Type C | Present or absent | Normal |
| Cholesteatoma | Type A, A$_D$ or B | Present or absent | Normal |
| Perforated tympanic membrane | Cannot | Be          Measured | |
| Functional hearing loss | Type A | Present | Normal |

**Figure 3–6**  Diagnostic information from tympanometry.

stimuli. The reflex decay test measures the decrease in the muscle contraction with a sustained auditory signal. In patients free of pathology, the acoustic reflex is elicited at approximately an 85 decibel hearing level, and there is less than 50 per cent decay of the reflex over a 10 second period at 500 and 1000 Hz.

Patterns of tympanometric and acoustic reflex results provide diagnostic information about a variety of disorders. Typical patterns are summarized in Figure 3–6.

## Tone Decay Tests

There are a variety of tone decay tests that measure the ability of a patient to hear a continuous tone for a specified period of time, usually one minute. If the patient is unable to detect a tone for a full minute, that is, if the tone fades away or decays, it is indicative of auditory adaptation or fatigue. Decay of a tone that is more than 30 decibels above threshold suggests a retrocochlear lesion.

## Performance-Intensity Function

In the performance-intensity function, the patient's ability to discriminate phonetically balanced words (PB) at increasing intensity levels is measured. The results are plotted as a function of performance versus intensity (PI) and referred to as the PI–PB function. For patients with cochlear lesions, PB scores rise to a maximum and then reach a plateau or decrease slightly as the intensity of the words is increased. For patients with retrocochlear lesions, PB scores decline rapidly (rollover) as the speech intensity is increased above the level of maximum discrimination. A rollover index (PB maximum minus PB minimum, divided by PB maximum) of greater than 0.45 suggests a retrocochlear lesion.

### Alternate Binaural Loudness Balance Test (ABLB)

The ABLB requires the matching of loudness of tones presented alternately to each ear. If recruitment is present, the change in intensity needed to balance the loudness in the two ears diminishes as the intensity increases, and suggests a cochlear lesion. Decruitment, an increase in intensity needed to balance the loudness of tones, is associated with central disorders.

### Short Increment Sensitivity Index (SISI)

The SISI test assesses the patient's ability to detect very small (1 decibel) changes in intensity of a tone presented continuously at a 20 decibel sensation level. A patient with normal hearing, pure conductive hearing loss or a retrocochlear lesion can detect few of the intensity changes, while the patient with a cochlear lesion is able to detect a large percentage of the changes. The SISI test may also be conducted at an 80 to 90 dB hearing level. Patients with normal hearing or conductive losses, as well as those with cochlear losses, can detect the changes in the high level SISI test, but patients with retrocochlear losses still cannot.

### Békésy Audiometry

Békésy audiometry, with the patient recording his own threshold automatically, first for interrupted tones and then for a continuous tone, produces four types of tracings (Fig. 3–7).

In Type I, the interrupted and the continuous tone tracings overlap, and the excursions are about 10 decibels wide. This type occurs in normal hearing and in pure conductive losses.

In Type II, the continuous tone tracing "C" breaks away from the interrupted tone tracing "I" at about 500 to 1000 Hz, with narrowed excursions for the continuous tone. This type occurs in many, though not quite in all, cochlear disorders, such as endolymphatic hydrops.

In Type III, the threshold for the continuous tone drops rapidly below the interrupted tone, until it is not heard at all. This type is highly characteristic of an eighth nerve lesion, such as acoustic neurinoma.

In Type IV, the continuous tone tracing runs well below the interrupted tone. This type is also highly characteristic of an eighth nerve lesion.

### Central Auditory Tests

Central auditory tests make use of difficult speech tasks to provide information about the functioning of the central auditory system. Some of the commonly used

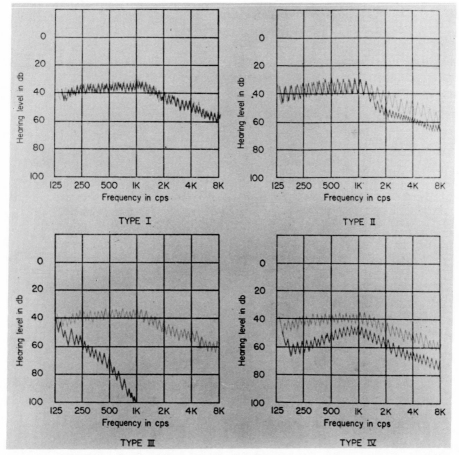

**Figure 3–7** The four types of Békésy audiograms. Type I occurs in normal ears and in disorders of the middle ear. Type II occurs in disorders of the cochlea. Type III and Type IV occur in disorders of the eighth nerve. (From Jerger, J.: Hearing tests in otologic diagnosis. A.S.H.A., 4:139, 1962.)

listening tasks include (1) dichotic tests, such as the staggered spondaic word test (SSW) and the synthetic sentence identification test (SSI); (2) binaural fusion tests, such as low and high band-pass filtered speech tests, and masking level differences for speech (MLD); and (3) low redundancy tests, such as time compressed speech, faint speech, and low-pass filtered speech.

## Evoked Response Audiometry (ERA)

Evoked response audiometry (ERA) is based on the measurement of electrical potentials of the auditory system that are elicited by sound stimuli (clicks, tone pips or tone bursts). The potentials resulting from this stimulation are picked up by electrodes, amplified and delivered to an averaging computer.

There are three types of ERA, which are described in terms of their measured potentials, their latencies and their differing anatomical sources. These three are (1) electrocochleography (E-Co-G), (2) brainstem evoked response audiometry (BER or BSER), and (3) cortical evoked response audiometry. In E-Co-G, the cochlear microphonic summating potential and action potentials arising 1 to 2 msec. following sound stimulation are measured via a needle electrode placed in the ear

## CLASSIC TEST RESULTS in THREE SITES of HEARING LOSS

| SITE | ACOUSTIC REFLEXES | TONE DECAY | PI-PB | ABLB | HIGH LEVEL SISI | BEKESY |
|---|---|---|---|---|---|---|
| CONDUCTIVE | Absent or present with normal reflex decay | Little or no decay | No rollover | No recruitment | 85 - 100% | Type I |
| COCHLEAR | Present except in profound hearing losses, with normal reflex decay | Less than 30 dB decay | Rollover Index of less than 0.45 | Recruitment | 85 - 100% | Type II |
| RETROCOCHLEAR | Absent or elevated with abnormal reflex decay | Greater than than 30 dB decay | Rollover index of greater than 0.45 | No recruitment | Less than 90% | Type III or Type IV |

**Figure 3–8**   Special test battery for site of hearing loss.

canal or passed through the tympanic membrane to the promontory. In BER and cortical evoked response audiometry, surface electrodes are placed on the vertex and mastoid process. The potentials arising in the eighth nerve and brainstem nuclei during the first ten msec. following auditory stimulation are measured in BER. The potentials arising above the brainstem, 10 to 500 msec. following the stimulation, are measured in cortical response audiometry.

The amplitude, latency and inner wave latencies of the potentials yield information regarding hearing levels, type of hearing loss and the integrity of the auditory system. The results can be beneficial in medical-legal cases, infants, and difficult-to-test adults, as well as in patients suspected of retrocochlear or central lesions.

*Diagnostic Significance of Special Auditory Tests.*   The special auditory tests, used as a battery, are far more reliable in indicating the site of an auditory lesion than any one used alone. Figure 3–8 displays the test results expected for six special tests in three sites of hearing disorders.

## VESTIBULAR TESTS

There are two basic procedures utilized in otology offices to test vestibular function. One is a modification of the Kobrac minimal caloric test, which is simple and practical for office use and is sufficient for determining the vestibular labyrinthine response for the routine diagnosis of many ear diseases. The other procedure is electronystagmography (ENG), which consists of a battery of tests during which nystagmus is permanently recorded by means of special ENG equipment.

### Cold Water Caloric Test

*Technique.* With the patient's head inclined backward at a 60 degree angle to place the horizontal semicircular canals in a vertical plane, 5 cc. of tapwater, to which an ice cube has been added, is introduced into the external meatus through a short length of soft rubber tubing on a 10 cc. glass hypodermic syringe (Fig. 3–9). If nystagmus does not appear after one minute, the test is repeated with 10 cc. of ice water, then with 20 cc. and finally with 40 cc. As soon as definite nystagmus appears, the head is inclined 30 degrees forward to lessen the disagreeable vertigo and no further water is instilled. In this position a rotary nystagmus from the vertical semicircular canals may be observed.

An alternative method giving similar results is to turn the head to the side with the external auditory meatus pointing upward, and to place 2.0 cc of ice water in the meatus for 20 seconds, after which the ear canal is emptied and the head placed 60 degrees back to elicit nystagmus from the horizontal canal, and 30 degrees forward to elicit nystagmus from the vertical canals.[6] If there is no response, the amount of ice water is doubled each time until nystagmus results.

### Interpretation of the Caloric Test

No nystagmus after 40 cc. of ice water is interpreted as complete absence of vestibular response. It is seen in "dead labyrinth" after suppurative labyrinthitis, skull fracture or meningitis. It occurs bilaterally after large doses of streptomycin. It

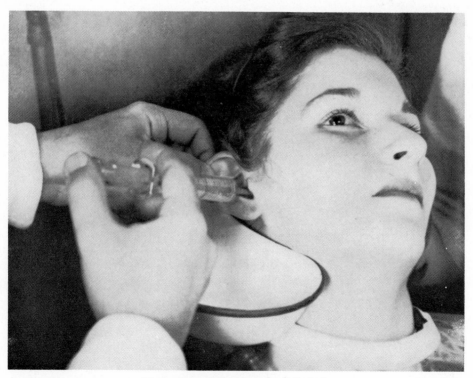

**Figure 3–9**   Technique of caloric test.

occurs unilaterally after labyrinthectomy or section of the eighth nerve and in some cases of acoustic neurinoma.

No nystagmus after 5 cc. of ice water but a response to 10 cc. or larger amounts indicates a hypoactive or depressed vestibular response. This occurs after smaller doses of streptomycin, in serous labyrinthitis, in endolymphatic hydrops, in labyrinthine concussion, in early acoustic neurinoma and sometimes after mumps.

Nystagmus after 5 cc. of ice water is interpreted as a normal vestibular response.

If the sensation produced by the caloric test is exactly the same as the vertigo experienced by the patient, the vertigo is probably of labyrinthine origin. If the patient's dizziness is unlike the sensation produced by the caloric test, the dizziness is probably not due to an ear lesion, but is of central cerebral origin.

If, instead of the expected horizontal nystagmus with the quick component toward the opposite ear, the caloric test produces a perverted nystagmus either toward the ear being tested, or oblique, vertical or rotary in direction, an intracranial lesion is probably present. For further consideration of the use of vestibular tests for the diagnosis of intracranial lesions the reader is referred to the excellent chapter by the Drs. Benjamin and Allen Shuster.[7]

### Electronystagmography[8]

*Technique.* Electronystagmography (ENG) requires 45 to 90 minutes for completion of the test battery. An electrode is placed lateral to each eye with a ground electrode placed on the forehead. Because of voltage differences between the cornea and the retina, eye movements can be graphed on a strip chart recorder.

The test battery consists of seven basic procedures:

1. *Saccade Test (Calibration).* Calibration of the equipment is accomplished by having the patient look back and forth between two calibration points placed 20 degrees apart. The recorder is adjusted until the pen deflects 20 mm. for 20 degrees of eye movement.

2. *Gaze Nystagmus Test.* The patient visually fixates on points, usually lights or dots at 20 degrees and at 30 degrees to the right and to the left.

3. *Sinusoidal Eye Tracking Test.* The patient visually follows a point moving back and forth along a slow pendular path.

4. *Optokinetic Test (OPK).* The patient observes a pattern of vertical stripes moving horizontally across the visual field. The test is conducted at two to three different speeds, with the stripes moving right-to-left and left-to-right.

5. *Positional Tests.* The patient is monitored while in a variety of head and body positions. Eye movements are recorded with eyes open and with eyes closed for 30 seconds each in each position. The patient is first observed when seated erect with the head straight and eyes closed. Nystagmus present in this position is called spontaneous nystagmus, as there are no nystagmus-inducing stimuli. Nystagmus present in other positions is called positional nystagmus. Common positions tested are:

    a. Supine with head straight, with head right and with head left.

    b. Supine with the whole body right and the whole body left.

    c. Sitting with the head left, with head right, with head hanging down and with head extended backwards.

6. *Positioning Test.* The patient is rapidly moved from a sitting to a supine

with head hanging right position, returned to sitting, then rapidly moved to a supine with head hanging left position, and returned back to a sitting position.

*7. J. B. Causse's Vertebro-Basilar Insufficiency (Deprivation) Nystagmus Test (VBI).* The patient is placed in the position for spontaneous nystagmus with eyes open in the dark. The head is bowed backwards as much as possible and then turned to the right or left as far as possible. This position is held for three minutes. If vertigo and nystagmus begin, the test is positive. The head is then returned to normal position, and the vertigo and nystagmus should promptly subside.

*8. Bithermal Caloric Test.* With the patient's head inclined backward 30 degrees and with eyes closed, each ear is irrigated separately with cool and warm water or air. Approximately 30 seconds after the response to the caloric stimulation begins, the patient is asked to fixate on a stationary spot or point for about ten seconds and then close his eyes again. When an ear is irrigated with the cool stimulus, the fast phase of the nystagmus should beat in the opposite direction of the ear that is irrigated. With the warm stimulus, the fast phase should beat toward the irrigated ear. Observations of the nystagmus resulting from the four stimulations are made in terms of its direction, duration, frequency and speed of the slow component.

### Interpretation of Electronystagmography

Electronystagmography is valuable because it permits monitoring of nystagmus with the eyes closed when suppression is less likely. It also provides a permanent record of nystagmus for medical-legal cases, for accurate objective calculation of the test results, and for the monitoring of treatment.

The results of the tests in the ENG battery aid the clinician in differentiating normal from abnormal vestibular systems. The analysis of the results can also differentiate between central and peripheral pathology, and in the latter case, it can help determine if the disorder is in the right or left ear. A brief interpretation of the test results follows. The reader is encouraged, however, to study recent texts on ENG for detailed information on specific procedures and interpretation before attempting a diagnosis from test results.

*1. Saccade Test (Calibration).* A normal calibration has the appearance of a square wave with no calibration overshoots (spikes). In conjunction with other signs, abnormal calibration suggests central pathology. This applies, however, only to tracings recorded by the direct current (DC) method. Recordings made with alternating current (AC) may appear similar to overshoots simply as a function of the recording method. Eye blinks may also look like overshoots.

*2. Gaze Nystagmus Test.* Nystagmus that appears when the patient gazes 20 to 30 degrees to the right or left or both is abnormal and indicative of central pathology if sedation effects and spontaneous nystagmus have been ruled out.

*3. Sinusoidal Eye Tracking Test.* Tracking responses can be categorized into four classes, Rubin Types I–IV (Figure 3–10). A tracking abnormality is supportive of central pathology.

*4. Optokinetic (OPK).* An abnormal optokinetic response is asymmetry of the recordings in the two directions, in terms of either appearance or speed of the slow component. Asymmetry indicates central pathology if spontaneous nystagmus and ocular disorders have been ruled out.

*5. Spontaneous and Positional Nystagmus Test.* The presence of spontaneous or positional nystagmus suggests pathology; however, it does not differentiate a

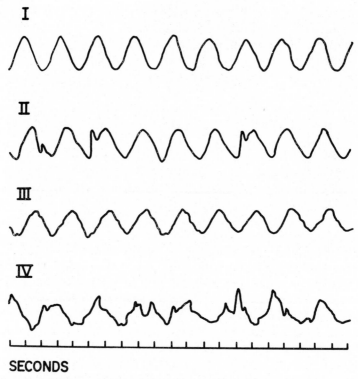

**SECONDS**

**Figure 3–10**  Sinusoidal eye tracking test responses: Rubin types I to IV. (From Rubin, Wallace, and Norris, Charles: Electronystagmography: What is ENG? 1974. Courtesy of Charles C Thomas Publisher, Springfield, Illinois.)

central from a peripheral disorder. When nystagmus is present, the following should be noted: (1) its direction and whether it is direction fixed or direction changing, (2) its average slow phase speed and (3) its fatigability and latency.

6. *Positioning Nystagmus Test.*  Nystagmus present in the positioning test suggests peripheral pathology if it meets the following classical criteria: (1) There is a latency of the response after assumption of the test position by one to eight seconds. (2) The nystagmus is transient, increasing rapidly, then declining rapidly. (3) It is not repeatable. (4) It is accompanied by dizziness.

7. *J. B. Causse's Vertebro-Basilar Insufficiency (Deprivation) Nystagmus Test (VBI).*  This test is positive only when a nystagmus appears after the third minute of the test. The competence of the vertebral artery that is being tested is the one opposite the rotation side.

8. *Bithermal Caloric Test.*  Caloric nystagmus test results allow comparison of the right and left vestibular systems. The most common measure is the speed of the slow component (SCC). From SCC calculations, differences between the ears can be obtained (unilateral weakness), as well as differences between the two right and the two left beating calorics (directional preponderance).

When interpreting the results, a 30 per cent difference is necessary to demonstrate unilateral hypoactivity or directional preponderance. Directional preponderance suggests pathology of the vestibular system, but it has no localizing or differentiating value. Unilateral weakness suggests a peripheral lesion. Bilateral hypofunction is a sign of an abnormality, but it has limited localizing value. Failure of fixation suppression (FFS) when the eyes are open during the peak of the caloric response is a strong indicator of a central nervous system disorder.

The proper interpretation of all these test results is quite complex. A thorough knowledge of the procedure for the administration of the test, the range of test results and possible causes is essential for the appropriate diagnosis.


## OTOSCOPIC INSPECTION

The general practitioner and pediatrician usually employ an electric otoscope, but for the practicing otologist a head mirror is preferable, as it leaves both hands free for instrumentation.


### Technique of Otoscopy

To expose to view the tympanic membrane, the external auditory meatus is conveniently straightened by grasping the auricle with the same hand that holds the ear speculum (Fig. 3–11). The largest speculum that can be introduced without pain should be used, and time should be taken to remove gently any obstructing cerumen or epidermal debris using a blunt ear hook or syringe. **Never syringe the ear** if there is a history suggesting a skull fracture or a perforation of the drum membrane.

The magnifying pneumatic speculum should be used to delineate minute lesions, such as a tiny perforation or one healed with a very thin transparent scar, and to test for a fluid level in the tympanic cavity. The office microscope is a valuable aid.

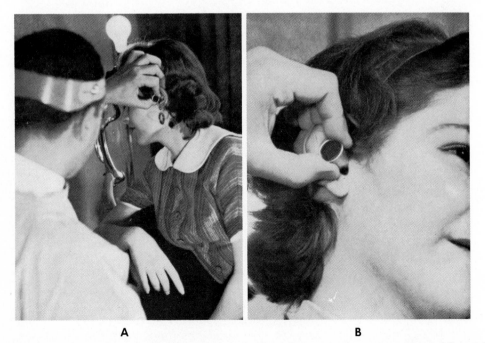

**A**                                                        **B**

**Figure 3–11**  Technique of holding ear speculum. *A*, Technique of grasping patient's left auricle between index and middle fingers. *B*, Technique of grasping auricle between middle and ring fingers of the hand holding speculum in patient's right ear.

*Interpretation of Otoscopic Picture* (See Figs. 7–1, 7–5
and 7–6)

Moderate and sometimes even marked changes, such as thickening, scarring, sclerotic deposits, atrophic areas and retracted position, should be recorded but do not necessarily mean interference with normal functioning of the sound-conducting mechanism.

The examiner should be alert to the tympanic membrane changes of secretory otitis media, a condition that is frequently overlooked. Typically the drum membrane in this condition has a yellowish color and an "oiled" look imparted by the clear amber or straw-colored fluid within the tympanum. The manubrium of the malleus stands out as a contrasting chalky white line. With the pneumatic speculum a fluid level or bubbles may be seen which shift with changes in the meatal air pressure, or on eustachian tube inflation. The diagnosis of secretory (serous) otitis media is more difficult in the presence of a thickened opaque tympanic membrane. In case of doubt, diagnostic myringotomy followed by inflation is indicated.

The hyperemic mucosa overlying an active otosclerotic focus is visible in a small percentage of patients with stapedial, cochlear or histologic otosclerosis as a positive Schwartze's sign.[9] A similar appearance may be produced by a crying child or by a recent eustachian tube occlusion with hyperemia ex vacuo of the tympanic mucosa.

Rarely a congenital cholesteatoma may be seen behind the intact tympanic membrane of a child as a doughy white cyst.[10]

The location of any perforation of the drum membrane should be observed carefully, for it is of great diagnostic value. If the perforation is confined to the pars tensa of the tympanic membrane, and mucous membrane is observed to line the visible portions of the tympanic cavity, it is termed a "central perforation," because a small intact margin of sulcus and annulus tympanicus is preserved in such cases. If the perforation includes portions of the sulcus and annulus tympanicus or of the pars flaccida, with skin lining portions of the visible middle ear cavity, it is termed a "marginal perforation." A perforation confined to the pars flaccida may not be a perforation at all, but an invagination of the pars flaccida into the attic. Invariably such an attic invagination or "attic perforation" is associated with an active or inactive cholesteatoma of the primary acquired or attic retraction variety (Chapters 7 and 10).

The character of any aural discharge is of diagnostic significance. A **mucoid** "benign" type discharge always means a perforation of the pars tensa of the tympanic membrane with infection or allergic reaction of the tympanic mucous membrane. A very tenacious rubbery type of mucus strongly suggests an allergic disturbance of the middle ear mucosa, analogous to and frequently associated with a chronic allergic rhinitis. The finding of eosinophiles in the mucus confirms the allergic etiology, but their absence does not rule out an allergic factor.

When the aural discharge is devoid of mucus it often has a foul odor and is coming from either an external otitis or a cholesteatoma in the attic or antrum. In either case the foul odor is due to decomposing desquamated squamous epithelial cells.

A polyp in the external meatus may protrude through a drum membrane perforation or, rarely, arise from the meatus. In most cases a polyp is the result of a chronic suppurative otitis media. The polyp is sometimes the result of the benign type of chronic suppurative otitis media and sometimes the result of a cholesteatoma. Because in some cases it is of neoplastic origin, **a polyp of the ear should always be examined microscopically after removal.**

A diagnostic procedure of value in distinguishing between a chronic suppurative otitis media of the benign mucous membrane type and a cholesteatoma is to irrigate through the attic cannula inserted into the perforation and directed upward into the attic. Warmed rubbing alcohol, 50 per cent, may be used, but the patient should be warned of possible pain. If the material obtained by irrigation contains flakes or lumps of epidermal debris, the diagnosis of an active cholesteatoma is confirmed and surgery may be required. If the material contains only mucus or mucopus, the otitis media is of the benign type and surgery for cholesteatoma is not indicated.

## EXAMINATION OF THE EUSTACHIAN TUBE

The walls of the cartilaginous eustachian tube normally lie in apposition and part momentarily to admit air only on swallowing or yawning or when there is a slight increase in nasopharyngeal air pressure. The levator and tensor muscles of the palate pull apart the posterior and anterior lips of the torus and simultaneously close the nasopharynx from the oropharynx.

The eustachian tube is examined by inspecting its nasopharyngeal orifice and by inflation.

### Inspection of Eustachian Orifice

A very satisfactory view of the eustachian orifice may be obtained by the experienced examiner using a small (size 0) postnasal mirror. If the patient gags easily, preliminary application of 10 per cent cocaine or 2 per cent Pontocaine to the soft palate and anterior pillars will facilitate the examination. Occasionally a palate retractor will be needed.

The nasopharyngoscope may be used instead of the postnasal mirror or in addition to it, after the inferior nasal meatus has been anesthetized by passing a cotton-tipped applicator along it moistened with 5 per cent or 10 per cent cocaine solution.

### Inflation of the Eustachian Tube

This is used to determine the presence of abnormal occlusion of the tube, with or without a secretory otitis media. Abnormal patency of the eustachian tube is a rare but interesting condition easily confused with abnormal occlusion. The patent tube causes a very disagreeable resounding of the patient's own voice in his ear, termed **autophonia**, and he complains that his ear feels "stopped up." Insufflation through the eustachian catheter of salicylic acid powder 1 part with boric acid powder 4 parts causes enough irritation and secretion to close the tube and relieve the symptoms for several days.[11]

Abnormal occlusion of the eustachian tube may be due to one of the following, listed in the order of their relative frequency in otologic practice:

1. Hypertrophy of nasopharyngeal adenoid tissue. This is a frequent cause of impaired hearing of mild to moderate degree in school children. It also causes occasional cases of impaired hearing in adults.

2. Allergic tubotympanitis. This is usually but not always associated with

allergic rhinitis. It is more frequent than hypertrophy of the adenoid as a cause of impaired hearing in children and adults and is often associated with lymphoid hypertrophy in the nasopharynx.

3.   Acute viral or bacterial nasopharyngitis.

4.   Descent in plane, train or mine-shaft, or ascent from caisson or deep-sea diving, when the patient fails to open his eustachian tubes at regular intervals because of head cold or allergy, or because he is asleep. The result is termed barotrauma or aero-otitis.

5.   Cleft palate, both before and after surgical repair, due to deficient structure and function of the tensor and levator muscles of the palate, is very often complicated by tubotympanitis, which is frequently allergic.

6.   Tumor of the nasopharynx. Persistent unilateral eustachian tube occlusion may be the first symptom of nasopharyngeal carcinoma.

7.   Scarring of the tubal orifice after adenoidectomy, or from healed syphilis or tuberculosis.

8.   Malocclusion of the mandibular joint (Costen syndrome).[12] This is an infrequent cause of impaired hearing due to tubal occlusion.

The effect on the hearing of abnormal occlusion of the eustachian tube is due to absorption by the lining mucosa of the oxygen from the air within the tympanic cavity, until a slight to moderate negative pressure develops. The tympanic membrane becomes sharply retracted and, owing to the resulting increased stiffness of the sound-conducting system, there is a mild conductive hearing loss, greater for the frequencies of low pitch (see Chapter 13). If the occlusion of the tube persists, the oxygen, then nitrogen is slowly absorbed from the air within the tympanic cavity, the middle ear mucosa becomes hyperemic from the increasing negative pressure and a clear amber or straw-colored transudate begins to accumulate to produce a secretory (serous) otitis media. The addition of the mass of this fluid to the increased stiffness produced by the negative pressure results in an increased moderate conductive hearing loss involving both high- and low-pitched tones. In some cases of secretory otitis of allergic origin a tenacious mucoid fluid fills the middle ear spaces, with little or no negative pressure ("glue ear"). The conductive hearing loss in these cases is the result of increased mass alone, with a greater loss for the frequencies of high pitch resembling and sometimes mistaken for a sensorineural loss.

In the initial stages, and in some cases even after many months or several years of a secretory otitis media, the middle ear changes remain reversible, and normal hearing may be restored by removing the source of the abnormal occlusion of the eustachian tube. However, in other cases, particularly when there is an allergic factor complicated by recurring attacks of inflammatory bacterial otitis media, a long-standing secretory otitis leads to permanent fibrotic changes in the middle ear. One of the most frequent causes of invagination of the pars flaccida, with eventual formation of an attic cholesteatoma, is a prolonged secretory otitis of allergic origin.[13]

A detailed discussion of the treatment of abnormal occlusion of the eustachian tube is beyond the scope of this *Surgery of the Ear*. Suffice it to mention that the great majority of cases will respond satisfactorily to careful surgical removal of excess nasopharyngeal adenoid tissue, with recognition of and attention to any associated nasal allergy, with a few tubal inflations and a myringotomy to evacuate accumulated clear fluid, and insertion of a ventilation tube into the myringotomy incision for long-standing cases. Radiation of the nasopharynx is no longer used, especially in children, because of the danger of late development of carcinoma of the thyroid.

The diagnosis of abnormal occlusion of the eustachian tube is made by:

1. A significant, measurable hearing improvement when the eustachian tube is inflated.

2. Demonstration of a clear nonpurulent fluid within the tympanic cavity.

For routine office diagnosis the author favors the Politzer type of inflation while the tympanic membrane is inspected. This has several advantages over catheter inflation: It is quicker and less painful for the patient; otoscopic inspection during inflation is one of the best ways to determine the presence of fluid, indicated by bubbles or a shifting fluid level; a very slight but definite visible outward movement of the tympanic membrane at the moment of inflation without a subjective or objective change in the hearing and without visible evidence of fluid very quickly rules out the eustachian tube as a factor in a conductive hearing loss. When the tube cannot be inflated by the Politzer method or when for some reason it is desired to introduce a medication into the tubal orifice, catheter inflation is resorted to.

### Technique of Politzer Inflation

The method used by the author requires an assistant. The examiner places the head of the patient in proper position to view the tympanic membrane through an ear speculum (Fig. 3–12). The assistant then introduces compressed air through a snugly fitting olive-shaped nasal tip while holding the nostrils tightly closed as the patient swallows or says, "K, K, K." Initially air under 10 pounds of pressure is used, and if the tubes do not inflate the pressure is gradually increased to a maximum of 20 pounds. Care must be taken not to rupture a thin or atrophic drum membrane. To protect the drum membrane of the opposite ear from possible damage from overinflation it is well to have the patient hold the tragus of this ear tightly against the meatus while the ear being watched is inflated. Should inflation cause accidental rupture of a thin tympanic membrane, prompt splinting by the application of a patch of cigarette paper, moistened on one side with 1 per cent phenol in glycerine to make it adhere, will result in rapid healing.

### Technique of Catheter Inflation

The floor of the nasal passage through which the catheter will be passed is first anesthetized by passing along it two or three times a cotton-tipped applicator moistened with 5 per cent or 10 per cent cocaine solution or 2 per cent Pontocaine solution.

The examiner stands at the same side of the patient as the tube to be catheterized and adjusts the auscultation tube between his meatus and the meatus of the patient. Facing in the same direction as the patient, the examiner rests his forearm nearest to the patient on the patient's head and gently lifts the tip of the nose with that hand (Fig. 3–13). The beak of the eustachian catheter, held in the free hand, is gently introduced into the vestibule and slid along the floor of the nose to the posterior wall of the nasopharynx. It is then withdrawn an average of 1.5 cm. (⅝ inch), and the curved beak is turned outward and directed toward the outer angle of the eye. The end of the catheter protruding from the nose is pushed gently against the septum and inward, engaging the tubal orifice. With the hand of the arm resting on the patient's head the catheter is held in place while the Politzer bag or compressed air is applied to the catheter with the other hand. A soft blowing sound is heard when

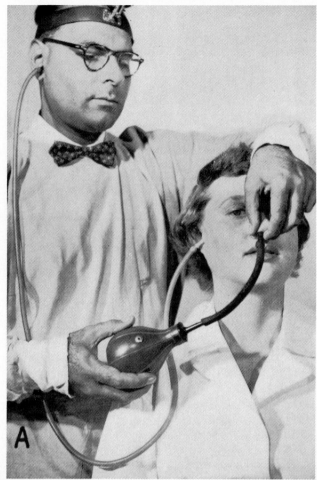

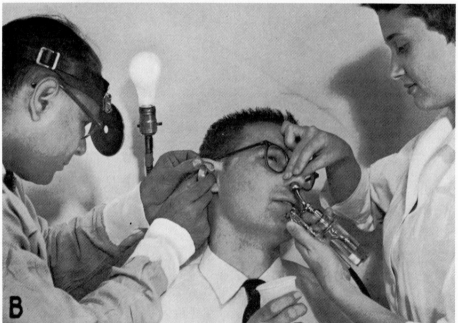

Figure 3–12  *A*, Traditional method of Politzer inflation of eustachian tube using auscultation tube. *B*, Simplified method of Politzer inflation for determining patency of eustachian tube and presence of fluid.

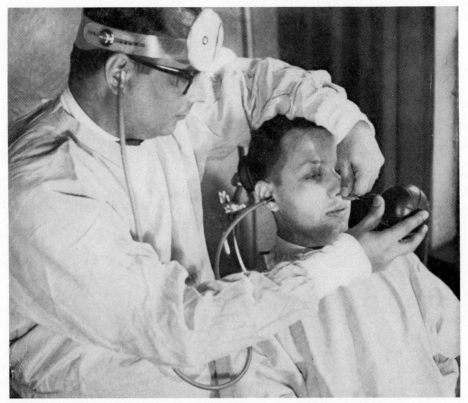

**Figure 3–13**   Technique of eustachian catheterization and inflation.

the catheter is in the tubal orifice and the latter is normally patent. A rough harsh flutter like the wings of a bird is heard when the beak of the catheter is in Rosenmüller's fossa instead of in the eustachian tube. A moist bubbling or squeaky sound is heard when there is fluid within the tympanic cavity. Inability to inflate the eustachian tube by catheter may be due to marked septal deviation. It is unusual for the tube to be permanently and completely occluded by scar tissue so that it cannot be inflated with the catheter.

*Interpretation of Eustachian Tube Inflation*

A great many incorrect diagnoses of abnormal occlusion of the eustachian tube have been made, and followed by months and even years of fruitless inflations, especially in patients with otosclerosis and endolymphatic hydrops. Such diagnostic errors can and should be avoided by these simple rules:

1.   Pure sensorineural hearing losses with a positive Rinne test to the 256 tuning fork and a shortened Schwabach test are never the result of eustachian tube occlusion.

2.   Successful inflation of the eustachian tube without evidence of fluid and without a measurable hearing improvement rules out the eustachian tube as a factor in a conductive hearing loss. Mention should be made of the occasional case of early beginning otosclerotic stapes fixation in which inflation may loosen the partially

fixed stages with a definite gain in hearing. Later, as the otosclerotic ankylosis advances farther, inflation no longer influences the hearing.

3.  Eustachian tube occlusion, nearly always accompanied by clear fluid in the tympanic cavity, is the **only** type of chronic hearing impairment that receives lasting benefit from inflation and for which inflation is indicated.

4.  In the absence of secretory otitis and a measurable hearing improvement after inflation, irradiation of the nasopharynx or opening of the mandibular "bite" cannot be expected to influence the hearing.

5.  A permanent adhesive process may follow a prolonged tubal occlusion. If the process is inactive and there is no longer fluid within the tympanum, further inflations are not indicated.

6.  If there is doubt as to the presence of a secretory otitis, a diagnostic myringotomy and inflation is indicated. If there is no fluid, the condition is not due to abnormal occlusion of the tube.

7.  Otosclerosis is a far more frequent cause of a conductive hearing loss in adults than is eustachian tube occlusion.


## DIFFERENTIAL DIAGNOSIS OF HEARING LOSSES

Complete diagnosis of a hearing impairment should begin with an exact estimate of the conductive and sensorineural components of the loss, proceed to a determination of the particular pathologic lesion and probable etiology of each component and end with the prognosis as to future progression or future maintained stable level of hearing, and the degree of improvement (if any) to be expected from therapy.

In many sensorineural losses the exact pathologic lesion and etiology remain obscure, and the final diagnosis must be: "perceptive loss, cause unknown." Conversely it is seldom that the exact pathologic lesion and etiology of a conductive loss cannot be determined with comparative ease and accuracy. This is fortunate, for **the great majority of conductive losses can be improved by therapy**, whereas with the exception of cases of endolymphatic hydrops, syphilis of the inner ear and cochlear otospongiosis, **sensorineural losses cannot be influenced by medical or surgical treatment**.


## ETIOLOGIC TYPES OF SENSORINEURAL LOSS

A list of 20 common types of sensorineural loss follows.

1.  Congenital nerve deafness in which the loss apparently dates from birth. As a rule the loss is stable and any residual hearing will remain unchanged. Two etiologic varieties can be distinguished:

    a.  Endogenous congenital nerve deafness, due to an inherited defect of the cochlea, usually with a positive family history and sometimes with consanguinity of the parents. Bilateral symmetry of the loss is characteristic, often with a "cookie-bite" type of audiometric curve.

    b.  Exogenous congenital nerve deafness, due to damage to the cochlea during intra-uterine life or at the time of delivery. Rubella or other virus in the mother during the first trimester of pregnancy, quinine taken during pregnancy, erythroblastosis due to Rh factor and anoxia at the time of delivery are possible causes of exogenous congenital nerve deafness. The loss is bilateral, usually greater for high frequencies and usually symmetric.

2. Toxic (febrile) nerve deafness occurring most often in childhood but occasionally later in life during the acute toxic febrile stage of a severe general infection such as measles, scarlet fever, influenza, pneumonia and typhoid fever. The history is very typical: normal hearing up to the time of the severe illness and a marked loss of hearing noted immediately after the severe toxic febrile stage of the disease, followed by a partial recovery of hearing in the next few months, after which the loss remains stable. The loss is bilateral, greater for high frequencies and usually symmetric.

3. Toxic nerve deafness from drugs, especially quinine, occasionally sali- cylates and more recently from streptomycin, neomycin, kanamycin, or other ototoxic drug. All but dihydrostreptomycin produce a bilaterally symmetric high-tone loss that comes on **during** the administration of the drug, with partial recovery of hearing when the drug is withdrawn, after which the residual loss remains stable. Dihydro- streptomycin produces a peculiar type of delayed loss of hearing that may not begin until 2 to 6 months after the drug is given.[14] This particular drug etiology therefore frequently escapes recognition.

4. Toxic nerve deafness from chronic osteomyelitis (not of the temporal bone) is bilateral and progressive and may lead to profound deafness.

5. Congenital syphilitic nerve deafness. The typical picture is that of a fairly rapidly progressing asymmetric sensorineural loss sometimes with vestibular symp- toms occurring several to many years after a childhood interstitial keratitis. The syphilitic nature of the hearing loss is determined by the history, since as a rule the blood and spinal fluid serology are negative as the result of previous antisyphilitic treatment. The pathologic lesion is a gummatous osteitis and periostitis of the laby- rinthine capsule and gummatous labyrinthitis.[15] Intensive treatment with penicillin for 6 weeks to 3 months, 2.4 million units of long acting penicillin (LABP) weekly with prednisone, 30–60 mg. every other day for 4 to 8 days, decreasing to 10 mg. every second day may arrest the progressive cochlear deterioration.

6. Acquired syphilitic nerve deafness. The perceptive loss may appear during the secondary stage, but more often it occurs in late tertiary syphilis. The positive blood serology test determines the diagnosis. Active treatment with penicillin and prednisone arrests and may improve an early hearing loss.

7. Progressive hereditary nerve deafness. This interesting and relatively uncommon bilateral symmetric high-tone sensorineural loss begins in late child- hood or early adult life; the loss is progressive and there are others in the family with the same condition.[16] The onset, progression and pattern of hearing loss resemble presbycusis except for the earlier age of onset.

8. Skull fracture that passes through the osseous labyrinth produces a sudden, severe, permanent and usually total loss of cochlear and vestibular function confined to the affected ear.

9. Concussion without fracture can produce a perceptive loss similar to that of a skull fracture, but usually less severe. It may be bilateral and asymmetric, and sometimes is accompanied by vestibular symptoms.[17]

10. Serous labyrinthitis secondary to an acute or chronic suppurative otitis media, or to surgical trauma during fenestration or stapes operation, produces a unilateral depression of cochlear function, with vertigo and often with diplacusis. If the labyrinthitis is mild, it may be reversible, with a return of normal function after several weeks. If it is severe, there may be a permanent residue of perceptive loss; in

some of these cases a slowly progressive deterioration of cochlear function eventually occurs.

11.  Suppurative labyrinthitis produces an abrupt loss of cochlear and vestibular response in one or both ears. Infection may gain access to the labyrinth from a suppurative otitis media, from imperfect aseptic technique during fenestration or stapes operation, rarely from an infected fenestration cavity, or via the internal auditory meatus from meningitis.

12.  Acoustic neurinoma produces unilateral progressive loss of vestibular and cochlear response, followed by involvement of the seventh (facial) and fifth (trigeminal) cranial nerves and then by cerebellar and brain stem symptoms, with x-ray evidence of bone erosion in or around the internal auditory meatus. Although it is usually unilateral, it may be bilateral in von Recklinghausen's multiple neurofibromatosis (see Chapter 23).

13.  Excessive noise produces two types of hearing loss:
   a.  A single sharp sound of high intensity, such as an explosion or the static "click" of early telephones, produces a permanent sensorineural loss in the exposed ear, with a variable audiometric pattern, usually with diplacusis. This is termed "acoustic trauma."
   b.  Prolonged exposure to industrial or aircraft noise or to gunfire produces the more common progressive notching of the audiogram in the region of 4000 cycles. In some cases the notch continues slowly to deepen and widen long after the noise exposure has ceased. This is termed "noise-induced hearing loss."

14.  Mumps or other virus may produce a unilateral, rarely a bilateral, severe sensorineural loss, with no impairment or a slight loss of vestibular response.

15.  Sudden labyrinthine unilateral deafness occurring in young or middle-aged adults who are otherwise in good health, sometimes with vestibular symptoms, may be due to interruption of the blood supply to the inner ear by vasospasm, embolus or thrombus, or to viral cochleitis such as the deafness from mumps.

16.  Endolymphatic hydrops or Meniere's disease is, as a rule, easily recognized by the **fluctuating** sensorineural hearing loss, accompanied by roaring tinnitus, attacks of vertigo, a sense of fullness in the ear, recruitment and diplacusis. In the early stages the low-pitched frequencies are usually affected more than the high-pitched tones. It usually begins in one ear but may become bilateral. Particularly characteristic of this common condition is the moderate impairment of discrimination producing difficulty in understanding speech that is out of proportion to the degree of loss. Békésy audiometry is Type II, and the SISI score is 60 to 100 per cent.

Endolymphatic hydrops is one of the few types of nerve deafness that sometimes can be improved by therapy. Others are psychogenic deafness, syphilis and cochlear otospongiosis. The medical and surgical treatment of labyrinthine hydrops is described in Chapter 21. The reader is referred to a useful summary of its medical management by Derlacki.[18]

17.  Sensorineural loss of central origin. Multiple sclerosis sometimes produces a sensorineural type of hearing loss probably due to interruption of the auditory pathways within the brain stem. Some cases of presbycusis with disproportionate loss of the ability to understand speech (phonemic regression) may be of central origin. Cases of recognizable central deafness are uncommon, and many are due to cerebral arteriosclerosis. Central nervous system diseases are usually **not** accompanied by a loss of hearing.

18.  Psychogenic deafness is not always easily differentiated from malingering,

the latter presupposing conscious deception. A true psychogenic (unconscious) hearing loss is often superimposed upon a previous organic loss and is termed "psychogenic overlay." A marked discrepancy between the pure tone loss and the speech reception threshold, an atypical history of sudden unexplained onset or unexplained fluctuations in hearing ability related to emotional stress, a positive Doefler-Stewart[19] test and finally unexpected improvement in hearing following therapy, such as in the untreated ear after fenestration or stapes surgery, all point toward a psychogenic loss. Most, but not all, cases of psychogenic deafness can be improved or relieved by psychotherapy. Acoustic reflex tests and Brainstem Evoked Response help to verify a psychogenic or malingering deafness.

19. Cochlear otospongiosis (otosclerosis) without stapes fixation may be suspected in patients with a positive family history of otosclerosis who develop in early or middle adult life a progressive sensorineural loss of unknown etiology. If, later on, stapes fixation occurs in one or both ears, the suspicion of cochlear otospongiosis is verified. A strongly positive Schwartze's sign (pinkish glow from the promontory) and tomographic visualization of osseous changes in the cochlear capsule (see Chapter 5) are confirmatory evidence of cochlear otospongiosis. Cochlear otospongiosis is probably more common than is generally appreciated. See Chapter 17 for further diagnostic criteria and therapy of cochlear otospongiosis.

Otospongiotic (otosclerotic) stapes fixation is accompanied by varying degrees of sensorineural loss in most but not all cases, the sensorineural loss presumably being of otospongiotic origin. The sensorineural loss that may accompany stapes fixation bears no constant relationship to the time of onset of the fixation or to the degree of fixation. Thus the sensorineural loss may precede, it may begin at the same time or it may follow after several years the onset of stapes ankylosis. Typically it is a high-tone loss, but it may involve the middle frequencies in a localized notching on the air and bone audiograms. Rarely it may affect the lower frequencies as much or more than the high frequencies. Symmetry of the loss between the two ears is frequent but not invariable in cochlear otospongiosis.

20. Prebycusis is the progressive bilaterally symmetric perceptive hearing loss that occurs with age. The age of onset and the rapidity of progression vary greatly among patients. The audiometric pattern of the loss also varies somewhat, from a sloping high-tone loss to a flatter audiogram with a loss for all frequencies, with variable impairment of speech discrimination.

## ETIOLOGIC TYPES OF CONDUCTIVE LOSS

1. Occlusion of the external auditory meatus may be the result of congenital atresia or absence of the meatus, acquired atresia from external otitis or trauma, foreign body or impacted cerumen, furuncle, polyp, exostosis, osteoma or other neoplasm. Restoration of normal hearing can be expected after removal of the obstruction, provided the tympanic membrane, ossicular chain and cochlear function are normal.

2. Perforation of the pars tensa of the tympanic membrane may be the result of trauma, following removal or extrusion of a ventilation tube or after an acute necrotic otitis media (Chapter 7). Closure of the perforation improves or restores the hearing to normal provided the ossicular chain is intact and mobile and the cochlear function is normal.

3. Occlusion of the eustachian tube may be caused by the conditions listed on pages 73 and 74.

Restoration of hearing to normal may be expected by evacuation of fluid from the tympanum with relief of tubal obstruction, provided the cochlear function is normal and adhesive changes have not complicated a long-standing secretory otitis.

4.   Suppurative otitis media of the ordinary acute variety (Chapter 7) produces a reversible hearing loss with restoration of normal hearing to be expected when the inflammation subsides. On the other hand, suppurative otitis media of the acute necrotic variety (Chapter 7) produces varying degrees of permanent fibrotic and destructive changes in the middle ear with varying degrees of residual conductive loss (chronic adhesive otitis media) after the acute inflammation subsides.

Chronic suppurative otitis media is associated with varying degrees of fibrotic and destructive changes in the middle ear, with resultant permanent conductive loss (chronic adhesive otitis media). An exception is the occasional primary acquired (attic retraction) cholesteatoma with intact ossicular chain and normal hearing (Chapter 10).

5.   Chronic adhesive otitis media may be the residue of an earlier acute necrotic otitis or of a no longer active chronic suppurative otitis or the result of a long-standing secretory otitis. The history of hearing loss following an otitis media and the absence of progression after the active process has subsided, with more or less pronounced changes of thickening and scarring in the tympanic membrane, serve to differentiate these cases from otosclerosis. A special variety of conductive hearing loss remaining after subsidence of an otitis media is that due to necrosis of the long process of the incus with ossicular interruption. Surgical reconstruction of the sound-conducting mechanism results in a useful improvement in hearing in most of these cases (Chapter 16).

6.   Congenital malformation of the ossicular chain resembles otosclerosis in that there is a conductive hearing loss without occlusion of the meatus, without perforation or scarring of the tympanic membrane and without obstruction of the eustachian tube or history of antecedent otitis media. It differs from otosclerosis in that the hearing loss dates from birth and **it is not progressive** (see Chapter 14). The malformation causing the impairment varies from an ankylosis of one or more of the ossicles to absence of part or all of an ossicle. Most of these cases are discovered during fenestration or stapes operation for supposed otosclerotic stapes fixation. The hearing can be improved or restored by appropriate surgical correction of the defective sound-conducting system.

7.   Stapedial otospongiosis (otosclerosis) produces a conductive hearing loss due to ankylosis of the stapes that comes on insidiously in early or middle adult life (rarely in childhood) and is progressive, without evidence of preceding otitis media or eustachian tube occlusion.

Rarely diagnosed during life prior to 1938, these cases were commonly called "chronic catarrhal otitis media." The fenestration and stapes operations, affording the opportunity to inspect and to test the mobility of the stapes footplate during life, have demonstrated beyond any doubt that **otospongiosis (otosclerosis) with primary stapes fixation is the most frequent cause of progressive conductive deafness during early and middle adult life**, and that it **can** be diagnosed during life with a high degree of accuracy.

Although the tendency is toward progression of the hearing loss in stapedial otospongiosis (otosclerosis), many cases become inactive and the hearing loss stabilizes after an initial active stage of progressive impairment of the hearing. In other cases the loss progresses for a time, stabilizes for several years and then progresses again, presumably as the otospongiotic focus becomes mature or actively enlarges.

The majority of hearing losses due to otospongiotic stapes fixation can be improved by stapes surgery or formerly by classic fenestration.

## *Acknowledgment*

Mr. Roger Larose, M.A., audiologist of the Shambaugh Ear Institute, and Mrs. Mary Evans, M.S., audiologist of Hinsdale, were a great help in revising Chapter 3.

## REFERENCES

1. Weiss, E., and English, O. S.: Psychomatic Medicine. 3rd Ed. W. B. Saunders Co., Philadelphia, 1957, p. 4.
2. Adapted from Nash, C. S., In Coates, G. M., et al. (editors): Otolaryngology. Vol. I. Prior, Hagerstown, Md., 1955, Chap. 7.
3. Ventry, I. M., Chailkin, J. B., and Boyle, W. F.: Collapse of the ear canal during audiometry. Arch. Otol., *73*:727, 1961.
4. Shambaugh, G. E., Jr.: Diplacusis: a localizing symptom of disease of the organ of Corti. Arch. Otol., *31*:160, 1940.
5. Katz, J. (editor): Handbook of Clinical Audiology. 2nd Ed. Williams & Wilkins Co., Baltimore, 1978.
6. Pulec, J. L., House, W. F., and Hughes, R. L.: Vestibular involvement and testing in acoustic neuromas. Arch. Otol., *80*:677, 1964.
7. Shuster, B., and Shuster, A., In Coates, G. M., et al. (editors): Otolaryngology. Vol. I. Prior, Hagerstown, Md., 1955, Chap. 5.
8. Rubin, W., and Norris, C. H.: Electronystagmography: What is E.N.G.? Charles C Thomas, Springfield, Ill., 1974.
9. Schwartze, H. H.: Handbuch der Ohrenkeilkunde, Leipzig, 1837.
10. Derlacki, E. L, and Clemis, J. D.: Congenital cholesteatoma of the middle ear and mastoid. Ann. Otol. Rhin. & Laryng., *74*:706, 1965.
11. Shambaugh, G. E., Jr.: The continuously open eustachian tube. Arch. Otol., *27*:420, 1938.
12. Costen, J. B.: Syndrome of ear and sinus symptoms dependent upon disturbed function of the temporomandibular joint. Ann. Otol. Rhin. & Laryng., *43*:1, 1934.
13. Jordan, R. E., discussion in Derlacki, E. L., and Shambaugh, G. E., Jr.: Allergic management of some common ear conditions. Tran. Am. Acad. Ophtha., *57*:311, 1953.
14. Glorig, A.: The effect of dihydrostreptomycin on the auditory mechanism. Ann. Otol. Rhin. & Laryng., *60*:327, 1951.
15. Mayer, O., and Fraser, J. S.: Pathologic changes in the ear in congenital syphilis. J. Laryng. & Otol., *51*:683, 1936.
16. Manasse, P.: Über chronische, progressive, labyrinthäre Taubheit. Ztschr. Ohrenh., *52*:1, 1906.
17. Schuknecht, H. F., and Davison, R. C.: Deafness and vertigo from head injuries. Arch. Otol., *63*:513, 1956.
18. Derlacki, E. L.: Non-surgical management of Meniere's disease. Laryngoscope, *64*:271, 1954.
19. Doefler, L., and Stewart, K.: Malingering and psychogenic deafness. J. Speech & Hearing Disorders, *11*:181, 1946.

# Chapter 4

# Conventional Radiologic Examination of the Temporal Bone

W. E. COMPERE, JR., M.D.
*La Mesa, California*

POSITIONS
TECHNIQUE OF ROUTINE FILMING OF THE DIAGNOSTIC
  POSITIONS
INTERPRETATION
ACUTE MASTOIDITIS
PETROSITIS
CHRONIC MASTOIDITIS
CONGENITAL CHOLESTEATOMA
ATRESIA
OTHER DISEASES OF THE TEMPORAL BONE

Radiologic studies are a valuable aid for the diagnosis of ear diseases associated with changes in the osseous structure. Routine films must be taken in positions designed to reveal pathologic lesions in the area most frequently involved in **chronic** ear disease, namely the attic-aditus-antrum or "key area." The otologic surgeon, who not only knows the clinical course of the disease in the particular patient but who can best correlate the radiologic changes with the pathologic lesion seen at surgery, is in a particularly favorable position to be able to interpret x-ray films of the ear.

## POSITIONS

Various positions have been described for radiologic study of the temporal bone. Some of these, like the Law position (Fig. 4–1) devised in the preantibiotic era

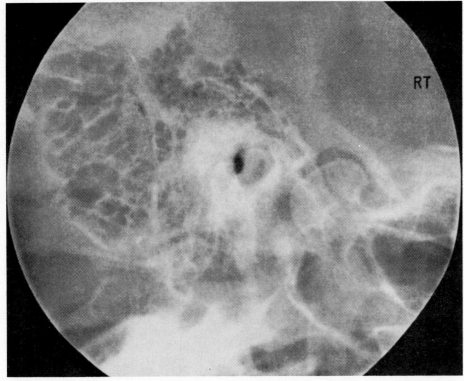

**Figure 4–1**  Law position. The external canal, tympanic cavity, vestibule and internal canal are shown by an area of diminished density behind the mandibular condyle. The attic-aditus-antral area is obscured entirely. The pneumatic cells of mastoid process are well visualized.

for acute coalescent mastoiditis, are unsuited for today's needs because they fail to visualize the key attic-aditus-antrum area. More useful are the Schüller (Fig. 4–2), Mayer (Figs. 4–3 and 4–4), Owen (Figs. 4–5 and 4–6), Stenvers (Fig. 4–7) and Chausse III (Figs. 4–8 and 4–9) positions, the five views that should be employed routinely. These positions will be better understood after a brief review of the evolution—as it occurred—of positions designed to visualize the key area.

In the first film, the x-ray beam is directed downward from a 15 degree elevation and anteriorly 15 degrees as described by Law in 1920. The ossicles are superimposed on the dense arcuate eminence of the superior (anterior) vertical semicircular canal, and so are not seen.

Schüller's position, described in 1905, displaces the arcuate eminence downward by increasing the elevation of the beam to 30 degrees. A good part of the antrum is now exposed, with a beginning exposure of the attic (Fig. 4–2). A portion of the head of the malleus may now be seen, but the remainder of the ossicles are still obscured by the dense osseous labyrinth. Thus the Schüller position differs from the Law position in that it opens up the antrum and part of the attic by the increased elevation of the beam. With this advantage it loses none of the remaining landmarks of the Law position: the root of the zygoma; condyle of the mandible; temporomandibular joint; external auditory canal superimposed on the tympanic cavity; vestibule of the labyrinth and internal auditory canal; the cellular structure of the mastoid process; the sinus plate; and the tegmen plate.

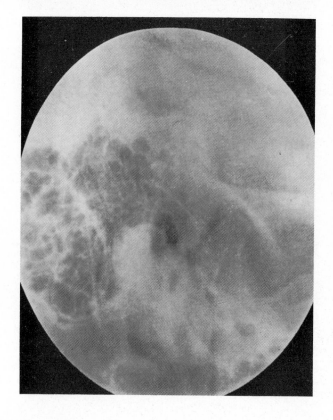

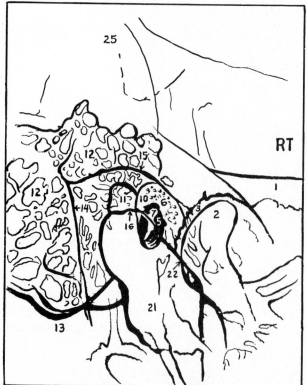

**Figure 4–2**   Schüller position. By increasing the elevation of the beam, the labyrinth is depressed and the head of the malleus is visible above the crest of the petrosa. Compare with Fig. 4–1.

By a still further elevation of the beam to 45 degrees from directly laterally, the labyrinth is further depressed. In this position, which we call the "primary Mayer," an increased amount of cellular area in the antrum, aditus and attic is freed from the dense shadow of the labyrinth. The head of the malleus and part of the incus are now clearly seen (Fig. 4–3).

The primary Mayer position is not generally used in diagnosis, the "conventional Mayer" being utilized instead. In the "conventional Mayer" (usually referred to simply as the "Mayer position") the same 45 degree elevation of the beam is maintained, but in addition the head is rotated so that the face turns away from the cassette about 30 degrees. This rotation combined with the elevation of the beam effectively frees the key area from the dense shadow of the labyrinth.

The malleus and incus are well seen in the upper tympanic and epitympanic cavities (Fig. 4–4). The cellular pattern of the osseous outer attic wall is well indicated. The antrum is less well visualized because it is partially obscured by the arcuate eminence. Observe that the ridge of the petrosa is almost vertical owing to the elevation of the beam and the rotation of the head.

The obliquity of the Mayer position, although necessary to free the key area from the shadow of the labyrinth, produces a distortion that may confuse the surgeon. Notice in Figure 4–5 that progressive elevation of the beam produces progressive elongation and distortion of the key area. To lessen this distortion the Owen position has been devised. The elevation of the beam is lessened to 30 degrees, but the

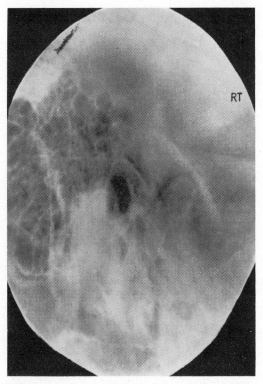

**Figure 4–3** "Primary Mayer" position. The dense labyrinth has been further depressed but still partially obscures the antrum and tympanic cavity.

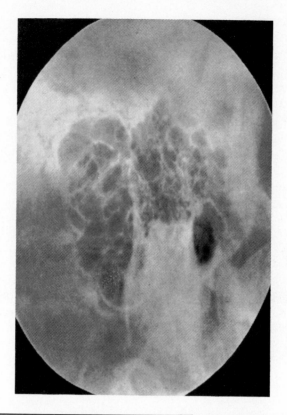

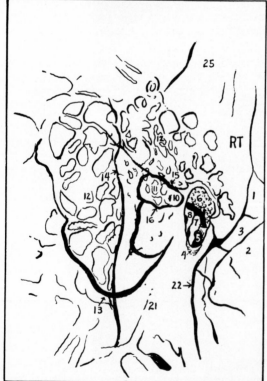

KEY TO THE LINE DRAWING

1. Root of the zygoma
2. Condyle of the mandible
3. Temporomandibular joint
4. External auditory canal
5. Tympanic cavity
6. Epitympanic cavity
7. Malleus
8. Incus
10. Area of the aditus
11. Area of the antrum
12. Mastoid cells
13. Mastoid tip
14. Anterior plate of the lateral sinus
15. Tegmen plate
16. Arcuate eminence
21. Petrosa
22. Anterior crest of the petrosa
25. Auricle

**Figure 4–4** Conventional Mayer position showing malleus and incus in tympanic cavity with cells of attic. The antrum is partially obscured by the arcuate eminence.

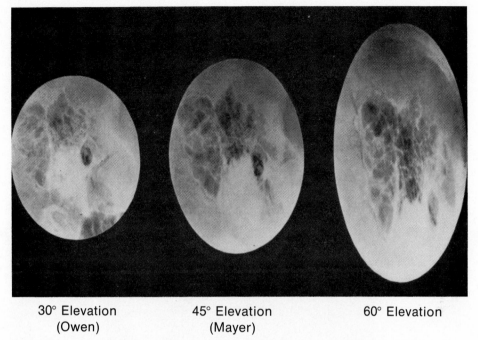

30° Elevation          45° Elevation          60° Elevation
(Owen)                 (Mayer)

**Figure 4–5**  Distortion of the "key area" produced by progressive elevation of the x-ray beam to depress the shadow of the labyrinth.

rotation of about 30 degrees is maintained. All the anatomic landmarks of the Mayer are retained, but the malleus and incus are "put back into the tympanic cavity where they belong," the short arm of the incus extending into the aditus (Fig. 4–6). The lateral wall of the attic with its pneumatic pattern is clearly visible, and the antrum is in a more normal position for the surgeon, just above the arcuate eminence.

The next routine diagnostic position is the Stenvers. This is taken with the central ray depressed, with a rotation of the face toward the cassette so as to bring the petrosa perpendicular to the beam. This position is best for the antrum, cellular structure of the petrous apex, internal auditory canal, cochlea, horizontal and vertical semicircular canals and vestibule of the labyrinth (Fig. 4–7). This position also shows the tegmen plate, tympanic cavity, ossicles, condyle of the mandible and mastoid air cells lateral to the antrum and in the mastoid tip.

The third projection of Chausse (Chausse III, Figs. 4–8 and 4–9) is a modified frontal projection useful for the study of the attic, aditus, mastoid antrum and especially of the lateral wall of the attic. This wall runs from back to front and slightly outward, forming an angle of 10 to 15 degrees with the sagittal plane of the skull. In the Chausse III projection the head of the patient is rotated so as to bring the lateral attic wall perpendicular to the plane of the film.

Additional positions sometimes employed are the **Chamberlain-Towne** position (Fig. 4–10) and the **submento-vertex** position (Fig. 4–11). These are used to view the petrous apex and the mastoid antrum but have no advantage over the Stenvers position, with the disadvantage of loss of clarity and detail because of increased antrum-to-film distance. Therefore they are not included in the recommended positions for routine diagnostic studies of the temporal bone.

*Text continued on page 94*

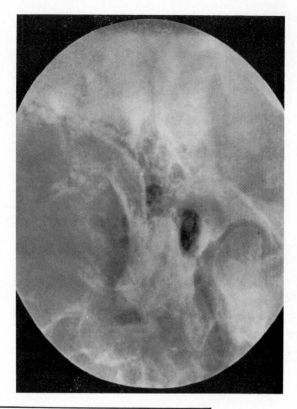

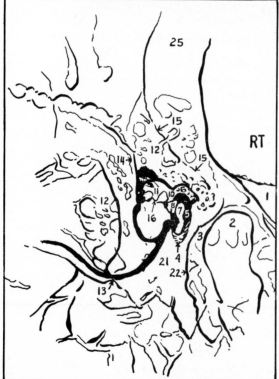

KEY TO THE LINE DRAWING

1. Root of the zygoma
2. Condyle of the mandible
3. Temporomandibular
   joint
4. External auditory canal
5. Tympanic cavity
6. Epitympanic cavity
7. Malleus
8. Incus
10. Area of the aditus
11. Area of the antrum
12. Mastoid cells
13. Mastoid tip
14. Anterior plate of the
    lateral sinus
15. Tegmen plate
16. Arcuate eminence
21. Petrosa
22. Anterior crest of the
    petrosa
25. Auricle

**Figure 4–6**  Owen position. Incus and malleus are clearly seen in tympanic cavity, with epitympanum and antrum in normal relationship.

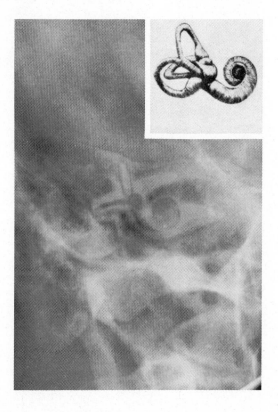

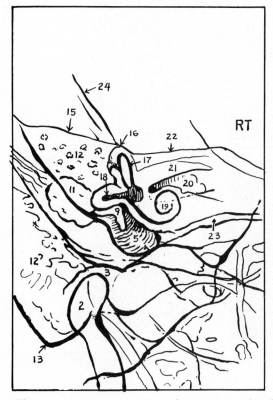

KEY TO THE LINE DRAWING

2. Condyle of the mandible
3. Temporomandibular joint
5. Tympanic cavity
9. Combined shadow of malleus and incus
11. Area of the antrum
12. Mastoid cells
13. Mastoid tip
15. Tegmen plate
16. Arcuate eminence
17. Superior semicircular canal
18. Horizontal semicircular canal
19. Cochlea
20. Internal auditory canal
21. Petrosa
22. Anterior crest of the petrosa
23. Petro-occipital suture
24. Sagittal crest of the occipital bone

**Figure 4–7**  Stenvers position, showing internal auditory canal, labyrinth and antrum.

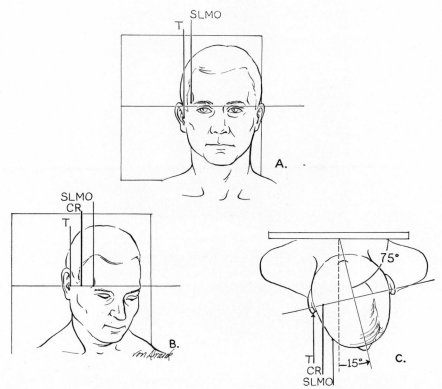

**Figure 4–8**  Chausse III projection. Positioning of patient. *A,* Patient's occiput on film. *B,* Head rotated 15° with chin flexed on chest. *C,* Same, as viewed from patient's vertex. *T,* tragus. *SLMO,* superior lateral margin of orbit. *CR,* central ray.

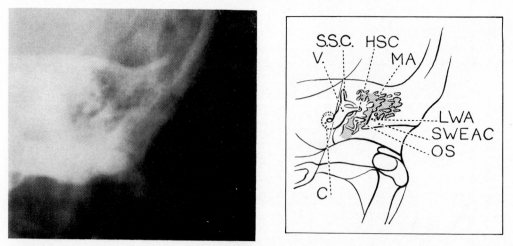

**Figure 4–9**  Chausse III projection. *LWA,* lateral wall of attic. *SWEAC,* superior wall of external auditory canal. *V,* vestibule. *C,* cochlea. *SSC,* superior semicircular canal. *HSC,* horizontal semicircular canal. *MA,* mastoid antrum. *OS,* ossicles (malleus and incus).

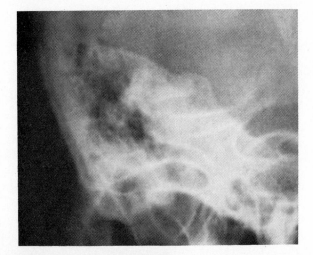

**Figure 4–10** Chamberlain-Towne position for petrous apex.

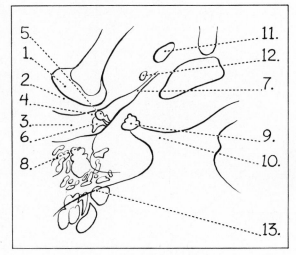

KEY TO THE LINE DRAWING

1. Condyle of mandible
2. Temporomandibular joint
3. External auditory canal
4. Attic
5. Head of malleus
6. Incus
7. Eustachian tube
8. Area of antrum
9. Cochlea
10. Internal acoustic meatus
11. Foramen ovale
12. Foramen spinosum
13. Anterior plate of sigmoid sinus

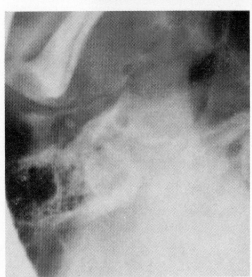

**Figure 4–11** Base view of skull (submento-vertex position).

## TECHNIQUE OF ROUTINE FILMING
## OF THE DIAGNOSTIC POSITIONS

Proper positioning of the patient is of paramount importance. The patient must be comfortable and not strained, in order to maintain the position. Two fixed points in the skull are utilized, one visible through the cassette holder, the other from the position of the x-ray tube. The transparent window of the cassette holder should be marked as follows: The verticle line is marked at 1 cm. and at 2 cm. above the center for use in the Mayer, Owen and Schüller positions. In each lower quadrant a mark is made 2 cm. below and 3 cm. lateral to the center for use in the Stenvers position (Fig. 4–12). The central beam is focused on the cross in the center of the window. The diaphragm and cone to be used for the Stenvers position should expose a 5 inch circle on the film, and the cone to be used for the Mayer, Owen and Schüller positions should expose a 3 inch circle on the film. For the last three positions the auricle is held forward with a piece of adhesive tape placed level with the external auditory meatus; where the tape crosses the postaural fold is the point used for positioning as will be described.

### Stenvers Position

The patient is seated erect facing the cassette. For the left temporal bone the external canthus of the left eye is placed over the mark in the right lower quadrant of

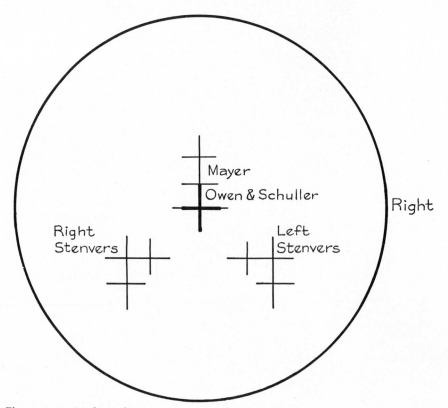

**Figure 4–12**   Markings for transparent area of cassette holder to insure exact positioning.

the transparent window. The skull is then rotated to place the midline of the occiput in the plane of the central beam. This brings the petrosa perpendicular to the beam, and the sagittal crest of the occipital bone is superimposed on the arcuate eminence in the center of the film. The central ray is depressed 12 degrees.

### Schüller Position

The patient is seated erect with the left shoulder (for the left mastoid) under the cassette. The point on the postauricular area where the adhesive crosses the postaural fold is placed against the mark made 1 cm. above the center of the transparent window of the cassette holder. The central ray is elevated 30 degrees so that it passes through the plane of the postauricular fold of the opposite (right) ear.

### Owen Position

The patient remains in the same position as for the Schüller, but with the face rotated about 30 degrees away from the cassette, maintaining a close approximation of mastoid to cassette. The central ray is directed 2 cm. posterior to the external canthus of the right eye. A wooden block cut at an angle of 30 degrees helps to keep the head in this rotation. The beam is elevated 30 degrees.

### Mayer Position

The patient remains seated as before, but the point on the postauricular area is now placed against the mark made 2 cm. above the center of the transparent window, and the central ray is elevated 45 degrees. In most cases the rotation of the face away from the cassette is a little less than the 45 degrees commonly recommended, usually about 30 degrees to 35 degrees, thus more nearly like the Owen position. Too much rotation throws the anterior border of the mastoid process on top of the external meatus, tympanic cavity and attic, destroying the diagnostic usefulness of the view.

### Third Projection of Chausse (Chausse III)

The patient is positioned with the occiput on the film (Fig. 4–8A), the head rotated approximately 15 degrees toward the side opposite the one under examination, and the chin is flexed on the chest (Fig. 4–8B). The central x-ray beam should be directed just above and lateral to the orbital process of the frontal bone of the side under examination and run in a plane crossing the external auditory canal (Fig. 4–8C).

The lateral wall of the attic seen on end casts a well defined linear density which meets inferiorly the superior wall of the external auditory canal. Medial to the lateral wall of the attic the ossicles are recognized as a triangular density. The prominence of the horizontal semicircular canal is well outlined and above the radiolucency of the antrum with the tegmen antri (Fig. 4–9).

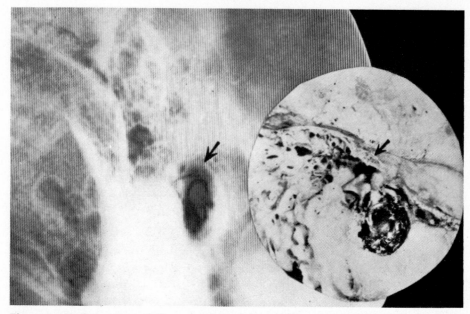

**Figure 4–13**  Comparison of Owen position of film with anatomic specimen to emphasize the normal pneumatic pattern of the epitympanic space.

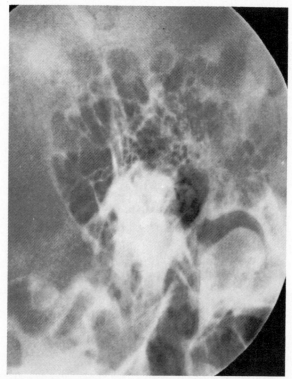

**Figure 4–14**  Normal mastoid pneumatization. Owen position. Well-pneumatized temporal bone. Cells still extend into arcus zygomaticus and squamosa.

## INTERPRETATION

A definite sequence should always be followed in order that nothing be left out in reading x-ray films. The **cellular structure of the mastoid process** is studied first and the **tegmen** and **sinus plate** are described. The **external auditory canal, tympanic cavity, ossicles, attic, aditus** and **antrum** are next examined. Finally the petrosa is studied, and the **internal auditory canals, pneumatic cells of the petrous apex,** the **cochlea** and the **semicircular canals** noted.

Especial attention is paid to small cells surrounding the attic. In the Mayer and Owen positions the inferior edge of the lateral attic wall is visible. Between this and the tegmen are the small cells of the epitympanum (Fig. 4–13). Loss of this osseous pattern of the epitympanum is the earliest manifestation of bone destruction in chronic otitis media.

The landmarks of the conventional Law and Schüller positions (Figs. 4–1 and 4–2) should be familiar to all otologists. To develop familiarity with the Mayer, Owen and Stenvers positions, the reader should study Figures 4–4 and 4–16 (Mayer position), Figures 4–6, 4–13, 4–14, and 4–15 (Owen position) and Figures 4–7, 4–17, and 4–18 (Stenvers position) and compare them with the following films showing pathologic lesions.

## ACUTE MASTOIDITIS

Acute mastoiditis occurs in most cases of acute suppurative otitis media in pneumatized temporal bones (see Chapter 7). The earliest radiologic finding is increased opacity (clouding) of the mastoid air cells due to the replacement of air by

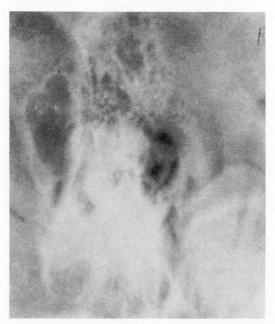

**Figure 4–15**  Normal mastoid pneumatization. Owen position. Pneumatization confined to the mastoid process.

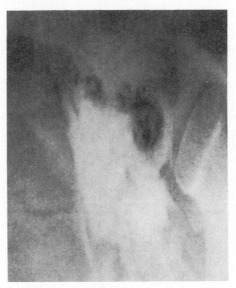

**Figure 4–16**  Limited mastoid pneumatization. Mayer position. Pneumatization of periantral area only. No history or clinical evidence of previous ear disease.

edema of the mucosa and fluid (Fig. 4–19), and is seen best in the Schüller position.

The Stenvers position gives an additional view of the cells of the mastoid process, as well as an excellent demonstration of the petrosa. A roentgenogram of the petrosa must always be obtained early in the course of acute mastoiditis because of the possibility of petrositis.

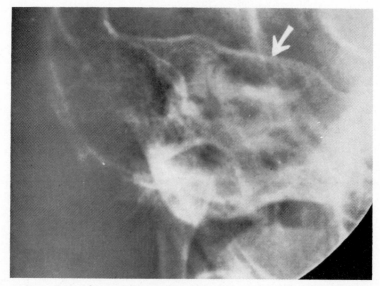

**Figure 4–17**  Normal mastoid pneumatization. Stenvers position. Pneumatic petrosa.

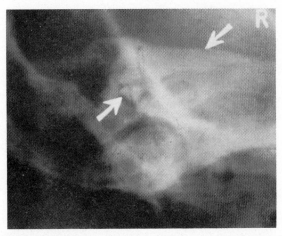

**Figure 4–18**  Limited mastoid pneumatization. Stenvers position. Sclerotic petrosa. The lower arrow indicates the ossicles.

If the infection progresses to a coalescent mastoiditis with beginning decalcification of the cell walls, these become blurred and indistinct. This is followed by a discontinuity of the cell walls, at first patchy and then diffuse. With the loss of calcium the radiolucency of the mastoid process **increases,** more nearly approaching that of the normal side but **lacking the sharp clear cell outlines** (Fig. 4–20).

In children under 2 years of age the pneumatized area may be confined to the periantral cells, requiring the Mayer and Owen positions to demonstrate the pathologic changes.

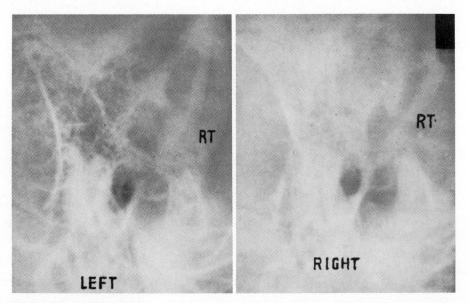

**Figure 4–19**  Acute mastoiditis, right ear, Owen position. Diffuse clouding of mastoid cells. Normal left ear for comparison. (Courtesy of Dr. Robert Scanlon, St. Vincent's Hospital, Los Angeles.)

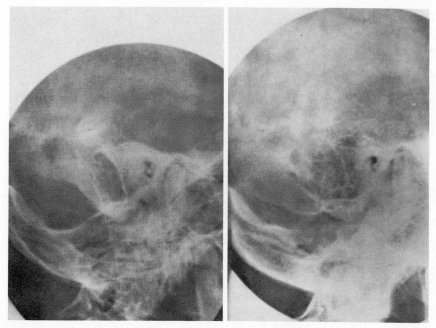

**Figure 4–20**   Acute mastoiditis of 5 weeks' duration, right ear, Law position. Demineralization of intercellular walls, beginning coalescence. Normal left ear for comparison on right side. (Courtesy of Drs. Shambaugh, Derlacki and Harrison.)

## PETROSITIS

Roentgenologically the pneumatic petrous pyramid, like the mastoid, shows a change from normal with almost every otitic infection. The petrous apex is particularly variable in the type and degree of pneumatization (Fig. 4–17 and 4–18). Every change in the density or apparent air content of the petrous apex is **not** a suppurative lesion. Decalcification of the bone, discontinuity of the cell walls and increased radiolucency of the pneumatic area are indicative of purulent coalescent petrositis, but this does not necessarily indicate surgical intervention.

## CHRONIC MASTOIDITIS

For radiologic purposes, chronic mastoiditis may be divided into two groups: that occurring in well pneumatized temporal bones and that occurring in temporal bones with underdeveloped cell systems.

Chronic infection develops infrequently in pneumatized temporal bones, and cholesteatomas are rare. Long-standing disease in a pneumatized mastoid, however, may produce sclerosis to the point of obliteration of the pneumatic spaces. Because of the surrounding air cells, small areas of bone destruction in the aditus and antrum are difficult to visualize on routine films. Tomograms **may** prove to be of value in these cases.

In the typical case of chronic otitis with cholesteatoma, the infection develops in a poorly pneumatized temporal bone, and the disease process is limited to the tympanic cavity, epitympanic cavity, aditus and antrum. In this type of ear, the

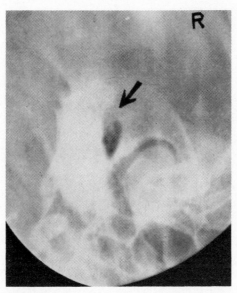

**Figure 4–21**   Chronic mastoiditis. Owen position showing clean-cut area of absorption in the epitympanic space. A typical attic cholesteatoma.

lateral projections are of little value. The diseased area is shown to the best advantage in the Mayer and Owen positions.

The bone of the mastoid process is usually sclerotic, and the few cell walls very thick. The first evidence of bone destruction is the loss of the normal osseous pattern of the attic (Fig. 4–21). As the disease progresses the aditus is widened (Fig. 4–22),

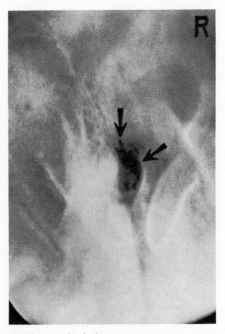

**Figure 4–22**   Chronic mastoiditis with cholesteatoma. Mayer position showing intact ossicles but definite area of absorption in the attic and extending into the aditus.

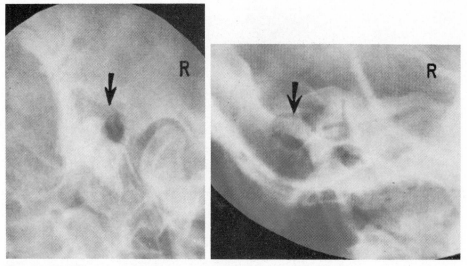

**Figure 4–23**   Chronic mastoiditis with cholesteatoma. Left: Owen position with ossicular remnant in tympanum, and cholesteatoma cavity extending through aditus into enlarged antrum. Right: Stenvers position with definite cavity in antral area.

and finally antral enlargements can be demonstrated, especially in the Stenvers projection (Fig. 4–23). These findings may be caused by granulation tissue as well as cholesteatomatosis.

The typical large cholesteatoma consists of a radiolucent bone defect in the antral area surrounded by a thin osteitic shell. Large cholesteatomas may cause erosion of the dural or sinus plates, with or without sequestration (Fig. 4–24). Erosion of the semicircular canals sufficient to produce a labyrinthine fistula may sometimes be demonstrated in the Stenvers and Chausse III projections.

In patients who have been previously operated on, the type of operation can be identified in the Mayer and Owen positions. After simple mastoidectomy, the

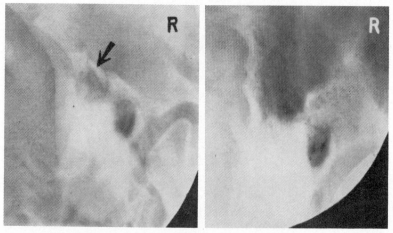

Fig. 4–24                          Fig. 4–25

**Figure 4–24**   Chronic mastoiditis with cholesteatoma. Owen position showing resorption in antral area with fracture and sequestration of tegmen plate.
**Figure 4–25**   Postoperative cavity. Mayer position showing large mastoid cavity, but intact bridge, posterior canal wall and ossicles.

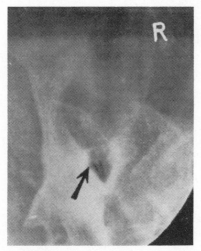

**Figure 4–26** Postoperative cavity. Mayer position showing malleus and incus present with clean-cut bone removal, including bridge. Bondy modified radical mastoidectomy.

posterior canal wall and ossicles are intact (Fig. 4–25). After modified radical operations the ossicles are present but the posterior canal wall is absent (Fig. 4–26), and after radical surgery both the ossicles and the posterior canal wall may be seen to have been removed (Fig. 4–27).

It is impossible to diagnose recurrent cholesteatoma in patients previously operated on unless serial films are available showing progressive enlargement of the cavity. Such complications as sequestration (Fig. 4–28) and bone absorption adjacent to the cavity can, however, be demonstrated.

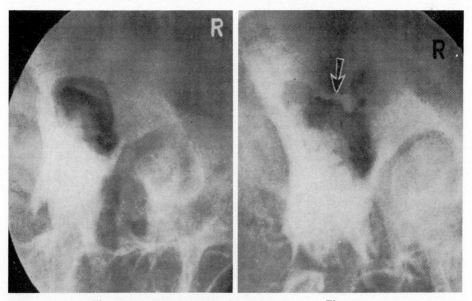

Fig. 4–27                    Fig. 4–28

**Figure 4–27** Postoperative classic radical mastoid cavity. Owen position with clean removal of ossicles, bridge, posterior canal wall and mastoid cells.

**Figure 4–28** Postoperative cavity. Mayer position showing radical mastoidectomy cavity with sequestration of tegmen and active bone resorption anterior to sequestrum.

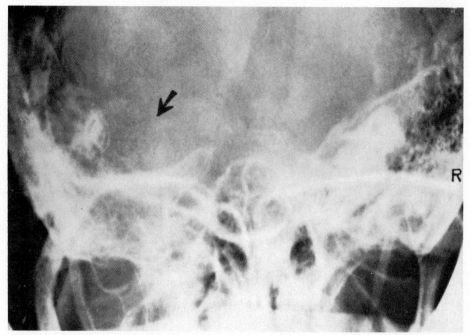

**Figure 4–29** Congenital cholesteatoma. Towne position showing complete loss of petrosa medial to the labyrinth.


## CONGENITAL CHOLESTEATOMA

The usual congenital cholesteatoma produces a sharply demarcated area of bone destruction with a sclerotic margin, but without evidence of chronic ear disease such as is present in secondary or acquired cholesteatoma. Congenital cholesteatoma may occur in the skull outside of the temporal bone, as well as in this bone without otitis media (Fig. 4–29).

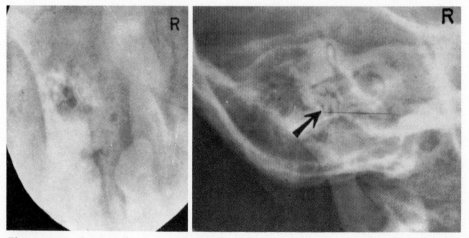

**Figure 4–30** Congenital atresia. Left: Mayer position with absent external canal, deformed auricle and moderate pneumatization. Right: Stenvers position showing normal labyrinth and normal malleus and incus in the tympanic cavity.

## ATRESIA

### Congenital Atresia

The radiologic findings in congenital atresia may vary from almost complete pneumatization with normal-appearing ossicles, to entirely absent pneumatization with no visible ossicles, and deformity of the mandibular condyle (Fig. 4–30). If the bony atresia is complete, ossicles cannot be demonstrated in the Owen and Mayer positions. If ossicular tissue is present, however deformed, it can frequently be visualized in the Stenvers projection. If ossicular tissue can be demonstrated, one may assume that there is an air space to house it, and feel more confident about the chances of surgical success. In bilateral cases, visualization of ossicles in one ear only will dictate the decision to operate on that ear.

## OTHER DISEASES OF THE TEMPORAL BONE

### Secretory Otitis Media

The radiologic findings of secretory (serous) otitis media are those of diminished air content of the mastoid cells due to the presence of fluid in the pneumatic spaces. It is interesting to note, however, that in many cases the temporal bones show evidence of previous disease, such as underdeveloped cell systems and sclerosis of the cell walls (Fig. 4–31).

Eustachian tube function can be determined by introducing not more than 1 cc. of radiopaque material, such as Pantopaque, into the tympanic cavity through an intact or perforated drum membrane. A film is taken immediately in the Stenvers

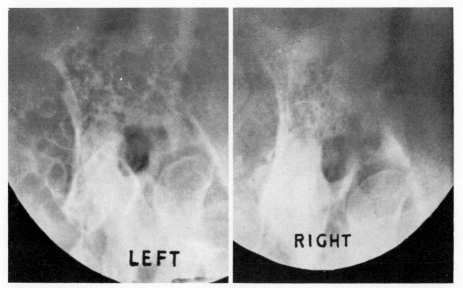

**Figure 4–31** Chronic secretory otitis media. Right ear, Owen position, reveals cloudy tympanic cavity and mastoid cells without bone destruction. Normal left ear for comparison.

position. After 10 minutes a second film taken in the same position will fail to show any contrast medium in the tympanic cavity if the eustachian tube function is normal. Retention of the dye indicates tubal disease[1] (Fig. 4–32).

## Paget's Disease

The radiologic examination in Paget's disease discloses variable osseous changes that depend upon the stage of the disease. Irregular areas of osteosclerosis are interspersed within areas of osteoporosis. In the petrosa, where the resorptive process is more pronounced, the semicircular canals and cochlea may be unusually well visualized (Fig. 4–33).

## Benign Tumors

The x-ray is very helpful in the diagnosis of benign tumors of the temporal bone, such as bone cysts or osteomas (Fig. 4–34).

## Fractures

Fractures through the temporal bone may be demonstrated by x-ray studies. The best position depends upon the direction of fracture (Fig. 4–35).

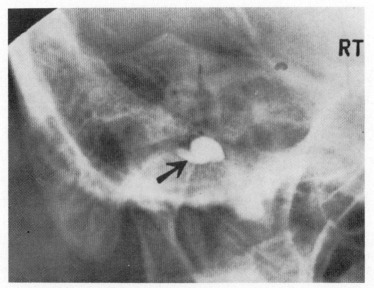

**Figure 4–32**  Chronic secretory otitis media. Stenvers position with tympanic cavity filled with contrast medium. The eustachian tube is not visualized because of obstruction in the osseous portion.

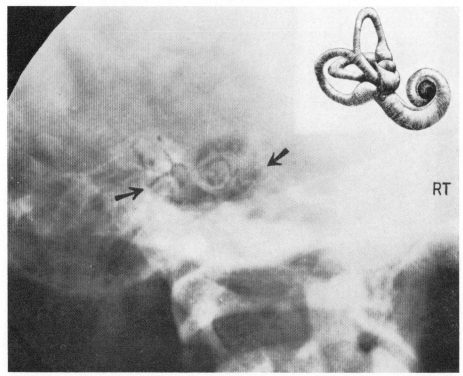

**Figure 4–33**  Paget's disease. Stenvers projection showing unusually distinct labyrinth due to osteoporosis.

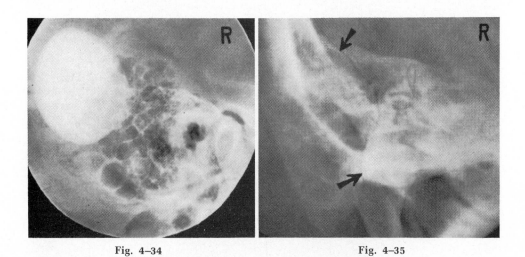

Fig. 4–34                            Fig. 4–35

**Figure 4–34**  Osteoma. Large osteoma arising from the mastoid process.
**Figure 4–35**  Fracture. Stenvers position. Fracture line extends from middle fossa through mastoid process lateral to the horizontal semicircular canal.

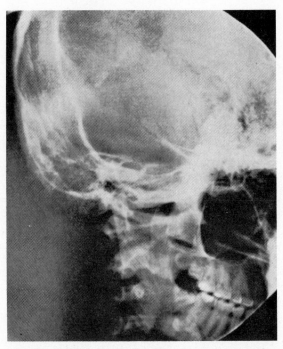

**Figure 4–36** Stenvers view of right side showing enlarged internal acoustic meatus due to neurinoma, removed at surgery. (Figures 4–36 to 4–38 courtesy of Drs. Shambaugh, Derlacki and Harrison.)

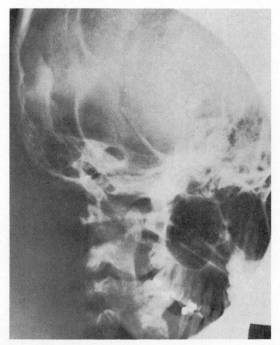

**Figure 4–37** Stenvers view of left side—same case as Figure 4–36—showing enlarged internal acoustic meatus, tumor subsequently removed. Multiple neurofibromatosis (von Recklinghausen's disease.)

## Otosclerosis (Otospongiosis)

Conventional radiography cannot be utilized to diagnose otosclerotic changes in the oval window or cochlear capsule unless these are extreme.

## Acoustic Neurinomas

The development of trans-temporal bone surgery for the removal of acoustic neurinomas has increased interest in early diagnosis of these tumors. The general dissatisfaction with radiologic demonstrations of acoustic neurinomas stems from overreliance on Towne's projection. In Stenvers' projection the internal auditory porus is parallel to the film, whereas the canal is foreshortened. Although all enlargements of one internal auditory canal should be reported (Figs. 4–36 through 4–39), early diagnosis depends upon Pantopaque myelography of the internal acoustic meatuses which should be done in all suspect neurinomas, whether or not the Stenvers' view and tomography show an enlarged or eroded meatus.

## Glomus Jugulare Tumors of the Middle Ear

Glomus tympanicum tumors have no pathognomonic radiologic findings. Glomus jugulare tumors are recognized in conventional views only if the destruction is far advanced (Fig. 4–40).

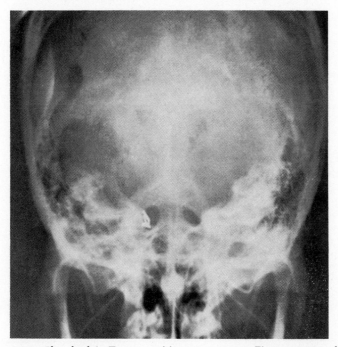

**Figure 4–38**   Chamberlain-Towne position, same case as Figures 4–36 and 4–37.

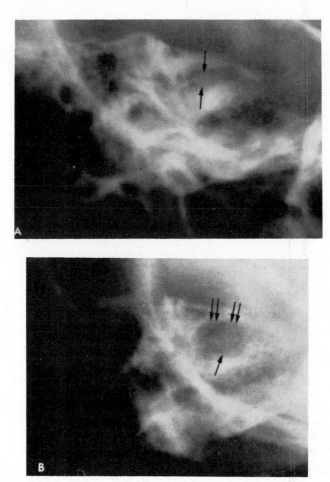

**Figure 4–39**  Acoustic neurinoma. *A*, Normal for comparison. Arrows indicate internal acoustic meatus. *B*, Arrow indicates internal acoustic meatus. Double arrows point to erosion of superior margin of meatus by neurinoma.

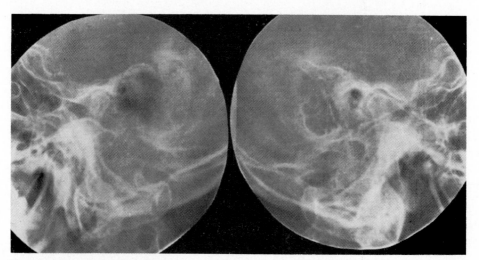

**Figure 4–40**  Glomus jugulare tumor. Law position showing destruction of floor of the osseous meatus and involvement of the mastoid process by large glomus jugulare tumor, right side, removed at surgery. Left side normal.

# REFERENCES

1. Compere, W. E.: Tympanic cavity clearance studies. Tr. Am. Acad. Ophth. & Otol., 62:444, 1958.
2. Law, F.: Radiography as an aid in the diagnosis of mastoid disease. Ann. Otol. Rhin. & Laryng., 22:635, 1913.
3. Taylor, H. K.: The roentgen findings in suppuration of the petrous apex. Ann. Otol. Rhin. & Laryng., 40:367, 1931.
4. Towne, E. D.: Erosion of the petrous bone by acoustic nerve tumor. Arch. Otol., 4:515, 1926.
5. Mayer, E. G.: The technique for the roentgenologic examination of the temporal bone. Translated by Isaac Gerber. Radiology, 7:306, 1926.
6. Owen, G. R.: The key area (attic-aditus-antrum) in the chronic mastoid. Tr. Am. Otol. Soc., 1951, p. 189.
7. Stenvers, H. W.: Roentgenology of the os petrosum. Arch. Radiol. & Electroth., 22:97, 1917.
8. X-ray Department, General Electric Company, 4855 Electric Ave., Milwaukee, Wisc.
9. Gianturco, C.: A device for sinus roentgenography with horizontal rays. Am.J. Roentgenol., 57:388, 1947.
10. The Franklin X-ray Corp., 500 Commerce Dr., Yeadon, Pa.
11. Rumstrom, G.: A roentgenological study of acute and chronic otitis media. Acta Radiol., Suppl. XVII, 1933.

# *Chapter 5*

# *Tomography of the Temporal Bone*

GALDINO E. VALVASSORI, M.D.
*Chicago, Illinois*

INTRODUCTION TO TOMOGRAPHY
NORMAL TOMOGRAPHIC ANATOMY
PATHOLOGIC CONDITIONS
    CONGENITAL MALFORMATIONS
    TRAUMATIC EFFECTS
    INFLAMMATORY PROCESSES
    NEOPLASTIC CONDITIONS
    OTODYSTROPHIES

## INTRODUCTION TO TOMOGRAPHY

Although surgical otology has made rapid advances since the introduction of the operating microscope, radiography of the temporal bone has not changed for over 30 years. All the classic views of the temporal bone — Law's, Schüller's, Towne's, Stenvers' and Mayer's — were devised by these authors in the decade between 1916 and 1926. Thereafter, except for some modifications, such as Chausse's and Owen's, nothing was added until the late 1950's. The refinement of surgical procedures that has resulted from use of the otomicroscope necessitates better radiographic demonstration of the fine anatomic details of the ear. Conventional radiography has the intrinsic defect of offering a picture that is the summation on a single plane of multiple structures located in different planes, so that the small structures under investigation are more or less obscured. The use of special projections, which might improve the visualization of a determinate structure, produces a certain degree of distortion of the structures because of the needed angulation of the patient's head or of the x-ray beam. The ideal technique of examination would be the one allowing visualization of the desired structure while obscuring the others in front of and behind it; the ideal projection is the one that offers the visualization of a structure under the same angle as seen by the surgeon during his operative approach. These conditions are fulfilled by body section radiography (tomography), which is the method of examining tissue structures by blurring out objects above and below the desired plane. Although this effect can be obtained by different techniques, the principle of body section radiography remains constant

112

and can be summarized as follows: It is a system in which focus and film move in opposite directions with constant ratio between their velocities with the film describing a translatory motion in relation to the object. In such a system, the rays incident on a fixed point on the film throughout the exposure will have a point of intersection that is stationary in relation to the object during the exposure. As each point of the film has a point of intersection, all the points of intersection will form a plane — the focal plane. The thickness of the plane in focus depends upon the angular opening of the scanning movement for a given focal film distance. The blurring of the structures outside the focal plane increases in proportion to the length of the scanning movement.

Unidirectional or linear body section radiography as used at the beginning of this technique proved unsatisfactory for the study of the small structures of the temporal bone because the short scanning movement produces inadequate blurring. Also, those structures whose long axis is parallel to the longitudinal axis of the trajectory are not effaced but merely elongated.

Multidirectional body section radiography or tomography overcomes these obstacles. The Polytome, made by Philips-Massiot Company, allows a thickness of the plane in focus as small as 1 mm. and a blurring effect about five times as great as the one obtained with a linear trajectory of the same angle.

The tomographic examination of the temporal bone consists of multiple sections in different positions, obtained 1 or 2 mm. apart. A small field is used, approximately 2 inches in diameter at the plane in focus. A movable cassette tray allows multiple exposures, usually six or nine on a 10 × 12 film.

An important consideration is the total x-ray exposure of the patient with this technique. Careful computation shows that owing to the small size of portal, the patient's gonads and bone marrow receive less x-ray exposure from 30 tomograms than from a single routine radiographic examination of the chest. The lens of the eye, which is included in the primary x-ray beam, is covered with a 2 mm.-thick lead shield or corresponding lead-containing glasses. This protection decreases the amount of irradiation of the eyes from 10–15 rads to 1–1.5 rads.

Computerized tomography is playing an increasingly important role in the radiological evaluation of the temporal bone and adjacent regions, in particular the posterior cranial fossa.

Computerized tomography is a radiographic technique that allows the measurement of small absorption differentials not recognizable by standard recording on x-ray films.

The scan is initiated at the chosen level and the x-ray tube, collimated to a thin or pencil beam, rotates around the patient. The transmitted x-rays are picked up by detectors arrayed along the circumference of the tube trajectory, converted into electronic currents, amplified and transmitted to the computer for storage and processing. The computer analyzes this data and develops an image on a 320 × 320 dots matrix, where the brightness of each point is proportional to the attenuation coefficient. The study is often repeated after intravenous injection of contrast agents, which produce an increase in density value or enhancement of several anatomical structures and pathologic processes.

## NORMAL TOMOGRAPHIC ANATOMY

Knowledge of the normal radiographic anatomy in the various projections is indispensable for the recognition and evaluation of pathologic conditions. The selection of the projections for the study of the temporal bone has been based by the author on the following principles: The projection should be simple and easily reproducible; it should visualize the ear structures under the same angle as the surgical approach; it should follow the same plane as that used in histologic sections; it should cut certain structures at right angles to their axis.

Six projections have been used. Two of them — frontal and lateral — are considered basic; the other four — Stenvers, semiaxial, axial and horizontal — are considered complementary, according to the area and pathologic condition to be studied.

### Frontal Projection

The patient may lie either prone or supine, with the line running from the tragus to the external canthus perpendicular to the table top. Because external, middle and inner ear structures are shown clearly at various levels, this single projection should be used in every case.

Figure 5–1 is a section obtained 1 mm. posterior to the anterior wall of the

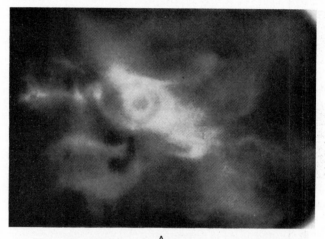

A

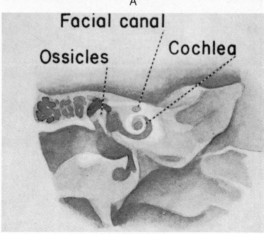

B

**Figure 5–1**   Frontal projection of normal ear. Section 1 mm. posterior to the anterior wall of the external auditory canal. *A*, Tomogram; *B*, explanatory drawing.

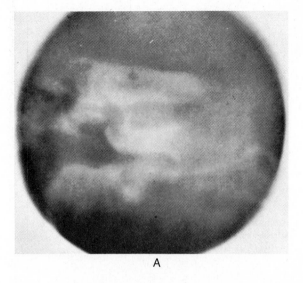

A

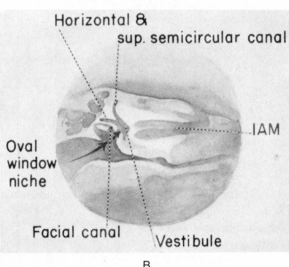

B

**Figure 5–2**  Frontal projection of normal ear. Section 5 mm. posterior to the anterior wall of the external auditory canal. *IAM*, Internal auditory meatus.

external auditory canal. The external auditory canal, tympanic cavity and epitympanic recess are well outlined. The slightly bilobar density seen in the epitympanic recess is the head of the malleus and part of the body of the incus. The proximal part of the handle of the malleus appears as a broad process, extending downward toward the tympanic membrane. Medial to the tympanic cavity one sees the apical and middle turns of the cochlea. Above the cochlea two holes are outlined. The medial one is produced by the petrous segment of the facial nerve canal and is larger because it contains the geniculate ganglion. The lateral hole, which has more the appearance of a groove than of a hole, is produced by the very proximal portion of the tympanic segment of the facial nerve canal. Below the cochlea the lower portion of the carotid canal and at the extreme medial end the petro-occipital fissure are outlined.

Figure 5–2 was obtained 4 mm. posterior to the previous one. Again the external auditory canal, middle ear cavity, epitympanic recess and tegmen tympani are clearly outlined. The superomedial lip of the external auditory canal, the so-called spur, is very prominent at this level. The ossicle, whose axis points downward and medially, is formed by the long process of the incus. The vestibule is clearly outlined, with the semicircular canals branching from it — namely, the ampullar limbs of the superior and horizontal semicircular canals. Just underneath the medial end of the horizontal semicircular canal the facial nerve canal is seen in section. A dehiscence is detectable on the lateral wall of the vestibule just beneath the horizontal semicircular canal between the facial nerve canal superiorly and the promontory inferiorly. This dehiscence represents the oval window (vestibular window). The reason for this opening is that the normal footplate of the stapes does not cast any linear density in this projection because it lies in an oblique direction to the plane of the film. Medial to the vestibule one sees the internal auditory canal, which is divided laterally by a horizontal crest — the crista falciformis (crista transversa). The upper smaller compartment contains the facial nerve and superior branch of the vestibular nerve. The lower larger compartment contains the cochlear nerve and the inferior branch of the vestibular nerve. Under the petrous pyramid the anterior portion of the jugular fossa becomes visible and medial to it the hypoglossal canal.

Six to twelve sections are usually obtained in the frontal projection, 1 or 2 mm. apart.

## Lateral Projection

The patient lies prone on the table with the side under examination away from the table top. This facilitates centering, particularly when the skull is asymmetric. The structures of the ear extend from 2 to 5 cm. from the outer surface. For orientation, the various portions of the ear are found in the following sections: (1) external auditory canal — from 1.5 to 2.5 cm.; (2) middle ear (ossicles) — from 2.5 to 3 cm.; (3) vestibule, most of the semicircular canals and the cochlea — from 3 to 4 cm.; and (4) internal auditory canal — from 4 to 5 cm. This projection is fundamental for the study of the middle ear.

Figure 5–3 was obtained at 2.6 cm. from the patient's skin surface. The external auditory canal, epitympanic recess, tegmen tympani and anterior tympanic spine are clearly seen. The malleus and incus are well demonstrated in this section. The anterior of the two ossicles is the malleus; its shape is that of a club. The head of the club corresponds to the head of the malleus. The vertical process underneath it is part of the handle of the malleus. The posterior ossicle is the incus; its base extends downward with a fine tail, the long process. It is extremely important to realize that these two processes, which extend downward from the head of the malleus and body of the incus, are seen in the same section and lie parallel to each other. Posteriorly, the vertical radiolucency of the mastoid portion of the facial nerve canal is easily recognizable. Anteriorly, the condyle of the mandible is seen. The sclerotic area posterior to the epitympanic recess is due to the bony capsule surrounding the horizontal or lateral semicircular canal.

Figure 5–4 was obtained at 3.2 cm. from the patient's skin surface. The tympanic cavity appears as a crescentic radiolucency crossed by fine lines owing to the walls of the pneumatic cells lining the cavity. The upper wall of the tympanic cavity is formed by the tegmen tympani. The posterior extension of the tympanic cavity underneath the sclerotic capsule of the cochlea and vestibule is termed the sinus tympani, or posterior sinus. The cochlea is sharply outlined in this cut. Posterior to

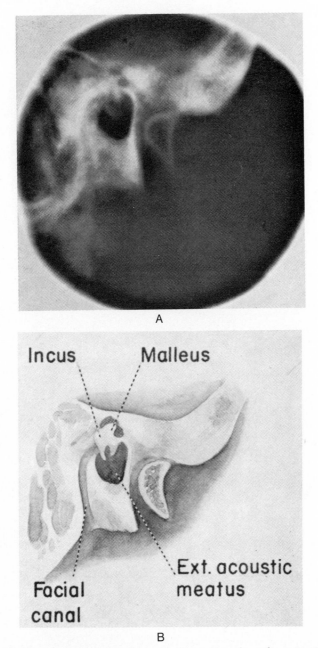

A

**Incus          Malleus**

**Facial
canal**

**Ext. acoustic
meatus**

B

**Figure 5–3**   Lateral projection of normal ear. Section 2.6 cm. from the patient's skin surface.

the cochlea, the vestibule and the crus commune are clearly seen. The bifurcation of the non-ampullated limbs of the superior and posterior semicircular canals is clearly outlined. Anterior and inferior to the tympanic cavity is the inferior portion of the carotid canal. The cleft on the posteroinferior aspect of the promontory represents the fossa of the cochlear or round window.

Between six and twelve sections are usually obtained in lateral projection, 1 or 2 mm. apart.

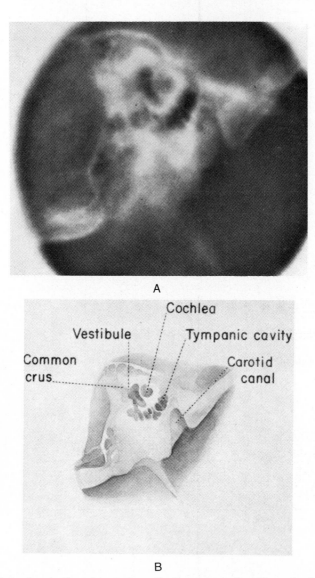

**Figure 5–4**   Lateral projection of normal ear. Section 3.2 cm. from the patient's skin surface.

### Stenvers Projection

The patient lies prone with his head rotated to a 45 degree oblique angle, bringing the petrous pyramid under examination parallel to the table top. The head is flexed 12 degrees. The structures of the ear are included in a 2 cm. thickness extending posteriorly from the external auditory porus. From front to back the structures best seen are: external and middle ear cavities, round window, vestibule and semicircular canals, especially the posterior, cochlea and, finally, internal auditory porus. This projection is most useful for the study of the relationship between the middle ear cavity and the carotid canal and for the study of the round window and of the petrous apex.

Figure 5–5 was obtained 1 cm. posterior to the outer opening of the external

auditory canal. Laterally, the section cuts across the mastoid air cells. The middle
ear cavity appears as a crescentic radiolucency whose superomedial wall is formed
by the promontory. The cleft in the superior part of the promontory is the round
window niche. The entire cochlea with its three turns is recognizable above the
promontory. Adjacent to these laterally, the vestibule is visualized with the entire
posterior semicircular canal seen as the radiolucent ring extending laterally from it.
The non-ampullated limb of the horizontal semicircular canal casts a linear band of
radiolucency within the bony capsule circumscribed by the posterior semicircular
canal. The carotid canal is seen in the medial part of this section as a curving band of
radiolucency. The styloid process projects inferiorly. The distal tract of the facial
nerve canal is outlined posterolaterally to it.

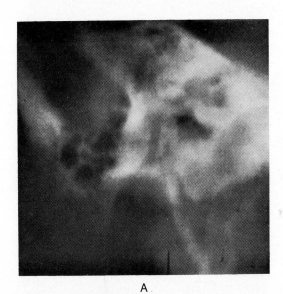

A

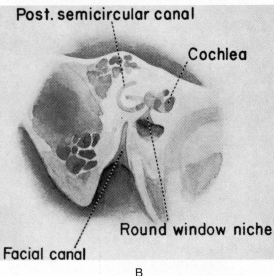

B

**Figure 5–5**  Stenvers projection of normal ear. Section 1 cm. posterior to the outer opening of the
external auditory canal.

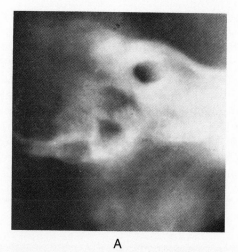

A

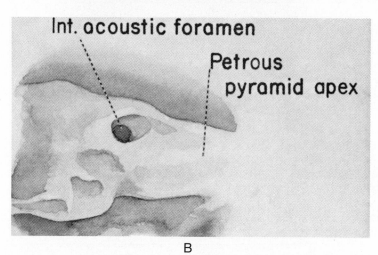

B

**Figure 5–6**   Stenvers projection of normal ear. Section at the posterior aspect of the petrous pyramid.

Figure 5–6 was obtained at the level of the posterior aspect of the petrous pyramid. The porus or medial opening of the internal auditory canal is sharply outlined and appears as a dense "C," open anteriorly because of the prominence of its posterior, inferior and superior lips. The petrous apex is completely outlined.

About six sections are usually obtained in the Stenvers projection, centered in the area of interest, 2 mm. apart.

### Semiaxial Projection of the Petrous Pyramid

The patient lies supine with his head turned 20 degrees toward the side under examination. In this way the medial or labyrinthine wall of the middle ear cavity, which normally forms an angle open posteriorly of approximately 15 to 25 degrees with the sagittal plane of the skull, becomes perpendicular to the plane of the film and to the plane of the section. This projection is used principally for the study of the oval window region in otosclerosis.

Figure 5–7 was obtained across the oval window. The external auditory canal appears oblique and shortened because of the obliquity of this projection. The entire tympanic cavity, including its roof, the tegmen tympani, is clearly outlined. The ossicle seen in the tympanic cavity is the incus, mainly the base of its long process. The vestibule and the superior and lateral semicircular canals are recognizable. Just underneath the lateral semicircular canal the facial nerve canal is seen in cross section. The promontory of the cochlea completes inferiorly the outline of the medial wall of the tympanic cavity. Between the prominent borders formed by the facial nerve canal superiorly and the promontory inferiorly, the oval window niche appears as a depression leading to the vestibule. The footplate of the stapes casts a fine line extending across the fenestra; the two crura are barely seen.

About six sections, 1 mm. apart, are usually obtained in this projection at and adjacent to the oval window.

### Axial Projection

The axial projection, called by European authors the Poschle projection, is obtained with the patient supine on the table and the head rotated, as for the Mayer view, 45 degrees toward the side to be examined. The long axis of the petrous pyramid becomes perpendicular to the plane of the film. We employ this projection for the study of the cochlear capsule, since the section or sections through the long axis of the modiolus allow good visualization on end of several segments of the cochlear coils. We also use this projection in combination with the lateral sections to visualize the vestibular aqueduct (Fig. 5–8). Six to nine sections, 1 mm. apart, are obtained, extending from the horizontal semicircular canal to the fundus of the internal auditory canal.

### Horizontal Projection

This projection is obtained by a submento-vertex direction of the x-ray beam. The line running from the tragus to the external canthus should be parallel to the table top. A 15 degree deflection of the head is advisable, however, when the jugular fossa and the adjacent posteromedial aspect of the petrous pyramid are under

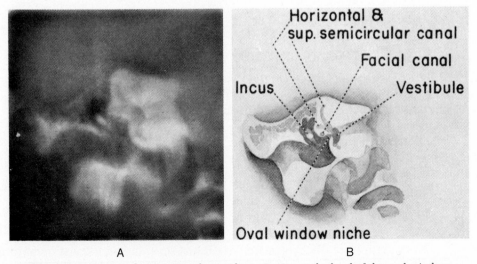

A                                              B

**Figure 5–7**   Semiaxial projection of normal ear. Section at the level of the oval window.

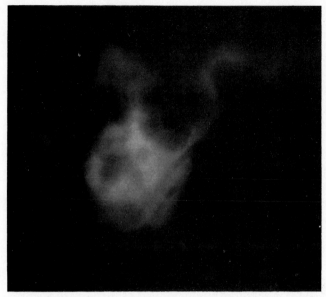

**Figure 5–8**   Axial projection of normal ear. The vestibular aqueduct is clearly visualized as it extends from the outer aperture on the posterior surface of the petrous pyramid to the common crus.

investigation. This projection is extremely valuable for the study of congenital malformations, fractures and tumors.

Figure 5–9 was obtained about 1 cm. below the arcuate eminence. The internal auditory canal is well defined medially. Anterior to its lateral portion, the cochlea starts to be in focus with its apical and middle turns. Anteromedial to these structures, the petrous apex is sharply outlined. Lateral to the base of the internal auditory canal the vestibule is now clearly seen, and is connected laterally to a circular band of radiolucency, the lateral semicircular canal. Posteriorly, the posterior semicircular canal is sectioned across. Anterolateral to the lateral semicircular canal the epitympanic recess is visualized, containing anteriorly the head of the malleus and just posterior to it the body of the incus, which extends posteriorly with its short process. Posterolateral to the epitympanic recess, the mastoid antrum casts a large area of radiolucency.

About six sections are usually obtained in this projection, 2 mm. apart.

## PATHOLOGIC CONDITIONS

The major categories of pathologic conditions involving the ear are congenital malformations, traumatic effects, inflammatory processes, neoplastic conditions and otodystrophies.

The otolaryngologist should learn as much as possible about the nature and the extent of the pathologic processes before deciding whether corrective surgery can be attempted.

### Congenital Malformations

The impossibility of a direct otoscopic examination of the middle ear in most of these conditions, owing to complete or partial atresia of the external auditory canal,

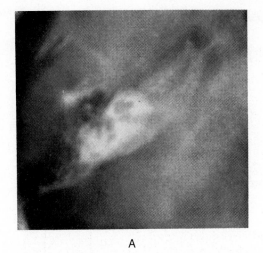

A

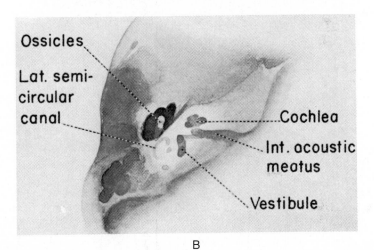

B

**Figure 5–9**   Horizontal projection of normal ear. Section 1 cm. below the arcuate eminence.

makes tomographic study more essential than in any other pathologic process. Conventional radiography is of limited value because of the more or less complete absence of the normal radiolucencies of the external auditory canal and middle ear cavity, the presence of a dense atretic block obscuring the superimposed structures and, finally, the distortion in axis and location of some of the structures, which makes the interpretation extremely difficult.

The abnormalities range from minor anomalies to complete aplasia of the entire ear. In order to perform corrective surgery with maximum safety and success the surgeon must know the following points:

    1.   Degree and type of abnormality of the tympanic bone.

    2.   Structure of the bony plate closing laterally the middle ear cavity (the so-called lamina or block of atresia) in cases of atresia of the external auditory canal (complete or incomplete, thick or thin).

    3.   Degree of development of the tympanic cavity.

    4.   Condition of the ossicular chain.

    5.   Degree and localization of the pneumatization of the mastoid antrum and mastoid cells.

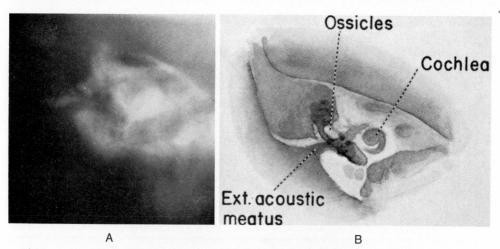

A                                    B

**Figure 5–10**  Incomplete atresia of the external auditory canal. Frontal section shows a small external auditory canal, measuring 3 mm. in diameter. The canal is filled with a soft tissue density, which at surgery was found to be cerumen and epidermal debris. Tympanic cavity and ossicles appear normal.

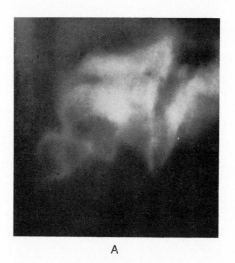

A

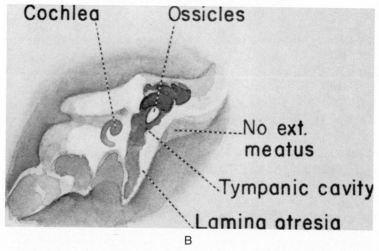

B

**Figure 5–11**  Complete atresia of the external auditory canal. Frontal section shows complete agenesis of the external auditory canal with a thick lamina of atresia closing laterally the hypoplastic middle ear cavity. There is a single ossicular mass.

**124**

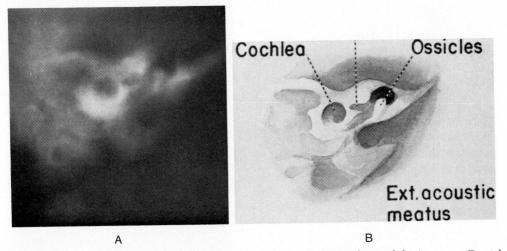

A               B

**Figure 5–12** Congenital absence of the oval window and abnormalities of the inner ear. Frontal section shows obliteration of the lumen of the basilar turn of the cochlea. The cavity seen lateral to the cochlea is the dilated lateral semicircular canal. External and middle ear appear normal.

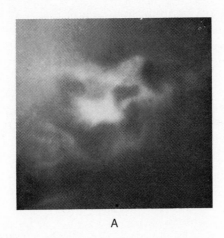

A

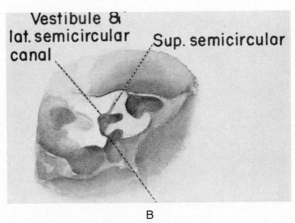

B

**Figure 5–13** (Same patient as in Figure 5–12.) Congenital absence of oval window and abnormalities of inner ear. Frontal section, 4 mm. posterior to that of Figure 5–12, shows absence of the oval window. The round window niche is instead quite prominent. The lateral semicircular canal is grossly abnormal and forms a single cavity with the vestibule.

6.  Route of the facial nerve canal.
7.  Status of the labyrinthine windows.
8.  Condition of the inner ear structures.
9.  Relationship of the meninges to the lateral aspect of the petrous pyramid, because frequently agenesis of the external auditory canal produces a large groove lateral to the petrous pyramid.

A properly done tomographic study can furnish all the above information. A few examples of congenital malformation have been selected for demonstration in Figures 5–10 to 5–13.

### Traumatic Effects

The petrous pyramids, mastoid and tympanic bone are unquestionably much more often involved in fractures following trauma to the skull than is demonstrated by the standard radiographic examinations. Fractures of these structures are, in fact, the most common fractures of the base of the skull. The demonstration of a fracture is important from the therapeutic approach and from the medicolegal aspect. There is no healing of fractures involving the labyrinth because of the endochondral structure of the otic capsule, so that the fracture tract forms an open route to the endocranium for any infection that might otherwise be innocuous. Fractures can be divided into three groups, according to the location — labyrinthine, tympanolabyrinthine and extralabyrinthine. The plane of the fracture can be longitudinal, following the long axis of the petrous bone, transverse or axial, following a plane perpendicular to the previous one, and oblique.

One should be aware that whereas fractures with separation or displacement of the fragments can be easily demonstrated by conventional radiography and tomography, smaller fractures without displacement and separation of the fragments can be detected only by tomography, if the plane of the fracture lies in or close to the direction of the x-ray beam. For this reason multiple projections are indispensible.

One or more of the three following clinical findings are present in patients referred for tomographic studies:

1.  Cerebrospinal fluid otorrhea usually is due to a fracture extending from the superior wall of the external auditory canal to the floor of the middle cranial fossa (Fig. 5–14) or to a fracture of the tegmen, when a tear of the tympanic membrane is present.

2.  Conductive hearing loss is present, resulting from a disruption of the ossicular chain, especially when the fracture involves the epitympanic area. The most common type of dislocation involves the incus, whose fixation by ligaments is looser than that of the malleus (Figs. 5–15 and 5–16). A rarer interruption of the ossicular chain is due to fracture of the stapes crura or separation at the incudo-stapedial joint. The diagnosis of this type of interruption can be made tomographically by direct visualization of the fragments or by detection of an abnormal rotation of the long process of an incus that has lost its normal relationship to the oval window. Fractures involving the labyrinth, large enough to be radiographically demonstrable, usually produce a complete nerve or vestibular loss or both. Longitudinal fracture of the petrous pyramid may involve one or more inner ear structures but often skips the labyrinth by running just in front or back of it. Transverse fractures of the petrous pyramid may occur at any level, although they tend to follow the plane of least resistance, which runs from the dome of the jugular fossa through the vestibule and basal turn of the cochlea to the superior petrous ridge.

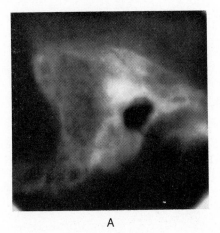

A

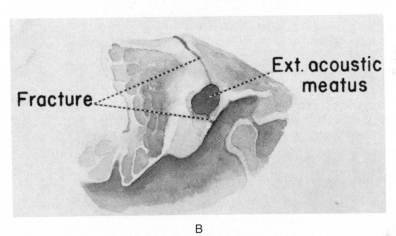

B

**Figure 5–14**  Extralabyrinthine fracture with cerebrospinal fluid leak from the ear. Lateral section shows a fracture extending from the superior wall of the external auditory canal to the middle cranial fossa. There is also fracture of the anterior wall of the external auditory canal.

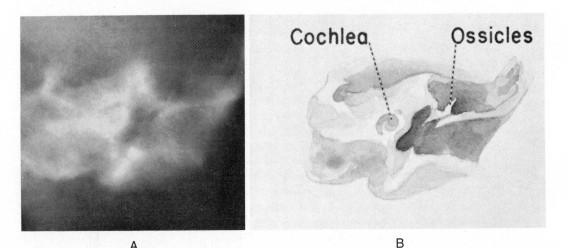

A                                                    B

**Figure 5–15**  Traumatic dislocation of incus. Frontal section shows the incus to be dislocated with its long process abutted against the promontory.

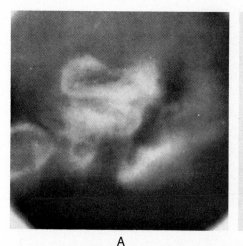

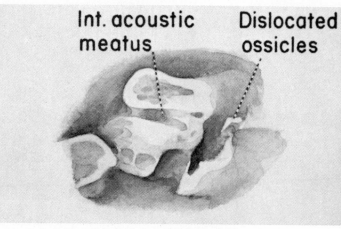

A

B

**Figure 5–16**  (Same patient as in Figure 5–15.) Traumatic dislocation of incus. Semiaxial view shows the lateral dislocation of the body of the incus. A fracture of the external auditory canal was also demonstrated in the lateral sections.

3.   Paralysis of the facial nerve results from involvement of the facial canal with consequent compression or tear of the nerve. The tomographic findings vary from complete disruption of a segment of the facial canal to transection of the canal by a fracture line and to separation and depression of a fragment of the canal wall (Fig. 5–17). The facial canal may be injured either by transverse fracture or by the more common longitudinal fracture of the petrous bone. The most common site of involvement is at or about the region of the superficial and poorly protected pyramidal turn of the canal.

### Inflammatory Processes

Tomography is of great help in evaluation of the extension of inflammatory processes. These can be roughly divided into three main categories: simple otitis media, otitis media with osteitis of the wall, of the ossicles or of both and otitis media with cholesteatoma. From the radiologic point of view, this classification seems much more logical than the clinical one of acute, subacute and chronic otitis, because the radiologic findings are often not characteristic of one phase.

In simple otitis media, one sees an abnormal haziness of all or part of the middle ear cavity due to fluid or mucosal thickening. When osteitis or cholesteatoma is present, the epitympanic recess is the area most commonly involved, especially its inferolateral wall: the so-called spur or surgical bridge. Destruction of the spur is usually associated with perforation of Shrapnell's membrane. The destruction may also involve the superior wall of the epitympanic recess, with consequent serious meningeal complications; the medial wall, with possible formation of a fistula of the horizontal semicircular canal; or the posterior wall, with erosion in the region of the aditus. The ossicles frequently are partially or completely destroyed. Necrosis of the long process of the incus, in our experience, is the most common finding (Fig. 5–18). The ampullar limb of the lateral semicircular canal is the usual site of a fistula. The diagnosis of a fistula is based on the detection of amputation of the lateral tip of the canal with absence of the otic capsule covering this, or flattening of the medial wall of the epitympanic recess due to erosion of the normal protuberance of the lateral semicircular canal (Figs. 5–19 and 5–20).

The differentiation between an otitis with osteitis and an otitis with cholesteatoma might be impossible because the density of a cholesteatomatous mass is identical to that of granulation tissue and the destruction of the surrounding bony structures might be the same in the two conditions. In our experience, however, destruction of the lateral attic wall and ossicles is nearly always the result of cholesteatoma. An exception is necrosis of the long process of the incus, which may be the result of simple osteitis without cholesteatoma. Tympanosclerotic plaques are occasionally demonstrated by tomography as irregular calcifications in the middle ear cavity and attic. Ankylosis of the ossicles, especially the head of the malleus, is best diagnosed in lateral tomographic sections by the filling in of the space between the anterior aspect of the head of the malleus and the attic wall.

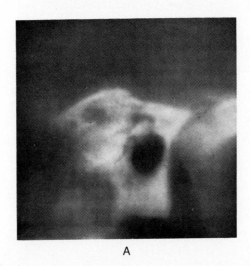

A

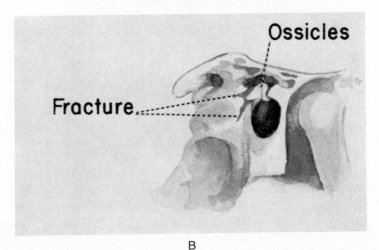

B

**Figure 5–17** Extralabyrinthine fracture with involvement of the facial nerve canal. Lateral section shows two fracture lines extending from the posterior wall of the epitympanic recess in the area where the facial nerve canal turns from its tympanic portion to its mastoid portion.

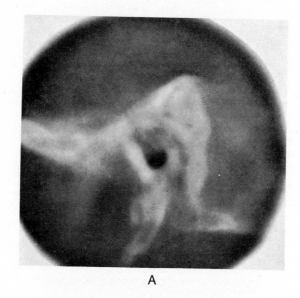

A

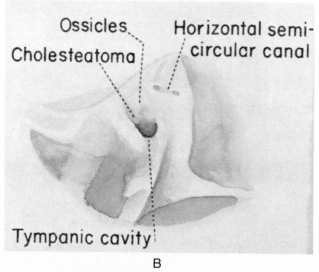

B

**Figure 5–18**　Otitis media with cholesteatoma. Lateral section shows a soft tissue mass in the epitympanic recess and upper part of the tympanic cavity. The ossicles are surrounded by the mass, and there is destruction of the long process of the incus.

## Neoplastic Conditions

The classification of neoplastic conditions involving the petrous pyramid and the ear is complicated by the frequent occurrence in this area of a group of lesions rarely seen elsewhere. We can divide the processes into four major groups: (1) histologically benign tumors with benign course; (2) histologically benign tumors with possible malignant clinical course because of the large destruction produced in the petrous pyramid and base of the skull by the growing tumor mass; (3) primary malignant processes; and (4) malignant tumors arising in structures adjacent to the petrous bone and involving it by direct extension, and metastatic lesions.

The first group includes conditions usually involving the external auditory canal, such as osteomas, fibromas and lipomas.

The second group includes neurinomas (from the seventh to the twelfth cranial nerve), glomus jugulare tumors, epidermoids (primary congenital cholesteatomas) and meningiomas. These lesions will be covered separately and deserve special attention not only because of their relative frequency but above all because of the fundamental role played by radiology in their diagnosis.

Carcinoma is the most common primary malignant tumor of the temporal bone. Carcinomas usually arise in the external auditory canal, where they produce a partial or total destruction of the canal walls (Fig. 5–21). The lesion may spread into the mastoid, involving the facial canal, extend into the middle ear cavity and from

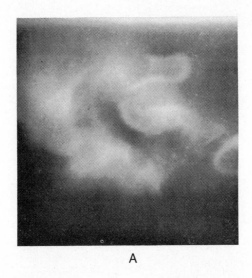

A

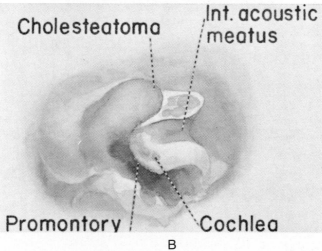

B

**Figure 5–19** Otitis media with cholesteatoma and fistula of lateral semicircular canal. Semiaxial view shows a large soft tissue mass in the region of the epitympanic recess which is expanded with thinning and partial erosion of the tegmen tympani. There is destruction of the ossicles, involvement of the facial nerve canal and extension of the destructive process into the petrous pyramid.

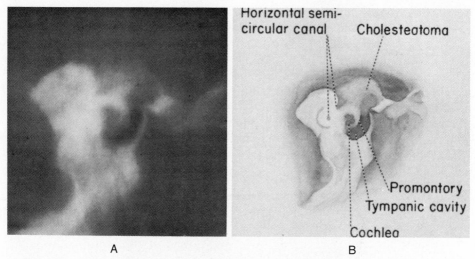

**Figure 5–20** (Same patient as in Figure 5–19.) Otitis media with cholesteatoma and fistula of lateral semicircular canal. Lateral section shows the large destruction in the region of the epitympanic recess and superior aspect of the petrous pyramid. The capsule surrounding the ampullar limb of the lateral semicircular canal is eroded, with formation of a fistula.

there involve the jugular fossa and petrous pyramid. Owing to their tendency to infiltrate rather than destroy, carcinomas produce a typical mottled or moth-eaten appearance of the involved bone. Sarcomas usually occur in young children and account for a destructive lesion of the petrous pyramid. Sarcoma may arise in the eustachian tube and spread by retrograde extension to the ear.

The fourth group of neoplastic conditions includes metastatic lesions such as from carcinomas of the breast, lungs or prostate, and involvement of the petrous bone by direct extension from malignant neoplasms arising in adjacent structures, such as the parotid gland and nasopharynx.

### Epidermoid (Congenital Cholesteatoma)

These tumors are derived from embryonic epidermal rests situated in the temporal bone or adjacent epidural space or meninges. The clinical and radiographic manifestations depend upon the site of the tumor.

*Primary or Congenital Cholesteatoma of the Mastoid and Middle Ear Cavity.* The otoscopic examination may reveal a characteristic whitish pearly mass behind an intact tympanic membrane. The tomographic examination demonstrates a well defined mass in the middle ear cavity which may erode the ossicular chain (Fig. 5–22). The inferior margin of the lateral wall of the attic is intact, but the lateral attic wall may be eroded from within, assuming a rounded defect concave medially. These two features are fundamental to the differential diagnosis of acquired and congenital cholesteatomas.

*Congenital Cholesteatoma of the Petrous Pyramid.* These lesions are characterized by facial paralysis as the first clinical finding. If the tumor arises within the petrous pyramid, the radiographic examination reveals an expansile cystic lesion (Fig. 5–23), usually accounting for elevation and thinning of the petrous ridge. The internal auditory canal is usually involved first, followed by the semicircular canal

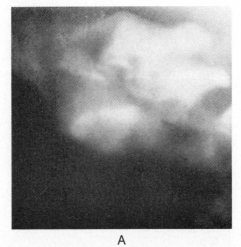

A

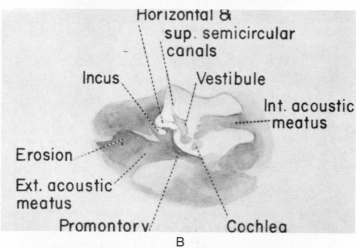

B

**Figure 5–21** Squamous cell carcinoma of external auditory canal. Frontal section shows destruction of the superior wall of the external auditory canal with involvement of the mastoid.

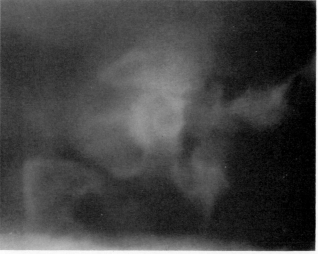

**Figure 5–22** Congenital cholesteatoma of the left middle ear cavity. The frontal tomographic section reveals a well defined soft tissue mass in the anterior portion of the left tympanic cavity medial to the malleus handle.

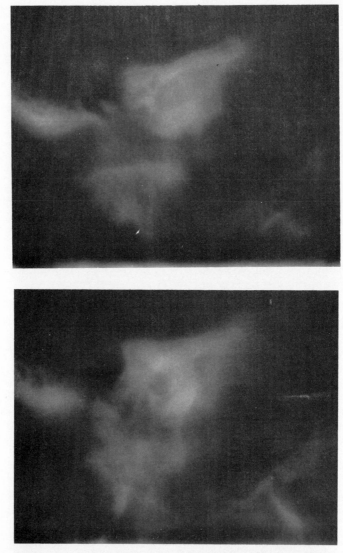

**Figure 5–23** Congenital cholesteatoma of the right petrous pyramid. The frontal tomographic sections reveal an expansile lesion in the petrous apex. The lesion erodes the posterior wall of the internal auditory canal and extends into the jugular fossa.

and the remainder of the labyrinth. If the lesion instead arises above the petrous pyramid in the epidural space or meninges, one finds a scooped-out appearance of the petrous ridge, not surrounded as in the previous case by a bony rim.

Congenital cholesteatomas may also be found in the cerebellopontine angle where they produce clinical symptomatology and radiographic features similar to those of an acoustic neurinoma. More rarely, congenital cholesteatomas may be found in the jugular fossa where they mimic both clinically and radiographically a glomus jugulare tumor.

### Meningioma

Primary meningioma originates from meningeal extension along the seventh and eighth cranial nerves within the internal auditory canal. It may expand the internal auditory canal and mimic an acoustic neurinoma. Clues to the diagnosis are calcifications within the mass and hyperostosis of the canal walls and of the crista falciformis.

Secondary meningioma involves the temporal bone by extension from overlying meningeal tumors. The radiographic findings vary from hyperostosis (Fig. 5–24) to moth-eaten erosion to frank destruction or to a combination of these. They may erode the labyrinth and break through the tegmen into the middle ear cavity.

### Glomus Tumors

Only radiography can demonstrate the extent of the glomus tumor and the presence or absence of other possible isolated multicentric lesions.

The tomographic findings depend on whether the lesion is a glomus tympanicum confined to the middle ear, a more extensive glomus jugulare involving the jugular foramen and the bone of the skull.

*Glomus Tympanicum.* In glomus tympanicum the tomographic findings are confined to the middle ear and are as follows:

1. There is a soft tissue mass of variable size usually in the lower portion of the middle ear cavity.

2. The floor of the middle ear, which forms the roof of the jugular fossa, is intact.

3. The internal carotid artery canal is intact and in its normal position.

4. Large glomus tympanicum tumors may fill the middle ear with a soft tissue mass, cause the tympanic membrane to bulge laterally and cause a concave indentation of the bony wall of the promontory. These tumors, as they enlarge, may extend posteriorly into the mastoid or inferiorly into the jugular fossa.

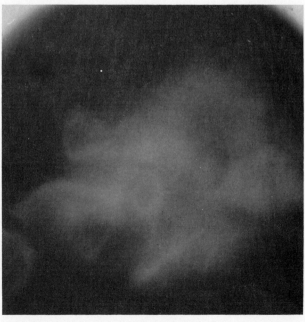

**Figure 5–24** Meningioma of the left petrous pyramid. This semiaxial section reveals marked hyperostosis of the superior aspect of the petrous pyramid. The lesion involves the tegmen tympani and extends into the middle ear cavity.

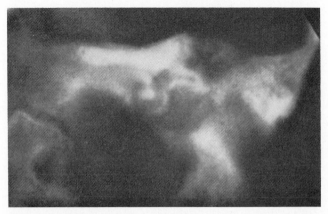

**Figure 5–25**   Glomus jugulare tumor. Frontal section shows a large destruction of the inferior aspect of the left petrous pyramid. The jugular fossa is enlarged and its cortical outline eroded. There is also erosion of the floor of the middle ear cavity and of the inferior wall of the internal auditory canal.

5.   The jugular venogram is normal, although this procedure is usually not necessary, since the floor of the middle ear is intact.

6.   In a glomus tympanicum, subtraction arteriography is indispensable for the demonstration of the vascular mass and the vessels feeding the tumor, if this information is needed.

*Glomus Jugulare.*   The radiographic findings of glomus jugulare tumors depend on the size and extension of the lesion. They may be summarized as follows:

1.   Enlargement of the jugular fossa with erosion of the cortical outline. A large jugular fossa without erosion of the cortical outline is not of diagnostic significance,

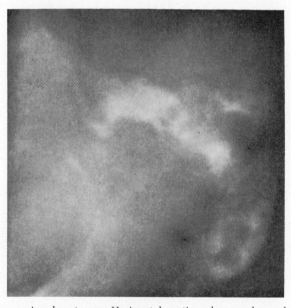

**Figure 5–26**   Glomus jugulare tumor. Horizontal section shows a large destruction of the posteromedial aspect of the left petrous pyramid. The jugular fossa, as best seen in other sections, is markedly enlarged. Same case as Figure 5–25.

since asymmetry of the two fossae of the same patient is extremely common (Fig. 5–25).

2.   Erosion of the bony septum between the jugular foramen and the outer opening of the internal carotid canal.

3.   Erosion of the floor of the middle ear cavity.

4.   Soft tissue mass of variable size in the middle ear cavity, which may extend into the mastoid and into the external auditory canal.

5.   Undermining or, in extensive lesions, frank destruction of the posteroinferior aspect of the petrous pyramid (Fig. 5–26).

6.   There may be erosion of the adjacent occipital bone extending to the hypoglossal canal.

7.   Retrograde jugular venography shows partial or complete obstruction of the jugular vein depending on the extent of the lesion (Fig. 5–27).

8.   Subtraction arteriography is indispensable for the delineation of the vascular mass and feeding vessels. The injection should be performed in the common carotid artery to visualize both internal and external carotid circulation. In our experience the ascending pharyngeal artery is the largest feeding vessel.

### Acoustic Neurinoma

Acoustic neurinomas account for approximately 10 per cent of unilateral sensorineural hearing loss and vestibular loss of unknown origin. They normally originate within the internal auditory canal and therefore produce osseous changes detectable by a proper radiographic study. The battery of radiographic tests for the diagnosis of acoustic neurinoma can be divided into three groups: (1) screening tests,

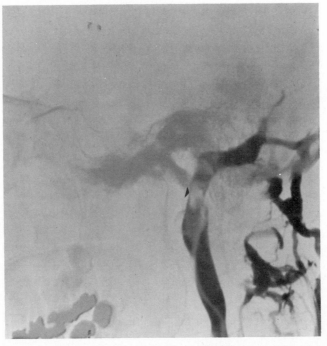

**Figure 5-27**   Right retrograde jugular venogram. A well defined oval-shaped mass is outlined in the internal jugular vein. The mass fills most of the lumen but does not obstruct the vein.

which include conventional radiography and tomography; (2) diagnostic tests, including opaque cerebellopontine cisternography and computerized tomography (CT); and (3) complementary tests, such as pneumoencephalography, angiography, and radioactive brain scan. Only the first two groups of tests, which are by far the most useful for the diagnosis of acoustic neurinoma, will be discussed.

*Screening Tests.*    Whenever conventional radiography is used, two projections are indispensable for the study of the internal auditory canal: the transorbital view, which shows the canal in its full length, and the Stenvers' view, for the study of the opening or porus of the canal, which is seen in this projection on face whereas the canal is quite foreshortened. A more precise study of the internal auditory canal can, of course, be obtained by tomography. This is particularly true whenever the petrous pyramids are extensively or asymmetrically pneumatized. Tomography should always be performed in two planes. The frontal sections are the most satisfactory for the study of the shape and size of the internal auditory canal and for the length of its posterior wall, whereas the lateral sections add details of utmost importance concerning the status of the cortex and porus of the canal. In addition, both sides should always be examined for comparison purposes. In fact, although there are slight variations in size and shape of the internal auditory canals of any one person, these variations are small when compared with the difference between subjects.

The following four parameters should always be examined for the detection of changes indicative of an acoustic neurinoma (all figures have been corrected for magnification):

1. *Vertical diameter.* This normally ranges between 2 and 10 mm., with an average of 4.5 mm. An enlargement of 1 to 2 mm. of any portion of the internal auditory canal under investigation in comparison to the corresponding segment of the opposite side should be considered questionable, and an enlargement of 2 mm. or more as definitely abnormal (Fig. 5–28).

2. *Length of the posterior wall.* This normally ranges between 4 and 12 mm., with an average of 8 mm. Shortening of the posterior wall of one canal by 2 to 3 mm.

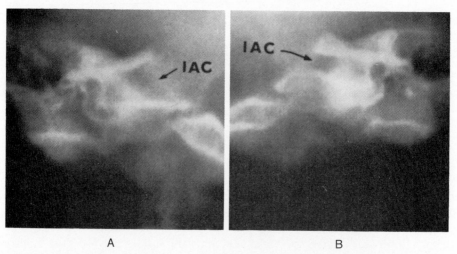

A                                         B

**Figure 5–28**   Acoustic neurinoma. *A,* Frontal section of the right ear shows extreme widening of the internal auditory canal. The shape of the canal, open medially, and the erosion of the posterior wall of the canal indicate that the tumor is extending largely outside of the canal into the cerebellopontine cistern. *B,* Frontal section of the normal left ear for comparison. *IAC,* Internal auditory canal.

should be considered questionable, and shortening by 3 mm. or more as definitely abnormal.

3. *Outline of the canal.* The lumen of the normal internal auditory canal is surrounded by a well defined white line made up by cortical bone that is denser than the surrounding bone of the petrosa. Destruction or demineralization of this cortical outline is a positive or suggestive indication, respectively, of a space-occupying lesion within the canal.

4. *Crista falciformis.* This structure divides the canal into two compartments but is always located at or above the midpoint of the vertical diameter of the internal auditory canal. A reverse of this ratio or an asymmetry by at least 2 mm. in the position of the crista is strongly suggestive of an intracanalicular mass.

*Diagnostic Tests.* Based on the results of the tomographic study, a decision can be made whether or not to perform additional diagnostic tests, i.e., opaque cisternography and computerized tomography. These studies are carried out when the tomographic examination has demonstrated an abnormal internal auditory canal; when the results of the audiometric and vestibular tests are strongly suggestive of a retrocochlear lesion, whatever the result of the tomographic examination; and when the borderline findings of a tomographic study are coupled with abnormal audiometric, vestibular or neurologic results.

**Opaque cisternography** is an invasive technique, since it requires a spinal puncture for the injection of the contrast material into the subarachnoid space. In proper hands it is a simple and conclusive study, but it becomes a useless and confusing examination in the hands of the inexperienced practitioner.

Two to three milliliters of isophendylate (Pantopaque) is injected into the subarachnoid space by lumbar puncture. Prior to the injection of the contrast material, the intracranial pressure is measured, and a few milliliters of cerebrospinal fluid are withdrawn for chemical testing. Under fluoroscopic control the contrast material is then moved into the posterior cranial fossa by tilting the table in the Trendelenburg position. During this maneuver the patient is kept in the lateral decubitus position so that the contrast material will collect in the dependent cerebellopontine cistern. The patient's head is then progressively rotated to an oblique, Stenvers-like projection and finally to a full face down view. This latter projection is extremely important for the visualization of the entire internal auditory canal without superimposition of the contrast material collected in the cistern (Fig. 5–29). During the study, multiple spot films are obtained at different angulations of the patient's head. Whenever the spot films show a very small or questionable intracanalicular defect, the patient is moved to a tomographic table, and multiple frontal and lateral tomographic sections are obtained. The absence of filling of the internal auditory canal (Fig. 5–30) and the demonstration of a filling defect in the cerebellopontine cistern (Figs. 5–31, 5–32 and 5–33) are positive evidence for a space-occupying lesion.

Opaque cisternography allows the recognition of masses as small as 2 to 3 mm. which appear as small filling defects (Fig. 5–34). Whenever the tumor is intracanalicular or the cisternal mass is small, opaque cisternography is by far the most satisfactory technique. The contrast material that infiltrates between the tumor, cerebellum and brain stem clearly outlines the entire lesion. However, if the tumor is larger and is adjacent or adherent to the brain stem and cerebellum, the contrast material will not outline the medial aspect of the mass, and therefore the determination of the tumor size becomes difficult. In these cases it is not unusual for the radiologist to underestimate the actual size of the tumor mass.

*Text continued on page 146*

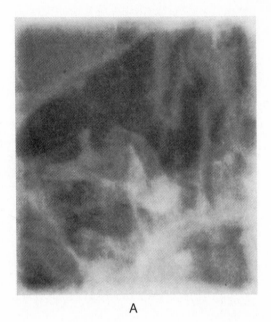

A

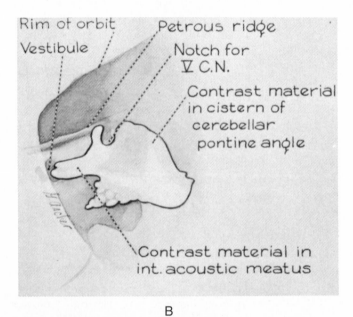

B

**Figure 5–29**  *A* and *B*, Normal opaque cerebellopontine cisternogram showing complete filling of the internal auditory canal. Note the well defined crista separating the superior and inferior compartments of the fundus of the canal. (Courtesy of Dr. G. Valvassori.)

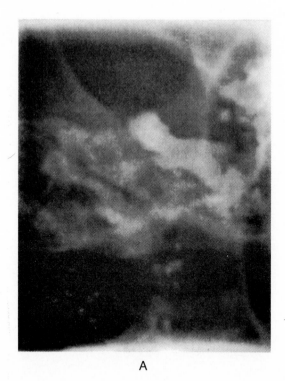

A

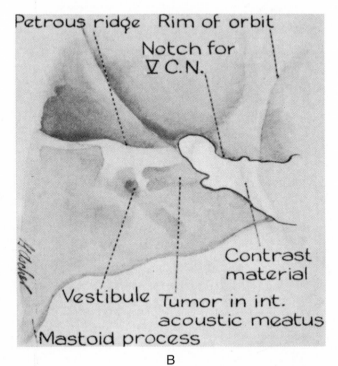

B

**Figure 5–30**  *A* and *B*, Opaque cisternogram showing a small tumor filling the internal auditory canal to the porus. The neurinoma was removed by the translabyrinthine approach without neurologic defect. (Courtesy of Dr. J. Clemis.)

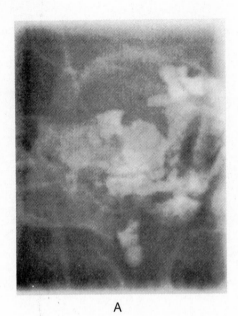

A

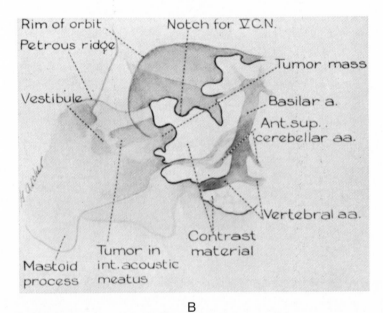

B

**Figure 5–31**  *A* and *B*, Opaque cisternogram of a larger but still small tumor filling the internal auditory canal and protruding 1 cm. into the cerebellopontine cistern. Translabyrinthine removal resulted in immediate facial paresis, with recovery beginning after 2 months. (Courtesy of Dr. J. Clemis.)

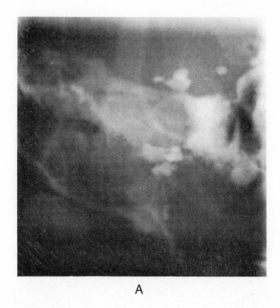

A

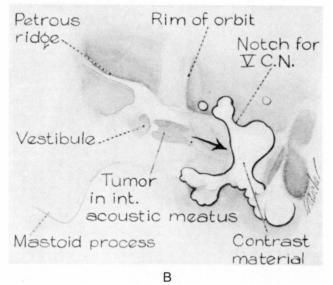

B

**Figure 5–32** *A* and *B*, Opaque cisternogram showing a medium-sized tumor filling the internal acoustic meatus and extending 1.8 cm. into the cerebellopontine angle (shown by arrow). It was removed by the translabyrinthine approach with immediate facial paresis, with the first evidence of recovery after 2 weeks. (Courtesy of Dr. J. Clemis.)

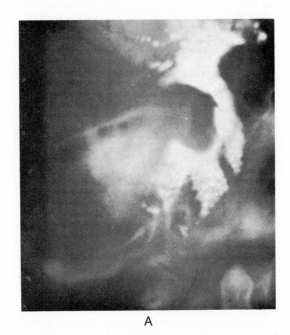

A

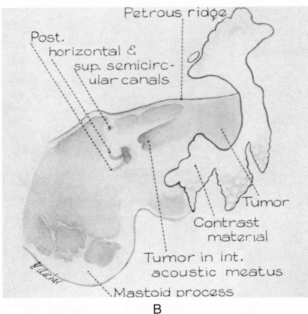

B

**Figure 5–33** *A* and *B*, Tomographic section of opaque cisternogram showing a medium-sized tumor filling the internal meatus and protruding 2.5 cm. into the cerebellopontine cistern. Death occurred 3 hours after translabyrinthine removal, as a result of a blood clot compressing the pons. (Courtesy of Dr. G. Valvassori.)

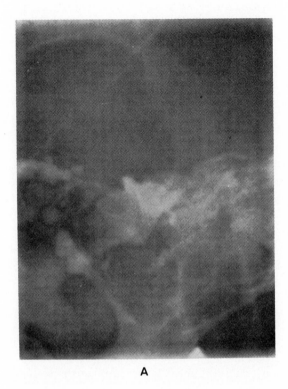

A

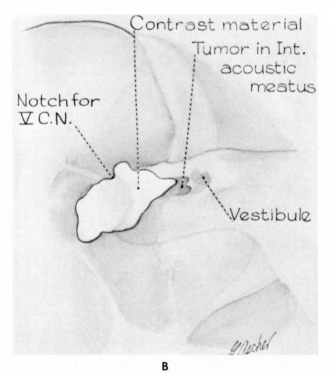

B

**Figure 5–34**  *A* and *B*, Opaque cisternogram of the opposite ear, in the same patient as in Figure 5–31, showing a small filling defect of the fundus of the internal acoustic meatus. It is probably a very small early tumor, not yet confirmed surgically. (Courtesy of Dr. G. Valvassori and Dr. J. Clemis.)

**Computerized tomography** is a non-invasive technique and as such can be performed on an outpatient basis. Two series of scans are usually obtained, the first prior to and a second during the drip infusion of contrast material. The first series shows the indirect signs of a tumor mass, such as the displacement of the fourth ventricle and the narrowing of the opposite cerebellopontine cistern by the displaced brain stem. The tumor mass may not be recognizable, since its density is quite similar to the surrounding brain structures. The second series demonstrates the actual tumor mass following enhancement of its density by the contrast material (Fig. 5–35). Computerized tomography allows a precise evaluation of the size of the lesion and of its extension, particularly in the region of the tentorial notch. It should be kept in mind, however, that in my experience and in the experience of other authors, small tumors (less than 1.2 cm. in diameter) may not be recognizable in the horizontal sections at present obtained by computerized tomography. For this reason additional coronal sections during drip infusion of contrast material should be obtained through the posterior cranial fossa (Fig. 5–36). Coronal sections will demonstrate extracanalicular tumors as small as 1 cm. in diameter.

At the present state of the art it is my belief that CT is the procedure of choice when:

1.   The neurological deficit is not limited to the eighth cranial nerve. (Fifth cranial nerve involvement, ataxia or other cerebellar or brain stem signs are present.)

2.   The neurological involvement is limited to the eighth cranial nerve but the tomographic study demonstrates a grossly enlarged internal auditory canal.

3.   In elderly patients.

Cerebellopontine cisternography is the procedure of choice in patients with

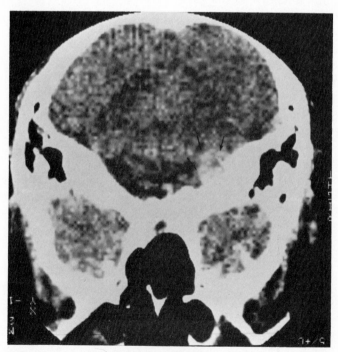

**Figure 5–35**   Right acoustic neurinoma: this CT horizontal section obtained after infusion of 300 cc. of 30 per cent Hypaque contrast material reveals the presence of a 1.2 cm. tumor in the region of the right cerebellopontine cistern.

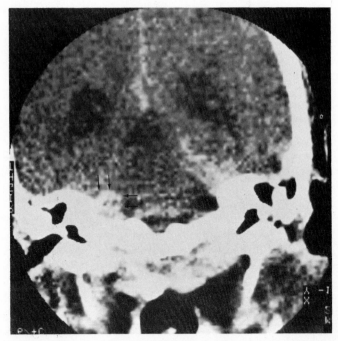

**Figure 5–36** Right acoustic neurinoma, same case as in Figure 5–35. Computerized tomography, coronal section: the contour of the lesion is more sharply outlined than in the horizontal section. In addition, this projection allows a more precise evaluation of the relationship between the tumor and adjacent structures such as the tentorium and 5th cranial nerve.

involvement limited to the eighth cranial nerve and minimal or moderate expansion of the internal auditory canal by tomography. It should also be performed in cases where the CT examination is negative, but the audiometric, vestibular and neurological tests are suggestive of a retrocochlear lesion.

*Results.* My series includes 6000 patients who underwent screening radiographic tests because of sensorineural or vestibular losses of unknown origin or other neurological symptomatology suggestive of a cerebellopontine angle lesion. Of these patients, 2000 (approximately 30 per cent) were selected for additional diagnostic tests. From approximately 10 per cent of the patients screened and 30 per cent of the patients who underwent diagnostic tests, 610 tumors of the cerebellopontine angle were found. Of the tumors, 90 per cent were acoustic neurinomas; the other 10 per cent were lesions such as meningiomas, primary cholesteatomas, gliomas, facial nerve neurinomas, artero-venous malformations, aneurysms and metastases. The tumor was confined to the internal auditory canal in 10 per cent, extended from the canal into the cerebellopontine cistern but without involvement of other cranial nerves or the brain in 57 per cent, involved the fifth cranial nerve or other structures in 33 per cent of the cases.

## Otodystrophies

Under this classification we include two groups of processes: (1) diffuse processes, such as Paget's disease, neurofibromatosis, osteogenesis imperfecta, and fibrous dysplasia, in which the involvement of the ear could be one of the pathologic manifestations; and (2) a localized ear disease, otosclerosis (otospongiosis).

In both groups, ankylosis of the stapes in the oval window can represent a feature of the process.

### Otosclerosis (Otospongiosis)

The diagnosis of fenestral otosclerosis is usually made by the otologist on the basis of the clinical history and audiometric tests. The role of radiographic assessment is therefore limited. Tomography may indicate the presence or absence of otospongiotic changes in cases where the diagnosis is otherwise in doubt and may enable the surgeon to decide which ear to operate in those cases with symmetrical hearing loss but asymmetric pathological involvement (Fig. 5–37). Tomography is, however, extremely helpful in evaluating postsurgical cases (Fig. 5–38) where an initial hearing improvement is subsequently lost. In these cases radiography may demonstrate partial or complete reobliteration of the oval window by recurrence of the otospongiotic focus and displacement or fixation of the prosthesis.

Cochlear otosclerosis may occur by progressive enlargement of the perifenestral foci or may be due to the presence of single or multiple foci in other locations of the cochlear and labyrinthine capsule. The diagnosis of cochlear otospongiosis is suspected by the otologist on the basis of the audiometric configuration, clinical history and clinical findings such as the Schwartze sign, but further confirmation is required. In this area the role of tomography is extremely helpful.

The normal cochlear capsule appears as a sharply defined, homogeneously dense bony shell outlining the lumen of the cochlea. The density of the capsule enhances the clearness of the lumen of the enclosed cavity, which because of an optic phenomenon appears more radiolucent than it would without the surrounding dense line. The portion of the capsule seen on end and therefore forming the outline of the capsule on the radiogram is more important from the interpretation point of view than the portion of the capsule seen on face and therefore superimposed upon the lumen.

A focus of otospongiosis can be visualized by tomography provided that (1) it is

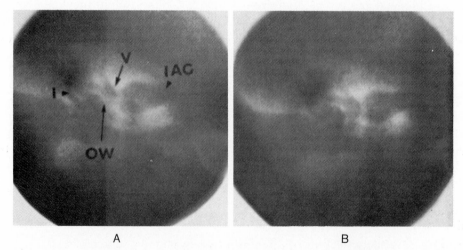

|     |     |
|-----|-----|
| A   | B   |

**Figure 5–37**  Otosclerosis. *A,* Frontal section shows complete obliteration of the oval window by a thick footplate of the stapes. *I,* Incus. *IAC,* Internal auditory canal. *OW,* Oval window. *V,* Vestibule. *B,* Frontal section of the same patient, obtained after stapedectomy and insertion of a polyethylene strut with vein graft, shows the oval window fully reopened.

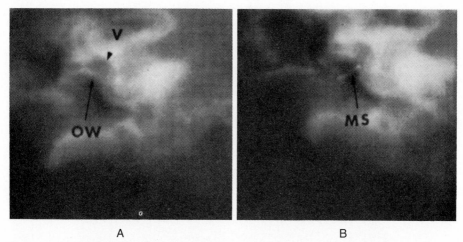

A                                                              B

**Figure 5–38**  Otosclerosis. *A,* Frontal section shows complete obliteration of the oval window by a thick footplate of the stapes. *OW,* Oval window. *V,* Vestibule. *B,* Frontal section of the same patient, obtained after stapedectomy and insertion of a tantalum prosthesis with fat graft, shows the oval window fully reopened and the metallic strut in good position. *MS,* Metallic strut.

sufficiently large, (2 mm. or more) and (2) the density of the otospongiotic focus is different from the surrounding normal capsule.

The location of the focus may also influence its detection. For instance, small foci are more easily detected in the capsule of the basal turn than in other portions of the cochlear capsule.

Whenever demineralizing or spongiotic changes involve the cochlear capsule, its outline becomes thinner, interrupted (Fig. 5–39) and finally may completely

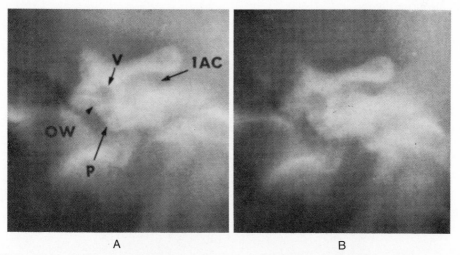

A                                                              B

**Figure 5–39**  Cochlear otosclerosis. Demonstration of foci in a patient with positive Schwartze sign. *A,* Frontal section shows a large focus of otosclerosis involving the basilar turn of the cochlea, the contour of which has become irregular. There are mixed areas of increased and decreased density producing a complete disruption of the normal structure of the otic capsule. The lumen of the cochlea seems encroached upon. *IAC,* Internal auditory canal. *OW,* Oval window. *P,* Promontory. *V,* Vestibule. *B,* Frontal section of the same patient, 2 mm. anterior to *A,* showing the same involvement of the basilar turn of the cochlea. There is marginal thickening of the footplate of the stapes.

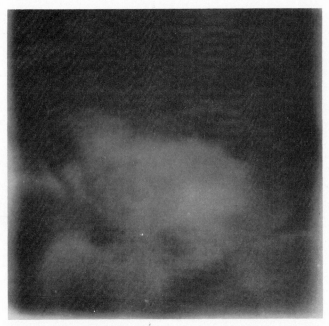

**Figure 5–40**  Active cochlear otosclerosis. This frontal tomographic section demonstrates a severe and diffuse involvement of the right cochlear capsule by otospongiotic foci. The contour of the capsule is disrupted and in several areas completely erased. Compare with Figure 5–1 showing the normal appearance of the cochlear capsule.

disappear (Fig. 5–40). As the involvement progresses, the ratio in density between the capsule and the lumen decreases so that the outline of the cochlea becomes indistinguishable from the surrounding bone of the petrosa. Because of the lack of differential absorption of the incident x-ray beam between the portion of the capsule seen on end and the portion seen on face, the lumen will appear less radiolucent than in normal cases.

As the otospongiotic focus matures and recalcifies, it becomes radiographically

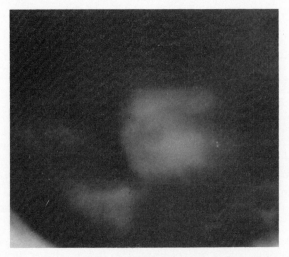

**Figure 5–41**  Mature cochlear otosclerosis. This semiaxial section of the right ear demonstrates irregular thickening of the cochlear capsule with scalloping of its outer and inner aspects.

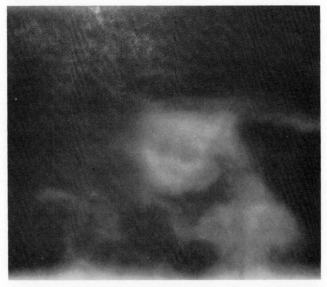

**Figure 5–42**  Forty-nine year old male who underwent successful fenestration at age 34. The hearing was stable for 13 years but showed a progressive sensorineural deterioration during the past two years. This frontal tomographic section of the left ear shows a severe involvement of the cochlear capsule by spongiotic changes. Sodium fluoride treatment was started.

undetectable if its density is similar to the density of the surrounding normal capsule. Sclerotic changes are the result of opposition of mature otosclerotic bone increasing the thickness of the capsule. Such foci are clearly recognizable in the portion of the capsule seen on end as areas of capsular thickening, roughening and scalloping of the outer and inner aspects (Fig. 5–41). However, the same foci involving the portion of the capsule seen on face may appear as areas of increased density superimposed upon the radiolucency of the lumen.

Follow-up examinations of the cochlear capsules are extremely important in patients with cochlear otospongiosis treated with sodium floride. The tomographic study will monitor the effect of the treatment by demonstrating recalcification or maturation of the otospongiotic foci (Fig. 5–42 and 5–43). The follow-up studies are

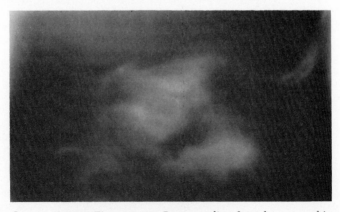

**Figure 5–43**  Same patient as Figure 5–42. Corresponding frontal tomographic section six years later showing a marked improvement in the definition of the cochlear capsule following remineralization of the spongiotic foci. The patient has been on sodium fluoride treatment since the first study and the hearing has been stable for the past three years.

performed one or two years apart only in the projection that best demonstrates the otospongiotic changes as revealed by the initial pre-treatment examination. The use of lead-containing glasses is mandatory in these cases to protect the lens of the eyes.

## REFERENCES

1. Agazzi, C., Cova, P. L., and Aenaldi, M.: Semeiotica stratigrafica dell' osso temporale. Relazione al XVI, Raduno del gruppo Otorinolaringologico dell' Alta Italia, Dic., 1958.
2. Brünner, S., Petersen, O., and Stoksted, P.: Tomography of the auditory ossicles. Acta Radiol., 56:20, 1961.
3. Brünner, S., Petersen, O., and Stoksted, P.: Laminography of the temporal bone. Am. J. Roentgenol., 86:281, 1961.
4. Buckingham, R. A., and Valvassori, G. E.: Tomographic and surgical pathology of cholesteatoma. Arch. Otolaryng., 91:464, 1970.
5. Clemis, J. D., and Valvassori, G. E.: Recent radiographic and clinical observations on the vestibular aqueduct. Otolaryngol. Clin. North Am. 339, October, 1968.
6. Compere, W. E., Jr.: Radiologic findings in otosclerosis. Arch. Otol., 71:150, 1960.
7. Cova, P. L., and Senaldi, M.: Anatomia stratigrafica del temporale. Parte 1, 2, 3, 4, 5. Audiol Prat., 1953–1954.
8. Francois, J., and Barrois, J. J.: Anatomie tomographique de l'os temporal normal. Ann. Radiol., 11:71, 1959.
9. Giraud, M., Bret, P., Anjou, A., Duquesnel, J., and Ogier, M.: L'exploration tomographique du rocher et de la mastoide. J. radiol. et electrol., 37:293, 1956.
10. Gross, J. P., Bloch, W., and Bourjat, P.: La paroi labyrinthique normale: aspects tomographiques. J. radiol., 5:253, 1962.
11. Juster, M., and Fischgold, H.: Etude Radio-anatomique de l'os temporal. Masson et Cie, Paris, 1955.
12. Langfeldt, B.: Tomography of the middle ear in columella operation. Acta Radiol., 53:129, 1960.
13. Monier-Kuhn, P., Heimendinger, E., Raber, R., and Klotz, G.: Etude tomographique de l'oreille moyenne. Ann. oto-laryng., 73:873, 1956.
14. Mundnich, K., and Frey, K.: Das röntgenschichtbild des Orhes. G. Thieme, Stuttgart, 1959.
15. Ombredanne, M., and Francois, J.: Etude tomographique des aplasies de l'oreille par balayage hypocycloîde. Ann. oto-laryng., 75:829, 1958.
16. Petersen, O., and Stoksted, P.: Tomography of normal temporal bone. Arch. Otolaryng., 73:37, 1961.
17. Portmann, M., and Guillen, G.: Radiodiagnostic en otologie. Masson et Cie, Paris, 1959.
18. Tarf, O.: Tomography of the temporal bone with the Polytome. Acta Radiol., 51:105, 1959.
19. Valvassori, G. E.: Laminography of the ear: Normal roentgenographic anatomy. Am. J. Roentgenol., 89:1155, 1963.
20. Valvassori, G. E.: Laminography of the ear: Pathologic conditions. Am. J. Roentgenol., 89:1168, 1963.
21. Valvassori, G. E.: Laminography of the ear in otosclerosis. Rev. Laryng., 60:770, 1963.
22. Valvassori, G. E.: Radiographic Atlas of the Temporal Bone. Book II. American Academy of Ophthalmology and Otolaryngology, 1964.
23. Valvassori, G. E.: Otosclerosis: A new challenge to roentgenology. Am. J. Roentgenol., 94:566, 1965.
24. Valvassori, G. E.: Radiologic diagnosis of cochlear otosclerosis. Laryngoscope, 75:1563, 1965.
25. Valvassori, G. E.: The interpretation of the radiographic findings in cochlear otosclerosis. Ann. Otol. Rhinol. Laryngol., 75(2):572, 1966.
26. Valvassori, G. E.: The abnormal internal auditory canal: The diagnosis of acoustic neuroma. Radiology, 92(3):449, 1969.
27. Valvassori, G. E.: Meniere's disease. Excerpta Medica International Congress Series No. 206, 612–613, August, 1969.
28. Valvassori, G. E.: Myelography of the internal auditory canal. Am. J. of Roentgenol. Radium Ther. Nucl. Med., 115:578, 1972.
29. Valvassori, G. E.: Benign tumors of the temporal bone. Radiol. Clin. North Am. 12(3):533, 1974.
30. Valvassori, G. E. and Buckingham, R. A.: Middle ear masses mimicking glomus tumors: Radiographic and otoscopic recognition. Ann. Otol. Rhinol. Laryngol. 83(5):606, 1974.
31. Valvassori, G. E. and Buckingham, R. A.: Tomography and Cross Sections of the Ear. W. B. Saunders Company, 1975.

32. Valvassori, G. E. and Clemis, J. D.: The large vestibular aqueduct syndrome. The Laryngoscope, 88:(5):723, 1978.
33. Valvassori, G. E. and Clemis, J. D.: Abnormal vestibular aqueduct in cochleovestibular disorders. Adv. Oto-Rhino-Laryng., 24:100, 1978.
34. Valvassori, G. E., Naunton, and Lindsay, J. R.: Inner ear anomalies: Clinical and histopathological considerations. Ann. Otol. Rhinol. Laryngol. 78(5):929, 1969.
35. Valvassori, G. E., and Pierce, R.: The normal internal auditory canal. Am. J. Roentgenol., 92:1232, 1964.

## Sir William Wilde

BORN 1815
DIED 1876

Described for acute subperiosteal mastoid abscess, the postaural incision formerly used for nearly all operations on the temporal bone and often employed today.

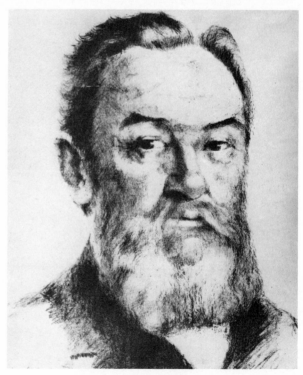

## Johannes Kessel

BORN 1837
DIED 1907

First performed endaural radical mastoidectomy, described by his chief resident in 1892. Performed in 1878, the first stapes mobilization and in 1879, described sound protection for the round window.

# Chapter 6

# Principles of Temporal Bone Surgery

SURGICAL ASEPSIS IN TEMPORAL BONE OPERATIONS
PROPHYLACTIC CHEMOTHERAPY AND ANTIBIOTIC
    THERAPY
ANESTHESIA FOR OPERATIONS ON THE EAR
INCISIONS TO EXPOSE THE TEMPORAL BONE
TECHNIQUES FOR SURGERY ON BONE IN EAR
    OPERATIONS
MAGNIFICATION IN EAR SURGERY
POSTOPERATIVE CARE

General principles that apply to all operations on the ear and temporal bone can be dealt with profitably before considering the individual surgical procedures. These include: the positive necessity for a flawless aseptic technique in operations on the temporal bone in a clean field; the optional use of sulfonamides or antibiotics for prophylaxis; preoperative sedation and anesthesia; the incisions used to gain access to the temporal bone; the special techniques for working on bone in ear operations; the use of the otomicroscope; and postoperative care after ear surgery.

## SURGICAL ASEPSIS IN TEMPORAL BONE OPERATIONS

In sharp contrast to otologic surgery prior to antibiotics, which was almost exclusively concerned with the evacuation of pus from the temporal bone, the majority of all operations on the ear today are undertaken in a clean field. In the old type of mastoid surgery the aseptic technique in the operation and postoperative care was perfunctory and decidedly imperfect. Although this may not often have done much harm when infection already existed, it certainly insured that surgery on previously uninfected ears was followed invariably by suppuration. It was expected as a matter of course that wounds would heal slowly, by second intention, with granulation formation and suppuration, and the careless operating room technique made sure that they did!

The same careless aseptic technique cannot be carried over into operations to restore hearing without the risk of wound infection and failure to improve hearing.

In operations on the labyrinth, endolymphatic sac and internal auditory meatus, infection of the meninges easily follows imperfect technique. Antibiotics and sulfonamides employed prophylactically **cannot substitute for a flawless aseptic technique** in the operating room and in the postoperative dressings. This is particularly true with the recent development of hospital strains of pathogenic hemolytic *Staphylococcus aureus* that are resistant to the common antibiotics.

For otolaryngologists accustomed to operating in the unsterile areas of the mouth, pharynx, nasopharynx and larynx, or for suppuration in the nasal accessory sinuses and middle ear cleft, the unlearning of established habits of careless aseptic technique and the acquisition of new habits of correct surgical asepsis are not at all easy tasks. First the surgeon must become convinced in his own mind of the necessity for strict adherence to a meticulous operating room ritual, and an equally careful aseptic technique for the postoperative dressings. If he will study the postoperative course and the final results that follow the employment of a precisely correct aseptic procedure he should be convinced. As just one example of many, in the well over 15,000 consecutive temporal bone operations in a clean field performed at the Chicago Wesley Memorial Hospital of Northwestern University during the past 42 years there has not been a known fatality within the first postoperative year, and not one case of meningitis or brain abscess occurring postoperatively. With freedom from introduced wound infection, healing proceeds by first intention without suppuration and without the development of troublesome granulations.

When he has become persuaded of the advantages of a flawless aseptic technique, the surgeon must then apply himself to learning the rules of correct aseptic surgical procedure. Careful observation and emulation of the precise technique of an experienced otologic surgeon will be helpful. Certain rules of sterile procedure, applicable to all surgery but especially to temporal bone operations in a clean field, are as follows:

1. Hands and arms of surgeon, assistant and sterile nurse are scrubbed for 10 minutes by the clock using a sterile brush and soap under running water. The two most commonly used soaps are pHisohex and Betadine. A three to four minute scrub may be used between cases if the gloves are not removed. After scrubbing, the arms are held upright to prevent water from the unscrubbed upper arm from trickling down over the scrubbed area.

2. The hands and arms are dried on a sterile towel handed to the person from the sterile table. Do not reach for the towel across the table with wet dripping hands, thus contaminating the entire table! First the hands are dried; then one arm is dried on one end of the towel and the other arm on the other end of the towel, so as not to carry contamination from the unscrubbed upper arm to a scrubbed area.

3. The headlight should be placed on the head and adjusted with a sterile towel before the scrub. The surgeon's back should be protected by a sterile vest or towel so that assistant, observer and sterile nurse standing behind him will not contaminate the front of their gowns.

4. Any observers must, like the surgeon, be clothed in operating room trousers and shirt, cap and mask, and then be covered with a sterile gown "mummy-fashion" (Fig. 6–1A). Two observers, and only one observer when the viewing tube is used on the operating microscope, are the maximum that can observe an operation on the temporal bone with profit to themselves and without increasing the risk of breaking the sterile technique. The most careful sterile preparations may be lost by one careless move of an observer. The advent of small color television cameras for the operating microscope has made it possible for larger groups to view microscopic surgery outside the operating room, reducing the chance of contamination.

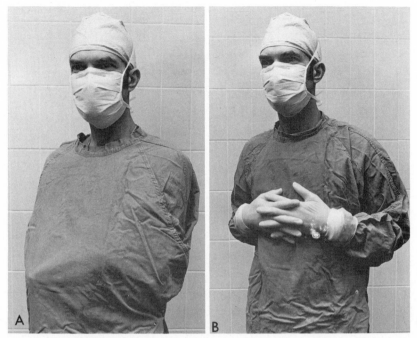

**Figure 6–1**  *A,* mummified observer. *B,* Surgeon's gloved hands must never be dropped to side or placed under the arms but should be held in front of chest.

5.    The gloved hands of surgeon, assistant and nurse must never be placed above the clavicle, below the waistline or posterior to the nipple line of the scrubbed person. When not engaged the hands should be held in front of the chest (Fig. 6–1*B*).

6.    Should a solution be spilled on the sterile drapes, the latter must be covered at once with fresh, dry, sterile towels to prevent the field from becoming contaminated from the underlying unsterile areas. Any tubing or instruments thus contaminated in the field must be resterilized.

7.    All operating room personnel must remain keenly alert to possible infringement of aseptic technique. If at any time the sterile nurse, assistant or surgeon so much as **suspects the possibility** that instrument, gown, glove or drape has touched an unsterile surface, the contaminated article must be discarded **immediately**. The surgeon should make a complete change of gown and gloves with a rescrub of his hands and arms if he or his sterile nurse suspects possible contamination at any time during the operation.

8.    The operating microscope must be covered with a sterile plastic disposable drape (Fig. 6–2). The dental-type drill should be capable of withstanding the autoclave (or gas sterilization) or should be wrapped in some type of sterile covering.

9.    Observers are not permitted to adjust or remove glasses by taking their hands from under their sterile gowns.

10.    The sterile nurse must be instructed and formally entrusted with the responsibility for maintaining a perfect aseptic technique in her operating room. Her reprimand or her admonition to discard an instrument or change gown and gloves must be accepted graciously and her instructions must be followed without question by the surgeon, his assistant and any observers.

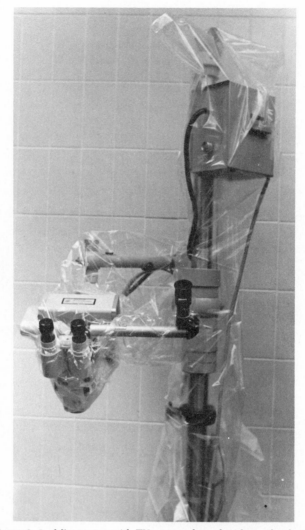

**Figure 6–2**   Microscope with TV camera draped with sterile plastic.

### Skin Sterilization

Staphylococci normally inhabit the superficial layers of stratified squamous epithelium. Absolute skin sterilization is not attainable, but a much reduced bacterial population will result from thorough cleaning of the skin surfaces as follows:

1. For the postaural incision and the endaural incision that extends upward from the meatus, the hair is clipped for a distance of 2 inches in front, above and behind the ear. It has been shown that shaving traumatizes the skin and increases the incidence of infection.

For the endomeatal incision, as for stapedectomy, the clipping may be confined to 1 inch in front and above the ear. Should temporalis fascia be utilized, the hair should be clipped for 2 inches.

2. The external auditory meatus is filled with Betadine, and with small sterile

sponges, the skin of the auricle and the adjacent skin are thoroughly scrubbed for 5 minutes using cotton applicators for the folds of the auricle.

3.  The skin is dried with sterile sponges, and a plastic ear drape is placed in proper position. This sticks to the skin and effectively protects the surgical field.

4.  The auricle and surrounding skin are wiped three times with 70 per cent alcohol using sterile sponges and cotton applicators; then the auricle and surrounding skin are painted with colorless tincture of Merthiolate, 1:1000.

An alternate method is to first apply plastic drapes to the clipped area, then scrub the auricle and drapes with Betadine soap. This is wiped clean by the circulating nurse using a sterile towel. Betadine solution is then placed into the ear canal by means of a small syringe and the auricle painted with the same solution. This is done three times and then removed.

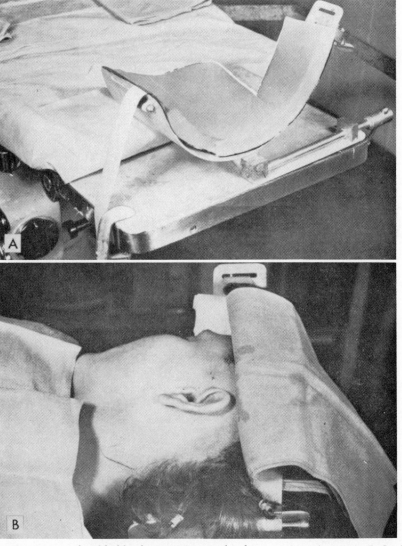

**Figure 6–3** *A*, Juers head holder for operations under the operating microscope. *B*, Sterile rubber sheet and towel protecting field from strap of head holder.

**Head Holder and Sterile Drapes**

A head holder, such as the one devised by Juers (Fig. 6–3), is preferred by the senior author and is a great convenience for temporal bone surgery under local anesthesia. It is invaluable for immobilizing the head and at the same time permits easy adjustment of the angle while the operating microscope is being used.

After completion of the skin sterilization, a sterile towel is placed over the ear, and a small sterile rubber sheet over this to prevent contamination of the surgical field by any moisture. The strap of the head holder is placed across the patient's head and forehead above the ear and fastened by the circulating nurse, who then carefully folds the sterile towel and rubber sheet upward across the unsterile strap, safely protecting the surgical field from it (Fig. 6–3*B*). A large sterile sheet covers the patient. Finally the surgical sheet with round hole for the ear 2 inches in diameter (5 cm.) is placed over the entire table and fastened to uprights connected with the table, so as to separate and shield the surgical sterile side of the table from the unsterile anesthetist's side (Fig. 6–4*A* and *B*). Green-colored drapes will appreciably lessen the reflected glare from the brilliant operating headlight or operating microscope, with lessened fatigue to the surgeon's eyes. A plastic sheet placed over the ear and the sterile drapes gives added protection from contamination by fluids and prevents lint from being carried by instruments into the ear.

An alternate method preferred by the junior author, using general anesthesia, is simply to turn the patient's head to one side and not depend upon a head holder. This allows the surgeon to move the head easily if necessary. In cases of obese individuals with short, thick necks, it is difficult to keep the head turned to one side without a holder. A 3M drape can be placed over the ear, followed by towels and a surgical sheet with a round hole two inches (5 cm.) wide (Fig. 6–5*A, B, C*). A waterproof paper "barrier" sheet is inserted between two regular sheets to effectively separate the patient from any fluids that might saturate the sterile sheets.

## PROPHYLACTIC CHEMOTHERAPY AND ANTIBIOTIC THERAPY

Because of the organisms that normally inhabit the superficial layers of stratified squamous epithelium, absolute skin sterilization is not a practical possibility. In addition, in every operating room there are a few bacteria floating on dust particles that may settle in a wound. The senior author found that the bacterial count on incubated blood agar plates that had been left exposed on the instrument table for an average of 2 hours during fenestration operations averaged 30 to 40 per plate; many of the organisms were staphylococci. When an ultraviolet light was installed in the ceiling of the operating room and kept on for one hour just preceding as well as during the operative procedure, the number of bacteria that settled on a blood agar plate was reduced by about half, but the visible air-borne bacteria were not eliminated.

Normally, healthy tissues are able, with their defense mechanisms, to resist infection by the few bacteria remaining in the skin after thorough skin preparation, and by the few bacteria that settle from the air. When there is traumatized, partially devitalized tissue or when a foreign body such as packing material is present, infection of the wound from these sources is more likely to occur. Prophylactic sulfonamide or antibiotic therapy may be helpful in protecting the wound from such infection, but some authors find that prophylactic antibiotics are not needed.

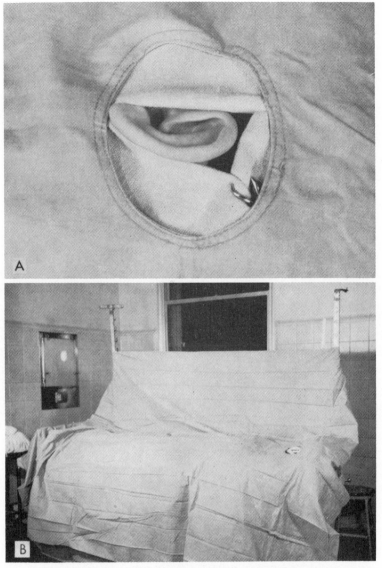

**Figure 6–4** Method of draping the ear and the patient.

For many years the senior author as a routine before every ear operation administered by intramuscular injection 600,000 units of penicillin before surgery and on each of 6 postoperative days that the average fenestration patient remained in the hospital. No untoward serious reaction occurred, other than that urticaria developed in an occasional patient a week to 10 days after the first dose of penicillin, or early in some patients who had received penicillin previously.

In the last few years, however, there has been a sharp rise in the incidence of severe and sometimes fatal anaphylactic shock following a single injection of penicillin in patients sensitized by previous administrations of this drug. Not all of these patients gave a history of allergic reaction from previous doses. Because of this increasing danger from injected prophylactic penicillin, along with the recent development of penicillin-resistant strains of pathogenic staphylococci, the senior

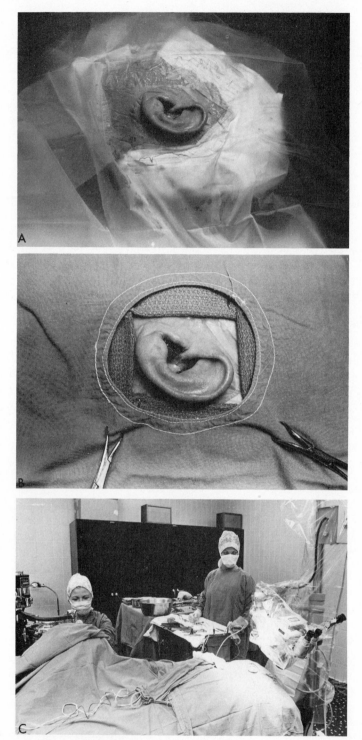

**Figure 6–5**  *A,* 3M® drape is placed over the ear and the ear is sterilized. *B,* Towels and a surgical sheet with a round hole 2 inches wide is placed over the plastic sheet. *C,* the patient is completely covered by a barrier sheet; the anesthesiologist and scrub nurse stand at opposite sides of the table. Note the sterile plastic drape over the microscope.

author now prefers to use a broad-spectrum antibiotic of relatively low toxicity that can be taken by mouth in effective therapeutic dosage. As a rule, erythromycin is administered by mouth as follows:

On the evening of admission to the hospital—250 mg.

On the day of surgery and for 2 or 3 postoperative days—250 mg. four times a day.

In recent years there has been a tendency by many surgeons to discontinue the routine use of prophylactic antibiotics. There remains at this writing some controversy concerning this entire subject. Certainly one should **never** substitute antibiotic coverage for aseptic technique.

## ANESTHESIA FOR OPERATIONS ON THE EAR

The senior author prefers local anesthesia with adequate preoperative sedation for nearly all temporal bone operations on adults. Many surgeons, however, will prefer general anesthesia for the majority of mastoid procedures and all neurotologic operations. Modern anesthetic agents and techniques allow local injection of adrenalin solution to reduce operative bleeding. While the noninfected mastoid can be opened under local anesthesia without pain, the sound and vibrations of the dental-type drill can be disagreeable to the wide-awake patient.

Local anesthesia for adults has these advantages:

1. On the average there is nearly always less bleeding with local anesthesia than with any type of general anesthesia. Lessened bleeding is particularly important for tympanoplasty and stapes operations.

2. The over-all safety of the patient is appreciably greater with local than with general anesthesia.

3. The slight but definite risk of injury to larynx and trachea by the intratracheal tube is eliminated by local anesthesia.

4. Postoperative nausea and vomiting are less and ambulation is earlier after local anesthesia.

5. Under local anesthesia the hearing can be tested if desired.

6. Reduced cost to the patient.

For children and adults who are extremely apprehensive, or react poorly to or become unruly from the preoperative sedation, general anesthesia is indicated in the form of intravenous Pentothal for adults and inhalation of a nonexplosive gas for children.

### Preoperative Sedation

In all cases local anesthesia should be accompanied by adequate sedation. Sedation should be sufficient to allay all apprehension so that the patient is completely relaxed and at ease, but it should not depress the respirations or blood pressure to a marked degree. Since the individual tolerance to sedatives, hypnotics and analgesics varies greatly, the only completely safe method of administering these drugs is fractionally, with enough time pause between doses to observe the full effect. A practical and safe routine that has been worked out by the senior author is as follows:

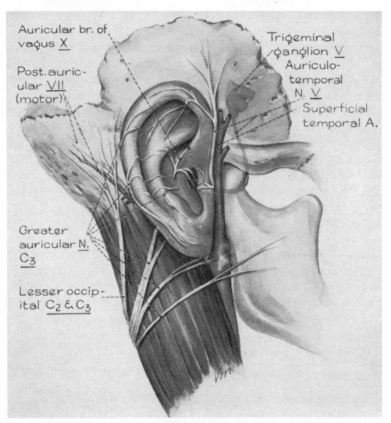

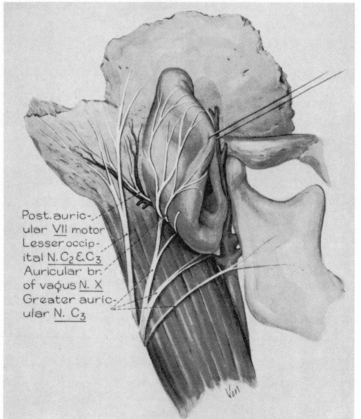

**Figure 6–6** Nerve supply of external ear.

An hour and half before the patient is taken to surgery he receives Valium 10 mg. by mouth.

One-half hour before he is taken to surgery he receives Talwin 30 mg., Phenergan 50 mg., and atropine 0.4 mg. by intramuscular injection.

If the patient is wide awake and apprehensive when placed on the operating table, additional sedation should be given at once, before he becomes agitated and begins to secrete his own alarm-reaction epinephrine. This additional medication may be an additional intramuscular injection of Talwin 15 mg. Should the patient become unruly toward the end of the operation the senior author prefers to give intramuscular Valium 5 mg. Morphine or Demerol should never be given late in the operation, since their maximal depressive effect on respiration will then occur after the patient has returned to bed. After the abrupt withdrawal of stimulation the patient may lapse into a deeply depressed coma with the possibility of a fatal respiratory failure if he is not under continuous observation.

When using local anesthesia many surgeons prefer to have an anesthesiologist or at least a nurse observer with the patient throughout the operation. Blood pressure, pulse, and respiration are monitored, and the patient's safety is ensured. Popular methods of sedation today include intravenous injections of Valium or Innovar by the anesthesiologist during the actual operative procedure.

## Local Infiltration for the Postauricular and Usual Endaural Incisions

In the absence of inflammation the mastoid bone is devoid of sensation except for its outer periosteum, and to a lesser degree its inner mucoperiosteum in the tympanum, epitympanum and antrum. Very satisfactory complete local anesthesia may be secured using 1 per cent Xylocaine containing 4 drops of 1:1000 Adrenalin to each 10 cc. for infiltration of the skin and periosteum so as to block the sensory nerve supply (Fig. 6–6) as follows:

1.   The tympanic branches of the auriculotemporal nerve (V) to the anterior meatal wall and tympanic membrane are blocked by injection of 1 or 2 cc. of solution into the anterior meatal wall at the junction of the cartilaginous and osseous meatus (Fig. 6–7A). The auricular branches of this nerve to the upper part of the auricle and skin above the meatus are blocked by injection of 1 cc. of solution at several points into the skin and periosteum of the incisura terminals, upward to the upper attachment of the auricle.

2.   The branches of the great auricular nerve ($C_3$) to the auricle and meatus are blocked by injection of 1 cc. of solution at several points behind the auricle over the mastoid process (Fig. 6–7B).

3.   The auricular branch of the vagus (X) is blocked by injection of the periosteum of the anterior surface of the mastoid process and of the skin of the floor of the meatus (Fig. 6–7A).

4.   Should the patient experience discomfort when the antrum, epitympanum or tympanum is entered, very good topical anesthesia of normal mucoperiosteum is obtained by instilling 2 per cent Xylocaine and then quickly withdrawing it by suction to prevent round window absorption.

Occasionally, for unexplained reasons, a vial of Xylocaine fails to induce adequate local anesthesia. Opening and injecting a fresh supply of this agent is nearly always effective.

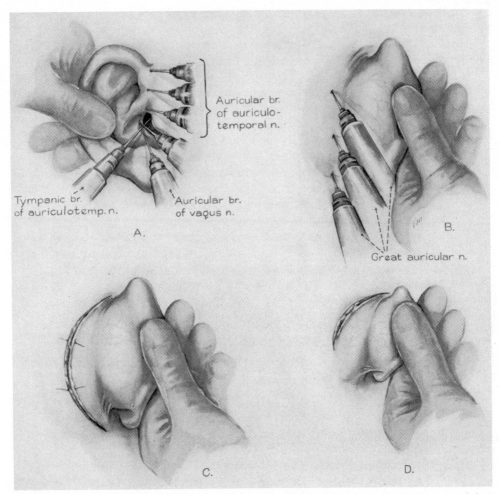

**Figure 6–7**  *A* and *B*, Points of injection for local anesthesia. *C*, Postauricular incision in adult. *D*, Infant's mastoid and line for incision.

## Local Anesthesia for Stapes Operations

In stapes operations, the patient should receive Valium 10 mg. by mouth two hours before surgery. One hour before surgery, Demerol 100 mg. or Talwin 30 mg., Phenergan 50 mg., and atropine 0.4 mg. intramuscularly.

For the incision within the meatus, about 1 cc. of a solution of 2 per cent Xylocaine, 6 parts, to Adrenalin 1:1000, 1 part, is infiltrated as follows:

1.   About 0.4 cc. is injected slowly, so as not to cause a bleb, into the posterior meatal wall just lateral to where the skin becomes closely adherent to the periosteum (see Fig. 18–3).

2.   About 0.2 cc. is injected into the anterior meatal wall at about the same depth.

3.   About 0.2 cc. is injected into the superior meatal wall and the same amount into the inferior meatal wall at about the same depth.

4.   If there is pain from the tympanic mucoperiosteum, the Xylocaine and Adrenalin solution may be instilled into the tympanic cavity or applied to the tympanic mucosa on small pieces of Gelfoam.

## INCISIONS TO EXPOSE THE TEMPORAL BONE

The four types of incisions commonly used to gain access to the temporal bone are: the postauricular, the usual endaural incision that extends upward from the meatus, the endomeatal incision within the meatus and the middle fossa incision that extends superiorly one finger breadth anterior to the tragus from the level of the zygomatic arch.

The postauricular or Wilde incision is generally employed to expose the mastoid process for a simple mastoidectomy in a well pneumatized mastoid process, for operations on the endolymphatic sac and internal auditory meatus and sometimes for tympanoplasty and radical mastoid operations (Chapter 17).

The endaural approach to the temporal bone, popularized by Lempert, was first employed by Kessel, who in 1885[1] described an endaural incision with removal of the lateral attic wall so as to enter the antrum by probe and curet.

In 1907 the elder Thies[2] perfected the endaural radical mastoid operation, which he subsequently employed in 1500 cases without a fatality.

In 1929 Lempert[3] advocated the extracartilaginous endaural incision for the simple mastoidectomy and radical mastoid operations, and in 1930 H. Heermann[4] began to describe endaural radical operations. In 1937 Lempert utilized the endaural approach for his petrosectomy operation, and in 1938[5] he applied it to the one-stage fenestration operation for otosclerosis. Largely through the teaching and example of Lempert the endaural approach was adopted until recent years for the majority of temporal bone operations.

The endaural incision has these advantages over the postaural incision:

1.  More direct access to the external osseous meatus, tympanic membrane, tympanic cavity, epitympanum, hypotympanum, labyrinth and facial nerve.

2.  Generally less trauma to soft tissue, with less bleeding into the operative field during surgery and less soft tissue reaction and discomfort after surgery.

3.  More accessibility and therefore simplified after-care in radical mastoid, modified radical mastoid and tympanoplasty operations, since the cavities are constructed through the same angle of approach from the meatus that will be used for future inspection and care.

Its disadvantages are poorer exposure of posterior and inferior mastoid cells in extensively pneumatized and infected temporal bones and poorer exposure of the anterior edge of the tympanic membrane and eustachian tube orifice. This last can be overcome by taking down the anterior osseous meatal wall as described by Wright.[6]

The middle fossa incision was first described by Frazier for tic douloureux operations on the fifth nerve. It represents the standard neurosurgical incision for access to the middle cranial vault.

### Technique of the Postauricular Incision

The postauricular incision for exposure of the mastoid process follows the curve of the postaural fold beginning at the upper attachment of the auricle, and continuing either in or ½ cm. behind the postaural fold downward to the tip of the mastoid process. Since the incision usually cuts across the posterior auricular artery or its larger branches, digital pressure by the finger tips of the surgeon's left hand on one side of the incision and the finger tips of an assistant on the other side will help to control excessive bleeding. The incision may first be lightly scratched with two light cross scratches to aid in accurate approximation when the wound is sutured

(Fig. 6–7C). The blade of the scalpel is held perpendicular to the surface so as not to bevel the incision while skin, subcutaneous tissue and periosteum are incised.

Should a dehiscence of the cortex from a previous mastoidectomy or from disease be suspected, the incision should not be made in one stroke, but should be deepened very slowly and cautiously to avoid possible injury to sigmoid sinus or dura.

Remember that the newborn infant does not have a mastoid process and that the usual postauricular incision will sever his facial nerve. In the infant and child under 2 years of age the incision should be almost horizontal just above the auricle, for the antrum in the infant lies almost directly above and only slightly behind the meatus, and there is as yet no mastoid process (Fig. 6–7D).

After any very large bleeders have been controlled with hemostat and electro-cautery, a broad periosteal elevator is used to expose the lateral surface of the mastoid process as far forward as the beginning of the posterior root of the zygoma and the suprameatal spine. However, care is taken not to strip the skin and periosteum from the superior and posterior osseous meatal wall as this may induce postoperative stenosis. A self-retaining mastoid retractor is inserted under the periosteum and is spread carefully to avoid stripping the skin from the meatus. The attachment of the sternocleidomastoid muscle to the outer surface of the mastoid tip is cut across cleanly with a scalpel and these muscle fibers with any remaining shreds of periosteum are scraped from the lateral surface of the mastoid process. Any remaining soft tissue bleeding points are controlled before the bone work is begun.

For surgical procedures requiring exposure of the skull base, the postauricular incision is carried into the neck along the anterior border of the sternocleidomastoid muscle (see Chap. 22). The incision line is kept within a natural crease to camouflage the postoperative scar. It is usually necessary to extend an anterior limb that has its superior extension at the lower level of the tragus. This produces a Y-shaped wound with an incision line in front of and behind the auricle and allows the surgeon to identify the facial nerve as it exits the stylomastoid foramen. The neck may be thus opened to expose the great vessels and nerves as well as the base of the temporal bone.

### Technique of the Usual Endaural Incision

The endaural incision employed by the senior author for many temporal bone operations is a slight modification of Lempert's extracartilaginous endaural incision.[7] The incision is made in two steps, with either the Lempert triangular knife or a Bard-Parker scalpel with No. 15 blade, as follows:

1. Beginning at "12 o'clock" on the superior meatal wall were the patient upright, and about ⅜ inch (1 cm.) in from the outer edge of the meatus, the first incision extends at about the same depth down the posterior meatal wall in the incisura terminalis nearly but not quite to "6 o'clock," then at right angles outward about ⅛ inch (2 or 3 mm.) to the edge of, **but not into,** the conchal cartilage (Fig. 6–8).

2. Beginning again at "12 o'clock" on the superior meatal wall where the first incision began, the second incision extends directly upward, still in the incisura terminalis, to a point about halfway between the meatus and upper edge of the auricle. For greater exposure this vertical incision can be extended as far upward as desired without encountering any important structure except for the temporal muscle and branches of the superficial temporal artery and vein.

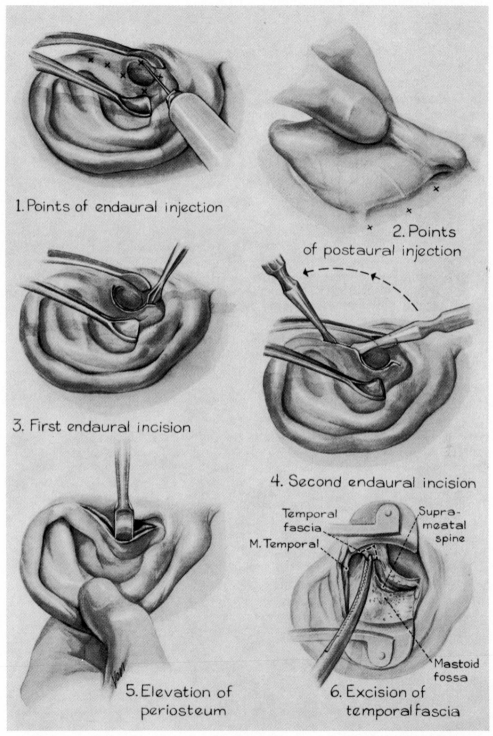

1. Points of endaural injection

2. Points of postaural injection

3. First endaural incision

4. Second endaural incision

5. Elevation of periosteum

6. Excision of temporal fascia

Temporal fascia

M. Temporal

Supra-meatal spine

Mastoid fossa

**Figure 6–8** Endaural incisions extending beyond meatus, and removal of temporal fascia.

The two incisions, now continuous and at first through the skin only, are deepened to include periosteum, with the knife held at an angle so that it will not plunge into the osseous meatus. A broad periosteal elevator is inserted into the incision, directed posteriorly, and the periosteum over the entire mastoid process is elevated posteriorly, and anteriorly only over the posterior root of the zygoma. Failure to elevate the periosteum sufficiently widely is a common cause of failure to obtain adequate exposure by this approach (Fig. 6–8).

Any free bleeding is controlled with hemostat and electrocautery, and the self-retaining endaural retractor is inserted beneath the periosteum. A small triangle of temporal fascia over the root of the zygoma is excised to complete the endaural exposure (Fig. 6–8).

### Technique of the Endomeatal Incision within the Meatus

Originally designed by Lempert for his tympanosympathectomy operation, the endomeatal incision within the meatus was adopted by Rosen for stapes operations and is now used almost exclusively for these procedures.

The incision for stapes operations as employed by the authors is as follows:

The incision begins at "6 o'clock" on the inferior meatal wall (were the ear viewed with the patient standing) close to the annulus tympanicus; it slopes outward and upward to a point 6 or 8 mm. from the annulus at "9 o'clock" for the right ear, and then extends forward to about 2 mm. above the short process of the malleus (Fig. 6–9). The incision is made first by intermittent pressure with the special angled knife (Fig. 6–10), and then by a sweep of the knife along the incision to cut any remaining fibers of periosteum. The upper extremity of the incision is through the thicker skin and vascular strip of the superior meatal wall and is best made by the alligator-type scissors (Fig. 6–10).

With the same knife, the periosteum and skin of the meatus are elevated inward to the annulus and sulcus tympanicus. Before the tympanic cavity is opened, all bleeding is controlled by the application of suction to small cotton balls moistened in the Xylocaine and Adrenalin solution that was used for infiltration. Any persistent troublesome bleeding point in the incision or bone is controlled by light electrocautery.

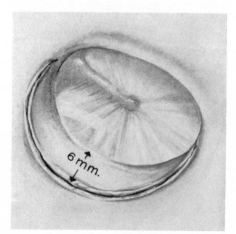

**Figure 6–9**   Line of endomeatal incision within the meatus.

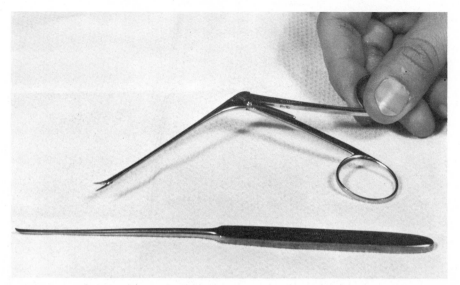

**Figure 6–10** Angled knife and alligator-type scissors for endomeatal incision within the meatus.

The same angled knife (Figs. 18–3E and 18–4, in the chapter on stapes surgery) is then used to elevate the annulus tympanicus from the sulcus tympanicus by pushing the instrument over the edge of the sulcus at separate points. The freed posterior half of the tympanic membrane is folded across the manubrium onto the anterior half, exposing the posterior portion of the tympanic cavity.

### Technique for the Middle Fossa Incision

A Bard-Parker No. 15 blade is used to make the incision, which is placed one finger breadth anterior to the tragus. It is important to start the incision at the level of the zygomatic arch and not below, as the frontalis branch of the facial nerve could be severed. The skin and subcutaneous tissue are incised in a superior direction for approximately 6 to 7 cm. (Fig. 6–11). Bleeding is controlled with the Bovie cautery. A forceps is used to lift the skin edges, and a knife is placed into the avascular plane over the temporalis fascia. The wound is thus undermined anteriorly and posteriorly for about 3 cm. Next, using the cutting cautery, the temporalis fascia and muscle are incised from the root of the zygoma superiorly to correspond with the skin incision. A self-retaining retractor is put into position to hold the muscle apart once the bleeding has been brought under control (Fig. 6–11). A "T" incision is made at the zygoma to "free up" the muscle in order that the root of the zygoma can be exposed. Once this has been accomplished, the squamous portion of the temporal bone has been exposed, and the craniectomy can be performed as described in Chapter 23.

### TECHNIQUES FOR SURGERY ON BONE IN EAR OPERATIONS

The physical properties and the biologic response of bone require special instruments and techniques for dealing with this tissue surgically. Compared to the

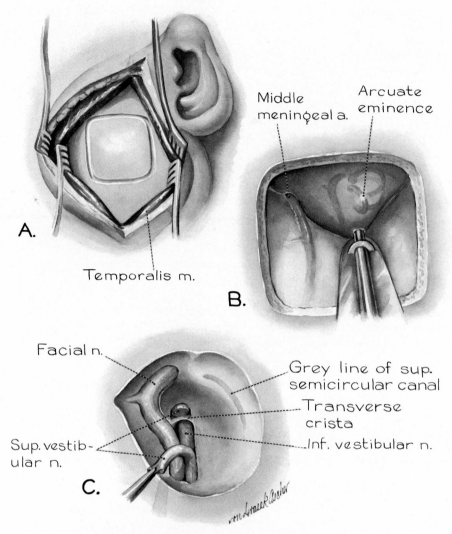

**Figure 6–11**    Middle fossa exposure for vestibular nerve section.

ear, bone surgery elsewhere is gargantuan in size and comparatively free from risk of injury to important contained or adjacent structures. The extremely minute and delicate bony structures that must be dealt with in the ear, always skirting close to the vital structures that crowd this area, have necessitated the development of highly specialized techniques for work on this bone, techniques that differ from those suitable for bone work elsewhere. The addition of magnification for most of the operations done today on the ear has further specialized the techniques in otologic surgery. Many of the technical details will be considered with the individual surgical procedures. It will suffice at this point to consider only general principles for working on bone in the ear.

### Instruments for Bone Removal

Previous generations of otologic surgeons brought the use of the mallet and gouge to a high state of artistic perfection for removal of cortical and cellular bone, and for the more delicate steps of taking down the bridge and facial ridge in the radical mastoid operation. The adoption of the loupe and operating microscope was accompanied by the use of the electrically driven dental-type burr, and as otologic surgeons have become accustomed to the rotating burr they have gradually substituted it for the mallet and gouge. Today the burr is used almost exclusively for the removal of cortical and hard cellular bone; the curet is used for soft cellular bone and the rongeur and curet for thin bony plates.

It might be well at this point to mention some of the wide variety of drills available to the otologic surgeon. These can be divided into two groups: pneumatic (commonly referred to as "air drills") and electric drills. There are two categories of the latter: those in which the motor is contained in the handpiece and those in which the motor is separate from the handpiece.

There are a wide variety of pneumatic drills on the market. They are all similar in their characteristics. By and large, they are powerful (high torque) and fast (over 20,000 rpm). There are three electric drills that contain the motor in the handpiece — the Kerr and original Shea Stapes Drill as well as the Shea Mastoid Drill. The time-tested Jordan-Day apparatus has its power supply separate from the handpiece and works off of a belt drive similar to a dental drill.

For large areas of bone removal, the authors currently favor the Glasscock air drill or the Shea drill with irrigation attachment. For small bone removals through the ear speculum, we favor the Kerr drill, or a similar instrument (Fig. 6–12).

A few simple rules will help the student and beginning surgeon to learn the proper use of the common bone-removing instruments.

### Technique of Using the Burr

1. Hold the handpiece of the drill like a pen and use the side of the burr as the cutting edge rather than its end.

2. Use a large burr whenever possible, to lessen risk of injury to dura, sigmoid sinus or facial nerve.

3. Avoid "running" of the burr across the bone by the use of an intermittent light pressure rather than a continuous pressure.

4. Avoid overheating and local devitalizing of bone by using continuous irrigation and an intermittent rather than continuous pressure in one spot. Overheating near the facial canal may induce facial paralysis.

5. Keep the burr teeth clean of bone dust. The coarse-toothed burr (Fig. 6–13) clogs less easily than the usual bone-cutting burr, but is more difficult to control and "runs" across the bone more easily. A field continuously flooded with sterile Tis-U-Sol or Ringer's solution leads to less clogging of the burr than a slightly moist or dry field. Because so-called normal physiologic saline damages living cells, it should not be used for irrigation.[8]

6. Never use the burr blindly to make a hole or to work in a hole, but always keep the field beveled and as wide open as possible. The curet is safer for work in a hole if it is necessary to follow a small cell tract.

7. Do not use a burr to enter the antrum blindly from the posterior superior osseous meatal wall. Although this is usually safe and always dramatic, even the most experienced surgeon may inadvertently wound the sigmoid sinus or facial nerve by this method.

8. Remember the potent osteogenic property of bone dust and avoid creating bone dust unless it is removed simultaneously by irrigation in areas where osteogenesis is to be avoided, such as in stapedectomy, tympanoplasty and endolymphatic sac or fenestration operations.

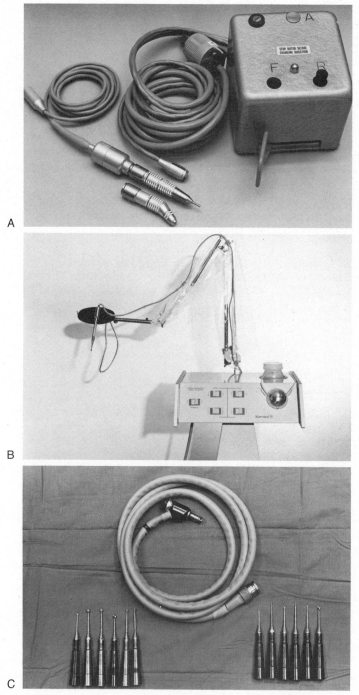

**Figure 6–12**   *A*, Kerr electric drill. *B*, John Shea electric drill with continuous irrigation. *C*, Glasscock air drill. (Kerr Drill from V. Meuller & Co., Chicago, Illinois; Shea Drill from Xomed Inc., Jacksonville, Florida; and Glasscock Drill from Edward Weck, Long Island, New York.)

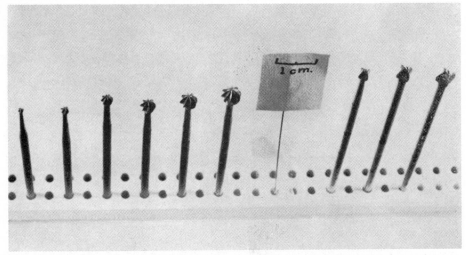

**Figure 6–13** Surgical bone cutting burrs (left). Coarse-toothed cutting burrs (right).

9. Diamond burrs, introduced to ear surgery in 1942 by the senior author, have several advantages over their cutting counterparts. The diamond burr cuts much more slowly; it does not tear into, but pushes soft tissues away; is less likely to run or jump and can be rotated forward or backward as needed. It can be used to obtain a blue line on one of the semicircular canals or to safely expose dura, the sigmoid sinus or jugular bulb. Furthermore, this burr helps to control bleeding from bone by pushing the vessel down into its channel and filling the channel with bone dust.

## Technique of Using the Curet

1. Hold the curet so that the cutting edge is always in full view and not obscured by the hand (Fig. 6–14).
2. Use the side of the curet rather than its tip as the cutting edge.
3. Employ the curet in sweeping strokes parallel with and not perpendicular against any important structure such as dura, sinus wall or facial nerve.
4. Always use sharp curets. They cut with less pressure and are much safer, as well as more effective, than dull curets.
5. Always use a large curet whenever possible, to lessen risk of injury to dura, sinus wall or facial nerve.

## Technique of Using the Rongeur

1. The heavy rongeur or Kerrison type of rongeur may be used to remove cortical overhang. For removing dural or sinus plate or taking down the osseous meatal wall and bridge use a narrow Juers-Lempert rongeur.
2. Be sure to separate the periosteum of the meatus, dura or sigmoid sinus from the bone before grasping the latter in the rongeur.
3. Take small bites with the rongeur, especially when taking down the bridge,

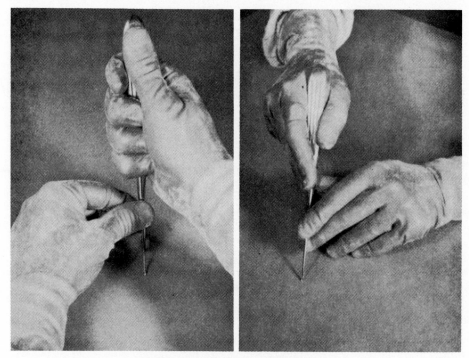

**Figure 6–14**   Methods of holding curet.

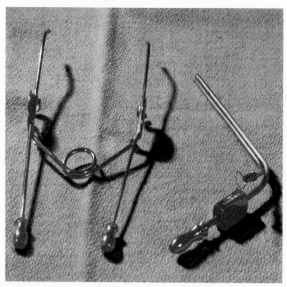

**Figure 6–15** Shambaugh continuous irrigator-suction attachment for self-retaining retractor (left). House suction irrigator (right).

as a large bite may fracture a larger piece of bone than anticipated, tearing the chorda tympani or even the facial nerve.

4. Take clean bites with a minimum of twist. If the bite does not come off easily, disengage and take a smaller bite, but do not hang on "like a bulldog," twisting and straining until the bone fractures.

## Control of Bone Bleeding

One of the secrets of competent temporal bone surgery is the ability of the surgeon to control operative hemorrhage. There are several methods available, and the one chosen will most often depend upon the situation at hand.

The diamond burr is particularly helpful in controlling bleeding from bone, as mentioned previously.

For dural bleeders, the bipopular cautery is of particular value, as the current goes only between the tips of the bayonet forceps and not through the body to an indifferent electrode. This characteristic makes this instrument invaluable in the control of bleeding from the sheath of the facial nerve. The regular Bovie cautery should never be used on this nerve but may be employed for dural bleeders if the current is turned down to a minimum. Failing to follow this "rule" may result in a postoperative leak of cerebrospinal fluid.

Copious amounts of irrigation will wash away blood and tend to lessen hemorrhage from the bone as well as from the cut edges of canal incisions (Fig. 6–15). This practice has the added advantage of washing out bone dust and bacteria in chronically infected ears. The colony counts are lessened considerably by this practice.

Bone wax is a foreign body and must be employed with care; however, it is a valuable adjunct when used properly in a clean field. It is of particular value in controlling bleeding from bone marrow that one often encounters in the mastoid tip and retrofacial cell tract.

Absorbable gelatin (Gelfoam) and absorbable gauze (Surgicel) can both be used to advantage in the mastoid. It is possible to obtain pressure with Surgicel and this material is helpful when there is an area it can be packed into, such as the hypotympanum. Surgicel must **not** be placed against facial nerve or brain stem as it causes local coagulation of tissue. Gelfoam has "clinging" properties that make it very useful in patching tears in the sigmoid sinus.

Avitene is a synthetic collagen sponge that can be left in the wound, and when moistened with topical thrombin will stop venous bleeding. Ordinary gauze, cotton or cottonoids must **never** be left in place, as they act as foreign bodies.

A useful technique for soft tissue and bone bleeding is to place a cotton ball soaked in topical thrombin against a pledget of compressed Gelfoam, which is thus carried to the bleeding point and held there for one to several minutes by alligator forceps and suction tip. The cotton ball is then removed, leaving the Gelfoam in place over the now dry bleeding point.

## MAGNIFICATION IN EAR SURGERY

Holmgren was the first to introduce the loupe and the binocular operating microscope for operations on the labyrinth in otosclerosis. Sourdille and Lempert employed the loupe but not the microscope for the fenestration operation. The

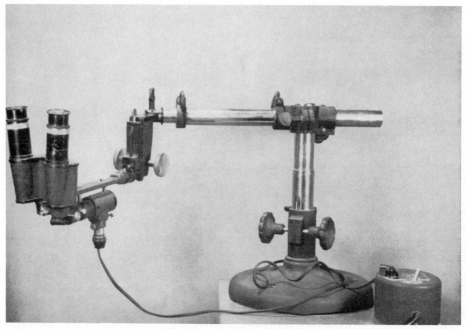

**Figure 6–16**   Shambaugh operating microscope introduced in 1940 for fenestration surgery. This, like the original operating microscopes of Holmgren, Cawthorne and Simpson-Hall, was a converted dissecting microscope with added light source and was mounted on a movable table.

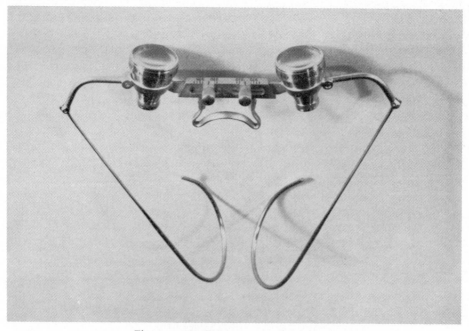

**Figure  6–17**   Zeiss 2× magnifying loupe.

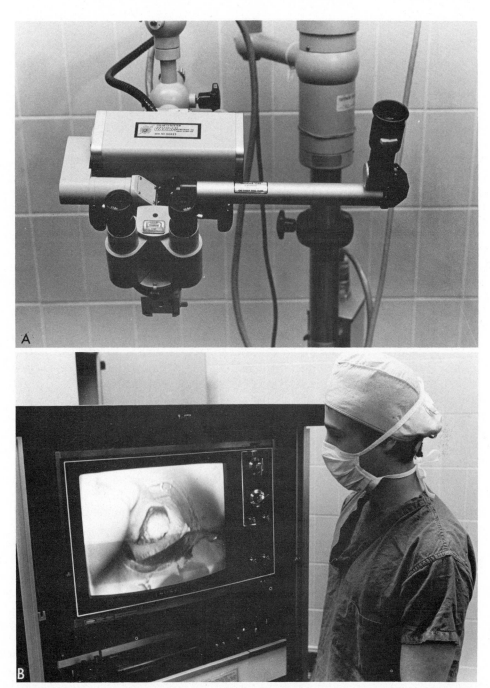

**Figure 6–18**  *A*, Small color television camera attached to the microscope with viewing tube. *B*, Operative procedure can be visualized outside of the operating room by more than one observer at a time.

author in 1940 and Simpson-Hall at about the same time applied the operating microscope to the one-stage fenestration operation (Fig. 6–16). Cawthorne had already used the microscope for operations on the facial nerve. The advantages of 6, 10, 16 or 25 × magnification rather than the 2 to 4 × afforded by the loupe have caused otologic surgeons to adopt the operating microscope for fenestration, stapes operations, tympanoplasties and myringoplasties, facial nerve surgery, labyrinth and endolymphatic sac operations, for middle fossa and skull base operations, and for translabyrinthine removal of acoustic neurinomas. The Zeiss oto-microscope for ear surgery combines the advantages of adequate working distance, excellent illumination that enters the field through the objective, and therefore at the same angle as the vision of the surgeon, and selective magnification of 6, 10, 16, 25 and 40 ×.

The Zeiss operating microscope has virtually replaced the headlight and loupe for most modern temporal bone surgery. Some still prefer to start the procedure with the loupe (Fig. 6–17) and then switch to the microscope for the middle ear work. However, many otologic surgeons prefer to use the microscope from the very beginning of the procedure.

The microscope is rendered sterile by means of a disposable plastic drape that covers the entire instrument as well as any attachments, such as the color TV system, 35mm or 16mm cameras and viewing tubes (Fig. 6–18).

## POSTOPERATIVE CARE

The immediate postoperative care after general anesthesia or local anesthesia with heavy sedation is directed toward any respiratory depression. Until the patient is awake and responding he should be under continuous observation, by a nurse if possible or by a relative if a nurse is not available.

Dehydration from persistent vomiting is seen occasionally after operations that open the labyrinth and requires 1000 cc. of 5 per cent glucose intravenously.

Postoperative femoral thrombophlebitis, though not at all as common as after abdominal operations, nevertheless constitutes a potentially dangerous complication of ear surgery. If the patient cannot be out of bed within 24 hours, a routine of massage and elevation of his legs at half-hour intervals until he is ambulatory is a very simple and effective prophylactic measure that prevents stagnation of blood in the pelvic and femoral veins.[9]

Postoperative facial palsy that is noted immediately after surgery and that does not disappear in an hour or two must be assumed to be due to surgical trauma with the possibility of a depressed fracture or severance of the nerve. Immediate (within 24 hours) exploration and decompression or repair of the facial nerve is indicated.

Facial palsy that begins after an interval of several days may be assumed to be due to edema of the nerve in the fallopian canal with the probability of spontaneous recovery without further surgery. Since the time of onset of facial paralysis is a determining factor in whether or not to explore, the facial nerve function must be determined after every temporal bone operation as soon as the patient can respond.

Intact canal wall types of procedures, such as the routine stapedectomy, myringoplasty, tympanoplasty with and without mastoidectomy and endolymphatic sac procedures, only require a mastoid-type dressing for approximately 24 hours (Fig. 6–19). After that either a sterile cotton plug or a postauricular "Band-Aid"–type

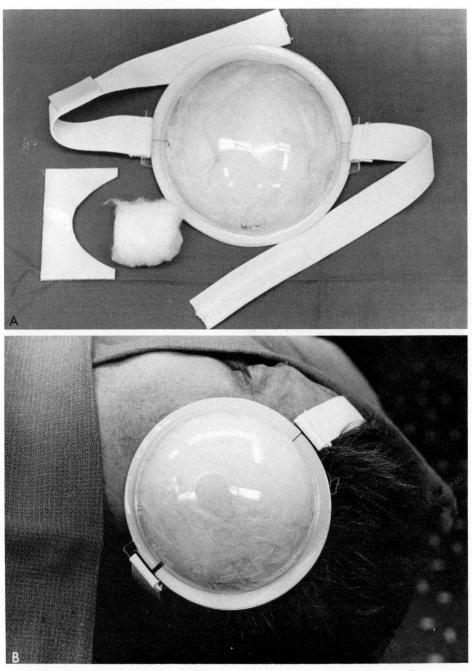

**Figure 6–19** *A*, prepackaged disposable mastoid dressing designed by junior author. *B*, mastoid dressing in place following tympanoplasty.

of dressing, or both, are all that is required. Tumor surgery and modified and radical mastoidectomy procedures should require the following postoperative regimen.

All postoperative dressings for the first month must be carried out with complete aseptic precautions. Many a skillfully performed ear operation with correct operating room aseptic technique has been followed by contamination by carelessly performed postoperative dressings. A great convenience and necessity for proper sterile dressing technique in the office or clinic is to have autoclaved sterile dressing packs containing a towel, cotton, ear speculum and applicators.

The outer dressing for most ear operations is not changed until the seventh day, when the packing may be removed, along with any sutures. This dressing should be done using sterile instruments, towels and cotton exactly as for a minor operation.

Postoperative dressing changes will be at various intervals, depending upon the procedure, but each, until the incision is healed, should proceed as follows:

1. The surgeon scrubs his hands and arms with brush and soap containing pHisoderm.

2. He dries his hands on the sterile towel from the autoclaved pack, and may adjust his headmirror or headlight with the same towel.

3. The outer edge of the meatus is cleaned with 70 per cent alcohol using a sterile applicator and cotton from the autoclaved pack.

4. The sterile speculum is introduced and the cavity inspected. If there is no infection, nothing is introduced beyond the speculum and the less done to the cavity the better.

5. If there is beginning infection, there will be an increase in the drainage, which begins to appear cloudy (instead of clear and serous) before it becomes frankly purulent. In this event the cavity must be cleaned thoroughly **each day** using sterile cotton applicators so that purulent material will not have a chance to dissolve the fibrin barrier by the action of proteolytic enzymes liberated by degenerating polymorphonuclear leucocytes. In addition the patient should use Gantrisin or Chloromycetin otic solution twice daily in his ear, and should receive parenterally an appropriate antibiotic determined by the culture and sensitivity tests. With such prompt and intensive treatment the infection should subside quickly before it can penetrate deeply into pneumatic cells to become chronic.

6. In the absence of infection, medicaments in the cavity are not needed and probably retard epidermization. An exception is the case in which the vertical portion of the endaural incision tends to close too rapidly. Aqueous gentian violet, 2 per cent, applied to the incision every 4 to 7 days retards adhesion of the cut surfaces and promotes epidermization of any unhealed areas.

Further details of postoperative care will be considered with the individual surgical procedures that follow in subsequent chapters.

## REFERENCES

1. Cited by Babbit, J. A.: The endaural surgery of chronic suppurations. *In* Kopetsky, S. J.: Loose-leaf Surgery of the Ear. Thomas Nelson & Sons, New York, 1947.
2. Thies, F., Jr.: Die Radikaloperation durch den äusseren Gehörgang. Ztschr. Hals-Nasen- u. Ohrenh., 33:459, 1933.
3. Lempert, J.: Mastoîdectomie sous-corticale. Ann. mal. oreil. larynx, 48:111, 1929.
4. Heermann, H.: Zur Frage der Plastik bei Gehörgangradikaloperationen. Ztsch. Laryng. Rhin. Otol., 39:304, 1930.
5. Lempert, J.: Improvement of hearing in cases of otosclerosis: new one stage surgical technic. Arch. Otol., 28:42, 1938.

6. Wright, W. K.: Repair of chronic central perforations of the tympanic membrane by repeated acid cautery; by skin grafting. Laryngoscope, 66:1464. 1956.
7. Whitaker, C. F., Juers, A. L., and Shambaugh, G. E., Jr.: A modified endaural incision with nerve block anesthesia for fenestration and mastoidectomy. Arch. Otolaryng., 45:662, 1947.
8. Kerth, J. D., and Shambaugh, G. E., Jr.: Irrigation of open vestibule in stapes surgery. Arch. Otol., 80:392, 1964.
9. Ochsner, A.: Prevention and treatment of postoperative thrombophlebitis. S. Clin. North Am., 33:993, 1953.

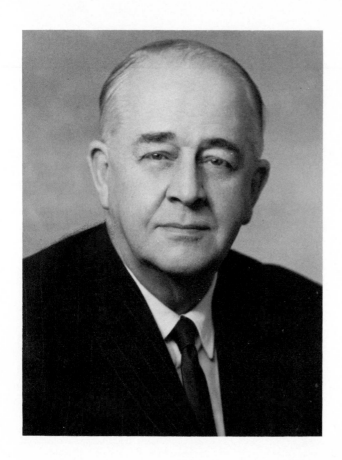

*Sir Terence Cawthorne*

BORN 1902
DIED 1970

Eminent London aural surgeon who helped to bridge the transition from surgery for the evacuation of pus to surgery in a clean field under the operating microscope.

# Part Two

> "It is essential to regard chemo- and biotherapy on the
> one hand and surgery on the other not in any way as
> rivals but as being complementary to one another."
>
> CAWTHORNE

# Surgery of
# Infections of the
# Ear

# Chapter 7

# Pathology and Clinical Course of Inflammatory Diseases of the Middle Ear

STRUCTURE AND DEFENSE MECHANISMS OF THE
  MUCOPERIOSTEUM OF THE MIDDLE EAR
CLASSIFICATION OF INFLAMMATORY MIDDLE EAR
  DISEASES
VIRAL OTITIS MEDIA
ACUTE SUPPURATIVE OTITIS MEDIA
ACUTE NECROTIC OTITIS MEDIA
ALLERGIC OTITIS MEDIA
TUBERCULAR OTITIS MEDIA
CHRONIC SUPPURATIVE OTITIS MEDIA
    BENIGN CHRONIC SUPPURATIVE OTITIS MEDIA
    SECONDARY ACQUIRED CHOLESTEATOMA
    ATTIC (EPITYMPANIC) RETRACTION
      CHOLESTEATOMA
    CONGENITAL CHOLESTEATOMA
    CHRONIC SUPPURATIVE OTITIS MEDIA DUE TO
      CHRONIC OSTEITIS OR OSTEOMYELITIS
DIFFERENTIAL DIAGNOSIS OF OTITIS MEDIA

Because of the strategic location of the middle ear cleft and its adjoining pneumatic cells, which are separated by the merest shell of bone from large areas of dura mater of the middle and posterior cranial fossae, every inflammatory otitis media due to a pathogenic microorganism carries with it the potentiality of intracranial extension. Hippocrates[1] said: "Acute pain of the ear, with continued strong fever, is to be dreaded, for there is danger that the man may become delirious and die."

Fortunately today this need not happen, for with a clear understanding of the pathology of the various types of middle ear infection, a clear-cut and sharp distinction can be made between infections controllable by antibacterial medications and those for which, because of their particular pathologic features, surgery alone can be effective. The ability to make this distinction is possessed by the ear surgeon, but the general practitioner and pediatrician who first see the patient and, armed with potent antibacterial weapons, undertake to treat otitis media must recognize that there is this distinction. Hazy or mistaken views of the pathologic process have led in the past to unnecessary and sometimes even harmful surgery, but may lead today to an equally disastrous failure to recognize a bone-invading process that surgery alone can arrest.

## STRUCTURE AND DEFENSE MECHANISMS OF THE MUCOPERIOSTEUM OF THE MIDDLE EAR

The structure and properties of the mucoperiosteal lining of the middle ear and its pneumatic cells determine the particular microorganisms that have a tendency to invade it, and its manner of response to infection.

The lining of the middle ear spaces is an extension and modification of the **respiratory mucous membrane** that lines the nasal cavity and its accessory sinuses, the nasopharynx and eustachian tube, part of the larynx, the trachea and the bronchi, down to the smallest terminal bronchiole. In all this area the mucous membrane consists of a layer of ciliated columnar epithelial cells with a subepithelial layer of connective tissue. A film of mucus clothes the membrane, replenished by goblet cells scattered among the ciliated epithelial cells and by mucous glands strategically located to combat the drying effect of inspired air, particularly in the anterior ends of the nasal turbinates, in the roof of the nasopharynx and mouth of the eustachian tube and in the larynx and trachea. The mucus film is kept in constant motion by the continuous action of the cilia, the direction of movement being always the same: from the nasal passages and tympanic cavity toward the nasopharynx and upward from the bronchi and trachea to the larynx.

Just as the lining epithelium of the terminal bronchioles becomes cuboidal and then loses its cilia and flattens to a pavement epithelium as it spreads out to line the alveoli of the lungs, so the ciliated columnar epithelium of the eustachian tube becomes cuboidal and loses its cilia as it reaches the floor of the tympanum, and then changes to a flat pavement epithelium in the epitympanum, antrum and pneumatic cells. As one progresses from the cartilaginous to the bony portion of the eustachian tube and from the tympanum to the antrum and air cells, the subepithelial connective tissue becomes progressively thinner until the pavement epithelium and periosteum together form a thin delicate membrane. Normally the non-inflamed mucoperiosteum of the pneumatic cells is so extremely thin as to be scarcely visible to the naked eye.

The mucosa of the respiratory tract, the gastrointestinal mucosa and the outer skin are the three usual routes by which pathogenic microorganisms attempt to gain entrance to the body. As should be expected, the tissues of these areas are endowed to a high degree with defense mechanisms against infection.

The defense mechanism of the respiratory mucous membrane begins with the constantly renewed mucus film that contains lysozyme, a potent bacteria-dissolving enzyme first described by Fleming, the discoverer of penicillin. In response to an invading organism that penetrates the mucus film the production of mucus is increased. Large numbers of phagocytic polymorphonuclear leucocytes with their potent proteolytic enzymes migrate from the dilated capillaries into the subepithelial connective tissue, and then through the epithelium to mingle with the mucus and form the **mucopus** so characteristic of respiratory infections. At the same time, specific antibodies against the invading microorganism begin to form rapidly, this being a highly developed property of respiratory mucous membrane, gastrointestinal mucosa and skin. However, these epithelial tissues do not always distinguish between a dangerous live parasite and a harmless inanimate protein. As a consequence, antibodies against pollen, dust, chemicals or foods, as well as against pathogenic bacteria, may be produced, making the respiratory mucosa, along with the skin and gastrointestinal mucosa, particularly subject to allergic non-bacterial disorders. Superficially at least, the allergic reaction may resemble and be confused with the inflammatory reaction to a bacterial invader.

The terminal mucosa of the respiratory tract in the middle ear spaces with which we are especially concerned resembles in a number of ways the terminal mucosa in the alveoli of the lungs. Both end in a flattened, non-ciliated, pavement epithelium with a remarkable ability to absorb inflammatory exudate and to absorb oxygen rapidly and nitrogen more slowly. The ciliated cuboidal epithelium of the tympanum and terminal bronchioles produces mucus, but this property is largely lost in the pavement epithelium of the pulmonary alveoli and the pneumatic cells of the temporal bone.

## CLASSIFICATION OF INFLAMMATORY MIDDLE EAR DISEASES

Six distinct clinical types of inflammatory reaction occur in the mucoperiosteum of the middle ear spaces:

1. Acute **viral otitis media.**

2. The usual acute bacterial infection producing the **usual acute suppurative otitis media.**

3. A special form of acute bacterial otitis media, occurring chiefly in small children with severe measles or scarlet fever, in which the tissues of the middle ear become necrotic and slough, producing an **acute necrotic otitis media.**

4. **Allergic otitis media,** with a sterile serous or mucoid **secretory otitis,** which may be combined with a bacterial otitis media.

5. **Tubercular chronic otitis media.**

6. **Chronic (non-tubercular) infections of the middle ear mucosa,** which behave quite differently from the usual acute otitis media.

The same group of microorganisms that have a predilection for respiratory mucosa elsewhere have a tendency to invade the mucoperiosteum of the middle ear. These are, in their order of importance in the middle ear: beta hemolytic streptococcus, pneumococcus, *Staphylococcus aureus*, and other respiratory organisms such as the non-hemolytic streptococcus and Pfeiffer's bacillus, viruses of the common cold and influenza, and the tubercle bacillus. The latter is comparatively rare in the United States today and produces an indolent type of chronic infection that will be considered under chronic suppurative otitis media.

## VIRAL OTITIS MEDIA

The effect of the common cold virus on the middle ear may be compared with its effect on the nasal mucosa. The most distinctive pathologic change is in the ciliated columnar cells, which degenerate in a characteristic and diagnostic manner and slough in large numbers, leaving a basal germinal layer of non-ciliated cuboidal cells. From these the ciliated columnar epithelium regenerates, and after 10 to 14 days, the nasal mucosa returns to normal.[2]

In the eustachian tube it is likely that a similar sloughing of the ciliated epithelium may be produced by the common cold virus. The temporary loss of ciliary activity and the hyperemic swelling and increased production of mucus combine to produce temporary closure of the tube with resulting oxygen absorption, negative intratympanic pressure and a tendency toward accumulation of transudate, so that a frequent otitic complication of the common cold is a non-inflammatory sterile secretory (serous) otitis media.

In many cases the common cold virus doubtless invades the mucosa of the tympanum. Its effect on the non-ciliated pavement epithelium of the antrum and air cells, as of the pulmonary alveoli, appears to be less drastic than on ciliated epithelium, so that clinical signs of an otitis media may be lacking. A subclinical involvement of the mucoperiosteum by the common cold virus is suggested by the observation—made by the senior author during fenestration operations on patients with an acute head cold—of hyperemia and excessive bleeding from the mucosa and bone of the epitympanum and antrum despite absence of symptoms or otoscopic signs of an otitis media. This subclinical mucoperiosteal hyperemia probably accounts for the temporary worsening of hearing during head colds so often mentioned by patients with stapedial otosclerosis (otospongiosis).

**Bullous myringitis** is a special form of viral otitis media that occors often in epidemics, involving especially young children in the family unit. If not complicated by a simultaneous invasion by hemolytic streptococci, pneumococci or *Hemophilus influenzae* (Pfeiffer's bacillus), the visible pathology may be confined to serous or hemorrhagic blebs on the tympanic membrane and adjacent meatal wall. Absence of fever and normal hearing indicate the absence of exudate within the middle ear. Simple bullous myringitis is painful but self-limiting, the blebs drying up and disappearing after a few days. Puncture of the blebs may be done to relieve pain, without perforating the entire thickness of the tympanic membrane. Sulfonamides or antibiotics are not effective against the common cold or influenza virus and are not indicated for bullous myringitis unless there is an accompanying bacterial otitis media with fever and hearing impairment.

The bacterial complications of the common cold and influenza are important and frequent. The virus, by destroying the ciliated epithelium, removes the first line of defense and permits bacterial invasion of the tissues, most often by the beta hemolytic streptococcus or pneumococcus in adults and by *Hemophilus influenzae* (Pfeiffer's bacillus) in young children. It seems likely that the bacterial invasion is not always previously present in the pharynx to which the host has become immune, but rather that in certain epidemics the virus and the hemolytic streptococcus, pneumococcus or *Hemophilus influenzae* are acquired simultaneously or successively by air-borne contagion.[3] The acute bacterial otitis media that may complicate a viral head cold or influenza can be differentiated from an uncomplicated viral otitis by the fever, hearing impairment and positive culture that occur with the bacterial infection.

## ACUTE SUPPURATIVE OTITIS MEDIA

The usual acute otitis media with fever encountered in clinical practice is of bacterial origin. The term "acute suppurative otitis media," also called acute purulent otitis media, will be used for all acute pyogenic bacterial infections of the middle ear even when they are mild and subside before they have progressed to the stage of suppuration. This will distinguish them from sterile allergic and secretory otitis media, and from viral and tubercular infections. Acute suppurative otitis media must also be distinguished from acute necrotic otitis media.

### Frequency

Acute suppurative otitis media is an extremely common condition, occurring at all ages but especially in the young. Routine examination of the middle ear cleft in autopsies on infants and children under the age of 3 revealed an otitis media in 4 out of 5, although not all showed clinical evidence of the infection.[4] The great frequency of clinical or subclinical otitis media in sick infants may be accounted for in part by their short, wide eustachian tubes, which permit the entry of vomitus.

### Etiology

Except for the rare cases of otitis media following traumatic rupture of the tympanic membrane or following surgery on the ear in a clean field but with imperfect sterile technique, infection of the middle ear practically always comes through the eustachian tube from the nasopharynx. In some cases forcible blowing of secretions into the tube or the entry of water carries the organism through the lumen of the eustachian tube to the middle ear. Probably in most cases the streptococcus extends in the subepithelial connective tissue of the tube exactly as it spreads in the layers of the skin in erysipelas.

The bacteria most often found on culture of an acute otitis media are the streptococcus and the pneumococcus. The latter, especially type III, and *Hemophilus influenzae*, predominate in infancy, the type III pneumococcus in diabetes and in old age; the beta hemolytic streptococcus is far more common at all other periods of life. In the otitis medias so often seen in measles and other childhood diseases, as in bacterial otitis media complicating the common cold and influenza, the beta hemolytic streptococcus is the usual invader, rather than the specific microorganism of the systemic disease, as one might expect. In children under 5 years of age, *Hemophilus influenzae* (Pfeiffer's bacillus) is the most frequent cause of acute otitis media, while after the age of 5 this organism is rarely found. The non-hemolytic streptococcus, staphylococcus, *Pseudomonas aeruginosa (Bacillus pyocyaneus)*, and other bacteria sometimes found in cultures from an acute discharging ear may, in some cases, be contaminants from the meatus, or they may be secondary invaders of the middle ear from the meatus after the primary hemolytic streptococcus has yielded to a sulfonamide or antibiotic.

Anything that interferes with the normal functioning of the eustachian tube predisposes to an acute bacterial otitis media. This includes: tamponade of the nasopharynx for nasal or nasopharyngeal hemorrhage, hypertrophied adenoid, allergic edema of the eustachian tube, viral salpingitis and cleft palate.

Hemolytic streptococcal pharyngitis and scarlet fever are, of course, particularly often complicated by streptococcal invasion of the middle ear.

### Characteristics

Certain general characteristics of acute suppurative otitis media help to differentiate it from acute necrotic otitis media, allergic otitis media, viral otitis media and chronic suppurative otitis media.

The first is that acute suppurative otitis media runs a **characteristic clinical and pathologic course** with successive stages that may be recognized and distinguished by particular symptoms and the otoscopic findings of each stage. Depending upon the virulence of the infecting organism and the resistance of the host, and today depending upon specific antibacterial therapy, the acute infection of the middle ear mucoperiosteum may pass through all the stages, or it may resolve after any stage.

The second characteristic of acute suppurative otitis media is that from the onset it tends to be a **self-limiting disease.** Just as pneumonia infecting the terminal respiratory mucosa in the lungs tends toward spontaneous resolution with return of the tissues to normal, provided the patient does not die of the infection, so acute suppurative otitis media tends toward eventual resolution and return of the tissues to normal even after severe infections, provided the patient does not succumb to a complication. Owing to this fact, and to the fact that acute suppurative otitis media is most often due to the hemolytic streptococcus, an organism that is especially susceptible to sulfonamides or the common antibiotics, this disease is especially controllable by antibacterial therapy. Nevertheless, cases are still encountered in which, because of absent or inadequate medication or because the organism is resistant to the particular medication used, the pathologic lesion progresses to the stage of bone erosion and mastoid cell coalescence requiring surgery to prevent intracranial extension. Therefore the physician who treats acute suppurative otitis media must understand clearly the successive stages through which the disease may advance.

## 1. The Stage of Hyperemia

*Pathology*

The first reaction of the mucoperiosteum of the middle ear spaces to an invading microorganism is a simple **hyperemia.** Beginning in the eustachian tube and tympanum, the hyperemic swelling **in most cases** extends to the mucoperiosteum of the antrum and pneumatic cells, though the symptoms and clinical findings may be confined to the tympanum.

*Symptoms*

**Earache** is the presenting symptom, usually accompanied by a sense of **fullness** due to hyperemic closure of the tube. **Fever** is an important symptom of all but the mildest infections, serving to differentiate a bacterial from a viral or sterile secretory otitis media. The hearing may be very slightly altered by a decrease or increase in intratympanic air pressure, depending upon the rapidity of development of the hyperemic swelling, but at this early stage **the hearing is very nearly normal.**

*Findings*

Otoscopy reveals loss of luster and **injection of the vessels of the tympanic membrane** but without enough thickening to cause loss of landmarks. The injection begins along the manubrium, around the periphery of the pars tensa and in the pars flaccida (Fig. 7–1B).

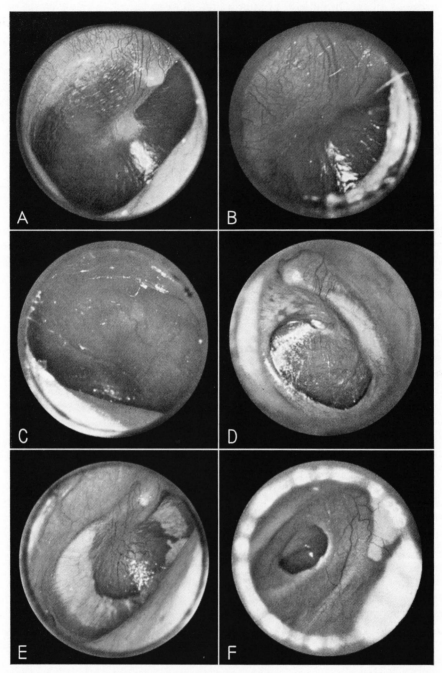

**Figure 7–1**   *A*, Normal tympanic membrane. *B*, First stage of acute otitis media. *C*, Second stage of acute otitis media. *D*, Large healed central perforation. *E*, Tympanic membrane showing scar. *F*, Tympanic membrane showing a small central perforation. (Courtesy of Dr. Richard A. Buckingham.)

*Therapy*

If there is **fever,** antibacterial medication in adequate dosage should be given. For fulminating infections, most of which are due to the beta hemolytic streptococcus, penicillin by injection is the agent of choice **provided there is not a history of sensitivity.** For milder infections, a sulfonamide or oral antibiotic such as erythromycin may be used. For *Hemophilus influenzae* in young children, Bactrim Suspension Pediatric, one teaspoonful t.i.d. is preferred to chloromycetin. Absence of fever indicates an allergic nonbacterial reaction, a viral otitis or a mild bacterial infection that will clear without antibiotic medication.

Local heat, analgesics and rest in bed in a warm room are indicated. Ear drops, such as Auralgan, may be comforting but are not curative. A mild nasal shrinking solution such as 0.25 per cent Neo-Synephrine in normal saline used 3 or 4 times a day may help to re-establish the patency of the eustachian tube.

## 2. Stage of Exudation

*Pathology*

Hyperemia of the mucoperiosteum is soon followed by an outpouring — from its dilated permeable capillaries — of serum containing fibrin, red cells and polymorphonuclear leucocytes, both into the subepithelial connective tissue and into the middle ear spaces. Very soon in virulent infections and after 12 to 24 hours in milder infections the middle ear and pneumatic cells become filled with **exudate under pressure.**

*Symptoms*

**Increased pain and fever** are accompanied by toxicity due to the rapid absorption by the mucoperiosteum of toxic products in the exudate. In infants a very high fever may be accompanied by vomiting, convulsions and meningismus (see Chapter 11). There is now a marked hearing impairment of the conductive type due to the increased mass of fluid on the conductive apparatus. The audiogram may show a greater loss for high-pitched frequencies than for low (see Chapter 13, p. 369).

*Findings*

Otoscopy reveals a **red, thickened, bulging** tympanic membrane with **loss of landmarks and light reflex** (Fig. 7–1C). **Mastoid tenderness** may be noted owing to the exudate under pressure filling the pneumatic cells. In infants **edema and hyperemia** may appear over the cribriform cortex of the antrum. In infections that develop more slowly, such as pneumococcal type III otitis media, the bulging tympanic membrane with loss of landmarks may appear pale instead of red, owing to thickening and desquamation of its outer stratified squamous epithelium.

An x-ray will reveal diffuse clouding of the mastoid cells as their air becomes replaced by fluid, but the experienced clinician who comprehends the pathology of this stage will not be alarmed or misled into premature mastoid surgery by the severe symptoms, the x-ray findings and the mastoid tenderness. Other than a simple myringotomy to release the exudate under pressure, surgical intervention is contraindicated in this early bacterial infection until there has been an opportunity for localization and "walling off." Operation on the mastoid at this early stage can only aggravate and spread the infection, with increased rather than lessened probability of serious complication.

### Therapy

If pain and toxicity are severe, immediate myringotomy to release the exudate under pressure is indicated, combined with specific antibacterial therapy, penicillin being the antibiotic of choice. Many cases subside with penicillin or other antibiotic without a myringotomy.

### 3. Stage of Suppuration

### Pathology

Following myringotomy or spontaneous perforation the ear begins to drain, at first a **hemorrhagic** or **serosanguineous** fluid, and then a **mucopurulent** discharge. The mucoperiosteum of the middle ear and air cells becomes progressively thickened by the new formation of many capillaries and young fibrous tissue, and infiltrated with lymphocytes and plasma cells and some polymorphonucelar leucocytes to form a very thick mucosal lining resembling granulation tissue. This and the local production of specific antibodies constitute the "walling-off" process that localizes and eventually resolves the infection. The blood vessels that nourish the extremely vascular, thickened mucosa reach it through the bony partitions of the pneumatic cells, which therefore partake of the increased hyperemia with the new formation of vascular channels, but **as yet the pneumatic cell walls are intact.**

### Symptoms

The release of the exudate under pressure when the ear begins to drain relieves the severe pain; the lessened absorption from the thickening mucoperiosteum and the local production of specific antibodies combine to **lessen the toxic absorption and fever.** The hearing impairment is somewhat greater as increased stiffness of the sound-conducting mechanism, due to the markedly thickened mucoperiosteum, is added to the mass of the purulent exudate. There is now impairment of low and high frequencies alike (see Chapter 13).

### Findings

Otoscopic examination reveals a discharge of mucopus, coming from a perforation in the **pars tensa** of the tympanic membrane. Whether the perforation occurs by myringotomy or spontaneously it is always **small** — just large enough to permit the escape of secretions—and it **never** enlarges. These invariable characteristics are important, for they help to differentiate acute suppurative otitis media from acute necrotic otitis media with its large pars tensa perforation, and from an attic retraction cholesteatoma with a pars flaccida perforation. (An exception is the rapid dissolution of a large atrophic healed perforation.)

With the lessening of pain and improvement in the patient's general condition the mastoid tenderness diminishes, and any redness and edema over the antrum of infants subsides. Radiography will show the pneumatic cells to be filled with fluid and therefore "cloudy," but the bony cell partitions are intact (see Fig. 4–19).

### Therapy

Culture and sensitivity tests with the various antibacterial agents should be done to select the one most effective against the particular organism. The ideal method for obtaining a culture free from contamination from the external meatus is to streak a blood agar plate with the tip of the myringotomy knife used to open the tympanic membrane.

The outer ear should be kept clean by frequent changes of cotton wicks. If the discharge begins to macerate the skin, the latter should be protected with cold cream and the meatus should be irrigated several times a day with warm boric acid solution from a soft rubber ear syringe. Ear drops at this stage are of no curative value, as they cannot reach the seat of the infection. Eustachian tube inflation is of no value until the acute inflammation begins to subside.

### 4. Stage of Coalescence and Surgical Mastoiditis

### Pathology

Depending upon the virulence and variety of the infecting organism and the resistance of the host, when the infection is severe and continued beyond 2 weeks, the progressive hyperemic thickening of the mucoperiosteum begins to obstruct the free drainage of mucopurulent secretions. The obstruction occurs in the epitympanum, where the ossicles and their swollen mucous membrane folds soon fill the narrow space, and in the smaller periantral pneumatic cells. The reaccumulation of pus under pressure in the larger peripheral cells combines with the marked hyperemia to cause venous stasis, local acidosis and dissolution of calcium (halisteresis) from the adjacent bony walls. The continued formation of many new blood vessels in the bone and the decalcification combine with the activity of numerous multinucleated osteoclasts to soften and finally remove the decalcifying bony partitions (Fig. 7–2). As a consequence, separate pneumatic cells **coalesce** into larger cavities filled with purulent exudate and markedly thickened vascular mucoperiosteal granulations. By this time in the otitis media the formation of specific antibodies is well advanced, and histologic studies will show that the areas of coalescent bone erosion are combined with adjacent areas of beginning healing by bone deposition (Fig. 7–3). Thus the tendency toward spontaneous resolution is particularly striking in the stage of coalescent or surgical mastoiditis. The erosion of bone, however, is not confined to the cell partitions within the mastoid process and other portions of the temporal bone. It proceeds in the thicker outer cortex and in the thin inner plate that separates the pneumatic cells from the sigmoid sinus and dura.

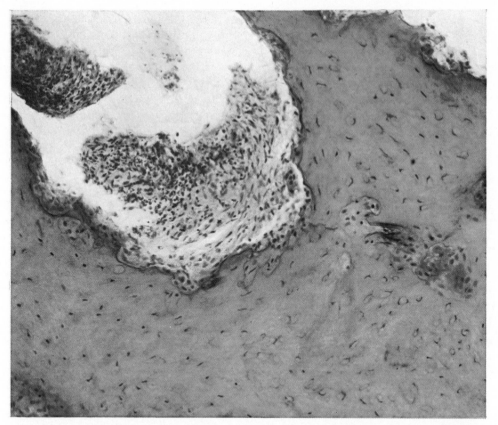

**Figure 7–2**   Acute coalescent mastoiditis showing osteoclastic erosion of mastoid cell partition. Bone specimens removed by senior author during mastoidectomies after scarlet fever.

The risk that intracranial extension by bone erosion will intervene before spontaneous healing occurs is such that surgical evacuation of the abscess cavity is indicated.

Much confusion in the minds of otologists was produced by the customary description of the surgical findings when a coalescent mastoiditis was treated by surgery; this description usually stated that in the mastoid there was "extensive necrosis with pus and granulations." Actually the softened and partially removed bony cell partitions are not necrotic at all: the tissues, though infected, are very much alive and the progressive decalcification and osteoclastic removal of bone need only the release of the pus retained under pressure to return to an active recalcification and osteoblastic repair. The very accurate description of the pathology of coalescent mastoiditis given by Scheibe[5] 76 years ago cannot be improved upon and is worth repeating to clarify the picture:

The lining of the cells contains very many blood vessels, is 40 to 80 times as thick as in the normal and changed into a lobulated granulation tissue rich in lymphocytes. The bony inner surface of the cells is eroded all over by small dimples, and in each one there is a multinuclear giant cell (osteoclast). These erosions extend over the adjoining bony canals and cavities containing marrow. They become enlarged and contain more cells than normal. Little by little in all directions an excentrical enlargement of the cavities filled with pus is thus effected, until it reaches the dura inwardly, or most frequently the protruding wall of the sinus, and outwardly the periosteum at some place of the mastoid process. Thus a fistulous

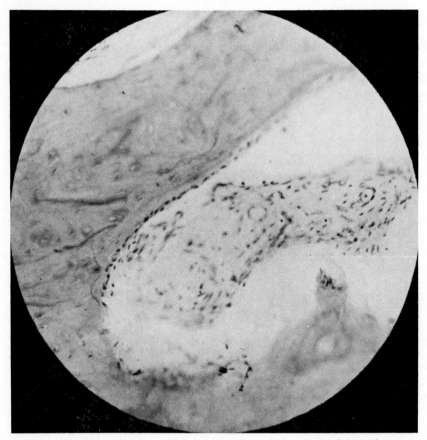

**Figure 7–3**    Acute coalescent mastoiditis—same patient as in Figure 7–2, but another area—showing beginning healing by osteoblastic bone deposition.

perforation occurs on the lateral surface if the process is not interfered with. The formation of osteoclasts and their bone-wrecking occupation comes to a standstill as soon as the pus is evacuated, and a layer of cells containing one nucleus takes their place on the walls of the diseased spaces. They are the osteoblasts which at once form osteoid substance and this later on becomes ossified all around the focus. At a greater distance from the focus of suppuration the occupation of the osteoblasts and the formation of osteoid tissue begins long before the evacuation of pus.

### Symptoms

The experienced clinician will not be lulled into a false sense of security by the fact that the patient's **symptoms in the stage of coalescence** are usually **much milder than in the earlier stage of exudation.** Now these **same symptoms have a much graver portent.** The accumulation of pus under pressure in the pneumatic cells causes a **recurrence of pain,** usually nocturnal, with **fever,** nearly always low grade, and **mastoid tenderness,** generally slight. Meanwhile, the ear continues to drain, the amount of the discharge varying with its intermittent obstruction. The discharge may become less mucoid as the infection improves in the tympanum, and more purulent as the infection persists and increases in the obstructed pneumatic cells.

*Findings*

The characteristic and diagnostic findings of a coalescent or surgical mastoiditis are:

**Continued profuse purulent discharge** from the ear for longer than 2 weeks in an acute suppurative otitis media. **Mastoid tenderness and thickening of the periosteum** to palpation as the cortex thins and the abscess approaches the surface. **"Sagging" of the posterosuperior wall of the osseous meatus** due to periosteal thickening adjacent to the antrum. A **nipple-like protrusion** of the tympanic membrane perforation due to the marked thickening of the tympanic mucosa. If the outer cortex perforates, a **fluctuant subperiosteal abscess** appears over the mastoid with outward and downward displacement of the auricle.

**Leucocytes and increased sedimentation rate,** with a low-grade, often intermittent, **fever,** indicate toxic absorption from pus under pressure in an abscess cavity. In the case of hemolytic streptococcus infections **secondary anemia** may be present.

Radiographic studies now show, in addition to diffuse clouding due to replacement of air by fluid, definite rarefaction and loss of distinctness of the bony cell partitions within the mastoid process and other pneumatized areas. These changes due to decalcification and coalescent bone removal are not uniform but are greater in one or several areas, usually at a distance from the antrum (see Fig. 4–20).

The physician must keep in mind that all of the symptoms and most of the findings of coalescent surgical mastoiditis are exactly the same as those of the earlier stage of acute otitis media when there was exudate under pressure behind the intact tympanic membrane. The **time** at which these symptoms reappear (or persist) in an acute middle ear infection **is more critical than their severity** in the diagnosis of a surgical mastoiditis with coalescent bone erosion.

*Therapy*

It is possible for antibiotic therapy alone, if not previously used in an acute infection, to cause resolution of a coalescent mastoiditis. As stated earlier, some patients with coalescent mastoiditis in the presulfonamide era who did not succumb to a sigmoid sinus thrombophlebitis with septicemia, or to a generalized meningitis or a brain abscess, did eventually recover, even without any form of treatment, with a return of the ear to normal. The risks of temporizing in the hope of spontaneous recovery are, however, so much greater than the negligible risk of a properly executed mastoidectomy done at the proper stage of the acute otitis media that **surgical evacuation of the abscess is indicated in any acute suppurative otitis media that reaches the stage of coalescence.** Today, with early and adequate antibacterial medication it is rare indeed, except among patients not receiving good medical care, for an acute otitis media to reach the stage of coalescent surgical mastoiditis.

## 5. Stage of Complication

Extension of infection beyond the mucoperiosteal lining of the middle ear and pneumatic cells to an adjacent structure produces a complication. This may be a manifest postaural subperiosteal abscess, extension to the facial nerve or labyrinth within the temporal bone, a symptomless but potentially dangerous perisinus or extradural abscess or the dreaded intracranial extension to produce a sigmoid sinus thrombophlebitis, a brain abscess or meningitis. Not infrequently a coalescent process in the pneumatic cells of the petrous apex accompanies a coalescent mastoiditis, as may be demonstrated by careful radiographic studies. When the process in the petrous pyramid begins to cause special symptoms, it is termed a "petrositis" and will be considered as one of the special complications of acute suppurative otitis media (see Chapter 12).

## Pathology

The pathologic process by which infection extends beyond the pneumatic cell system by coalescent bone erosion was so well described by Scheibe (see p. 196) that it does not require repetition.

A second important way in which extension of infection may take place is by a spreading **thrombophlebitis** of venules that may carry infection from the tympanic mucoperiosteum through intact bony walls of the middle ear and pneumatic cells to the jugular bulb, sigmoid sinus, dura, brain, facial nerve and possibly the perilymphatic labyrinth (see Figs. 12–1 and 12–2). Complication by thrombophlebitic extension occurs **through intact bone,** and it often occurs early in the otitis media, sometimes even before the ear has begun to drain,[6] as well as soon after the onset of otorrhea. Later in an otitis media, when coalescence begins to be evident, the process of localization of the infection has proceeded to the point at which thrombophlebitic extension is less likely to occur. As would be expected, certain strains of streptococci and pneumococci are more likely to cause complication by thromophlebitic extension than other varieties of infecting organisms.

At one time certain writers[7] explained complication by thrombophlebitic extension as the result of a special form of otitis media quite different from the usual acute suppurative process leading to a coalescent mastoiditis. The name "acute hemorrhagic mastoiditis" was applied to this hypothetical disease because marked hyperemia and vascularity of soft tissue and bone characterized the operative findings within the mastoid, rather than the decalcification and coalescence with abscess formation of the usual mastoidectomy performed later in an acute otitis media. It is now generally believed that acute hemorrhagic mastoiditis was merely an unusually severe, early acute suppurative otitis media, caused by a virulent hemolytic streptococcus, in which surgical intervention was undertaken before the process had reached the stage of coalescence. If early mastoidectomy was performed only because of the severity of the symptoms of acute otitis media, it probably did more harm than good. In some cases, however, surgical intervention was necessitated before the stage of coalescence because of a manifest complication by thrombophlebitic extension, such as sigmoid sinus infection or meningitis.

## Symptoms and Findings

The symptoms and the findings of a complication of acute suppurative otitis media will be very nearly the same whether the extension occurred through intact bone by thrombophlebitis or by coalescent bone erosion. They will also be similar to the symptoms and findings of a complication of chronic suppurative otitis media of the bone-eroding type. They will depend upon the structure involved and will be considered in detail in Chapters 11 and 12.

*Therapy*

Complication by coalescent bone erosion calls for **antibacterial therapy** for the complication **combined with surgical evacuation** of the abscess cavity. Medication through the blood stream does not reach organisms in a collection of pus satisfactorily and should not be relied upon to sterilize the coalescent focus causing the complication. Before the advent of sulfonamides and antibiotics the only hope for saving the life of a patient with beginning meningeal infection by thrombophlebitic extension through intact bone was to remove the focus of infection with its adjacent thrombophlebitic venules as thoroughly as possible. An immediate mastoidectomy with extensive resection of the inner plate so as to expose both the middle and posterior fossa dura adjacent to the middle ear and mastoid cells was performed upon the first evidence of headache, stiff neck and increased number of cells in the spinal fluid. Such a procedure carried out before the meningitis became generalized did seem to arrest the process in a good proportion of cases.[8] Today we may rely upon antibiotics to control the thrombophlebitic process and the complication without the need for surgery on intact mastoid cells.

## 6. Stage of Resolution

The end result of an acute suppurative otitis media, if the patient survives, is eventual resolution and healing of the ear, usually with normal hearing.

*Pathology*

As the resistance of the host overtakes the virulence of the infecting organism, or as an effective antibacterial medication reaches the organism, the acute infection begins to subside. A coalescent abscess may need to drain itself by an external fistula or may need to be drained by surgical mastoidectomy before healing can proceed.

The first evidence of resolution of the infection is diminution and cessation of the aural discharge. The small central perforation closes almost immediately. Remaining exudate in the tympanum, antrum and pneumatic cells is absorbed rapidly and completely. The marked granulation-like thickening of the mucoperiosteal lining recedes more slowly. The conductive hearing loss due to the mass of fluid recovers first; that due to the stiffness imparted by the thickened mucoperiosteum recovers last; but nearly always the hearing eventually approaches normal. Any partial decalcification and osteoclastic erosion of pneumatic cell partitions are repaired by deposition of calcium and osteoblastic activity. A large coalescent cavity fills first with vascular connective tissue which later becomes pale — sometimes described at surgery as "chicken-fat granulations" — and finally is partially replaced by osteoid tissue; or the pneumatic cells may re-form.

It is rare for an acute suppurative otitis media to leave any permanent residue. This is in contrast to acute necrotic otitis media, which **always** leaves permanent residues.

## ACUTE NECROTIC OTITIS MEDIA

The special form of acute bacterial otitis media that is accompanied by true necrosis and sloughing of considerable areas of tissue in the middle ear and adjacent region is known as "acute necrotizing otitis media" or "acute necrotic otitis media." It is very different from the usual acute suppurative otitis media in its clinical symptoms, findings and course, in its pathologic changes within the ear and in its sequelae.

Acute necrotic otitis media occurs for the most part in infants and young children who are acutely ill and toxic from scarlet fever, measles, pneumonia, influenza or some other systemic febrile infection. As a rule, the attending physician or pediatrician is too preoccupied with the severity and gravity of the systemic infection to pay close attention to the ear until an otorrhea appears. Even then, unless he has the necessary instruments, skill and patience to clean out the profuse discharge from the meatus so as to obtain a really good view of the drum membrane and tympanum, he will not be aware of the necrotic nature of the otitis media. Moreover, the otologist who has not attended the early stages of otitis media in a contagious disease hospital but is called in only for surgical indications rarely has the opportunity to see the early stages of this unusual but important condition. Thus we find that acute necrotic otitis media is hardly mentioned in many texts on ear disease, and it was poorly understood by Bezold,[9] who stated that: "The origin of the large majority of chronic suppurations of the middle ear with persistent perforation remain therefore unexplained."

Nevertheless, the distinctive clinical picture of acute necrotic otitis media and the early diagnostic pathologic changes in the tympanic membrane and tympanic mucosa are there to be seen* in a certain number of children severely ill from a systemic infection, most often scarlet fever or measles. These are the children who will be observed later in life with a chronic otorrhea coming from a large permanent perforation of the tympanic membrane, or who will present an intact tympanic membrane, the central portion of which is a thin transparent scar closing an old large perforation.

Before proceeding with the pathology of this interesting and serious form of otitis media, it will be worthwhile to recount observations the senior author made at the Chicago Contagious Disease Hospital in the years immediately preceding the introduction of the sulfonamides and penicillin. Many hundreds of cases of acute middle ear infection complicating the exanthemas were observed, and many of them were followed to their ultimate termination in a chronic suppurative otitis media.

The majority of the otitis medias that complicated measles and scarlet fever, and to a lesser extent other childhood diseases, were of the usual type seen in otherwise healthy persons. Earache and fever were followed by a small perforation in the pars tensa of the tympanic membrane, spontaneous or produced by myringotomy, with a discharge that became mucopurulent. The perforation remained small, never enlarged, and closed as soon as the drainage ceased. After several weeks of otorrhea several of the patients developed the signs and symptoms of a coalescent mastoiditis and were operated on. A very few developed a sigmoid sinus thrombophlebitis or signs of beginning meningitis and were operated on, and one developed a cerebellar brain abscess and was operated on. In all of these patients the lesion eventually healed with an intact drum membrane and good hearing.

A second variety of acute middle ear infection, less common than the usual variety, was encountered at this Contagious Disease Hospital in patients very severely ill and toxic from their contagious disease. Most were infants and small children, but one was a nurse who contracted scarlet fever while working in the

---

*"Were there to be seen" would be more accurate, since acute necrotic otitis media fortunately appears to be a vanishing disease.

hospital. In these patients the tympanic membrane perforated spontaneously very soon after the onset of earache, and when first inspected a few hours or days after the onset of otorrhea there was **already a large perforation.** In some especially sick children the aural discharge was thin and foul, and a day or two after the onset the tympanic membrane was found to be gone entirely with bare white bone visible on the medial wall of the tympanum. Surprisingly, most of these patients did not develop the symptoms and signs of a coalescent mastoiditis, but a few did develop meningitis and at operation white bloodless necrotic bone was found in the mastoid process.

Many of these children with large perforations of the drum membrane left the hospital with ears that were still draining after many weeks. The policy was not to send children home with a positive culture from the ear for hemolytic streptococcus. By the time of discharge from the hospital the bacteria in the otorrhea had changed from the original pure culture of hemolytic streptococcus to a mixed flora of staphylococcus, *Pseudomonas aeruginosa,* and other organisms derived from the external meatus. In some children a persistent mucopurulent otorrhea from a large central perforation dried up after removal of large tonsils and adenoids. In a few cases the suppuration continued for several years after return home, at the end of which time the patient was seen again with a cholesteatoma that had developed in the antrum and mastoid by ingrowth of skin from the meatus to replace the mucoperiosteum that had been destroyed in the first few days of the original necrotizing otitis. In two of these children, an operation was performed a year or two after the original acute necrotic otitis because of continued profuse purulent discharge, a good sized sequestrum being found in a mass of infected granulations. Varying degrees of permanent hearing impairment were observed in all of these patients, with a conductive loss due to destruction of portions of the sound-conducting apparatus, not infrequently complicated by a sensorineural loss due to a serous or a toxic labyrinthitis that occurred in early stages of their necrotizing otitis.

Particularly significant for the etiology of chronic suppurative otitis media was the consistent observation that **the loss of tissue** in the tympanic membrane, ossicular chain and surrounding mucoperiosteum and bone **always occurred within a few days** of the onset of the disease, and **was never a slowly progressive process.** Subsequent development of a cholesteatoma, or (rarely) a sequestrum, was the final result of the original early severe destructive process (see Fig. 7–4).

From these years of observing the early and late results of acute necrotic otitis and many years of observing acute suppurative otitis medias of the usual type, the author agrees entirely with Bezold,[10] who states of the usual "genuine" acute suppurative otitis media:

> The suppuration may have run its course in a few days, but it may also last several weeks or months with or without interruptions. I have seen it last even longer than a year in some cases, and yet it healed, the perforation closing and the normal function returning. I have **never** in an otherwise healthy organism, seen a **genuine** suppuration of the middle ear become chronic or develop a persisting or enlarging perforation.

Bezold then compares this usual picture with the acute otitis sometimes encountered during the exanthema:

> The clinical picture in the ear differs totally from the very beginning from that in genuine suppuration of the middle ear. I saw, for example, discolored fetid secretions in the meatus of an ear in which an extensive perforation had taken place during the previous night. . . . I saw another case where within six days the whole tympanic membrane was destroyed and the handle of the malleus became necrotic, at the height of the scarlet fever.

*Pathology*

The essential pathology of acute necrotic otitis media is a true necrosis or gangrene of considerable areas of soft tissue and sometimes bone due to a virulent microorganism, nearly always a beta hemolytic streptococcus, in a child whose general resistance has been lowered by a severe systemic infection. The necrotizing toxins produced by the streptococcus in the middle ear overwhelm the tissues before they have been able to react to the infection by increased vascularity and production of specific antibodies. The most vulnerable areas to the necrotizing process are those with the poorest blood supply. Thus the first tissue to succumb is the central kidney-shaped area of the pars tensa of the tympanic membrane; the portions with a better blood supply along the manubrium, near the annulus tympanicus, and the pars flaccida resist longer and may escape necrosis. The progressive necrosis of tissue probably occurs only during the first several days of the acute otitis media before the mucoperiosteum has begun to localize the infection by vascularization, granulation tissue and local production of specific antibodies. Thereafter, the process of actively spreading necrosis ceases, and the remaining living tissues of the ear proceed to react to the acute suppurative otitis media in the usual manner, but with this important exception: the necrotic tissue that sloughs is never replaced by perfectly normal tissue, but is replaced by cicatricial tissue which persists throughout the life of the person. This may be seen on otoscopic inspection as thickening and scarring of the tympanic membrane with sclerotic deposits. The patient may also have a permanent "adhesive" conductive hearing impairment, or a larger conductive loss due to ossicular necrosis and interruption, dating from the childhood infection.

The extent of the early initial necrosis of tissue varies greatly and determines the end result of this destructive and comparatively rare type of acute otitis media. The following are the usual degrees of pathology encountered:

In the **mildest** cases the necrotizing process is confined to a central area of the pars tensa of the tympanic membrane, frequently kidney-shaped. Thereafter the acute otitis proceeds as the usual acute suppurative process, including possible coalescence of pneumatic cells, but ending eventually in resolution and restoration of all tissues to normal with the single exception of the large tympanic membrane defect. The latter may eventually heal with a thin scar, or it may remain open, either dry or with a chronic "benign type" of otorrhea (Figs. 7–1D, E, and F and 7–5A).

In the **moderately severe** cases of acute necrotic otitis media, not only most of the tympanic membrane including its annulus succumbs and sloughs, but the tympanic mucoperiosteum becomes necrotic and is rapidly dissolved by the proteolytic enzymes released by degenerating polymorphonuclear leucocytes. Not infrequently the necrotic slough includes the bony sulcus tympanicus and portions of the ossicles that are exposed to the necrotizing toxins of the bacteria. When healing finally occurs, the denuded bone of the tympanum becomes lined either by the ingrowth of skin from the meatus or by the regrowth of respiratory mucosa from the eustachian tube. The result may be that the portion of the tympanum near the tube will be lined by mucous membrane and the posterosuperior area farthest from the tube will be lined by stratified squamous epithelium. Should the stratified squamous epithelium extend upward to line the epitympanum and antrum, its outer desquamating layers will collect as masses of debris, called "cholesteatoma" because of their content of crystals of cholesterol when examined microscopically.

In the **most severe** cases of acute necrotic otitis media not only do the entire tympanic membrane and tympanic mucoperiosteum slough, but also the mucoperiosteum of the antrum and pneumatic cells dissolves away leaving bare white bone. Areas of adjacent bone deprived of nutrition may die, leading to large sequestra or smaller areas of chronic bone necrosis, usually around the antrum.

The most extensive and severe case of acute necrotic otitis media encountered by the senior author is worth recounting briefly, to aid in a clear comprehension of the pathology of this disease. In the presulfonamide and preantibiotic era, the author was called to operate upon a small child desperately ill with scarlet fever who developed an otitis media with total loss of the tympanic membrane, and who, after some days, developed the symptoms and signs of meningitis. Surgery was undertaken to remove the suppurative focus in the mastoid. When the mastoid bone was exposed by the usual postaural incision, almost the entire mastoid process was found to consist of grayish-white completely bloodless bone, sharply demarcated from surrounding living inflamed bone covered with granulations, above and behind the mastoid process. When opened into, the mastoid cell walls were hard and bloodless, and completely devoid of granulations or a mucoperiosteal lining, being partially filled with a thin foul liquid pus (Fig. 7–4). The adjacent underlying dura of the middle and posterior cranial fossae was gray, bloodless and leathery, and sharply demarcated from the surrounded living and inflamed dura covered with

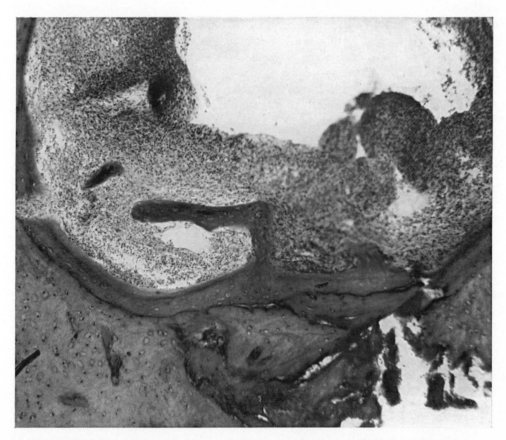

**Figure 7–4**  Bone from mastoid case of acute necrotic otitis media during scarlet fever, showing loss of mucoperiosteum with liquid pus in cell lumen. Note beginning sequestration of necrotic bone with empty lacunae adjacent to pneumatic cell lumen, with a beginning line of separation from living bone with osteocytes in lacunae.

granulations. In view of the extensive pathologic process it was not unexpected that this child succumbed to generalized meningitis.

## Symptoms

The symptoms of acute necrotic otitis media are the same as those of the usual acute suppurative otitis media, but with **these important differences:**

**Early spontaneous perforation** of the tympanic membrane occurs, so that the **first symptom of ear involvement may be the appearance of an otorrhea.** The **discharge is devoid of mucus and has a foul odor** whenever the necrosis includes the tympanic mucoperiosteum. **Profound or total sensorineural deafness** in the affected ear early in the otitis suggests the necrotic type of infection, although, in most cases, the hearing impairment is conductive and of moderate severity.

## Findings

The otoscopic findings are characteristic and diagnostic of this variety of otitis media:

Since the necrotic tympanic membrane melts away rapidly from the action of proteolytic enzymes liberated by degenerating polymorphonuclear leucocytes, the perforation may be large at the first otoscopic inspection, or it is observed to enlarge rapidly after the initial perforation. **A large tympanic membrane perforation always occurs** in this disease and **never** occurs in the usual acute suppurative otitis media, unless the latter is in an ear with a thin atrophic scar that breaks down with a middle ear infection.

In acute necrotic otitis media it may be difficult to see the tympanic membrane because of **granulations in the osseous meatus.** The cotton applicator may catch on **roughened bone** of the sulcus tympanicus. The physician may be startled to observe **naked white bone** of the promontory where he expected inflamed mucous membrane. Occasionally a **necrotic ossicle** may be seen projecting from the epitympanum. The physician will recognize that all of these findings are contrary to the odorless mucoid or mucopurulent discharge coming from a tiny perforation of the tympanic membrane that characterizes the usual acute suppurative otitis media. Wittmaack's[11] succinct description in 1907 of the clinical picture of acute necrotic otitis media is worth quoting:

> This type of lesion complicates the exanthemata. Otoscopically one observes, besides the defects in the membrana tympany, areas of necrosis in the bony walls and ossicles. The discharge, while not very profuse at the outset, later becomes so. It is frankly purulent and very foul.

Otoscopic examination weeks or months after the onset of the acute infection will begin to show the final end results of the necrotic process, as, for example, stratified squamous epithelium lining the tympanum and extending into the epitympanum, accompanied by the typical foul discharge of cholesteatoma.

## Therapy

The best hope of preventing or arresting the progressive necrosis and slough of tissues of the middle ear before severe and permanent damage has occurred is to give

**penicillin by injection as early as possible** in a child acutely ill with an infectious disease who begins to develop an otitis media. In fulminating infections the intramuscular (never intravenous) injection of gamma globulin to provide antibodies might also be considered.

Surgery has nothing to offer in the early stages of acute necrotic otitis media, and should certainly be delayed until the child has begun to recover from the

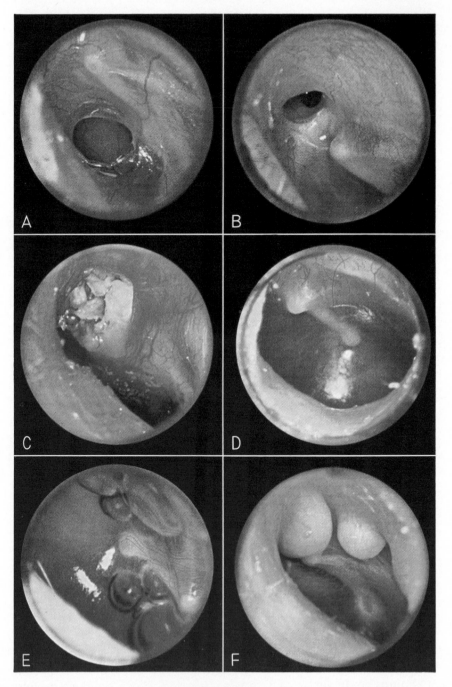

**Figure 7–5** *A*, Tympanic membrane showing a large central perforation. *B*, Dry attic perforation. *C*, Active attic cholesteatoma. *D*, Secretory otitis. *E*, Secretory otitis after inflation. *F*, Exostosis of meatus. (Courtesy of Dr. Richard A. Buckingham.)

debilitating effects of his systemic disease. The indications for mastoidectomy are then similar to the usual indications in acute suppurative otitis media with coalescent mastoiditis. Much later, when the processes of healing are far advanced, a chronic suppuration of the bone-invading type following the necrotic process may require operation.

The beneficial effects of antibacterial medication in preventing or controlling acute necrotic otitis media are already evident in the decreased number of cases of chronic suppurative otitis media with large perforations encountered in otologic practice. Nearly all of these that are seen today began with scarlet fever or measles during the presulfonamide and preantibiotic era. We may hope and expect that this frequent source of chronic suppurative otitis media will almost disappear, except among children in the most isolated areas deprived of medical care. In a visit by the senior author to a Navajo Indian Reservation more cases of recent necrotic otitis media were seen in one week than in several years of otologic practice in Chicago. Nearly all of these were in children from remote areas of the sparsely populated desert, who had had an acute middle ear infection during severe measles or scarlet fever without benefit of medical care.

### End Results of Acute Necrotic Otitis Media

The end results of the necrotizing form of acute middle ear infection depend upon the areas of tissue lost by necrosis and slough, with these various possibilities:

1. Healing of the large central perforation with a thin scar, but with essentially normal hearing (Fig. 7–1D).

2. Healing of the large central perforation but with a permanent conductive hearing loss due to scarring within the tympanum or loss of part of the ossicular chain (Fig. 7–1E).

3. A permanent large central perforation, often kidney-shaped, with a dry ear and a conductive hearing loss (Figs. 7–1F and 7–5A).

4. A permanent large central perforation with a chronic mucoid discharge.

5. A permanent perforation with skin lining the tympanum, a dry ear and a conductive hearing loss.

6. A permanent perforation with skin lining the tympanum and extending upward into the epitympanum to produce a cholesteatoma with a chronic foul otorrhea.

7. A permanent central perforation with a chronic otorrhea, usually foul and purulent rather than mucoid, due to an area of perilabyrinthine osteitis or osteomyelitis, or a sequestrum.

The surgical management of the various sequelae of acute necrotic otitis media will be considered in Chapters 10, 15 and 16.

## ALLERGIC OTITIS MEDIA

In recent years otologists trained in allergic diagnostic techniques have begun to recognize allergic otitis media as a definite and not uncommon clinical entity.[12] That there should be allergic disturbances of the mucoperiosteum of the eustachian tube and tympanum should not be a surprise, for as we have seen, the ready production of antibodies against a foreign protein, whether animate or inanimate, is one of the highly developed properties of respiratory mucous membrane. We should expect that allergic sensitization of the respiratory mucosa in the eustachian tube and middle ear would occur especially in the allergic type of person with an inherited predisposition and a nasal or bronchial allergy. We should also expect allergic sensitization of the middle ear mucosa to occur more readily in those anatomic-pathologic situations that permit repeated contact of an inanimate foreign protein with the mucous membrane, as for example in a large permanent tympanic membrane perforation permitting contact with dust and pollen, or in a patient with a cleft palate who repeatedly bathes his eustachian tube orifice with milk or other food material.

Several clinical varieties of allergic disease of the middle ear may be distinguished:

1.    When the sensitized mucosa is chiefly in the eustachian tube, usually as part of a nasal allergy, a very stubborn chronic or recurring **secretory (serous) otitis media** (otitis media with effusion) may result, which resists all therapy until the underlying allergic factor is discovered and controlled. In the experience of the author the **majority of cases of chronic secretory otitis media** in children that persist after adenoidectomy are the result of a perennial nasal allergy. Hemotympanum with a bluish color of the tympanic membrane imparted by old blood in the transudate is especially often of allergic origin. Reduction of the allergic edema of the tubal orifice by irradiation of the nasopharynx is not without risk of late undesirable sequelae, and it is no longer employed.

2.    Allergic edema of the mucosa of the eustachian tube may predispose to frequently **recurring bacterial invasions** of the tube and middle ear, just as perennial nasal allergy predisposes to frequent respiratory infections.

3.    When the allergic reaction includes both the tympanic and tubal mucosa, a painless, afebrile **allergic otitis media** results. The middle ear becomes filled with mucoid material that may contain eosinophiles. The tympanic membrane, though pale, may be thickened and bulging. Myringotomy releases a gummy or rubbery viscid mucus referred to as a "glue ear." Sometimes a mastoidectomy is mistakenly performed because of the stubborn process, in which case the mucous membrane of the middle ear spaces will be found to be thickened, edematous and pale. The eosinophilic infiltration of the mucosa found on histologic section betrays the true nature of the process. These cases resist all therapy, **including mastoidectomy,** until the allergic factor is finally recognized and controlled.

4.    Allergic sensitization of the tympanic mucosa exposed by a large permanent perforation to dust, pollens and molds from the outer air causes an extremely stubborn **benign type of chronic suppurative otitis media.** Again the large content of mucus and the occasional presence of eosinophiles point toward an allergic process. The prompt response to allergic management after all other forms of therapy have failed may be taken as proof of the allergic etiology. Methods of diagnosis and therapy[13] of the underlying allergic factor causing an allergic otitis media are beyond the scope of *Surgery of the Ear*. It should be emphasized that allergic disorders of the ear are more common than generally appreciated, and that unless the otologic surgeon is trained and equipped to make his own diagnostic allergic studies and to manage these cases himself, he usually fails to recognize their allergic nature.


## TUBERCULAR OTITIS MEDIA

Tubercular otitis media, like pulmonary tuberculosis, may be acquired by contact with infected sputum, but in the case of the middle ear the patient usually

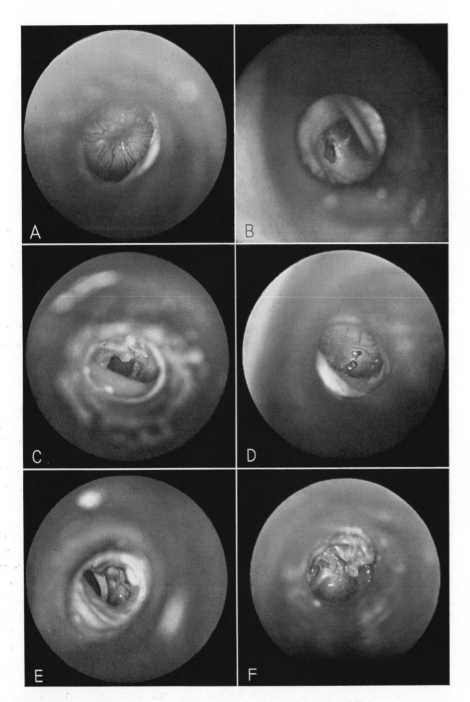

**Figure 7–6**    Appearance of tympanic membrane in tuberculosis of middle ear. *A*, Tympanic membrane thickened and bulging before perforation. *B*, Small perforation. *C*, Large central perforation. *D*, Two small perforations. *E*, Large perforation, which has destroyed three fourths of membrane. *F*, Complete destruction of tympanic membrane. (Courtesy of Dr. Linden J. Wallner.)

infects his own middle ear via the eustachian tube by coughing up sputum laden with tubercle bacilli. Tubercular otitis media also occurs in children without pulmonary tuberculosis from drinking unpasteurized milk from tubercular cows.

The infection in the middle ear, just as in the lung, is characterized by an **insidious and painless onset.** The tympanic membrane becomes thickened and **perforates spontaneously,** and there is a **scanty, thin, odorless discharge** (Fig. 7–6). From this point on the infection runs an **indolent and chronic course.** These peculiarities, especially the **painless afebrile onset** and a perforation that **enlarges or is multiple** with **pale granulations,** accompanied by **hearing that is depressed out of proportion** to the other symptoms, are highly suggestive of a tubercular process. When these occur in an adult with active pulmonary tuberculosis or in a child who has had unpasteurized milk, the presumption of tubercular otitis media is justified.[14] The conclusive diagnosis, as of tuberculosis in other areas of the body, depends upon finding the tubercle bacillus by stained smear, culture or guinea pig inoculation.

The treatment of tubercular otitis media with today's effective antitubercular medications is not a difficult problem. One no longer sees the progressive invasion of soft tissue and bone with extensive caseation necrosis and sequestration that formerly often led to facial nerve involvement and destruction of the labyrinth, and that required surgical mastoidectomy. In fact in the United States today one seldom encounters this condition outside of tuberculosis sanitariums.

## CHRONIC SUPPURATIVE OTITIS MEDIA

Chronic suppurative otitis media is a very different disease from the usual acute suppurative otitis media, not only in the duration of the discharge, but even more in the etiology, in the pathologic changes in the ear and in the clinical course. In fact, a neglected acute suppurative otitis media of several months' duration may still be essentially a self-limiting process that will tend toward complete resolution, whereas an epitympanic cholesteatoma **from the very first day of the otorrhea** should be classified as a chronic suppurative otitis media. Thus it is not the duration of the discharge in days, weeks or months but rather the particular pathologic changes that cause an otitis media to be classed as chronic rather than acute and self-limiting.

Chronic suppurative otitis media, as we have seen, may be due to the tubercle bacillus. Less than 1 per cent of cases of chronic otorrhea seen in the office practice of otology today are of tubercular origin. The vast majority of cases fall into two almost equally large pathologic and clinical groups: the **benign** non-dangerous chronic suppurations and the **dangerous** bone-invading chronic suppurations.

### Benign Chronic Suppurative Otitis Media

We have seen in the earlier part of this chapter how the special form of acute middle ear infection, known as acute necrotic otitis media, that occurs during the exanthemas frequently results in a permanent central perforation of the pars tensa of the tympanic membrane. The tympanic mucosa thus exposed to the outside air is easily sensitized by dust or infected by bacteria from the external meatus. Such an ear is also more easily infected via the eustachian tube than the normal ear. A chronic or recurring mucoid otorrhea results. Since the chronic discharge comes from the mucous membrane rather than from a deep-seated bone-invading disease, this is termed a "benign type" of chronic suppurative otitis media.

### Diagnosis

The following characteristics serve to differentiate the benign from the bone-invading types of chronic suppurative otitis media:

There is always a **central perforation** involving the pars tensa of the tympanic membrane, of varying size and shape but with a narrow margin of intact annulus, and usually with part or all of the manubrium of the malleus remaining, giving the perforation a kidney shape.

Just as important as the central perforation, there is always **mucous membrane** (rather than stratified squamous epithelium) lining the visible portions of the tympanic cavity. Depending upon the amount of recent infection, the visible mucous membrane may be bright red, thick and velvety, or pink and edematous, or very pale and thin. Occasionally there will be granulations or a large polyp arising from markedly thickened mucous membrane.

The discharge is **always mucoid or mucopurulent.** The amount of pus mixed with the mucus varies with the amount of recent infection. When the patient is first seen, the discharge sometimes has a foul odor, but with cleanliness and the local use of a mild antiseptic or antibacterial agent the odor quickly disappears, leaving the typical **odorless mucoid discharge.**

In some patients the otorrhea is constant, very stubborn and very mucoid, and tenacious or "rubbery" in character. In others the discharge is intermittent, recurring whenever there is a fresh head cold, or if water accidentally enters the ear.

These cases are all termed "benign" because the chronic discharge is coming from the mucous membrane of the tympanum and tube rather than from a deeper bone-invading process. Chronic benign otitis media probably never transforms itself into a chronic dangerous otorrhea. However, there is nothing to prevent a new virulent organism from entering such an ear and causing a fresh acute infection. Such an "acute exacerbation of a chronic otitis" is not immune to a serious complication by thrombophlebitic extension. In fact there may be a greater tendency toward a complication in such an acute exacerbation than in an acute otitis media in a well pneumatized mastoid without previous infection. This is explained by the presence of a pre-existing pathway for infection remaining from the initial acute necrotic otitis media in the form of an old inactive perisinus or extradural abscess which had healed with granulations and fibrous tissue but which is easily reinvaded by a fresh virulent microorganism. These acute infections superimposed on a chronic benign type of otitis media should be treated exactly like the usual acute suppurative otitis media. They will respond readily to appropriate antibacterial therapy given orally or parenterally, and they rarely require surgical intervention.

Attention should be called to the occasional atypical case of apparently benign chronic otitis with a central perforation and with mucous membrane lining the visible portions of the tympanic cavity, but with a concealed cholesteatoma encountered sufficiently often that Wullstein advises an exploratory inspection of the attic and antrum in every case through "control holes" before proceeding with a myringoplasty (see Chapter 15).

The **treatment** of the benign type of chronic suppurative otitis media is directed toward the local mucosal infection in the tympanum, and toward any pathologic lesion at the nasopharyngeal orifice of the eustachian tube. Locally the discharge from the ear is carefully removed by suction or dry wipes; the eustachian tube is inflated and mild antiseptic or antibacterial powder is insufflated. Sulzberger's powder of 1 per cent iodine in boric acid is very satisfactory. If there is a musty or foul-smelling discharge suggesting staphylococcus or *Pseudomonas aeruginosa* infection, the meatus and tympanum may be painted with tincture of Merthiolate 1:1000, and Aerosporin or some similar broad-spectrum antibiotic in boric acid powder may be insufflated. If the discharge is profuse and purulent, the patient should be given boralcohol, Gantrisin, Colymycin or Chloromycetin otic solution or some other antiseptic antibacterial medication in solution to use as ear drops twice daily for the first week. Thereafter the "dry" method of treatment with insufflated powder should be used once or twice a week until the ear is dry.

Adenoid hypertrophy obstructing the eustachian tube orifice should be removed. Many of these patients have a perennial nasal allergy of which house dust is the most frequent cause, and this should receive appropriate treatment, preferably by the dilute optimum dosage method of Hansel and Rinkel.[15]

Not infrequently a chronic benign type of otorrhea of many years' duration will respond quickly and dry up after as few as one or two local treatments. Other patients require a longer period of local treatment, and some will continue to have a persistent mucoid discharge that may contain eosinophiles and resists all treatment, including surgery, until an allergic factor is searched for and brought under control.

The fact that the chronic mucoid otorrhea persists or recurs despite local treatment **does not in itself** mean that there is, after all, a process requiring surgery. In fact it is in exactly these cases that misdirected surgery often results in a troublesome mucoid tubal discharge after a radical mastoidectomy.

Recurrences of the mucoid or mucopurulent discharge are very common in the benign type of chronic otorrhea, as long as the large perforation remains open. Closure of the perforation as soon as the ear becomes dry should be undertaken using the methods described in Chapter 15. Successful closure does not eliminate the possibility of reinfection from the eustachian tube, but it greatly reduces the susceptibility to tubal extension of infection from the nasopharynx, and it eliminates reinfection from the meatus. At the same time there is very often a useful improvement in hearing.

### Secondary Acquired Cholesteatoma

We have seen how an acute necrotic otitis media with sloughing of the tympanic mucoperiosteum may heal by the ingrowth of stratified squamous epithelium from the meatus to line the denuded tympanic cavity, epitympanum and antrum. Necrotic slough of the annulus and sulcus tympanicus, producing a **marginal perforation**, favors the ingrowth of skin, since skin grows with difficulty over a sharp annular edge. Occasionally, as noted before, epidermis will enter the tympanic cavity through a central type of perforation.

The normal desquamation of the outer cornified layers of skin proceeds to collect in the epitympanum and antrum in concentric onion-like layers of whitish debris containing crystals of cholesterol and hence called **cholesteatoma.** Although occasionally a large cholesteatoma may exist for a long time without bacterial contamination and resultant otorrhea, cholesteatoma debris offers a favorable culture medium for various pathogenic and putrefactive bacteria from the external meatus, producing the characteristic foul chronic discharge. The microorganisms commonly found on culture are a mixture including staphylococci, *Pseudomonas* *aeruginosa, Bacillus proteus,* colon bacilli, aerobic and anaerobic non-hemolytic streptococci, diphtheroid bacilli and aspergilli molds. The reader will recognize the very great difference between this mixed infection of organisms from the skin of the external meatus, many of them resistant to the usual antibiotics, and the pure infection with a pneumococcus or a hemolytic streptococcus that invades the respiratory mucosa of the middle ear in acute otitis media.

The pressure exerted by the accumulating layers of desquamating epidermal debris combines with the acid reaction produced by bacterial decomposition to cause a slow erosion of the surrounding bone. The erosion may eventually expose the lumen of a semicircular canal, the facial nerve, the dura or the wall of the sigmoid sinus. The pathogenic bacteria in the decomposing material may then invade the structure, causing labyrinthitis, facial paralysis, brain abscess, meningitis or sigmoid sinus thrombophlebitis.

Cholesteatomas such as these, acquired secondary to a childhood acute necrotic otitis media, are referred to as "secondary acquired cholesteatomas" to distinguish them from those that arise without a preceding acute otitis media.

### Therapy

A cholesteatoma cavity filled with infected debris is actively enlarging and is a mortal, though not necessarily immediate, threat. The aim of therapy is to arrest the bone erosion and the threat to life by removing the debris and exteriorizing the pocket, producing a clean, dry, odorless, inactive, skin-lined cavity open to the external meatus. Although this can be accomplished by local treatment in certain cases, the majority of secondary acquired cholesteatomas require a radical mastoidectomy, as described in Chapter 10. In some cases the entire sac-like cholesteoma can be removed intact from the attic and antrum, as described in Chapter 16. In other cases the cholesteatoma, including its epidermal matrix, can be removed by the intact canal wall technique, or by the osteoplastic epitympanotomy described in Chapter 10.

### Attic (Epitympanic) Retraction Cholesteatoma

Attic retraction cholesteatoma is the rather frequently encountered variety of chronic suppurative otitis media in which the perforation, often very small, is confined to the region of the pars flaccida of the tympanic membrane.

These are the cases sometimes referred to as "true cholesteatoma," "cholesteatoma verum," "genuine cholesteatoma" or "primary acquired cholesteatoma." The name "primary pseudocholesteatoma" was suggested by Day[16] to differentiate these cases on the one hand from the very rare congenital epidermal tumor, and on the other from the cholesteatomas that are secondary to an acute necrotic otitis media with a very large or total perforation of the tympanic membrane. The authors prefer the term suggested by Juers, attic retraction cholesteatoma.

### Etiology

The etiology of attic retraction cholesteatoma continues to be the subject of debate. Habermann[17] was the first to claim that cholesteatomas develop by an ingrowth of epidermis from the external meatus into the middle ear and attic. Bezold[18] explained the development of the attic retraction variety as the result of tubal occlusion leading to a retraction of Shrapnell's membrane into the attic, where its outer cornified layers proceeded to collect as a plug of epidermal debris. Wittmaack[19] enlarged upon this theory by showing that persistence of a hyperplastic embryonic-type of mucoperiosteum in the epitympanum could lead to adhesions walling off areas, especially between the head of the malleus and Shrapnell's membrane (Prussak's space). Since air from the eustachian tube could not reach these areas, the resulting negative pressure would have the same effect as a prolonged tubal occlusion. In these cases the hyperplastic mucosa that produced the retraction of Shrapnell's membrane also caused an arrest of pneumatization of the mastoid process, accounting for the frequency with which attic retraction cholesteatomas are seen in small, contracted, poorly pneumatized mastoids (see Fig. 4–21).

Although the explanations of Bezold and Wittmaack agree with the clinical observations of the authors, and have received widespread acceptance, other theories are still held. Tumarkin[20] believes that under the influence of infection the pavement epithelium of the epitympanum may undergo metaplasia, "throwing off paper-like squames," which, if there is not much discharge, can collect in sheets and "gradually roll up into a compact ball, the so-called cholesteatoma perle." McKenzie,[21] Diamant[22] and Teed[23] believe that a congenital epidermal rest causes most cases of attic cholesteatoma that occur with a perforation confined to the pars flaccida. Nager,[24] Lange,[25] Hellmann[26] and more recently Saxen and Ojala[27] and Ruedi[28] have modified Wittmaack's theory by stating that cone-like extensions from the basal layer of epidermis of Shrapnell's membrane can become invasive as the result of infection, producing first a cholesteatoma in the attic and then later a perforation of Shrapnell's membrane outwardly to the external auditory meatus.

The simplest explanation, that of Bezold and Wittmaack, namely that the entire process begins as a simple pouch-like invagination of Shrapnell's membrane in response to negative pressure in the attic, seems to be adequate for the clinical manifestations of the great majority of cholesteatomas that arise without a preceding necrotic otitis and without a pars tensa perforation.

As Day[16] points out, the retraction of Shrapnell's membrane initially induced by negative pressure is made permanent by adhesions to the walls of the attic. Unless the desquamation of cornified cells is stimulated by moisture or infection, such an attic retraction may remain dry and harmless for many years (Fig. 7–5 B). Moisture and desquamation cause the invaginated pouch to become filled with epidermal debris, producing an actively enlarging cholesteatoma (Fig. 7–5 C). The occasional reported case of attic cholesteatoma without a perforation may be either a case with a minute attic perforation not observed before operation or a previous attic perforation that later closed or a congenital epidermal rest.

If the reader will inspect carefully under magnified vision the pars flaccida of the tympanic membrane of every patient that he examines, he will soon have observed the successive stages in the development of this interesting and common condition, as follows:

The earliest and entirely asymptomatic first stage of an attic retraction cholesteatoma is a small dimple-like indentation of the pars flaccida of the tympanic membrane just above and either in front of or behind the projection of the short process of the malleus. Unlike the temporary and reversible retraction of the pars flaccida and pars tensa seen in tubal occlusion of recent origin, this retraction is confined to the pars flaccida, and it cannot be reduced by inflation of the eustachian tube. This initial dimple-like permanent pars flaccida retraction may arise in one of two ways:

1.  It may be the result of an infantile otitis media that occurred before the gelatinous fetal subepithelial connective tissue of the middle ear of the newborn child had time to recede. Aschoff[29] demonstrated in 1897 that the middle ear of the newborn infant may be filled with a non-bacterial mucopurulent secretion containing a mixture of amniotic fluid, vernix caseosa and meconium, causing an irritation and infiltration of the embryonic subepithelial connective tissue. Wittmaack[30] suggested in 1918 that this infantile sterile otitis media neonatorum or non-bacterial otitis media occurring soon after birth could lead to a permanent residual fibrosis and thickening of the embryonic subepithelial tympanic connective tissue before it has had time to resorb. This, in turn, would impede the normal process of pneumatization in the epitympanum and antrum, and would retard or arrest the ensuing pneumatization of the mastoid process and other normally pneumatized portions of the temporal bone. Not only would such a temporal bone remain apneumatic or very poorly pneumatized throughout life, but the tympanic and epitympanic mucoperiosteum will be permanently thickened with numerous fibrous adhesions especially between the folds of mucosa that envelop the ossicles and their ligaments. A localized pocket of negative pressure might easily result in the epitympanum of such an ear, causing a permanent pit-like retraction of the pars flaccida.

The correctness of Wittmaack's observations and deductions is borne out by the frequency of radiographic absence of pneumatization in patients who exhibit the various stages of attic retraction cholesteatoma. Further corroborative evidence is the senior author's observation during fenestration for otosclerosis on patients with absent pneumatization that the epitympanum and antrum are often lined by a thick, velvety, vascular mucoperiosteum, despite the absence of a history of acute otitis media.

2.  The second way in which a permanent pit-like retraction of the pars flaccida may develop is from long-standing secretory otitis media[31] usually occurring during childhood (Fig. 7–5 D and E). This may be from hypertrophied adenoids or from an allergic salpingitis.[13, 32] Recent tubal occlusion results in a temporary, reversible retraction of the pars tensa and pars flaccida that disappears on inflation. Long-standing tubal occlusion permits the sharply retracted pars flaccida to become irreversibly adherent to the underlying ossicles and their mucous membrane folds. Removal of the fluid from the middle ear and inflation of the tube then restores the pars tensa to its normal position, but not the pars flaccida. Radiography in such patients will show a well pneumatized mastoid process, in contrast to the radiographic findings in patients with infantile otitis media described before.

The **second stage** in the development of an attic retraction cholesteatoma occurs if the pit-like retraction of the pars flaccida becomes filled with a plug of desquamated epithelium. Once this happens the next stage soon follows: The pressure from accumulating layers of desquamating epidermis causes the pocket to enlarge, slowly at first, and more rapidly when the debris becomes contaminated by bacteria from the external meatus.

When the pocket reaches the walls of the attic, it proceeds to enlarge by bone erosion in exactly the same manner as secondary acquired cholesteatoma. In some cases the expanding sac-like cholesteatoma pocket remains above the ridge of the bony tympanic facial canal; in others it may project down into the tympanic cavity as a small epidermal sac filled with desquamated debris and entirely separate from the mucous membrane-lined air space of the tympanic cavity. Inflation of the eustachian tube in such a case will cause the pars tensa to bulge, without the escape of air from the epitympanic opening. Should the skin-lined sac rupture, spilling its infected contents into the tympanic cavity, an acute otitis media will occur. The physician should not conclude that the cholesteatoma is the result of the acute otitis media!

The opening from the external auditory meatus into the cholesteatoma cavity appears to the examiner as a hole or perforation of the pars flaccida (Fig. 7–5 B). As we have seen from the manner in which it develops, it is in reality not a perforation at all, but an **invagination of the pars flaccida** which expands as the cholesteatoma cavity enlarges.

In some cases the epitympanic "perforation" remains quite small and easily escapes detection in a cursory otoscopic examination, especially when it is obscured by a crust or tiny polyp. The use of the microscope or magnifying speculum and the introduction of a blunt ear hook into the "perforation" in the superior meatal wall above the short process of the malleus help to demonstrate its presence. In other cases the original small attic "perforation" enlarges as the outer bony wall of the epitympanum is eroded away, until there is a good sized epitympanic opening or "perforation," but the pars tensa of the tympanic membrane always remains intact.

The effect on the ossicles of an attic retraction cholesteatoma explains the variable effects on the hearing. As long as the ossicular chain remains intact and mobile, the hearing remains very nearly normal. As the cholesteatoma sac enlarges it frequently envelops the long process or all of the incus, depriving it of its blood supply, with resultant painless necrosis. The patient now exhibits a conductive hearing loss of considerable degree owing to interruption of the ossicular chain, unless there is contact between the head of the stapes and the upper edge of the pars tensa. In the latter event, the sound-conducting apparatus may function by nature's "myringostapediopexy" so well that the hearing is very nearly normal. Necrosis of the head of the malleus occurs less commonly than necrosis of the incus, but the effect on the hearing is similar.

The possibility should not be overlooked that the "perforation" in the pars flaccida may heal over after the establishment of an epitympanic attic retraction cholesteatoma. This unusual event does occur occasionally and might be easily misinterpreted by the surgeon as a cholesteatoma of congenital origin.

### Therapy

An actively enlarging attic retraction cholesteatoma filled with infected debris carries exactly the same risks of a serious complication as the secondary acquired variety. The aim of therapy is also exactly the same, namely, to render an active bone-eroding cholesteatoma cavity clean, dry and odorless by mechanical removal of its debris. There is this difference, however: The hearing in attic retraction cholesteatoma is often sufficiently good to be worth preserving by a modified rather than a classic radical mastoid operation or by an intact canal wall or osteoplastic epitympanotomy technique (see Chapters 10 and 16).

### Congenital Cholesteatoma

An epithelial rest of embryonal origin, occurring in one of the bones of the skull, is known as a congenital cholesteatoma or epidermoid cyst. Histologically the pathology is similar to that of the acquired varieties, namely, a bone-eroding skin-lined cavity filled with concentric layers of desquamated squamous epithelium,

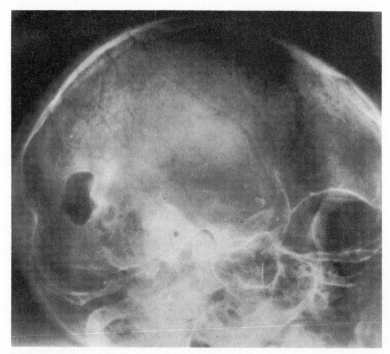

**Figure 7–7**   Congenital cholesteatoma of the skull just behind the mastoid process in a patient with acute coalescent mastoiditis. At operation, the cholesteatoma-filled bone defect was not connected with mastoid cells.

but there is this important difference: The pocket initially has no connection with the outer ear and therefore it remains sterile unless contaminated surgically or as a result of its eroding through into the external meatus.

Congenital cholesteatoma is usually a chance finding by radiography of the skull (Figs. 4–29 and 7–7), showing a sharply localized defect with smooth margins resembling a large trephine opening.

Slowly progressive facial palsy, deafness and loss of caloric response on the same side, with x-ray evidence of widespread bone erosion not beginning in the internal acoustic meatus, serve to differentiate congenital petrous cholesteatoma from acoustic neurinoma. Tympanic or attic cholesteatomas in childhood behind a perfectly normal intact tympanic membrane are of congenital origin (Fig. 7–8). For further consideration of congenital cholesteatoma, see Chapter 23.

### Chronic Suppurative Otitis Media due to Chronic Osteitis or Osteomyelitis

Acute necrotic otitis media when unusually severe and extensive may involve areas of bone around the antrum or in the petrous pyramid. A large necrotic area of bone will eventually sequestrate, becoming surrounded by a mass of infected granulations, a source of chronic otorrhea.

Occasionally an acute suppurative otitis media of the ordinary type results in a chronic osteomyelitis of non-pneumatized areas of the petrous portion of the temporal bone. This unusual sequel to an acute middle ear infection is attributable to

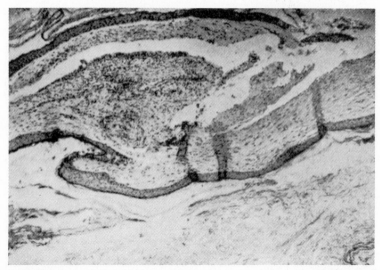

**Figure 7–8**  Low power view of pathologic specimen "epidermoid cyst" of tympanum. (From Derlacki, E. L., and Clemis, J. D.: Congenital cholesteatoma of the middle ear and mastoid. Ann. Otol. Rhin. & Laryng., 74:706, 1965.)

a staphylococcus or an anaerobic streptococcus and is less likely to occur in well pneumatized temporal bones than in those with poor pneumatization and consequently more residual marrow-containing diploic bone.

The tympanic membrane perforation in these comparatively rare cases of chronic osteitis or osteomyelitis may be either small or large, but there is no evidence of stratified squamous epithelium extending into the epitympanum to produce a cholesteatoma.

The **persistently purulent non-mucoid discharge,** often foul despite careful local cleaning and antiseptic medication, differentiates this type from the much more common benign type of chronic otorrhea. Pain or headache, low-grade fever and malaise associated with temporary cessation of discharge and relieved when the ear drains, with other symptoms of petrositis (see Chapter 12), all point toward a chronic focus of osteitis or osteomyelitis. Radiographic study is of little help for diagnosis in these cases unless there is a frank sequestrum.

### Therapy

A sequestrum, like any foreign body, needs to be removed surgically. Chronic osteitis or osteomyelitis also requires surgery, but when the focus is in the petrous pyramid it is difficult to eradicate and may recur or persist despite repeated extensive operations and antibiotic therapy.

## DIFFERENTIAL DIAGNOSIS OF OTITIS MEDIA

A clear understanding of the pathology of the various types of otitis media is so necessary for their intelligent management that a brief summary of their salient characteristics is indicated.

*Viral otitis media* with a common cold causes a non-inflammatory secretory (serous) otitis without fever. Bullous myringitis is a special form with pain but not fever.

**Acute suppurative otitis media** is an acute infection of the mucoperiosteum of the middle ear cleft by respiratory microorganisms, most often the pneumococcus or beta hemolytic streptococcus. The infection runs a typical and self-limiting course ending in resolution and return of the tissues to normal. The tympanic membrane perforation is **always small** and **always in the pars tensa.** The disease is especially responsive to appropriate antibacterial medication, as determined by culture and sensitivity tests. Pain, fever and impaired hearing are the symptoms.

**Tubercular otitis media** is a comparatively rare type of infection recognizable by its clinical peculiarities: the painless onset, the scant discharge, the progressive enlargement of the perforation, which may be multiple, and the profound impairment of hearing, in a patient with pulmonary tuberculosis or one who has had unpasteurized milk.

**Allergic otitis media** takes several forms; it is more common than is generally appreciated; and it is characterized by its mucoid discharge, stubborn chronicity and resistance to therapy unless the underlying allergy is recognized and brought under control.

**Acute necrotic otitis media,** rarely seen today, is a special form of acute middle ear infection that occurs in children severely ill with a systemic disease, especially scarlet fever and measles. It is characterized by necrotic sloughing of part or all of the tympanic membrane, often with mucosa and bone, and because of the loss of tissue the ear can never return to normal. The tympanic membrane perforation is **invariably large.**

Cases of **chronic otorrhea** with a large permanent tympanic membrane perforation are the result of an acute necrotic otitis media. Three types of chronic otorrhea occur from this disease, depending upon the extent of the original necrosis of tissue:

1.   A **benign** type of chronic suppurative otitis media with a **central perforation,** mucous membrane (not skin) lining the exposed tympanic cavity and an odorless mucoid discharge. Many of these patients have an allergic sensitization of the exposed mucosa.

2.   A bone-invading **secondary acquired cholesteatoma** with a marginal perforation, skin (not mucous membrane) lining the tympanic cavity and extending into the epitympanum, and a foul non-mucoid discharge.

3.   A bone-invading **chronic osteitis,** chronic osteomyelitis or sequestrum with a persistently foul purulent discharge.

Of these three sequelae of an acute necrotic otitis media, the benign type of chronic otorrhea is the most common, the secondary acquired cholesteatoma is next in frequency and chronic osteitis without cholesteatoma is comparatively rare.

A fourth variety of chronic suppurative otitis media is the bone-invading **attic retraction cholesteatoma** that arises insidiously in a previously normal ear by invagination of the pars flaccida of the tympanic membrane.

As acute necrotic otitis medias become more infrequent owing to antibiotic therapy of early acute otitis media, the relative proportion of chronic suppurative otitis medias due to attic retraction cholesteatoma increases. Today the majority of chronic otorrheas that require surgical intervention are cholesteatomas with attic perforations and an intact pars tensa of the tympanic membrane.

## REFERENCES

1.  Cawthorne, T.: The surgery of the temporal bone. J. Laryng. & Otol., 67:377, 1953.
2.  Hilding, A. C.: Summary of known facts concerning the common cold. Ann. Otol. Rhin. & Laryng., 53:444, 1944.

3. Badger, G. F., Feller, A. E., Hodges, R. G., Jordan, W. S., Jr., and Rammelkamp, C. H., Jr.: A study of respiratory infections in families. Tr. A. Am. Physicians, *62*:99, 1949.

4. Bezold, F.: Textbook of Otology. Translated by J. Holinger. E. H. Colgrove Co., Chicago, 1908, p. 157.

5. Scheibe, A.: Aetiologie und Pathogenese des Empyems im Verlaufe der akuten Mittelohreiterung. Ztschr. Ohrenh., *48*:1, 1904.

6. Faunce, C. B., and Shambaugh, G. E., Jr.: Abscess of the brain following mild transitory otitis media. Arch. Otol., *17*:673, 1933.

7. Kopetsky, S.: Otologic Surgery. Paul B. Hoeber, Inc., New York, 1929, p. 22.

8. Shambaugh, G. E., Jr.: The surgical treatment of meningitis of otitic and nasal originl J.A.M.A., *108*:696, 1937.

9. Bezold, op cit., p. 189.

10. Ibid., p. 173.

11. Wittmaack, K.: Diskussionsbemerkung zur Bakteriologie der akuten Mittelohrentzündung. Verhandl. deutsch. otol. Gesellsch., *16*:100, 1907.

12. Derlacki, E. L.: Aural manifestations of allergy. Ann. Otol. Rhin. & Laryng., *61*:179, 1951.

13. Derlacki, E. L., and Shambaugh, G. E., Jr.: Allergic management of some common ear conditions. Tr. Am. Acad. Ophth., *57*:304, 1953.

14. Wallner, L. J.: Tuberculous otitis media. Laryngoscope, *63*:1058, 1953.

15. Hansel, F. K., and Rinkel, H. J.: Clinical Allergy. C. V. Mosby Co., St. Louis, 1953.

16. Day, K. M.: Primary pseudocholesteatoma of the ear. Arch. Otol., *34*:1144, 1941.

17. Habermann, J.: Zur Entstehung des Cholesteatoms des Mittelohrs. Arch. Ohrenh., *27*:42, 1888.

18. Bezold, F.: Cholesteatom, Perforation der Membrana flaccida Shrapnelli und Tubenverschluss. Ztschr. Ohrenh., *20*:5, 1890.

19. Wittmaack, K.: Wie entsteht ein genuines Cholesteatom? Arch. Ohren-, Nasen- u. Kehlkopfh., *137*:306, 1933.

20. Tumarkin, A.: Middle ear suppuration and cholesteatoma. J. Laryng. & Otol., *53*:685, 1938.

21. McKenzie, D.: Pathogeny of aural cholesteatoma. J. Laryng. & Otol., *46*:163, 1931.

22. Diamant, M.: Chronic Otitis, a Critical Analysis. S. Karger, New York, 1952.

23. Teed, R. W.: Cholesteatoma verum tympani. Arch. Otol., *24*:455, 1936.

24. Nager, F.: The cholesteatoma of the middle ear. Ann. Otol. Rhin. & Laryng., *34*:1249, 1925.

25. Lange, W.: Tief eingezogene Membrana flaccida und Cholesteatom. Ztschr. Hals-, Nasen- u. Ohrenh., *30*:575, 1932.

26. Hellmann, K.: Studien über das sekundäre Cholesteatom des Felsenbeins. Ztschr. Hals-, Nasen-u. Ohrenh., *11*:406, 1925.

27. Saxen, A., and Ojala, L.: Pathogenesis of middle-ear cholesteatoma arising from Shrapnell's membrane. Acta Oto-laryng., Suppl. 100, 1952, p. 33.

28. Ruedi, L.: Pathogenesis and treatment of cholesteatoma in chronic suppuration of the temporal bone. Ann. Oto. Rhin. & Laryng., *66*:283, 1957.

29. Aschoff, L.: Die Otitis media neonatorum. Ztschr. Ohrenh., *31*:295, 1897.

30. Wittmaack, K.: Über die normale und die pathologische Pneumatisation des Schläfenbeines. Fischer, Jena, 1918.

31. Bagby, R. A., and Farrior, J. B.: The treatment of the chronic middle ear and the pathogenesis of cholesteatoma. South. M. J., *46*:712, 1953.

32. Jordan, R. E.: Role of allergy in otology. Arch. Otolaryngol., *55*:363, 1952.

33. Cawthorne, T., and Griffith, A.: Primary cholesteatoma of the temporal bone. Arch. Otolaryngol., *73*:252, 1961.

34. Derlacki, E. L., and Clemis, J. D.: Congenital cholesteatoma of the middle ear and mastoid. Ann. Otol. Rhin. & Laryng., *74*:706, 1965.

# Chapter 8

# Operations on the Auricle, External Meatus and Tympanic Membrane

ANATOMIC CONSIDERATIONS
SURGICAL CONDITIONS OF THE AURICLE
    FROSTBITE
    HEMATOMA
    LEPROSY
    PERICHONDRITIS
    ERYSIPELAS
    SEBACEOUS CYST
    KELOID
    LOP EARS
    CONGENITAL PREAURICULAR CYST AND FISTULA
SURGICAL CONDITIONS OF THE MEATUS
    EXOSTOSIS AND OSTEOMA
    CICATRICIAL STENOSIS AND ACQUIRED ATRESIA
    FURUNCLE
    FOREIGN BODY
    POLYP
    CARIES OR LOCALIZED NECROSIS OF THE
      OSSEOUS MEATUS
    CHOLESTEATOMA OF THE EXTERNAL AUDITORY
      MEATUS
    ACUTE AND CHRONIC INFECTIONS OF THE
      EXTERNAL AUDITORY MEATUS
SURGICAL CONDITIONS OF THE TYMPANIC MEMBRANE
    MYRINGITIS BULLOSA
    MYRINGOTOMY FOR ACUTE SUPPURATIVE OTITIS
      MEDIA
    MYRINGOTOMY AND VENTILATION TUBE FOR
      SECRETORY (SEROUS) OTITIS MEDIA
    TRAUMATIC PERFORATIONS
    CHRONIC MYRINGITIS

## ANATOMIC CONSIDERATIONS

The **outer or external ear** includes the auricle, external auditory meatus and tympanic membrane. These structures are clothed in skin with its outer **epidermis** of stratified squamous epithelium and its underlying **dermis** of dense connective tissue containing nerve endings, a rich capillary network, hair follicles and glands.

The skin of the outer ear is modified in specific areas as follows: The skin of the osseous portion of the external auditory meatus and of the tympanic membrane lacks hair and sebaceous glands, and it also lacks the rete pegs that help to anchor the epidermis to the dermis in other areas of the body. As a result the epidermis can be stripped from the dermis of the osseous meatus and tympanic membrane relatively easily for the operations of myringoplasty (Chapter 15) and tympanoplasty (Chapter 16).

The skin of the cartilaginous meatus contains large hair follicles and sebaceous glands that make this a frequent site for furuncle. It also contains the ceruminous glands that extend nearly to the notch of Rivinus in the skin of the superior osseous meatal wall. The skin of the auricle and cartilaginous meatus is tightly bound to the perichondrium, preventing diffusion and absorption of hematomas and causing the severe pain of furuncle.

The skin of the posterior (medial) surface of the auricle and adjacent surface of the mastoid process is thin and delicate, with a loose subepithelial connective tissue and without large hair follicles, making it particularly suitable, as well as conveniently accessible, for split or full thickness skin grafts to be utilized in plastic reconstructions of the meatus. For myringoplasty the postauricular skin is less suited as a free graft than skin from the osseous meatus because of postauricular sebaceous glands creating preformed pathways for cholesteatoma invasion of the middle ear.

The skin of the outer ear is subject to all of the diseases that afflict skin elsewhere. However, there is a special predilection for allergic reactions and for chronic inflammations and infections in the case of the skin of the meatus because of the tendency toward retention of moisture and debris.

Those conditions of the outer ear that have surgical implications will be included in this chapter, with the exception of congenital malformations, closure of chronic perforations of the tympanic membrane and carcinoma, which will be considered in Chapters 14, 15 and 22.

## SURGICAL CONDITIONS OF THE AURICLE

### Frostbite

The thinness and exposed position of the auricle make it the area most frequently involved by frostbite in civilian life. The tendency toward frostbite is influenced by wind, humidity and duration of exposure, as well as by temperature. The frozen area begins along the upper and outer edges of the auricle, which becomes yellow-white and waxy in appearance and cold and hard to the touch. This appearance combined with **loss of cutaneous sensation** is diagnostic of frostbite.

### Etiology and Pathology of Frostbite

True tissue freezing starts with the formation of miniscule particles of ice in the extracellular spaces and continues with the accretion of more ice crystals as water is drawn out of the surrounding cells and into the extracellular spaces. This ice crystal formation takes place at the time of freezing and again during thawing. This process of ice crystal growth causes cellular compression and cell membrane rupture, while the most serious effect of extracellular ice crystal growth may be the loss of intracellular fluid with resulting intracellular damage.

As long as a tissue part is frozen, it is in a state of metabolic standstill; many of the gross and cellular changes occur with thawing, when ice crystal formation is actually enhanced, with formation of larger extracellular crystals and further tissue damage. Slow thawing results in prolonged intravascular changes, with clumping of red cells and thromboses of small vessels occluding the distal vascular tree.

### Treatment of Frostbite

The extent of injury to the auricle may not be readily apparent. Only sometime after treatment will the true extent of damage be known. The current therapeutic approach to frostbite, which differs from traditional therapy, evolved from the experimental work of Dr. Harold T. Meryman[1] and the clinical trials of Dr. W. J. Mills.[2]

The treatment is designed to prevent the accretion of extracellular ice crystal formation during thawing and to pass the auricle through the thawing process with as little ice crystal formation as possible. The auricle is better left frozen until it can be **rapidly** thawed, taking care to prevent thawing and refreezing. This can be accomplished with rapid thawing in water at 100 to 108° F. This temperature is sufficiently warm to dissolve the ice rapidly but not so warm as to cause undue discomfort or tissue damage. The auricle should not be massaged as this will cause further mechanical damage and ice crystal formation.

With the rapid thawing a pink flush will appear, and it is not unusual for painful sensation to return. Analgesics may be required during this process. Blebs and blisters may form with the return of sensation (Fig. 8–1). These are sterile and should not be opened. Tetanus toxoid should be administered. Treatment should be open and non-occlusive. The ear should be washed gently with pHisoHex in warm water twice daily. The blebs generally break on the third to seventh day and will dry in a dark, firm eschar. The eschar should not be manipulated except for gentle washing,

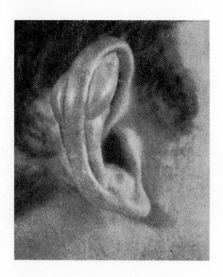

**Figure 8–1**    Frostbite of ear. (From Lederer, F. L.: Diseases of Ear, Nose and Throat, 6th ed., Philadelphia, F. A. Davis, 1952.)

and it generally falls off, with healing having taken place underneath. Antibiotics are not used unless infection develops; steroids are not used and may be contraindicated.

In summary, frostbite treatment consists of keeping the tissue frozen until it can be thawed **once** rapidly. It should then be kept clean and open. Allow for spontaneous separation of non-viable tissue.


## Hematoma

Trauma to the auricle with extravasation of blood beneath the skin and periosteum produces a hematoma of the auricle. The smooth rounded swelling of a hematoma (Fig. 8–2) is not likely to be confused with the diffuse indurated inflammatory swelling of perichondritis.


### Treatment

If it is not evacuated, a hematoma of the auricle proceeds to organize, producing the permanent deformity of "cauliflower ear." Evacuation of the blood clot should be carried out under **careful sterile precautions** by means of an incision along the fold of the helix. A curet may be needed to remove adherent clot; then a pressure bandage is applied for several days using rolls of vaselined cotton fitted to the contours of the auricle.

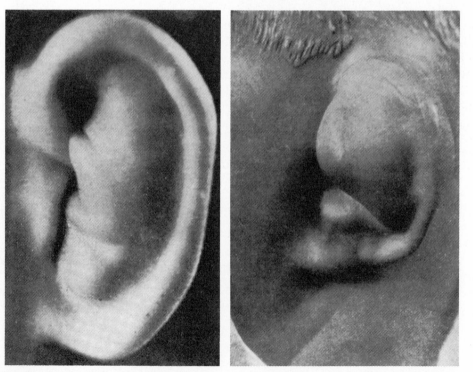

**Figure 8–2**    Hematomas of ear. (From Lederer, F. L.: Diseases of Ear, Nose and Throat, 6th ed. Philadelphia, F. A. Davis, 1952.)

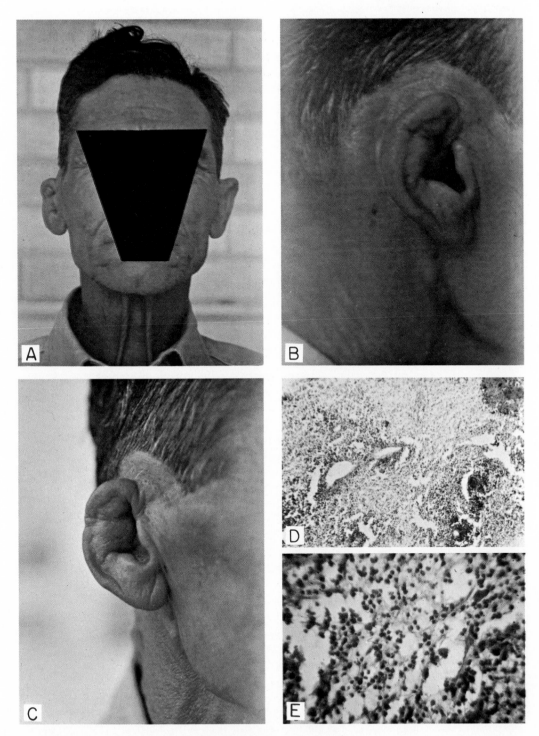

**Figure 8–3**   Leprosy of auricle. *A*, Appearance of patient after 375 days on sodium sulfoxone for leprosy of right ear. *B*, Lateral view of healed right ear. *C*, Oblique view of right ear. *D*, Biopsy from ear removed before treatment (×100) showing dense inflammatory infiltrate. *E*, Enlargement of biopsy showing large foamy "lepra" cells of lepromatous leprosy (×450). The finding of acid-fast bacilli in nests and clumps confirmed the diagnosis. (From Storrs, L. A.: Hansen's disease of the external ear. Arch. Otol., 79:530, 1964.)

**Leprosy**

A rare cause for chronic inflammatory enlargement of the auricle with ulceration and discharge is Hansen's disease or **leprosy.** Tissue biopsy showing large, foamy lipoid-containing cells and giant cells in a dense inflammatory round cell infiltration containing acid-fast bacilli in nests and clumps establishes the correct diagnosis.[3]

Sodium sulfoxone (Diasone), 330 mg. orally daily for as long as a year to prevent recurrences, has resulted in healing of an ulcerated auricle with contraction and deformity (Fig. 8–3).

**Perichondritis**

Perichondritis of the auricle may follow an operation such as a radical mastoidectomy or it may occur as a complication of hematoma or of external otitis, especially that caused by swimming in contaminated water. The causative organism is *Pseudomonas aeruginosa* (B. pyocyaneus), commonly found in cholesteatomas and cases of external otitis.

*Diagnosis and Treatment*

An indurated, tender, dusky-red thickening of the auricle to two or three times its normal thickness beginning several days after an operation on the ear or during an external otitis, with a greenish or brownish musty-smelling discharge from the meatus and a positive culture for *Pseudomonas aeruginosa*, is diagnostic of perichondritis. Perichondritis untreated tends to run a protracted and indolent course, often ending in a thickened contracted deformity of the auricle. It should not be confused with leprosy of the auricle, which causes a chronic deforming inflammatory thickening and is diagnosed by biopsy.[3]

The pseudomonal external otitis causing perichondritis should be treated by irrigations of the meatus several times daily with 1 per cent acetic acid in 70 per cent alcohol, followed by Colymycin ear drops. Exposure of the auricle to ultraviolet irradiation, twice the mild erythema dose, repeated two days later, has been effective in all four cases encountered by the senior author, without the need for surgical intervention, and without resultant deformity. Carbenicillin (Geocillin) administered by mouth, two tablets 4 times a day, is a valuable adjunct to treatment. Garamycin intramuscularly according to body weight and kidney function is ototoxic, and if used, must be administered cautiously, observing the patient for vertigo, tinnitus and hearing loss (Fig. 8–4).

Surgical management should be used if response to ultraviolet irradiation, carbenicillin, meatal irrigation and Colymycin drops is not prompt (within 48 hours) and consists of incision and drainage of the auricle.

The incisions are made in such a manner as to allow the insertion of small polyethylene catheters under the perichondrium (Fig. 8–5). Perforations have been made in these in order to allow the nurse to irrigate the wound several times a day with 1.5 per cent acetic acid followed by Garamycin. A large mastoid dressing is applied over the auricle to allow it to soak in these solutions.

Prompt attention to perichondritis should result in a resolution of the infection without deformity (cauliflower ear).

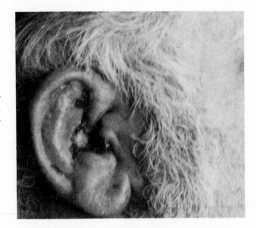

**Figure 8–4**  Perichondritis secondary to a neglected pseudomonas-infected fenestration cavity. Resolved with 1% acetic acid irrigations of the meatus, ultraviolet irradiation and carbenicillin.

## Erysipelas

Erysipelas of the auricle or surrounding skin, like erysipelas elsewhere, is due to a spreading hemolytic streptococcus infection of the dermis. It may follow an operation on a hemolytic streptococcus otitis media, or it may be due to contamination of a surgical or accidental wound in a previously uninfected ear.

### Diagnosis and Treatment

A slowly advancing, red, slightly tender, indurated area of skin, with a rather sharp, slightly elevated border that is redder than the older central area, which becomes brownish, is sufficiently characteristic to leave little doubt of the diagnosis. Except in the mildest infections, malaise, toxemia and fever are prominent symptoms of erysipelas.

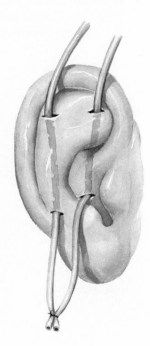

**Figure 8–5**  Incisions are made in the skin of the auricle to allow insertion of small catheters in the perichondrium.

Formerly a dreaded surgical complication because of its considerable mortality rate, this hemolytic streptococcus infection responds quickly to penicillin or erythromycin. Cases occurring in the hospital are contagious, and the patient should be isolated.

## Sebaceous Cyst

The loose skin behind the lobule of the auricle is rich in sebaceous glands and is a frequent site for a sebaceous cyst. Other common sites are the concha or floor of the meatus and the skin below the auricle.

### Diagnosis and Treatment

A sebaceous cyst produces a soft, slightly fluctuant, rounded swelling in the dermis and offers little difficulty in diagnosis. If it is merely incised and evacuated, it always recurs. It is necessary to enucleate the cyst with its walls and contents intact, using a fine scissors and a microscope or magnifying loupe to aid in this meticulous dissection. If the cyst is acutely infected, excision of it and its walls should be deferred until the acute inflammation has subsided.

## Keloid

Keloid formation around the ear is not uncommon in dark-skinned people, especially Negroes. The overgrowth of connective tissue follows any sort of trauma to the skin, and frequently occurs in the lobe as the result of piercing for earrings (Fig. 8–6). It may also occur in the scar of a postaural or endaural incision. An elevated, slightly reddened and slightly tender indurated scar that becomes more protuberant with time, rather than less prominent as normally happens with healing, is due to keloid formation. When it occurs following an endaural incision, it often causes a stenosis or atresia of the meatus.

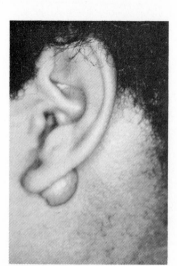

**Figure 8–6**  Keloid of ear.

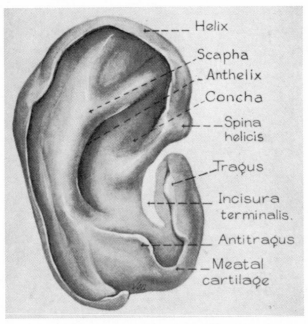

**Figure 8–7**   Auricular cartilage.

## Treatment

A keloid that is unsightly or that causes stenosis or atresia of the meatus should be excised; excision should be followed immediately by 300 r of roentgen irradiation of the area to prevent a recurrence.

## Lop Ears

Abnormal protrusion of the auricle, known as **lop ear,** is a common anomaly of the external ear, with a definite hereditary predisposition.[4] In this respect it differs from congenital atresia with microtia, which is rarely hereditary. Its importance is in its psychic effect on the person, since it produces reactions of mirth in other people

The degree of protrusion of the auricle is determined by the angle between the scapha and the concha produced by the anthelix (Fig. 8–7). When the fold of the anthelix is absent or poorly developed, the auricle protrudes away from the head. Any surgical procedure for lop ear that fails to construct a normal-appearing anthelix will fail to produce a normal-appearing auricle.

### Indications for Surgical Correction

Surgical correction of lop ear is indicated when the deformity is sufficient to cause a psychologic disturbance in the patient. As a rule a child is especially bothered by such a deformity, and correction will be indicated during childhood.

## Technique

The method described by Becker[4] is preferable to previously described, somewhat simpler techniques.[5] It creates a normal-appearing auricle by creating an anthelix at the same time as it corrects the abnormal protrusion. Simply "pinning the auricle back" by excising a strip of postauricular skin and connective tissue will be doomed to failure because the uncorrected spring of the cartilage again pulls the member away from the side of the head.

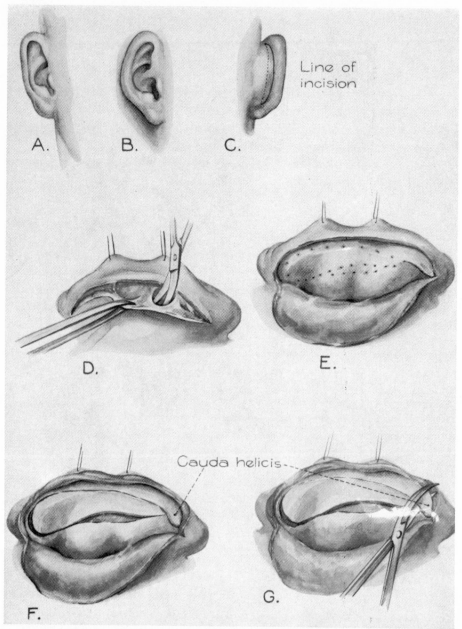

**Figure 8–8**  Surgical technique for correction of lop ears. *A*, Ear from in front before correction. *B*, Same, lateral view. *C*, From behind, with skin incision, solid line. Dotted line indicates area of skin removal. *D*, Elevation of skin and perichondrium. *E*, Needle punctures marked by gentian violet to indicate borders of new anthelix. *F*, Cartilage incision with small semilunar excisions. *G*, Excision of cauda helicis. (Continued on opposite page.)

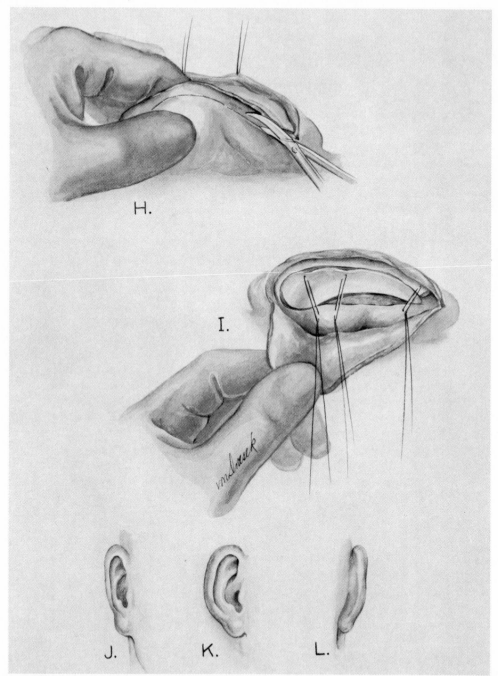

**Figure 8–8** (*Continued*)    Surgical technique for correction of lop ears. *H*, Excision of excess strip of skin behind ear. *I*, Sutures through perichondrium, to be tied after ear is in corrected position. *J*, Corrected ear from in front. *K*, Same, lateral view. *L*, Same, from behind. (Operation by Dr. Ira J. Tresley.)

**Anesthesia and Skin Incision.** Following the usual preoperative sterilization of the auricle and surrounding area, as described in Chapter 6, the skin surrounding the auricle on all sides is infiltrated with 1 per cent Xylocaine containing 1:5000 Adrenalin. Additional solution is injected into the skin of the posterior surface of the auricle and on the anterior surface of the anthelix, for hemostasis.

A curved vertical incision through skin and perichondrium, but not through the cartilage, is made on the posterior surface of the auricle near its outer edge, from the junction of the auricle and the scalp above to the base of the antitragus close to the mastoid region (Fig. 8–8C). The skin and perichondrium are then elevated backward from the entire auricular cartilage almost to the postauricular fold (Fig. 8–8D).

**Creation of Anthelix.** If the auricle is folded back against the head into a normal position, a new anthelix is observed on the anterior surface. A hypodermic or straight skin suture needle dipped in methylene blue or brilliant green is then used to make two vertical rows of punctures from the anterior to the posterior side, marking the anterior and posterior borders of the new anthelix (Fig. 8–8E). At the upper end the punctures converge to a curved apex, and also at the lower end. An incision is then made through the cartilage along each row of punctures from the posterior aspect, avoiding going through the skin on the anterior surface. By means of additional incisions a narrow diamond-shaped piece of cartilage is outlined and then removed (Fig. 8–8F). This is to overcome the spring of the auricular cartilage; the width of the piece removed varies from 6 to 9 mm. In most cases the lower end of the cartilage of the helix, the cauda helicis, should then be removed to complete the breaking of the spring of the auricular cartilage (Fig. 8–8G). In some cases a small section of cartilage must also be removed from the upper and lower ends of the rows of punctures. If the auricle does not now fold back smoothly and without spring, partial crosshatching of the remaining cartilage between the two rows of punctures may be needed to weaken it.

**Sutures.** Three or four surgical gut mattress-type sutures are now placed through the edges of the cartilage on either side of the rows of punctures (Fig. 8–8I) and tied just tightly enough to form a new anthelix fold. A strip of excess skin is removed from the reflected postaural flap (Fig. 8–8H) and the skin is closed with interrupted fine black silk sutures. Sterile wet cotton strips are placed along the convolutions of the auricle on the anterior surface, and a fairly snug pressure bandage is applied and left for a week, when the silk skin sutures are removed and a light mastoid bandage is applied for another week. For the third week the patient wears a tight-fitting stocking cap at night to hold the ear back (Figs. 8–8J, K and L and Fig. 8–9).

A more recent variation of this procedure has been described by Tardy.[6] An incision is made on the posterior surface of the auricle with minimal undermining; to facilitate postauricular scar formation in the posterior trough formed by the neoanthelical fold, the periosteum is not stripped bare of subcutaneous tissue. This postauricular scar produces the strength of the repair. The neoanthelical fold is produced with thumb and index finger and outlined with temporary marking sutures (4-0 black silk) passed from anterior to posterior to indicate the precise position for the permanent mattress sutures. (This eliminates the need for ink marking.) (Figs. 8–10, 8–11, 8–12, 8–13)

Using the black silk sutures as a guide, transperichondrial horizontal mattress sutures (4-0 braided white nylon) are positioned sequentially along the neoanthelical fold from caudal to cephalic (Figs. 8–14 and 8–15). The suture must encompass both the anterior and posterior perichondrium in order to prevent ultimate tearing through of the suture. In most cases, at least four horizontal mattress sutures are required.

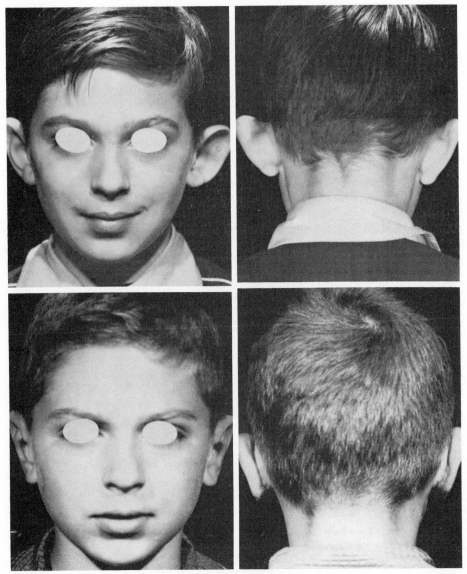

**Figure 8–9**    Bilateral lop ears before and after correction. Observe absence of preoperative anthelix especially on patient's left ear. (Courtesy of Dr. Ira J. Tresley.)

Each suture must be test-tightened to assess its effect, and each can be readjusted to produce the most natural effect.

An auricle that has deep cavum conchae may require the excision of a semilunar segment of cartilage at this point to properly construct the neoanthelix.

Following meticulous hemostasis, a continuous running intradermal monofilament nylon suture is used to close the postauricular incision (Fig. 8–16). This is removed in 10 to 14 days. Drains are not used, but a light compression bandage comprised of mineral oil-soaked cotton, gauze fluffs and Kerlex wrap-around gauze is employed. The initial bandage is changed the morning following surgery, and another is applied for 36 to 72 hours. A nylon stocking cap is recommended for sleep over the ensuing weeks.

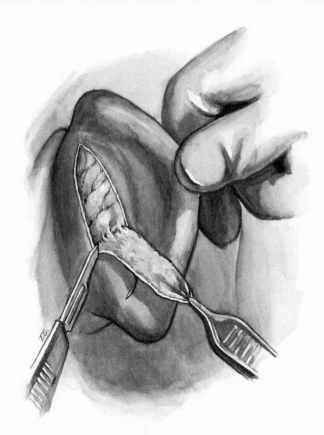

## DORSAL SKIN EXCISION
### Figure 8–10

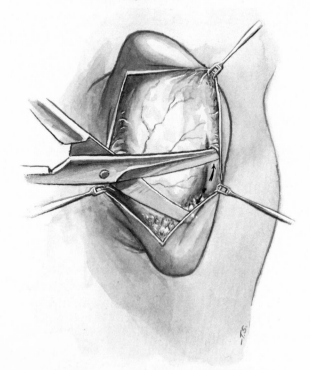

## DORSAL SKIN UNDERMINING
### Figure 8–11

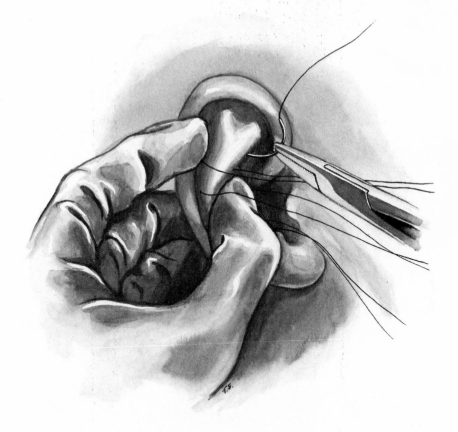

## PREPLACED SUTURES
### Figure 8–12

### Congenital Preauricular Cyst and Fistula

A pit-like depression just in front of the helix and above the tragus is a common remnant of the embryonic fusion of the first and second branchial arches to produce the auricle (see Chapters 1 and 14). Not infrequently the depression leads to a cyst, or there may be an epidermal-lined fistulous tract with an intermittent or continuous scant foul discharge (see Fig. 14–5). The condition is often bilateral and has a familial predisposition.

### Treatment

Treatment consists of surgical dissection and excision of the epithelial-lined tract and cyst. This is easiest if the cyst is not expressed for several days before surgery, and if the fistula is first closed by a suture to prevent extrusion of the cyst contents. A vertical and horizontal incision is made just behind and above the fistula, forming a triangular flap that when pulled down reveals the entire cyst structure, which is excised intact to the fistulous opening.

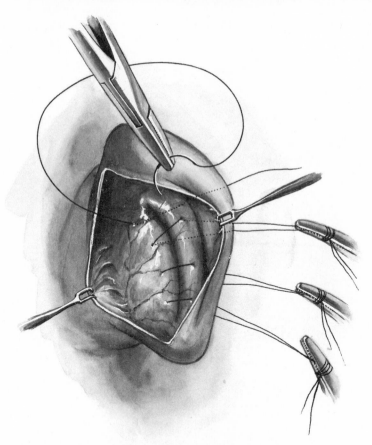

PREPLACED SUTURES

Figure 8–13

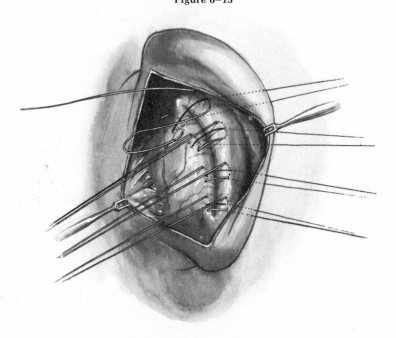

TRANSPERICHONDRIAL

MATTRESS SUTURES

Figure 8–14

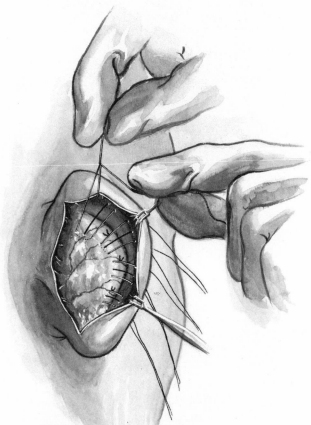

TRANSPERICHONDRIAL
MATTRESS SUTURE LIGATION
Figure 8–15

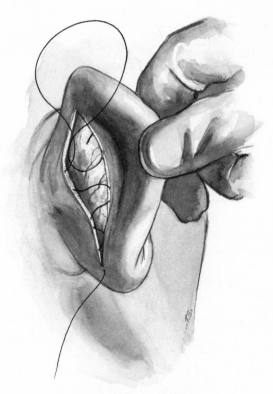

## WOUND CLOSURE
### Figure 8–16

## SURGICAL CONDITIONS OF THE MEATUS

### Exostosis and Osteoma

Nodular bony outgrowths from the osseous meatus, usually sessile, multiple and bilateral, are a common incidental finding on otoscopic inspection, and are known as **exostoses** or **hyperostoses;** the former name is usually applied to discrete nodules, and the latter is used for more diffuse bony elevations of the wall of the osseous meatus. Since there is not a clearly defined distinction between exostosis and hyperostosis of the meatus, and since both have a common etiology, the term **exostosis** will be used in this text. **Osteoma** of the meatus is the relatively rare occurrence of a unilateral, single and sometimes pedunculated bony tumor of the osseous meatus.[7]

### *Etiology*

Exostoses of the meatus were first related to swimming in cold water by van Gilse.[8] Fowler and Osmun[9] confirmed this observation and were able to produce new

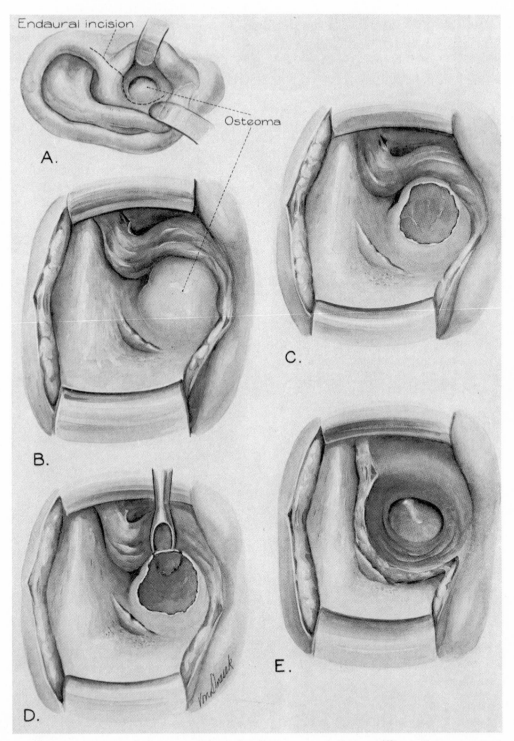

**Figure 8–17** Removal of osteoma of external auditory meatus. *A*, Osteoma filling entire osseous meatus. *B*, Skin and periosteum reflected forward to expose the osteoma. *C*, Osteoma hollowed out with dental burr; only a thin shell is left. *D*, Remaining walls of osteoma fractured inward by curet; skin of meatus is preserved. *E*, Skin replaced after removal of osteoma.

formation of bone on the most exposed portion of the promontory of guinea pigs by two to nine weekly irrigations of the external auditory meatus for 1 hour with water at 19° C. (67.5° F). So close is the relationship between cold water exposure and exostoses of the inner end of the osseous meatus that the otologist will seldom be mistaken in surmising (to the patient's amazement) that he has been an ardent swimmer in relatively cold water (see Fig. 7–5F).

### Diagnosis and Treatment

Multiple exostoses are nearly always bilateral and appear as hard, smooth, rounded whitish nodules that lie close to the sulcus tympanicus, resulting in a greater or lesser narrowing of the osseous meatus, and rarely in occlusion of the meatus. An osteoma appears as a single bony nodule on one side only, and it may occur near the outer portion of the osseous meatus and may have a covering of somewhat thickened skin.

When exostoses or an osteoma causes atresia or sufficient stenosis of the osseous meatus to produce retention of epidermal debris and a conductive hearing impairment, they should be removed surgically. This is best accomplished through the usual endaural incision extending upward above the meatus (Fig. 8–17A). The skin and periosteum covering the bony tumor should be carefully elevated from it (Fig. 8–17B) and the tumor removed with a small, round cutting dental-type burr, until the normal contour of the bony canal has been restored. To prevent injury to the underlying tympanic membrane or even to the facial nerve in the case of a large bony tumor, the latter may be hollowed out with the dental-type burr until only a shell remains (Fig. 8–17C). With a small No. 000 curet the walls may then be fractured inward as the skin and periosteum are separated and preserved (Fig. 8–17D and E). Should the preservation of sufficient skin and periosteum to cover the denuded area be unsuccessful, a small split thickness Thiersch skin graft from the posterior surface of the auricle may be applied (Fig. 8–18).

### Cicatricial Stenosis and Acquired Atresia

Cicatricial stenosis or atresia of the meatus may follow external trauma; it may be the result of a simple mastoid operation in which the skin and periosteum of the

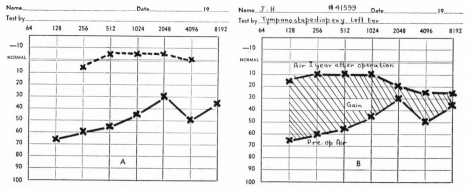

**Figure 8–18**  *A*, Preoperative audiograms of patient with osteoma illustrated in Figure 8–17. *B*, Four weeks postoperative audiogram of the same patient, showing gain.

osseous meatus were elevated and not reapplied with pressure packing; it may follow an endaural operation in which the incision was allowed to close too rapidly; and it may be due to a keloid in the scar of an endaural incision. An interesting type of cicatricial atresia of the bony meatus follows a prolonged external otitis in which the epidermis of the osseous meatus and outer surface of the tympanic membrane has ulcerated and sloughed. Healing eventually occurs as a blind skin-lined pouch that ends lateral to the tympanic membrane, the intervening space being filled with loose or dense fibrous tissue.

## Diagnosis and Treatment

The history will indicate whether the atresia is congenital or acquired. Congenital atresia is often associated with other developmental malformations of the outer and middle ear and will be considered in Chapter 14.

The only symptom of acquired atresia is the conductive hearing impairment, unless, of course, there is persistent discharge from an active external otitis.

The treatment of cicatricial atresia of the meatus is surgical removal of the pathologic fibrous tissue without injury to the tympanic membrane, followed by the application of skin grafts to the denuded area. The outer edge of the osseous meatus is first exposed by the usual endaural incision extending upward from the meatus. The skin of the atresia is incised vertically, permitting the elevation of two triangular skin flaps and exposing the osseous meatus filled with fibrous tissue (Fig. 8–19). The problem now is to remove this fibrous tissue down to the outermost circular fibers of the pars tensa of the tympanic membrane without destroying the latter. This may be accomplished by carefully elevating the mass of fibrous tissue from the upper posterior quadrant of the osseous meatus using a narrow periosteal elevator until the latter is felt to reach the notch of Rivinus. The notch is enlarged sufficiently by removal of a rim of bone to obtain a view into the upper part of the tympanic cavity (Fig. 8–19C), similar to the bone removal used to visualize the stapes footplate (see Chapter 18). With the medial surface of the pars tensa in view as the landmark, it is not difficult to peel the fibrous tissue of the atresia from the radial and circular fibers of the pars tensa (Fig. 8–19F). Should the osseous meatus thus exposed be found to be narrow, it may be widened safely by concentric removal of bone from the anterior and inferior meatal walls. The gap between the upper edge of the pars tensa and the bony meatal wall should be bridged with a small full thickness skin graft from behind the ear, using split thickness skin grafts to cover the remainder of the denuded osseous meatus and tympanic membrane. These grafts should be held in place with strips of surgical rayon and small cotton balls moistened in Gantrisin otic solution, placed **without pressure** against the grafts and left in place for a week to 10 days.

Immediate postoperative prophylactic roentgen irradiation — 300 r — retards fibrosis and thus helps to prevent a recurrence of the atresia.

## Furuncle

Furuncle occurs in the cartilaginous hair-bearing portion of the meatus owing to staphylococcus infection of a hair follicle, frequently after swimming in contaminated water.

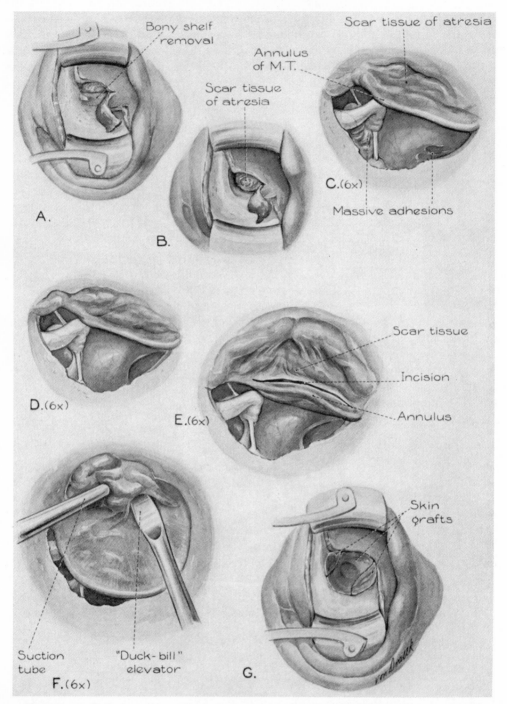

**Figure 8–19**   Technique of correcting recurrent acquired atresia. *A*, Incision through skin of atresia. *B*, Bony shelf removed, meatus enlarged. *C*, Middle ear and upper edge of tympanic membrane exposed under operating microscope. Scar tissue fills both window niches. *D*, Scar tissue removed from oval and round window niches. *E*, Incision between tympanic membrane and scar tissue of atresia. *F*, Dissection of scar tissue from fibrous layer of tympanic membrane. *G*, Split thickness grafts applied.

*Diagnosis*

Because of the tight adherence of skin to periosteum in the meatus, furuncle here is exceptionally painful, and may be confused with a surgical mastoiditis. The marked tenderness on compression of the cartilaginous meatus from below and the normal hearing as long as the meatus is patent serve to differentiate a furuncle from a mastoiditis.

*Treatment*

Rarely if ever does a furuncle of the meatus need to be incised. The application of dry heat and the use of Gantrisin otic solution ear drops may be supplemented by a cotton pack inserted into the meatus and kept moist with the same solution. If the furuncle begins to discharge, the purulent material should be carefully cleaned out and bor-alcohol ear drops used to prevent reinfection. Resistance to the causative staphylococcus may be enhanced by subcutaneous injections of staphylococcus toxoid 0.01 unit to 0.1 unit once a week.

## Foreign Body

Most foreign bodies in the external auditory meatus can be removed easily by instrumentation with a blunt ear hook, or by syringing with warm water. Should the foreign body become wedged at or beyond the isthmus, rather than traumatize the meatus and risk injury to the tympanic membrane, it is far better to hospitalize the patient and under local or general anesthesia to make an endaural incision extending upward from the meatus. The bony meatus containing the foreign body is thus brought to the surface, greatly facilitating removal of the object.

## Polyp

A polyp filling the external auditory meatus nearly always originates from the middle ear or a cholesteatoma in the epitympanum. In rare cases a polyp may arise from the bony meatus or outer surface of the tympanic membrane. A polyp may be the first evidence of carcinoma or a glomus jugulare tumor. It has been said that a polyp should never be avulsed forcibly, since it may arise from a fistula of the labyrinth and pulling on it may induce a suppurative labyrinthitis or might avulse an adherent stapes.

*Diagnosis and Treatment*

Until the polyp is removed it is impossible to determine its character and its source. Except in small children a polyp can be removed as an office procedure using topical anesthesia with 10 per cent cocaine in freshly prepared aniline. Using an ear snare, the polyp should be cut off as close to its base as possible, avoiding forcible avulsion. The physician should be prepared for profuse bleeding requiring a tight meatal pack in case the polyp arises from a glomus jugulare tumor. Having removed the polyp in one or several pieces, the physician can then determine whether it comes from the meatus, from the outer surface of an intact tympanic membrane or from the middle ear, and it should **always** be examined histologically so as not to overlook an early malignant tumor. Since a polyp may arise from the mucosa of the promontory in benign chronic suppurative otitis media, as well as from the attic in cases of bone-eroding disease, one is not justified in proceeding with a radical mastoidectomy in every polyp complicating a chronic otorrhea.

### Caries or Localized Necrosis of the Osseous Meatus

A chronic ulcer with a base of roughened bone is sometimes observed in the osseous meatus. It may complicate a chronic external otitis, follow a surgical procedure or occur spontaneously. Frequent and repeated cleaning and the application to the ulcer of 2 per cent aqueous gentian violet may result in healing by epidermization. If not, the roughened bone at the base of the ulcer should be gently curetted. An endaural incision extending upward from the meatus will facilitate the procedure in a narrow meatus. **Biopsy** of granulations from the margin of an ulcer should be done to exclude carcinoma.

### Cholesteatoma of the External Auditory Meatus

Keratitis obliterans is a rare and interesting condition of the osseous meatus, with the accumulation of layers of desquamated epithelium that gradually fill the meatus with a mass of cholesteatoma debris. Bone erosion results in a gradual enlargement of the osseous meatus exactly as occurs in cholesteatoma of the attic and mastoid. The cause of the condition is not known. By periodic removal of accumulated debris further bone erosion may be retarded. The simple application of three to four drops of baby oil twice daily will help prevent debris buildup and facilitate its removal. The ear canal should be thoroughly cleansed using magnification in the office at three-month intervals.

### Acute and Chronic Infections of the External Auditory Meatus

Acute infections (bacterial) of the external auditory meatus are commonly known as "swimmer's ear" and are usually very painful. These are seen most frequently in the summer months. The canal skin is swollen, and many times the meatus is occluded. Any motion of the auricle produces excruciating pain. Treatment consists of a cotton wick (or the new cellulose expanding wicks) inserted carefully into the canal. This wick is left saturated with Domeboro* solution for 24 hours. During this period the swelling subsides, and the pain is relieved. Antibiotic drops of Colymycin are then used for approximately one week. At this time the

---

*Chemical name: aluminum acetate and calcium acetate.

patient comes into the office to have the wick removed if it has not already fallen out of the ear of its own accord.

During treatment and for three weeks after the swelling has subsided, the patient is instructed to keep water out of the ear canal.

Chronic infections of the external auditory meatus are usually due to fungal organisms and have a tendency to recurrence. Many of these patients do not produce cerumen, and the skin of their canals is very dry and easily irritated. Also, many of these patients are chronic cotton swab users and often abrade the skin overlying the osseous meatus.

Once the infection has been brought under control with 2 per cent aqueous gentian violet or Colymycin antibiotic drops, the individual should be instructed as how best to prevent reinfection. These patients should not allow water to enter the ear canal at any time and should give up water sports or use "swimmer's drops."* When washing their hair, cotton covered with Vaseline should be inserted into the external auditory meatus. Twice a day a small amount of Vaseline should be placed into the canal, and the patient should refrain from using bobby pins, paper clips and cotton swabs to scratch the ear canal.

In older individuals and in any resistant case, the skin of the canal should be biopsied to rule out carcinoma of the external auditory meatus.

Skin testing for Trichophytin-Oidiomycin-Epidermophytin (T.O.E.) will often prove positive in resistant cases and will require skin titration and optimum dosage desensitization. These individuals will often have an accompanying fungus infection elsewhere on the body.

House dust and specific food allergies account for many cases of resistant severe external otitis, which respond dramatically to allergic management.

There are rare cases of chronic external otitis that will not respond to any medical regimen and require surgical intervention. The technique involves stripping the external auditory meatus of its skin down to the tympanic membrane and replacing it with a skin graft.

A very special category of infections involving the external auditory meatus is caused by pseudomonas in a diabetic. Known as malignant otitis externa,[10] the condition is fatal if proper therapy is not instituted as soon as it is recognized. Facial paralysis is often a presenting symptom and indicates involvement of the bone. The infection can spread through the skull base and become inoperable if the condition is not recognized.

Garamycin and carbenicillin in high doses must be administered for a sufficient period of time (usually 2 weeks) and continued for one more week after evidence of infection has cleared. Should the infection not respond to these drugs, then a radical mastoidectomy with wide debridement of the external auditory meatus and skull base must be carried out.

## SURGICAL CONDITIONS OF THE TYMPANIC MEMBRANE

### Myringitis Bullosa

Myringitis bullosa is caused by a virus, and may occur by itself or in association with an acute suppurative otitis media. The serous or hemorrhagic blebs on the

---

* Dow-Corning "200 Fluid," a silicone liquid.

tympanic membrane and adjacent meatal wall cause severe pain because of distention of the inflamed epidermis. Fever is mild or absent and the hearing is not affected, as long as there is not an accompanying otitis media.

### Treatment

Except for superficial puncture of the blebs to relieve severe pain, avoiding perforation of the tympanic membrane, bullous myringitis without suppurative otitis media requires no therapy.

## Myringotomy for Acute Suppurative Otitis Media

Myringotomy by incision of the pars tensa of the tympanic membrane is indicated for cases of acute suppurative otitis media with exudate under pressure in the tympanum (see Fig. 7–1). The etiology, pathology and symptoms of this condition were described in Chapter 7. When the pain and fever are mild, a preliminary trial on antibacterial therapy alone may be employed for 24 hours, and in many cases the acute infection will clear without a myringotomy. In all severe infections with a thickened, bulging drum membrane, severe pain, fever and mastoid tenderness, and in persisting or recurring infections that do not clear completely after antibacterial therapy, a myringotomy should be done.

### Technique of Myringotomy

For infants no anesthesia should be used; the arms and legs should be confined by being wrapped in a sheet or cotton blanket "mummy fashion" while an assistant holds the head. For children and adults a brief general anesthesia, using vinyl ether or nitrous oxide by inhalation or Pentothal by intravenous injection, will permit the operation to be done painlessly. The local application of 10 per cent cocaine in freshly prepared aniline is not very effective for an acutely inflamed and thickened tympanic membrane, but may be better than nothing.

Myringotomy should always be done under direct vision and **never blindly,** because of the risk of injuring the facial nerve or stapes. An incision 2 or 3 mm. long should be made in the **posterior inferior quadrant** of the pars tensa and should be deep enough to go entirely through a thickened membrane (Fig. 8–20). As a rule the bone of the promontory will be felt with the tip of the knife. The tip of the knife should immediately be cultured, with antibiotic sensitivity tests, for this is the best opportunity for determining the causative organism and the most appropriate antibacterial agent.

## Myringotomy and Ventilation Tube for Secretory (Serous) Otitis Media

Secretory (serous) otitis media is a non-bacterial accumulation of clear (rarely cloudy) straw-colored serous or tenacious mucoid fluid in the tympanic cavity and pneumatic cells, as a result of eustachian tube occlusion often with an allergic basis (see Fig. 7–5D). The etiology and pathology of this non-inflammatory otitis media were described in Chapter 7. Myringotomy may be indicated for both diagnosis and treatment.

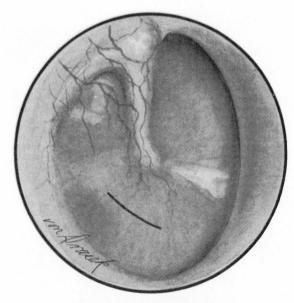

**Figure 8–20**   Site of myringotomy.

Diagnostic myringotomy for possible secretory (serous) otitis media should be considered whenever there is a conductive hearing loss and a thickened tympanic membrane preventing otoscopic visualization of a fluid level, or when otoscopy reveals the characteristic straw-colored fluid with a chalky white manubrium. Tympanometry will aid in the diagnosis of fluid in the tympanum (see Chapter 3).

Therapeutic myringotomy with insertion of a ventilating or grommet tube (see Fig. 8–21) is done whenever a secretory (serous) otitis media lasts more than a week and fails to clear after one or two eustachian tube inflations and with management of an accompanying food or inhalant allergic rhinitis.

### Technique of Myringotomy for Serous Otitis

Generally myringotomy is performed in conjunction with the insertion of a ventilating tube. Infants and small children are best managed by performing this procedure under a general anesthetic. In older children and adults, a local anesthetic may be employed. The best method for this technique is to use one of the new **electrophoresis** machines now available (Fig. 8–21).[11]

Four per cent Xylocaine with Adrenalin 1:1,000,000 is placed into the ear canal and an active electrode inserted. An indifferent electrode is attached to the arm and the machine turned on. An electrical current flows between the electrodes, driving the solution through the normally intact skin of the external auditory meatus and tympanic membrane. The whole procedure takes about 10 minutes and is quite effective.

The incision in the tympanic membrane can be made in the **anterior inferior quadrant** if the tube is to remain in place for a long period of time or in the **posterior inferior quadrant** if a short time is desired. There are a wide variety of ventilating tubes available through commercial sources. Depending upon the design of the tube, it will stay in the eardrum from 1 to 2 months up to 5 to 6 years. A straight polyethylene tube will seldom remain in the drum for over 2 months, while a

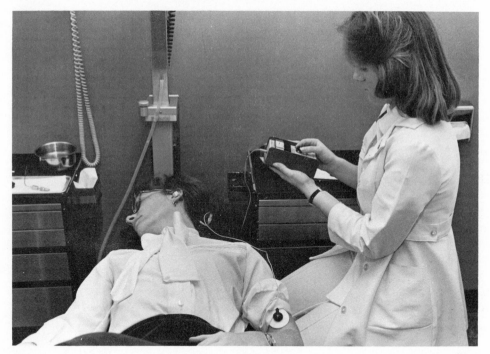

**Figure 8–21**　A patient's eardrum membrane is being anesthetized by means of electrophoresis.

grommet-type tube is more likely to stay in place for 8 to 12 months (Fig. 8–22). Perlee[12] tubes are known for their ability to function for years. The latter is used only in long-standing eustachian tube problems and is preferable to multiple myringotomies.

### Traumatic Perforations

Abrupt change in air pressure in the meatus produced by a blow with the cupped hand (of loving spouse), by an explosion, by strong eustachian tube inflation or by barotrauma may result in an irregular tear of the pars tensa. The symptom is a sudden "pop" in the ear followed by a hearing impairment. On inspection a jagged or linear, rarely a circular, tear is seen, sometimes with tiny points of hemorrhage along the margins. Traumatic perforation may also occur during stapes operations while the tympanomeatal flap is being elevated, or during fenestration, modified radical mastoidectomy or tympanoplasty while the head of the malleus is being amputated.

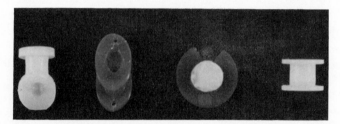

**Figure 8–22**　There are wide varieties of grommet tubes available.

*Treatment*

Immediate application of a disc of cigarette paper (or the blue paper that surgical cotton is wrapped in), moistened with Ringer's solution or 1 per cent phenol in glycerin to make it adhere, will act as a splint preventing the edges from curling under and promoting rapid healing of the tear. The paper should be allowed to fall out of the meatus by itself. An alternate method is to approximate the drum edges and apply a small disc of Steri-Strip tape.

## Chronic Myringitis

Chronic myringitis occurs as part of a chronic external otitis, but is also seen as an isolated lesion of the external surface of the tympanic membrane. A chronic, scant, non-mucoid otorrhea is the symptom. Flat granulations are seen on the thickened but intact tympanic membrane. The normal hearing, failure of air to escape on inflation of the eustachian tube and failure to find an epitympanic perforation serve to differentiate the rare case of otorrhea due to chronic myringitis from the much more frequent cases of chronic suppurative otitis media.

*Treatment*

Repeated cleaning of the meatus followed by the application of 2 per cent aqueous gentian violet to the granulations results in healing by epidermization.

## REFERENCES

1. Meryman, M. T.: Tissue freezing and local cold injury. Physiol. Rev., *37*:233, 1957.
2. Mills, W. J., Whaley, R., and Fish, W.: Frostbite: Experience with rapid rewarming and ultrasonic therapy. Alaska Med. *3*:28, 1961.
3. Storrs, L. A.: Hansen's disease of the external ear. Arch. Otol., *79*:530, 1964.
4. Becker, O. J.: Surgical correction of the abnormally protruding ear. Arch. Otol., *50*:541, 1949.
5. Davis, G. S., and Kitlowski, E. A.: Abnormal prominence of ears: method of readjustment. Surgery, *2*:835, 1937.
6. Tardy, M. E.: Otoplasty. *In* Ballenger, J. J., ed.: Diseases of the Ear, Nose, and Throat 12th ed. Lea & Febiger, Philadelphia, 1977.
7. Kline, O. R., and Pearce, R. C.: Osteoma of the external auditory canal. Arch. Otol., *59*:588, 1954.
8. van Gilse, P. H. G.: Des observations ultérieures sur la genèse des exostoses du conduit externe par l'irriations d'eau froide. Acta Oto-laryng., *26*:343, 1938.
9. Fowler, E. P., Jr., and Osmun, P. M.: New bone growth due to cold water in the ears. Arch. Otol., *36*:455, 1942.
10. Chandler, J. R.: Malignant external otitis. Laryngoscope, *78*:1257, 1968.
11. Echols, D. F., Norris, C. H., and Tabb, H. G.: Anesthesia of the ear by iontophoresis of lidocaine. Arch. Otol., *101*:418, 1975.
12. Perlee, J. H.: Experiences with a "permanent" wire flanged middle ear ventilation tube. Laryngoscope, *79*:581, 1969.

## SUGGESTED ADDITIONAL READING

Brownrigg, G. M.: Frostbite: classification and treatment. Am. J. Surg., *67*:370, 1945.
Lange, K., and Boyd, L. J.: The functional pathology of frostbite and the prevention of gangrene in experimental animals and humans. Science, *102*:151, 1945.
Lele, D. N.: Ultraviolet in hematoma and perichondritis of auricle. Arch. Otol., *79*:33, 1964.
Stevenson, E. W.: Bacillus pyocyaneus perichondritis of the ear. Laryngoscope, *74*:255, 1964.

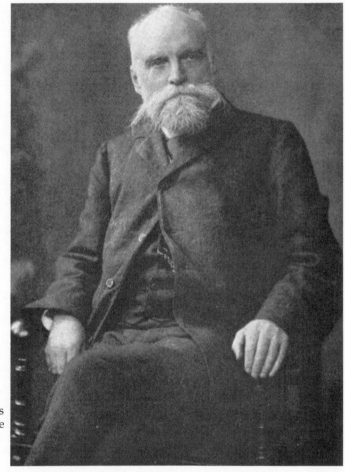

*Hermann Schwartze*

BORN 1837
DIED 1910

Established the indications
and technique of the simple
mastoid operation.

# Chapter 9

# *The Simple Mastoid Operation*

HISTORICAL NOTES
INDICATIONS FOR THE SIMPLE MASTOID OPERATION
TECHNIQUE OF THE SIMPLE MASTOID OPERATION
AFTER-CARE OF THE SIMPLE MASTOID OPERATION
ACCIDENTS DURING SIMPLE MASTOIDECTOMY

The simple mastoid operation to evacuate a coalescent abscess from within the mastoid process is seldom required today. This was formerly the most frequently performed operation upon the temporal bone, and the story of its rise and decline is an interesting one.

## HISTORICAL NOTES

The potential seriousness of ear suppuration was appreciated by Hippocrates, as we saw in Chapter 7, but the idea of operating to relieve the condition seems to have occurred for the first time about four centuries ago to the great medieval surgeon Ambrose Paré. Called to the sickbed of the young King Charles II of France, and finding him delirious, in a high fever and with a discharging ear, barber-surgeon Paré proposed an operation on the skull to drain away the pus. The boy-king's bride, Mary, Queen of Scots and of France, assented, but the king's mother, Catherine de' Medici, forbade an operation, so Mary lost her first husband and her first throne while she was still only 18 years old.[1]

The first recorded successful mastoid operation for the relief of aural suppuration was by Jean Petit[2] of Paris. Independently, a short time afterward in 1776, Jasser, a Prussian military surgeon, successfully operated upon a soldier's mastoid. But the new operation was doomed to a long period of eclipse when Baron Bergen, personal physician to the King of Denmark, hearing of Petit's successful operation, persuaded a surgical colleague to operate upon his mastoid to relieve deafness and tinnitus. It is not surprising that this operation, undertaken in a clean field before any knowledge of surgical asepsis, ended in infection. When Bergen died 12 days later in great pain from the mastoid operation for mistaken indications, the procedure fell into a disrepute that lasted nearly 100 years.[3]

In 1853 Sir William Wilde[4] of Dublin introduced his famous postaural incision for suppuration of the ear with postaural abscess. Still he advised against opening the bone unless there were symptoms threatening to life, and apparently he never carried out a mastoidectomy. It remained for Schwartze[5] in 1873 to describe the indications and technique of the mastoid operation thoroughly enough to overcome the century of prejudice against it. So well did Schwartze succeed that by the end of the nineteenth century the operation had attained general acceptance and such importance that Whiting[6] wrote of it: "As a life saving measure few surgical procedures equal and none surpass in efficiency the modern mastoid operation."

The dread with which a "mastoid operation" was often regarded by the laity came not from the timely interventions by qualified surgeons, but from their efforts to save patients whose infections had already extended beyond the mastoid process and who died despite, not because of, their mastoid operation.

It is true indeed that a skillfully performed and properly indicated mastoidectomy for a well localized coalescent infection proved remarkably effective not only in removing the risk of serious complication from the abscess within the mastoid, but also in very quickly bringing to an end the continued aural suppuration. It needed only the addition of criteria and techniques for dealing with a similar process in the less accessible apex of the petrous pyramid[7-10] to bring this triumph of otologic surgery to final fruition. And almost at that precise moment appeared the revolutionary antibacterial therapy destined to do more for acute coalescent mastoiditis and other complications of acute otitis media than all of the most elaborate and highly developed surgery.

Sulfanilamide was first employed in 1935 in the form of Prontosil for the serious complications of acute ear infection, especially for the almost invariably fatal otitic meningitis. The favorable results that began to follow its use in some of these cases encouraged its application to earlier stages of severe ear infections. At first otologic surgeons were loath to abandon the tried and proved surgical procedures, fearing and predicting that sulfonamides would mask the clinical picture and lead to late dire results. But very soon it became clear that the earlier the sulfonamide, and then the even more effective penicillin, could be given before localized collections of pus had begun to form, the fewer the complications and the indications for surgery.

The credit for the rapid decline of the need for the simple mastoid operation of Schwartze goes to Domagk and Fleming, the discoverers of sulfanilamide and penicillin. But credit should also go to the multitude of family doctors and pediatricians who put these antibacterial agents to such early and effective use that today few acutely infected ears ever drain, and even fewer reach the operating table.

## INDICATIONS FOR THE SIMPLE MASTOID OPERATION

The simple mastoid operation is **indicated** for cases of acute suppurative otitis media that fail to respond to sulfonamide or antibiotic therapy and that proceed to a **coalescent mastoiditis.** In the presulfonamide era the simple mastoid operation was sometimes required for certain early cases of acute suppurative otitis media with a beginning complication by osteothrombophlebitic extension. Today we may rely upon antibacterial medication for the latter group of cases, confining the simple mastoidectomy to cases of coalescent mastoiditis.

In Chapter 7 the pathology of acute suppurative otitis media in its various stages was described, including the stage of coalescent mastoiditis. At this point certain of the fundamental characteristics of mastoiditis in acute otitis media will bear repeating.

The physician should remember that the pneumatic cells of the mastoid process are lined by a continuation of the tympanic mucoperiosteum which is simultaneously involved to some degree in every acute bacterial invasion of the middle ear, with purulent exudate in the mastoid cells as well as the tympanum. This was never by itself an indication for surgery, for the normal processes of localization of the infection led to spontaneous resolution of the infection of the mucoperiosteum without bone involvement in the great majority of cases. In the presulfonamide era not more than 1 to 5 per cent of patients with acute suppurative otitis media required a mastoidectomy, the percentage depending upon the virulence of the organism in different epidemics.

The involvement of bone with development of areas of coalescent bone erosion requires at least 10 days to 2 weeks or more of a severe untreated middle ear infection; the average duration of the otitis media before mastoidectomy becomes necessary is 3 to 5 weeks.

Areas of coalescent bone erosion are always associated with adjacent areas of beginning healing, and only evacuation of trapped pus from involved mastoid cells is required in order to replace the coalescent process of bone removal with active osteoblastic bone repair. Mastoidectomy is performed in acute otitis media with coalescent mastoiditis to accomplish just this evacuation of pus. It is not done to remove "necrotic bone," for there is none in the usual acute coalescent mastoiditis. Nor is it done to prevent a chronic suppurative otitis media, for the latter rarely results from a neglected acute suppurative otitis media of the usual non-necrotizing variety.

### Symptoms and Signs of Surgical Coalescent Mastoiditis

It should be re-emphasized that many of the symptoms and signs of a coalescent mastoiditis requiring a simple mastoidectomy are exactly the same as those of an early severe acute suppurative otitis media, but with this essential difference: When the symptoms occur early in the first few days or week of an acute middle ear infection, they do **not** call for surgical opening of the mastoid process, but when they persist or recur after several weeks of an acute otitis media, they point toward a developing coalescent process in the mastoid air cells that may require a mastoidectomy. Failure to appreciate this difference in the significance of symptoms in the first few days of an acute otitis media, compared to the same symptoms after the ear had drained for several weeks, led to errors of both commission and omission in mastoid surgery. On the one hand some surgeons would open a mastoid process in an early "red hot" hemolytic streptococcus otitis media before any sort of localization of the infection had occurred. The result of such untimely surgery was an extraordinarily high incidence of intracranial and distant complications due to dissemination of the infection. At the other extreme, complacency toward persistent pain and low-grade fever from an ear that had drained for a month or more sometimes allowed a coalescent abscess to erode the inner plate, producing a fatal meningitis. The **time at which symptoms and signs appear is more important than their severity** in evaluating the need for a mastoidectomy in an acute suppurative otitis media. These symptoms and signs are:

**Persistence of aural discharge** for more than 3 weeks in an acute suppurative otitis media is the most constant symptom pointing toward a coalescent process, especially when the discharge is profuse or creamy (rather than thin and mucoid) or varies in amount with periods of profuse drainage alternating with periods of scant or absent drainage. With an understanding of the normal tendency toward localization and resolution of an acute infection of the middle ear, the physician will appreciate that the persistence of a purulent discharge beyond 3 or 4 weeks indicates that the normal tendency toward healing is being prevented by inadequate drainage from coalescing pneumatic cells.

As the mastoid abscess develops, the discharge not only persists but usually becomes more purulent and creamy and may begin to vary in amount as the pus forces its way from time to time out of the abscess cavity. In rare cases the discharge may actually cease and yet a walled-off abscess may remain to cause symptoms and radiographic changes. This occurs especially when a coalescent abscess develops in the petrous apex, in a pneumococcus type III otitis media or in acute otitis media partially arrested but not eradicated by inadequate or ineffective antibacterial medication.

**Pain,** localized deep in or behind the ear, is the next most common symptom of coalescent mastoiditis. The pain is due to the pressure of the trapped pus on the inflamed tissues and diminishes when drainage increases. Severe pain suggests an extradural abscess. The pain is typically worse at night, perhaps because of increased venous congestion in the recumbent position that increases the pressure. If the pain is felt deep behind the eye a coalescent process in the petrous apex is suggested.

Again the physician should remember that the time of appearance of pain after the onset of the otitis media is the factor that determines its surgical significance. The extreme, even excruciating, pain of an unruptured drum membrane in the first day or two of the otitis should not alarm the physician, whereas comparatively mild pain that recurs after several weeks of painless discharge should cause deep concern.

**Persistence of pain** for longer than 2 weeks after the onset of an otitis media has the same significance as recurrence of pain after several weeks of an acute otitis media.

Pain is not an invariable symptom of a surgical mastoiditis and may be absent in the presence of a well localized coalescent abscess.

**Tenderness** over the mastoid process is the most consistent physical sign of a coalescent mastoiditis. Again, tenderness in the first few days of an acute otitis media may be considerable and yet it does not indicate a surgical process, whereas after several weeks of draining of the ear even a slight detectable difference of sensitivity to deep pressure between the affected and the normal mastoid points toward a coalescing process.

The tenderness is greatest where the trapped pus is nearest to the periosteum — in adults over the tip of the mastoid process, in children with incomplete pneumatization more often over the fossa mastoidea near the antrum.

**Periosteal thickening** is due to edema where the abscess is approaching the lateral surface of the mastoid process by bone erosion. To demonstrate slight but significant degrees of periosteal thickening the examiner should stand behind the patient and palpate both mastoids at the same time. The irregularities of the bony surface will seem to be obscured or "ironed out" by a thickened periosteum on the involved side.

**Subperiosteal abscess** occurs when the eroding pus perforates the outer cortex. The usual perforation on the lateral surface of the mastoid process is above the

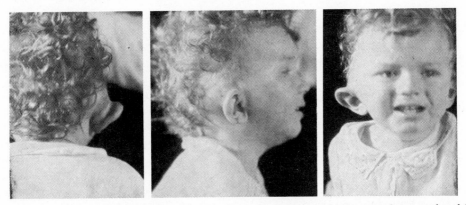

**Figure 9–1**   Subperiosteal abscess. Note the displacement of auricle downward, outward and forward. (From Lederer, F. L.: Diseases of Ear, Nose and Throat, 6th ed. Philadelphia, F. A. Davis, 1952.)

insertion of the sternocleidomastoid muscle and it produces the typical **displacement of the auricle** downward, outward and forward (Fig. 9–1). Owing to the thickness of the overlying tissues, fluctuation may not be easy to detect at first, but as the subperiosteal abscess enlarges, deep fluctuation can be demonstrated.

Less often the perforation occurs over the posterior root of the zygoma, producing a **zygomatic abscess.** The periosteum under the lower edge of the temporal muscle is elevated and the upper half of the auricle is displaced away from the skull by the abscess.

Perforation on the medial aspect of the mastoid tip into the digastric groove (incisura mastoidea) produces a deep abscess of the neck, known as Bezold's abscess. To quote from Bezold:[11]

Exceptionally large cells are often found in the adult . . . on the inner surface of the mastoid process, sometimes extending from the incisura mastoidea as far as the bulb of the jugular vein. Perforations at these places produce a very distinct clinical picture. . . . The pus cannot reach the surface. . . . No fluctuation can be felt. A moderately sensitive swelling develops rather suddenly in the lower surroundings of the mastoid process concealing its contours. . . . The suppuration spreads gradually in all directions . . . below the fascia of the neck. The pus may descend along the sheaths of the large vessels and may reach the larynx and even the mediastinum. The pus may descend . . . along the muscles of the vertebral column. A burrowing of pus leading to the formation of a retropharyngeal abscess was observed. . . .

A perforation of the tympanic membrane . . . did not precede the descensions of pus in the neck in 29 per cent of the cases I observed. Pneumococci were found most frequently to be the cause of the suppuration.

To this we may add that an empyema of the apex of the petrous pyramid can produce a similar deep abscess of the neck.

A very rare type of perforation of the outer cortex is from the cells of the root of the zygoma downward and forward into the mandibular fossa.[12] A tender fluctuant abscess appears just in front of the tragus, with a displacement of the mandible toward the normal side so that the teeth no longer meet in occlusion.

**Sagging of the posterosuperior meatal wall** is a very frequent and dependable sign of a coalescent mastoiditis. It is due to thickening of the periosteum of the osseous meatus adjacent to the antrum. Should the bone perforate at this point with the formation of a subperiosteal abscess, the sagging becomes so great as to nearly obliterate the lumen of the meatus. Today this is much less likely to happen in an acute otitis media than in a chronic otitis with cholesteatoma formation.

The tympanic membrane continues to be **markedly thickened** and red with loss of landmarks. A **nipple-like** protrusion of the small central tympanic membrane perforation, caused by the marked thickening of the tympanic mucoperiosteum, often accompanies a coalescent process within the mastoid. The purulent discharge may be seen coming from the tip of the conical elevation.

**Fever,** usually low grade and intermittent, is caused by toxic absorption from the trapped pus under pressure. Since by the third or fourth week of the middle ear infection the process of localization and production of specific antibodies is well advanced, any fever, leucocytosis and malaise due to toxic absorption are very much less than during the first week, yet they are now far more ominous as evidence of a dangerous bone-eroding process.

Fever may be absent, or so occasional as to escape detection unless the temperature is taken regularly every 4 hours.

**Leucocytosis and increased sedimentation rate** in an acutely diseased ear that has discharged for more than 3 weeks are indicative of retained pus, and may be present without fever.

**Secondary anemia** may develop in hemolytic streptococcus infections that persist, especially when they are complicated by a sigmoid sinus thrombophlebitis and septicemia. Anemia may also develop as a toxic reaction to sulfonamides and less often to an antibiotic; in these cases the anemia is associated with a leucopenia.

**The conductive hearing impairment** of an acute suppurative otitis media continues as long as the ear drains and the mucoperiosteal lining in the epitympanum and tympanum remains thickened. The presence of normal hearing speaks against a mastoiditis secondary to an otitis media and in favor of a large furuncle of the meatus which may cause signs and symptoms that simulate a coalescent mastoiditis.

**Radiographic changes** of a coalescent mastoiditis are very characteristic and diagnostic. To the clouding of the pneumatic cells, which always occurs in an acute suppurative otitis media as their content of air is replaced by exudate, are added a fading out and beginning fuzziness and indistinctness of the discrete bony cell partitions as decalcification and osteoclastic bone removal proceed. Serial x-rays made of the mastoid once a week during the course of an acute otitis media will help to demonstrate the progressive bone changes of coalescence.

## Differential Diagnosis of Coalescent Mastoiditis

**Suppuration of the mastoid lymph node and furuncle of the meatus** are two conditions that may be confusing and must be differentiated from a surgical mastoiditis. The mastoid lymph node, lying on the lateral surface of the mastoid process, drains the scalp and becomes inflamed in hair follicle infections or pediculosis capitis. The normal hearing and absence of history and symptoms of an otitis media should make the differentiation easy. Furuncle of the meatus secondary to an external otitis is easily differentiated from a surgical mastoiditis by the normal hearing, provided the meatus is patent. When a furuncle complicates an otitis media the diagnostic problem is more difficult. Extreme sensitiveness of the cartilaginous meatus to pressure suggests a furuncle, but absence of great discomfort when the cartilaginous meatus is manipulated speaks for a mastoiditis.

### Atypical Mastoiditis

The term "atypical," "latent," "silent" or "masked" mastoiditis has been applied to cases of coalescent mastoiditis without a draining ear or the other usual symptoms and signs of this condition. Cases of this sort were encountered in the preantibiotic era, especially in pneumococcus type III infections. The patient's symptoms might consist of slight stuffiness in the ear or tinnitus; the tympanic membrane was intact with only minimal thickening or inflammatory change; mastoid tenderness was slight or absent. Because of persistent fever or a meningitis or other complication an x-ray of the mastoid would be taken and would reveal extensive changes of decalcification and coalescence, and these x-ray findings would be confirmed at surgery.

The early use of antibacterial medication in acute otitis media modifies the clinical course in some cases, causing the otitis media to resemble a type III pneumococcus infection. When the antibacterial agent is given in insufficient quantity or for too brief a period of time, or when the antibiotic of choice for a particular organism has not been selected, or when the organism is one that has developed a resistance to all antibiotics, the infection in the middle ear is slowed down but not checked.

The acute symptoms subside, and the patient appears well for a time, but after a period of weeks fever of unknown origin, recurring attacks of acute otitis media or a meningitis, facial paralysis or labyrinthitis calls attention to a possible atypical mastoiditis. The only evidence of widespread suppurative disease within the temporal bone may be slight persistent inflammatory thickening of the drum membrane, persistent impaired hearing or slight deep bone tenderness over the mastoid. The x-ray may show definite changes, or it may be reported as normal.

Whereas cases of typical acute coalescent mastoiditis have become rare indeed, otitic complications from atypical mastoiditis continue and may even be on the increase.[13, 14] The diagnosis of atypical mastoiditis requires not only a careful history of an earache following a respiratory infection, but a complete otologic examination including hearing tests and radiographic studies of the temporal bone. In case of doubt, an exploratory mastoidectomy may be necessary to establish the diagnosis.

In every case of acute suppurative otitis media, including atypical cases without rupture of the tympanic membrane, when evidence of active infection persists beyond 3 or 4 weeks, the physician must weigh any symptoms and signs of a coalescent process against whatever evidence there is of spontaneous resolution. In case of doubt a period of watchful waiting is indicated, with the patient in the hospital, where he may obtain a maximum of rest, where he may be given a trial on a more appropriate antibiotic as determined by culture and sensitivity tests and where his signs and symptoms, temperature and radiographic and blood changes may be watched closely.

A simple mastoidectomy is not an emergency operation that must be performed immediately, unless there are signs and symptoms of a threatened complication.[15, 16] These will be considered in detail in Chapters 11 and 12.

## TECHNIQUE OF THE SIMPLE MASTOID OPERATION

The early operations on the mastoid process for an acute coalescent abscess consisted of removing the cortex from the lateral surface of the mastoid process, locating the antrum, opening the abscess cavity widely and scooping out adjacent softened cell remnants and granulations. Intact pneumatic cells were not disturbed. The wound was packed with a long strip of iodoform gauze and left open. The packing was replaced every few days for 3 to 5 weeks until the purulent drainage had ceased and the mastoid cavity had filled with healthy granulations.

As the technique of the operation improved, it was found that the more complete the exenteration of all accessible pneumatic cells from the mastoid process, the squama and the posterior perilabyrinthine petrous area medial to the antrum, the quicker the cessation of purulent discharge and the less often it became necessary to revise the operation to remove remaining coalescent foci of persistent suppuration. As the simple mastoidectomy changed to a complete anatomic dissection of all accessible pneumatic cells, the name "complete mastoidectomy" was proposed as being more appropriate. However, just as the name "otosclerosis" has persisted rather than the more accurate "otospongiosis," so the term "simple mastoidectomy" is still generally used for the operation for acute coalescent mastoiditis, although the complete removal of all accessible pneumatic cells is hardly a simple procedure.

### Anesthesia

General anesthesia is usually selected — intravenous Pentothal for adults, inhalation of non-explosive gas for children. If for any reason a general anesthetic is contraindicated, a very satisfactory and excellent local anesthesia may be secured as described in Chapter 6.

### Incision

The endaural incision may be used for the simple mastoid operation on a mastoid process with restricted pneumatization, as advocated by Lempert, but for the usual well pneumatized bone the postaural Wilde incision will give far better exposure (Fig. 9–2). The techniques for both the endaural and the postaural incision were described in Chapter 6. There is one word of caution: If there is a subperiosteal abscess or if the mastoid was previously operated on, a bold incision through skin, subcutaneous tissue and periosteum in a single stroke is contraindicated, and the tissues should be incised cautiously in layers to avoid possible injury to an exposed middle fossa dura or wall of the sigmoid sinus.

Remember that in the infant there is not yet a mastoid process, so that the usual postaural incision will section the facial nerve. Until the age of 2 years a modified incision should be used, as described in Chapter 6 (Fig. 6–7).

### Removal of the Cortex

The cortex of the lateral surface of the mastoid process, formerly removed by mallet and gouge, is conveniently removed with the dental-type electric drill using a large round cutting burr. The cortex should be removed from the entire lateral surface from the temporal line above to the mastoid tip below, and from the posterior osseous meatal wall in front to the probable extent of pneumatization behind as seen in the x-ray.

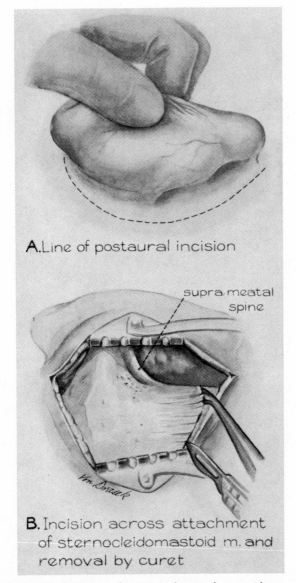

**A.** Line of postaural incision

supra meatal spine

**B.** Incision across attachment of sternocleidomastoid m. and removal by curet

**Figure 9–2**  Incision and exposure for simple mastoidectomy.

## Exenteration of Mastoid Cells

If a coalescent abscess is opened into when the cortex is removed, it should be examined carefully for exposed wall of the sigmoid sinus or middle fossa dura before pneumatic cells are removed with a curet and rongeur.

An orderly systematic removal of cell tracts will save a great deal of time and insure a complete exenteration of all accessible cells. Remembering that the pneumatic cells of the mastoid process developed in early childhood as outgrowths from the antrum, the removal of cell tracts is best accomplished in a similar manner, working from the antrum outward.

To locate the antrum, first remove the cells just above and behind the suprameatal spine; this removal is accomplished with a large-sized (No. 1 or No. 2)

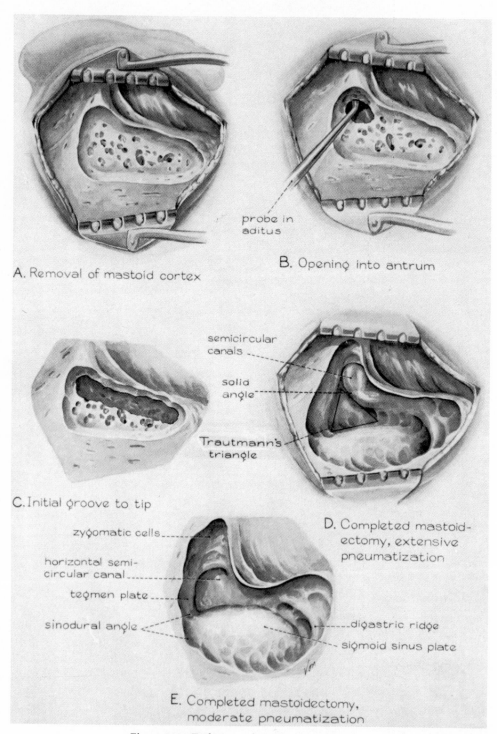

A. Removal of mastoid cortex

B. Opening into antrum

probe in aditus

C. Initial groove to tip

semicircular canals

solid angle

Trautmann's triangle

D. Completed mastoid-ectomy, extensive pneumatization

zygomatic cells

horizontal semi-circular canal

tegmen plate

sinodural angle

digastric ridge

sigmoid sinus plate

E. Completed mastoidectomy, moderate pneumatization

**Figure 9–3**　Technique of simple mastoidectomy.

sharp curet. The opening should be beveled and conical, rather than a relatively blind, narrow, deep hole. In the adult the antrum lies at an average depth of 12 to 15 mm. from the lateral surface. The cavity of the antrum may be completely filled with mucoperiosteal granulations. A blunt ear hook inserted into it will slip forward without resistance into the aditus and epitympanum.

The **most common error** in locating the antrum is to seek it too far below the temporal line. Sometimes when there is a very low middle fossa dura, it is necessary to proceed upward at an angle under the dura to enter the antrum.

In searching for the antrum remember that it always lies just above and behind the posterosuperior osseous meatal wall a few millimeters lateral to the annulus and sulcus tympanicus (Fig. 9–3). The surgeon while searching for the antrum should beware of:

1. Injuring a forward-lying sigmoid sinus.

2. Injuring a low middle fossa dura.

3. Injuring the pyramidal segment of the facial nerve where it curves downward to begin its vertical mastoid course.

4. A "false antrum," the result of a well developed Körner's septum between cells that grow outward in the squamous bone and those that grow down in the petrous bone to form the cells of the mastoid process (see Fig. 1–27).

The opening into the antrum is enlarged by removal of cells superiorly and posteriorly with a large curet. From the antrum the various cell tracts are followed to their termination in a systematic manner as follows:

1. The vertical tract of cells from the antrum to the tip of the mastoid process is removed; this establishes the "initial groove." Remember the position of the vertical portion of the facial nerve and keep away from it (see Fig. 2–14).

2. The sheet of cells that covers the sigmoid sinus is followed backward from the initial groove until the sinus plate is well defined and meets the outer cortex posteriorly, indicating the posterior limit of pneumatization. The mastoid emissary vein may be encountered in this area and injury to it should be avoided.

3. The tip of the mastoid process contains one or several large cells. These are cleaned out; the lateral wall of the tip is removed and within the mastoid the digastric ridge, which corresponds to the digastric groove or incisura mastoidea, is defined. Remember that the stylomastoid foramen containing the facial nerve lies at the anterior end of this ridge.

4. Cells that extend toward the jugular bulb medial to the digastric ridge between it and the sigmoid sinus are carefully excavated with the largest curet appropriate for the space. The lower half of the mastoid process has now been exenterated and the surgeon turns his attention to the upper half.

5. The sheet of cells against the tegmen plate is removed until the plate is defined and meets the cortex of the squama superiorly, indicating the limit of pneumatization in a superior direction.

6. The sinodural angle is cleaned out until the tegmen plate meets the sigmoid sinus plate at a sharp angle.

7. Remove any cells extending forward into the posterior root of the zygomatic process, without opening the epitympanum.

8. Last of all, very carefully clean out all small pneumatic cells medial to the antrum down to the hard bony posterior and superior semicircular canals. Define the posterior end of the bony horizontal semicircular canal very carefully, avoiding injury to or dislocation of the incus. The landmarks for the vertical portion of the facial nerve may now be located: the posterior end of the bony horizontal semicircular canal, the digastric ridge and the tympanomastoid suture in the posterior osseous meatal wall (see Chapters 2 and 20). The surgeon may proceed to remove

remaining cells along the posterior osseous meatal wall, carefully avoiding the course of the facial nerve.

In the completed simple mastoid cavity the osseous superior and posterior meatal wall has been left standing; the tegmen and sinus plates are defined but intact; the cell tracts have been followed to their termination from the antrum inferiorly to the tip, posteriorly to the junction of sinus plate and cortex, superiorly to the junction of tegmen plate and cortex, anteriorly to the limit of pneumatization in the posterior root of the zygoma and medially to the superior and posterior osseous semicircular canals. Removal of partially decalcified softened cells is accomplished with curets rather than with the burr. Overhanging cortex is removed with burr and rongeur.

Should the sinus plate or tegmen plate be softened by disease, it should be carefully elevated from the underlying sigmoid sinus or dura and removed in small bites, with a small rongeur or curet, until firm, healthy bone and healthy sinus or dura without granulations are encountered. Unnecessary exposure of sinus or dura under healthy bone should be avoided, as it only exposes fresh tissue to the infecting organism.

Coalescent mastoiditis occurs most often in a well pneumatized temporal bone. But it may occur in a partially pneumatized bone with peripheral areas of diploic marrow-containing bone in the mastoid process and petrous pyramid. A coalescent osteitis in such a bone may extend to adjacent diploic bone to produce a localized osteomyelitis. With the curet it is not difficult to determine when diploic bone is softened by disease, and when it is, it should be curetted away down to firm healthy bone exactly as is done with the coalescent pneumatized bone.

## Suture of the Wound

A complete mastoidectomy on a well localized coalescent mastoiditis no longer needs to be packed and left open but may be sutured with a small drain leading to the antrum left protruding from the lower end of the incision. With antibiotic coverage the wound may be sutured without any drainage in selected cases, but as a

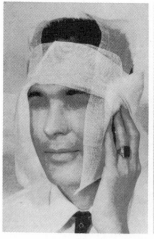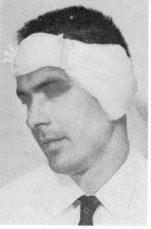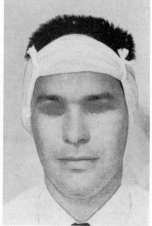

**Figure 9–4**   Technique for mastoid dressing.

rule the surgeon will prefer to leave a small, soft rubber tube drain from the antrum for 3 or 4 days. To keep the drain in position it may be sutured to the skin.

After the cavity is debrided of any loose fragments of bone, it is irrigated with warm sterile Tis-u-sol or Ringer's solution for hemostasis and removal of any remaining smaller particles of bone. The skin and periosteum are approximated by interrupted silk sutures. The meatus is packed firmly with a strip of petroleum jelly gauze to prevent stenosis. A mastoid dressing is applied (Fig. 9–4).

## AFTER-CARE OF THE SIMPLE MASTOID OPERATION

The patient should be ambulatory the day following surgery. The mastoid dressing is changed on the fourth postoperative day, with sterile technique (Chap. 6). If there is no purulent discharge from the drain, it may be removed; otherwise it should be left until the purulent drainage ceases. The appropriate antibiotic as determined by sensitivity tests for the organism cultured from the mastoid at the time of surgery should be administered until all aural or postaural discharge has ceased, and then for 5 more days. Other appropriate suggestions for postoperative care as described in Chapter 6 should be followed.

The patient usually leaves the hospital 4 to 6 days after the operation. The mastoid dressing may be dispensed with as soon as the wound is dry. As soon as the tympanic membrane perforation has closed, the patency of the eustachian tube should be re-established by an inflation or two until hearing is normal.

Persistence of discharge from the ear or mastoid may be due to one of the following:

1. Operation was performed too soon, before localization of the infection had occurred.

2. There was incomplete removal of mastoid cells.

3. There is a coalescent process in the petrous pyramid (petrositis).

4. A simple mastoidectomy was erroneously performed for an allergic otitis media or for a cholesteatoma.

## ACCIDENTS DURING SIMPLE MASTOIDECTOMY

The most common serious surgical accident during the simple mastoid operation is **injury to the facial nerve.** This occurs most often in operations by poorly trained or occasional operators, but **it can happen to the most skilled and experienced temporal bone surgeon** when the nerve has an anomalous course.

Facial paralysis occurring during the operation or noticed immediately afterward means a probable injury or severance of the facial nerve. An exception is transitory facial paralysis due to a local infiltrating anesthetic agent, in which case complete recovery occurs within a few hours. Prompt exploration with decompression and repair of the injured nerve is indicated within 24 hours of the operation before granulations and degeneration of the severed ends of the nerve make it difficult to identify (Chapter 20).

If the paralysis does not begin until several days after operation, an edema of the nerve is likely, with the probability of spontaneous recovery without surgical intervention. Thus the **time** after operation that the paralysis is first noted is of decisive importance in determining the therapy. Therefore, as soon after operation as the patient can respond, he should be asked to "show his teeth" so that the facial muscles can be observed for weakness or paralysis.

For further details of the management of facial nerve paralysis, see Chapter 20.

Injury to the sigmoid sinus, the superior petrosal sinus, the jugular bulb or the mastoid emissary vein results in an alarmingly profuse venous bleeding, which, however, is easily controlled by compressed Gelfoam moistened with topical thrombin held agains the vessel by iodoform gauze for at least 2 minutes by the clock. As soon as the field is dry the iodoform gauze may be removed, with the Gelfoam left in place, and the operative procedure may be resumed. Be sure that a spicule of bone is not left projecting into the sinus.

Bone wax to control bleeding may act later as a foreign body and should be avoided.

Injury to the dura with the escape of spinal fluid is less common and more dangerous. Carefully remove sufficient bone around the tear to expose a margin of intact dura all around and be sure there is not a fragment of bone holding the tear open. Place a piece of temporal muscle over the tear; the muscle should be held in place by compressed Gelfoam and then by iodoform gauze. If the escape of spinal fluid has stopped at the conclusion of the operation, the iodoform gauze should be removed. If clear fluid is still escaping the iodoform gauze should be left in place until the first dressing on the fourth postoperative day, and at that time if spinal fluid is still escaping, fresh iodoform gauze should be placed against the Gelfoam and muscle. Absolute sterility in these postoperative dressings is mandatory!

As a rule a tear of the middle fossa dura closes rapidly as fibroblastic proliferation of the adjacent arachnoid mesh walls off the area. Tears of the posterior fossa dura near the sinodural angle heal more slowly because of the arachnoid-free lateral prolongation of the basal cistern. Provided the surgeon observes the strict aseptic technique described in Chapter 6, supplemented by prophylactic antibiotic therapy, accidental tears of the dura should heal without producing meningitis or brain abscess.

Dislocation or removal of the incus results in a particularly severe permanent conductive hearing loss. Later on hearing may be restored very nearly to normal by a tympanoplasty operation (see Chapters 13 and 16).

## REFERENCES

1. Kemble, J.: Hero-Dust. Methuen, London, 1936.
2. Petit, J. L.: Traité des maladies chirurgicales. Paris, 1774.
3. Ballance, C. A.: Essays on the Surgery of the Temporal Bone. MacMillan, London, 1919.
4. Wilde, W.: Aural Surgery, Dublin, 1853.
5. Schwartze, H. H., and Eysell, C. G.: Ueber die künstliche Eröffnung des Warzenfortsatzes. Arch. Ohrenh., 7:157, 1873.
6. Whiting, T.: The Modern Mastoid Operation. Philadelphia, 1905.
7. Eagleton, W. P.: Unlocking of petrous pyramid for localized bulbar meningitis secondary to suppuration of petrous apex. Arch. Otol., 13:386, 1931.
8. Kopetsky, S. J., and Almour, R.: Suppuration of petrous pyramid: pathology, symptomatology and surgical treatment. Ann. Otol. Rhin. & Laryng., 39:999, 1930; 40:157, 396, 922, 1931.
9. Ramadier, J.: Les ostéites pétreuses profondes (pétrosites). Oto-rhino-laryng. Internat., 17:816, 1933.
10. Lempert, J.: Complete apicectomy (mastoidotympano-apicectomy), new technic for complete apical exenteration of apical carotid portion of petrous pyramid. Arch. Otol., 25:144, 1937.
11. Bezold, F., and Siebenmann, F.: Textbook of Otology. Translated by J. Holinger. E. H. Cosgrove and Co., Chicago, 1908.

12. Shambaugh, G. E., Jr.: Involvement of the jaw joint in acute suppurative otitis media. Arch. Otol., *33*:975, 1941.
13. Rosenwasser, H., and Adelman, N.: Otitic complications. Arch. Otol., *65*:225, 1957.
14. Courville, C. B.: Intracranial complications of otitis media and mastoiditis in the antibiotic era. Laryngoscope, *65*:31, 1955.
15. Shambaugh, G. E., Jr.: The surgical treatment of meningitis of otitic and nasal origin. J.A.M.A., *108*:696, 1937.
16. Kopetsky, S. J.: Otologic Surgery. Paul B. Hoeber, Inc., New York, 1929.

## Emanuel Zaufal

BORN 1837
DIED 1910

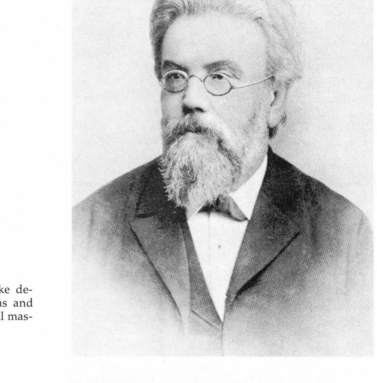

With Küster and Stacke developed the indications and technique of the radical mastoid operation.

## Fritz Thies

BORN 1873
DIED 1957

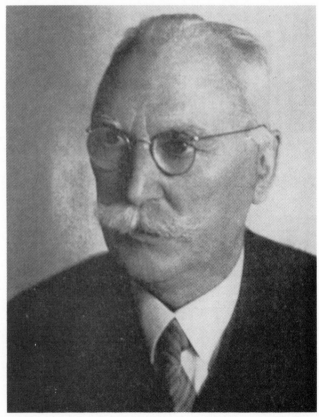

Rediscovered and used extensively the endaural approach for the radical mastoid operation.

266

# Chapter 10

# The Radical and Bondy Modified Radical Mastoid Operations

HISTORICAL NOTES

INDICATIONS FOR THE CLASSICAL RADICAL MASTOID
   OPERATION

INDICATIONS FOR THE BONDY MODIFIED RADICAL
   MASTOIDECTOMY

CONTRAINDICATIONS FOR THE RADICAL AND BONDY
   OPERATIONS

RADICAL MASTOIDECTOMY FOR CHRONIC OSTEITIS OR
   OSTEOMYELITIS

RADICAL OR BONDY MASTOIDECTOMY FOR ATYPICAL
   CHRONIC OTORRHEA

TECHNIQUE OF THE RADICAL MASTOIDECTOMY AND
   BONDY MODIFIED RADICAL MASTOIDECTOMY

     ANESTHESIA

     ATTICOTOMY BONE REMOVAL

     BONE REMOVAL BEYOND THE CHOLESTEATOMA

     TAKING DOWN THE BRIDGE AND THE FACIAL
       RIDGE

     PREPARATION OF THE MEATAL PLASTIC SKIN
       FLAP

     TOILET OF THE TYMPANUM

     FINAL INSPECTION OF THE CAVITY

     OBLITERATION OF THE RADICAL OR BONDY
       CAVITY

     TECHNIQUES OF OBLITERATION

     ATTICOTOMY FROM WITHIN THE MEATUS

     MYRINGOSTAPEDIOPEXY

     EXTENSION OF CHOLESTEATOMA INTO THE
       MESOTYMPANUM BEHIND THE PARS TENSA

     PLACEMENT OF THE MEATAL FLAP AND PACKING
       OF THE CAVITY

     SKIN GRAFTING THE RADICAL OR BONDY CAVITY

SECONDARY STAPES OPERATION, TYMPANOPLASTY OR
   FENESTRATION

POSTOPERATIVE CARE

COMPLICATIONS OF THE RADICAL AND BONDY
   MODIFIED RADICAL OPERATIONS

## HISTORICAL NOTES

In 1873 von Tröltsch[1] suggested a modification of the Schwartze simple mastoidectomy for cases of chronic otorrhea, having observed how the simple operation failed to cure the disease, as remnants of cholesteatoma in the attic, antrum or mastoid would invariably cause a recurrence of the chronic otorrhea. The name "radical" was applied by von Bergmann[2] to cases in which the posterior and superior osseous meatal walls were removed, leaving an open cavity. In 1890 Zaufal[3] described in detail the technique of the radical operation that gained access to and left open all areas of chronic disease, including the tympanic cavity. The next year Stacke[4] described the addition of a plastic meatal skin flap.

Just as the simple mastoid operation came to be known as the Schwartze operation, so the radical operation was often referred to as the Zaufal or Stacke operation. Essentially, the radical operation converted the attic, antrum, mastoid, tympanum and external auditory meatus into a common "radical cavity" that could be inspected and cleaned the rest of the patient's life, thus preventing recurrence of bone-invading life-threatening cholesteatoma.

In most cases that required the radical operation, the initial severe childhood necrotic otitis (see Chapter 7) had destroyed much of the tympanic membrane, ossicles and tympanic mucosa, allowing stratified squamous epithelium, as healing occurred, to extend from the external meatus into the tympanum, attic, antrum and mastoid. Hearing was poor, and was not made much worse when remnants of tympanic membrane and ossicles were extracted and remaining tympanic mucosa scraped out, with an attempt to close the eustachian tube.

There were, however, cases of cholesteatoma in the attic, with an intact pars tensa of the tympanic membrane, the perforation being confined to the pars flaccida. Some of these had quite good hearing. In 1899 Körner[5] had suggested that in certain cases of chronic otitis the tympanic membrane and ossicles could be left in place during the radical operation, thus preserving the good hearing. It remained for Bondy[6] in 1910 to describe the indications for and technique of a modification of the radical operation for cases of chronic otorrhea in which the pars flaccida perforation was accompanied by an intact pars tensa. Without disturbing the intact (except for the attic perforation) tympanic membrane, tympanic cavity and ossicles, the superior osseous meatal wall and part of the posterior were taken down, thus exteriorizing the attic and antral cholesteatoma into a permanently open "modified radical" cavity that could be kept clean safely through the external meatus.

Despite the very clear indications set forth by Bondy, his modification of the radical mastoid operation was very slow to receive widespread acceptance. As late as 1929, it was not even mentioned in a standard text of otologic surgery.[7] Otologic surgeons continued to be preoccupied with the prevention of intracranial complications in cases of chronic otorrhea, with scant regard for the hearing. The aim of surgery was to produce a *safe* ear, and incidentally, a *dry* ear, but not a functioning ear.

With the introduction of Lempert's one-stage fenestration operation in 1938,[8] otologic surgeons began to be more concerned with preserving or improving hearing as well as with preventing complications from chronic otorrhea. Soon the few earlier advocates of the Bondy operation (including the senior author of this text) were joined by numerous writers in America and abroad. Baron[9] pointed out that by 1944 the Bondy operation was indicated for more cases of chronic otorrhea with cholesteatoma than was the classical radical operation.

In 1951 another development further reduced the indications for the radical mastoidectomy. This was the introduction by Zöllner[10] and Wullstein[11] of tympanoplasties to reconstruct the sound-conducting apparatus of the middle ear. Successful tympanoplasty requires an open, functioning eustachian tube, normal mucosa in the tympanic cavity and utilization in the reconstruction of remnants of tympanic membrane and ossicles. The radical mastoid operation that attempted to close the eustachian tube and to remove remnants of tympanic membrane, tympanic mucosa and ossicles made subsequent tympanoplastic reconstruction impossible. As a result, the radical mastoid operation is rarely employed today, while the Bondy operation is used when it is desired to exteriorize a cholesteatoma without disturbing the tympanic cavity.

As early as 1885 Kessel[12] described the endaural approach for the radical mastoid operation, but this was forgotten along with other of Kessel's brilliant innovations. In 1907 the elder Thies[13] rediscovered the endaural approach and used it in 1500 mastoid operations without a fatality. In 1929 Lempert[14] advocated the endaural incision for all mastoid surgery. When he began to teach it to the hundreds of otologic surgeons who came to learn the fenestration operation, the endaural approach came to be preferred by most otologic surgeons for operations on chronic ears as well as for fenestrations. Recently, techniques have been developed for dealing with cholesteatomas without taking down the osseous meatal wall, the so-called "wall-up" or closed techniques (see Chapter 16). With these, the postaural approach is experiencing renewed preference.

The endaural approach, utilized for nearly all cases of cholesteatoma by the senior author, has the following advantages over the postaural incision for the radical and Bondy modified radical mastoid operations:

1. A plastic meatal skin flap to turn back over the facial ridge is more easily constructed.

2. Extensions of an attic cholesteatoma down into the tympanic cavity are more readily accessible.

3. Extensions of cholesteatoma into the sinus tympani are more directly accessible.

4. In most cases of attic retraction cholesteatoma the mastoid process is free of disease and need not be widely exenterated. Thus, with the endaural approach, the final open cavity can be kept quite small in most cases.

5. As a rule, the final open cavity constructed endaurally is more easily accessible for subsequent inspection and cleaning than when constructed through a postaural incision.


## INDICATIONS FOR THE CLASSICAL RADICAL MASTOID OPERATION

As cases of childhood necrotizing acute otitis media (see Chapter 7) are becoming scarce as a result of antibiotic therapy, the indications for surgery for the resulting secondary acquired cholesteatomas are diminishing in comparison with the far more frequent attic retraction cholesteatomas. Even in the few remaining cases in which a large tympanic membrane perforation is associated with ossicular destruction and cholesteatoma and when cochlear reserve is good as determined by bone conduction audiometry and speech discrimination, the eustachian tube should not be closed, tympanic mucosa should not be curetted nor should ossicular and tympanic membrane remnants be removed, as required in classical radical mastoidectomy, for these will be needed for future tympanoplasty.

Thus, today radical mastoidectomy is indicated only for the following unusual situations:

1. Chronic otorrhea due to secondary acquired cholesteatoma with profound sensorineural hearing loss.

2. Chronic otorrhea due to chronic perilabyrinthine osteitis with a scant foul discharge and chronic pain in and deep in the ear, in which the tympanum, hypotympanum and peritubal area, in addition to the mastoid, attic and perilabyrinthine areas, need to be explored.

3. Carcinoma of the external meatus and middle ear requires a radical mastoidectomy with removal of most of the temporal bone (see Chapter 22); while preservation of hearing is of secondary importance.

## INDICATIONS FOR THE BONDY MODIFIED RADICAL MASTOIDECTOMY

The Bondy type of modified radical mastoidectomy is indicated for cholesteatoma with chronic or recurring otorrhea in which cochlear reserve is sufficient for contemplation of future tympanoplasty, and where exteriorization of the cholesteatoma is desired. In recent years, the intact canal wall or "canal wall-up" technique of dealing with cholesteatomas has achieved some popularity, but unsuspected residual cholesteatoma or cholesteatoma recurrence due to recurrent attic retraction in as high as 30 per cent of operations has caused some leading otologic surgeons to return to the principle of exteriorization of the cholesteatoma cavity.[23, 24] The junior author prefers the intact canal wall technique, but always in a two-stage operation, as described in Chapter 16. The first operation is performed to remove all cholesteatoma and to repair the tympanic membrane perforation; the second operation six months later, to inspect the cavity in order to detect and remove any residue or recurrence of cholesteatoma, and to perform the ossicular reconstruction needed to improve hearing.

The senior author continues to favor the Bondy operation for all cholesteatomas except the tiny attic retraction pocket lateral to the incus and malleus that can be reached endaurally or endomeatally, the sac removed intact and the defect in the canal wall reconstructed with a cartilage graft as described in Chapter 16. S. Wullstein has perfected an "osteoplastic epitympanotomy" in which the superior osseous meatal wall is removed as a free bone graft, to be replaced after removal of cholesteatoma and its matrix from the attic.

For the occasional operator, the Bondy operation is recommended for all cases of cholesteatoma of the attic, antrum or mastoid, rather than the more difficult and less dependable intact canal wall or replaced canal wall techniques. The Bondy operation should be selected for patients who will not submit to a "second look" operation six months to a year later or who live far away or may move far away so that a "second look" is impractical.

The diagnosis of cholesteatoma in cases of chronic otorrhea requires brief mention. The great majority of cholesteatomas are associated with a pars flaccida or a marginal type of perforation, in which visibly stratified squamous epithelium extends into the attic. Rarely, there will be a central type of perforation and a mucoid discharge, but when the middle ear and attic are explored, cholesteatoma is found. An attic or pars flaccida perforation (actually an invagination) *always* means a cholesteatoma. Non-infected cholesteatoma debris may be present behind a dry attic perforation. A granulation or polyp protruding from an attic perforation means an infected cholesteatoma behind it.

The size of the attic perforation has little relation to the size of the cholesteatoma cavity. This is more easily determined by x-ray studies, both conventional and polytomographic, the latter being especially useful in demonstrating whether the cholesteatoma sac lies lateral or medial to the incus and malleus head, whether the bony horizontal semicircular canal has been thinned or fistulized by the cholesteatoma, whether the long process of the incus has been resorbed and whether the bony fallopian canal has been eroded. X-ray studies help to indicate when the cholesteatoma cavity is large enough to have eroded the tegmen plate, with possible dural exposure, or the lateral sinus plate, with possible exposure of the sigmoid sinus.

Retrieval of the typical flakes of cornified epithelium from the attic or mesotympanum by means of a small blunt ear hook or by attic irrigation is further diagnostic confirmation of cholesteatoma.

At this point, a word concerning the name cholesteatoma is necessary. This was applied many years ago when cholesterol crystals were found in the tumor-like mass of epidermal debris that desquamates from the skin-lined sac in the middle ear, attic or mastoid. Perhaps a better name would be keratoma, but this is commonly applied to corns on the feet, which are quite different from the skin-lined sac in the middle ear, attic and mastoid that erodes bone, becomes infected and, when neglected, leads to serious and sometimes fatal complications.

The conservative management of a cholesteatoma can be tried when the attic opening is large and the cholesteatoma sac is shallow, allowing the accumulated desquamated debris to be removed with a blunt ear hook or by irrigation with 50 per cent or 70 per cent alcohol through an attic cannula. Conservative management is contraindicated when:

1. Radiologic evidence of an enlarged smooth-walled antrum indicates a large cholesteatoma cavity.

2. Otorrhea persists after several attic irrigations.

3. A very small attic perforation renders attic irrigation painful, difficult and unsatisfactory.

4. Cholesteatoma is observed to extend down behind the pars tensa.

5. There are symptoms or signs of erosion of an adjacent structure, such as a fistula of a semicircular canal, facial nerve paresis or meningeal irritation.

6. The hearing is decreasing, indicating progression of the cholesteatoma.

7. The patient is uncooperative or lives far away, unable to return as necessary for conservative management.

In actual clinical experience, only very rarely will the otologist decide that an attic cholesteatoma can be treated safely without surgery.

## RADICAL MASTOIDECTOMY FOR CHRONIC OSTEITIS OR OSTEOMYELITIS

Most cases of chronic otorrhea in clinical practice are of the benign type described in Chapter 7, with an odorless mucoid discharge frequently associated with an allergic rhinitis, or are due to cholesteatoma secondary to either a childhood acute necrotic otitis or an attic retraction. The *least frequent* variety of chronic otorrhea is due to a chronic osteitis or osteomyelitis without cholesteatoma. Despite the usual conservative treatment of any allergic factor and an adequate course of antibiotic according to culture and sensitivity, the chronic, often foul smelling, and usually scant discharge from a small central perforation persists. Pain deep in the ear is a prominent symptom. Progressive sensorineural hearing loss with intermittent vertigo accompanies a perilabyrinthine osteitis.

The *treatment* of chronic osteitis or osteomyelitis is surgical. If a simple intact canal wall mastoidectomy does not find and remove the areas of softened osteitic bone, a radical operation permitting exploration of peritubal and hypotympanic, as well as perilabyrinthine, tracts toward the petrous apex may be required. As a rule, severe sensorineural hearing loss in such cases precludes eventual tympanoplasty, so there is no reason to preserve middle ear structures.

## RADICAL OR BONDY MASTOIDECTOMY FOR ATYPICAL CHRONIC OTORRHEA

The otologist will sometimes encounter a case of chronic otitis media that does not seem to fit the usual types described in Chapter 7. An example is the patient with a profuse mucopurulent discharge from a central type of perforation that resists all the usual treatments. Finally, in desperation the otologist may resort to a mastoidectomy of the simple or radical type. Pale granulations without osteitic softening of cell partitions are found packed into the epitympanum, antrum and mastoid cells. Just as chronic allergic sinusitis is helped for a time by surgery, the profuse aural discharge is diminished for a time, but then it returns just about as before. The finding of eosinophiles in the discharge or in a nasal smear finally directs the surgeon to the correct diagnosis. With competent allergic diagnosis of inhalant and food factors and management by the Rinkel techniques, the otorrhea is finally brought under control. Radical mastoidectomy in these cases is *not* indicated.

Occasionally, a cholesteatoma in the attic exists in the presence of a central perforation and an odorless mucoid discharge. One such case observed by the senior author was operated on because of vertigo with a positive fistula test. An unsuspected cholesteatoma with erosion of the horizontal semicircular canal was found and exteriorized with a Bondy operation. The small central perforation promptly closed as the otorrhea ceased.

When the physician is in doubt as to the nature of a particular case of chronic otorrhea, he should observe it for a period of time, employing conservative therapy. If the otorrhea persists, an exploratory atticotomy and antrotomy with preservation of the canal wall should be done, and converted to an open Bondy type cavity only if a cholesteatoma is found.

## CONTRAINDICATIONS FOR THE RADICAL AND BONDY OPERATIONS

These operations are never indicated in the benign type of chronic mucoid otorrhea with a central perforation and without cholesteatoma. They are never indicated for cases of acute otitis media with coalescent mastoiditis. They are not indicated for persistent secretory otitis media or cases of chronic allergic otitis media. With today's effective chemotherapy, they are not indicated for tubercular otitis media. Since they can be performed quite well under local anesthesia, age is not a contraindication.

## TECHNIQUE OF THE RADICAL MASTOIDECTOMY AND BONDY MODIFIED RADICAL MASTOIDECTOMY

The surgeon should keep in mind the purposes of the radical and Bondy mastoid operations: to remove all of the bone-invading disease, consisting of the cholesteatoma, its matrix and the osteitis surrounding it; to create a perfectly accessible exteriorized cavity that can be inspected and kept clean the rest of the patient's life; and to promote a dry ear by epithelialization of the cavity with healthy skin.

Contrary to the impression created by illustrations in many texts, a radical or Bondy mastoid operation should not begin with a preliminary exenteration of all mastoid cells, after which the superior and posterior osseous meatal walls are taken down to create the open radical cavity. Since many cholesteatomas with their adjacent osteitis and sclerosis do not extend beyond the antrum, it is best to confine the surgical exposure to the attic and antrum, and then to take down the superior and posterior meatal walls to construct the permanently open cavity. The resultant cavity, which must be kept clean the rest of the patient's life, will then be much smaller than if a complete mastoidectomy is first performed.

A second common misapprehension is that the bone-invading disease (cholesteatoma) requiring the radical operation involves the tympanic cavity. On the contrary, in the majority of secondary acquired cholesteatomas that require surgery, the tympanic cavity has long since recovered from the ravages of the initial childhood acute necrotic otitis media, with healing by epidermization of areas of the tympanum where the necrotic mucosa sloughed and left bare bone. Only occasionally will cholesteatoma extend into the eustachian orifice, sinus tympani or facial recess, requiring surgical exposure of these areas.

## Anesthesia

For all but unusually apprehensive adults, the senior author employs local anesthesia with adequate preoperative sedation, as described in Chapter 6. For children under the age of 14 to 16, general anesthesia is preferable. Advantages of local anesthesia include a more rapid recovery, the patient being ambulatory the afternoon after surgery and often ready to go home the next morning. Bleeding is less under local anesthesia, while vertigo, should a semicircular canal or a fistula be opened, and facial twitching, should the facial nerve be exposed, are helpful warning guides for the novice, as well as for the experienced surgeon, when anatomic landmarks are distorted by disease or by previous surgery.

## Atticotomy Bone Removal

The incision and atticotomy bone removal are the same for the classical radical mastoidectomy and for the Bondy modification. The usual endaural incision employed by the senior author for thousands of fenestrations, radical mastoid and Bondy modified radical mastoid operations is described in Chapter 6.

The self-retaining (Shambaugh) endaural retractor is inserted with retraction of periosteum, exposing the bone above and behind the osseous meatus, from the posterior root of the zygomatic process to 2 or 3 cm. posterior to the suprameatal spine of Henle and from the temporal line above to the lower portion of the mastoid process below (Fig. 10–1A). Wide retraction of periosteum is essential to "mobilize the incision," as emphasized by Lempert.

Atticotomy by means of a surgical cutting burr removes outer cortex just above and behind the meatus over a semilunar area (Fig. 10–1B). As the surgeon deepens the initial groove, he watches for the pink color shining through the bone, and then for a little bleeding as the middle fossa dura is approached. An effort is made to

*Text continued on page 277*

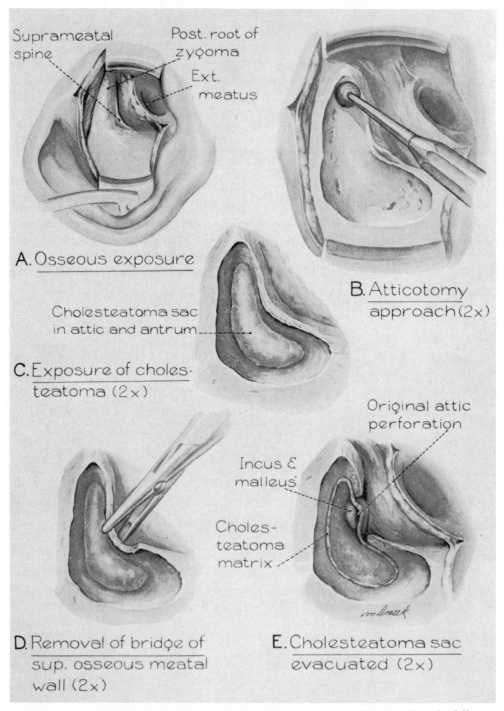

**Figure 10–1**  Technique for Bondy modified radical mastoidectomy. (Continued on the following page.)

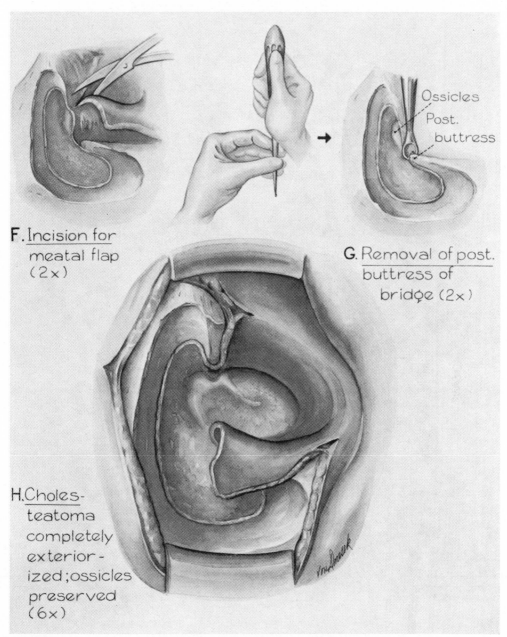

F. Incision for meatal flap (2x)

G. Removal of post. buttress of bridge (2x)

Ossicles
Post. buttress

H. Cholesteatoma completely exteriorized; ossicles preserved (6x)

**Figure 10–1** (*Continued*)   Technique for Bondy modified radical mastoidectomy. (Continued on the following page.)

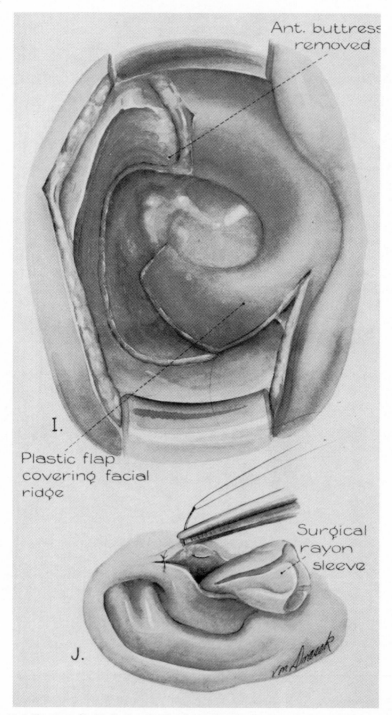

**Figure 10–1** (*Continued*)    Technique for Bondy modified radical mastoidectomy. *I*, Anterior and posterior buttresses of bridge taken down, the plastic flap turned back onto facial ridge. Any overlap of flap edge onto retained matrix must be trimmed away so as to exteriorize all portions of the cholesteatoma. *J*, Surgical rayon sleeve into which elastic sponge packing has been placed.

avoid unnecessary dural exposure as the groove between dura and superior meatal wall is deepened. The notch of Rivinus is located by passing a narrow periosteal elevator inward along the superior osseous meatal wall. The epitympanum will be encountered shortly before the groove reaches the depth of the Rivinian notch, and if the preoperative diagnosis was correct, the white smooth wall of the cholesteatoma sac will be identified (Fig. 10–1C). The middle fossa dura might resemble the wall of the cholesteatoma, requiring careful removal of bone anteriorly, inferiorly and posteriorly before the surgeon is sure.

The sac is opened cautiously (in case dura is mistaken for sac wall), the cholesteatoma contents removed by suction and instrumentation, and its furthest extensions anteriorly, superiorly and posteriorly explored by a blunt mastoid searcher. Bony cortex and overhang removal proceeds with cutting burr, curet and rongeur until the entire cholesteatoma sac lies exposed. In some cases, the cholesteatoma lining or matrix is smooth, with a thin layer of connective tissue between it and eburnated surrounding bone. More often, the cholesteatoma matrix is closely applied to bone with finger-like extensions into small cells and haversian canals. All cholesteatoma extensions must be followed to their end with the aid of the operating microscope. All matrix is removed with the following exceptions:

1.  Matrix firmly adherent to exposed dura or sigmoid sinus may be left rather than risk injury to these structures.

2.  Matrix over a fistula of a semicircular canal may be left to avoid postoperative serous labyrinthitis. Some surgeons prefer to dissect matrix from the fistula and immediately apply a thin fascial graft.

3.  Matrix firmly attached to exposed facial nerve may be left.

4.  Matrix extending into the mesotympanum and covering the stapes footplate may be left at the initial operation rather than opening the vestibule, with the risk of serous or suppurative labyrinthitis. At a second operation after the ear is dry and healed, cholesteatoma matrix can be dissected from the oval window and tympanoplasty can proceed as described in Chapter 16.

### Bone Removal Beyond the Cholesteatoma

Remembering that chronic otorrhea is the result of infected epidermal debris in the cholesteatoma sac; in most cases evacuation of the sac, removal of matrix (epidermal lining) and curettage of softened osteitic bone adjacent to the matrix will suffice to control the disease. The surgeon needs to exercise prudent judgment with regard to mastoid cells outside the cholesteatoma sac. These may be infected and osteitic (softened), with granulations requiring removal, but in many cases mastoid cells are intact and need not be removed. If cells beyond the cholesteatoma are removed, this portion of the cavity should be obliterated by a connective tissue-muscle pedicle flap, as described below.

### Taking Down the Bridge and the Facial Ridge

The remaining superior osseous meatal wall bridging across the notch of Rivinus is removed in small "bites" with a narrow rongeur (Fig. 10–1D) after first elevating the meatal skin from bone. With a small 000 curet, always working *outward* away from the fallopian canal and facial nerve, the anterior and posterior spines of the notch of Rivinus, comprising the anterior and posterior buttresses of the bridge, are taken down (Fig. 10–1G). The tympanic segment of the facial canal is identified and kept in view, while ossicles or remnants of ossicles are inspected. Wherever cholesteatoma envelops or extends onto the medial surface of malleus head or incus, these ossicles must be removed. When cholesteatoma matrix lies against and lateral to these ossicles, the matrix may be left (Fig. 10–1H) or carefully removed and the ossicles left undisturbed. When the long process of the incus is absent and matrix lies against the mobile stapes head, with excellent hearing producing nature's myringostapediopexy, this portion of matrix is undisturbed.

The step in the radical and Bondy operations most often accomplished poorly is taking down the posterior osseous meatal wall, which, deeper in, houses the posterior bend and vertical facial nerve, and thus is called the facial ridge. The approximate position of the facial nerve is located by three usually dependable landmarks: the bony horizontal semicircular canal above, the tympanomastoid suture in the posterior meatal wall, clearly evident by adherence of the meatal skin posteriorly to the suture line, and the digastric ridge in the mastoid tip. Since the tip cells rarely require removal in radical and Bondy mastoidectomies, the surgeon will need to dispense with the latter dependable landmark.

The bony facial ridge is taken down slowly and carefully with drill or curet, working under the operating microscope, always parallel to and never across the direction of the facial nerve, until the bowl of the surgical cavity after removal of disease is flush with the intact (or perforated) tympanic membrane. A pinkish color and bleeding will be encountered when the facial nerve is approached. It is better not to expose the nerve unnecessarily, for a Bell's palsy type of paresis occurs more often when this nerve is exposed than when not. While the paresis, beginning one to six or seven days postoperatively, generally recovers completely in a matter of weeks, residual weakness with synkinesis and spasm can ensue, just as occurs after recovery of some cases of Bell's palsy.

As the facial ridge is carefully lowered, the patient's face should be watched by the anesthesiologist or circulating nurse for any telltale twitching, indicating exposure of the nerve. The statement attributed to Lempert that "there is no use in watching the face for by the time it twitches the nerve has been cut" is incorrect unless the surgeon is unusually heavy-handed or completely lost anatomically.

### Preparation of the Meatal Plastic Skin Flap

The plastic pedicled skin flap that will be turned back to cover the facial ridge and the floor of the completed operative cavity consists of the skin and periosteum of the entire superior osseous meatal wall and most of the posterior meatal wall. As the atticotomy proceeds and the bridge is being taken down, a narrow periosteal elevator separates the skin and periosteum from the superior and posterior meatal walls. With a curved meatal knife and iris scissors, an incision along the anterosuperior angle of the meatus (Fig. 10–1F) frees the plastic flap anteriorly. The connective tissue band that enters the tympanosquamous suture will need to be cut, and posteriorly, similar but less pronounced connective tissue in the tympanomastoid suture will need to be separated, beginning at the annulus and working outward. The outer edge of the meatal flap may need to be thinned to make it lie smoothly over the facial ridge (Fig. 10–1I).

### Toilet of the Tympanum

In the classical radical mastoidectomy, the tympanic cavity is inspected minutely under the operating microscope as originally advocated in 1921 by Nylen,

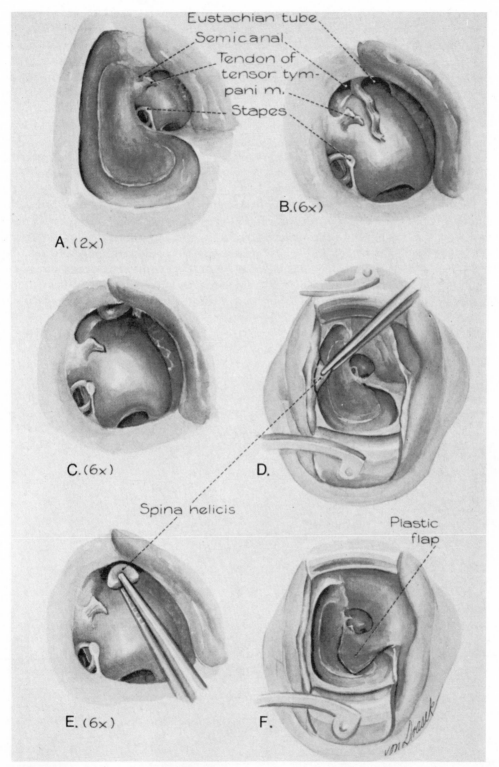

**Figure 10–2** Classical Radical Mastoidectomy. *A*, Tympanum exposed. *B*, Tensor tympani muscle elevated from its semicanal. *C*, Posterior end of tensor tympani muscle folded and inserted into eustachian tube. *D*, Line of excision of spinal helicis. *E*, Closure of eustachian tube with spina helicis. *F*, Plastic flap covering the facial ridge.

the first to use a microscope for ear surgery. Healthy skin and remnants of tympanic membrane closing off the eustachian tube are not disturbed, but any polyps, granulations or remaining mucosae are removed (Fig. 10–2). Instrumentation in the oval window and round window niches should be avoided because of the possibility of opening the labyrinth. If the eustachian tube orifice is open and mucosal-lined, an attempt is made to close it in the classical radical operation after curetting its mucosa, as depicted in Figure 10–2C and D. Another method is to use a small full thickness skin graft from behind the ear. In curetting the mouth of the eustachian tube, remember that the internal carotid artery is separated from it only by a thin plate of bone. Should curettage produce brisk bleeding, this is usually from the venous plexus that surrounds the carotid in its journey through the temporal bone and not from the artery.

In removing a mass of granulations from the stapes and oval window, start at the pyramidal eminence and strip the granulations in a forward direction parallel with the stapedius tendon to keep from dislodging the stapes. However, in many hundreds of radical mastoid and Bondy operations, the senior author has found that in the majority, very little needed to be done to the tympanum. Once the bone-invading infected cholesteatoma in the attic, antrum and sometimes the mastoid has been removed, any small granulations in the middle ear caused by the purulent drainage soon dry up with local conservative treatment.

### Final Inspection of the Cavity

The completed open radical or Bondy cavity is irrigated with warm Tis-U-Sol or Ringer's solution for hemostasis and for removal of any bone particles or other debris. Under the operating microscope, the cavity is inspected minutely for any remaining osteitis or cholesteatoma remnants. There must be no cortical overhang

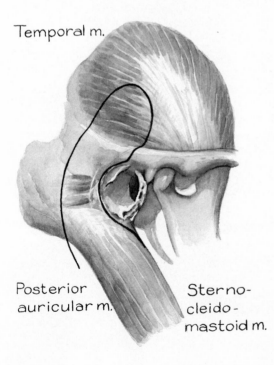

Temporal m.

Posterior
auricular m.

Sterno-
cleido-
mastoid m.

**Figure 10–3** Outline of incision for pedicle graft attached inferiorly, including temporal muscle, mastoid fascia and posterior auricular muscles and upper end of sternocleidomastoid.

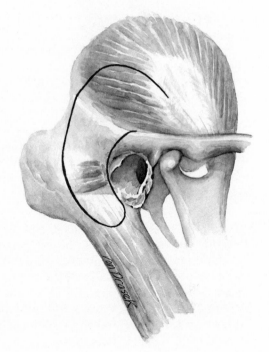

**Figure 10–4** Outline of incisions for pedicle graft attached superiorly and anteriorly.

and no part of the cavity not perfectly accessible and exteriorized from the external meatus.

## Obliteration of the Radical or Bondy Cavity

A pedicle muscle flap was first described by Passow in 1908[15] to close a postoperative mastoid fistula and then by Kisch[16] in 1928 to reduce the size of the radical mastoid cavity. Meurman in 1949[17] and then Guilford[18] and Palva,[19] described similar techniques, all utilizing pedicled flaps of muscle and fascia turned in to reduce the size of the postoperative cavity.

The surgeon may feel that with the aid of the operating microscope, he can remove every vestige of cholesteatoma matrix when cholesteatoma has invaded mastoid cells, and that he may then safely obliterate the entire mastoid cavity. The report of Adams[20] of recurrent cholesteatomas under fascial grafts one to nine years later, and the more recent reports of Cody[21] and Wright[22] of cholesteatoma residues and recurrence after closed wall techniques emphasize the advisability of obliterating only those parts of the operative cavity that did not contain cholesteatoma.

## Techniques of Obliteration

The use of proplast to reduce the size of the radical or Bondy cavity has not been satisfactory in the long run in the experience of the authors because of a tendency toward extrusion months or years later. Autogenous tissues are best used and may be of fat, cartilage, bone, muscle and fascia. Most convenient are pedicled flaps of fascia and muscle, as depicted in Figures 10–3 and 10–4. These are used to obliterate the lower portion of the mastoid process that was not involved in cholesteatoma.

### Atticotomy from Within the Meatus

For a small cholesteatoma sac lateral to the incus and malleus head and with a large external meatus, it may be possible to perform an endomeatal atticotomy as follows: a stapes type of meatal flap extended forward superiorly and outwardly is followed by removal of the meatal rim to exteriorize the small attic cholesteatoma sac. The surgeon may then dissect the sac and remove it intact, or he may leave the matrix and exteriorize the sac as a small Bondy radical cavity. Should he find that the cholesteatoma pocket is larger than anticipated, he should proceed with an endaural incision and atticotomy as described previously.

### Myringostapediopexy

In attic retraction cholesteatomas in which the sac-like skin-lined pouch lies lateral to the incus and head of the malleus, the ossicular chain may be intact and functioning with normal or nearly normal hearing. In other cases, the cholesteatoma has enveloped and partially destroyed these ossicles, yet the patient has normal or nearly normal hearing because of adherence of the upper edge of the pars tensa to the head of the stapes, "nature's myringostapediopexy." Such an adherence should not be disturbed provided cholesteatoma has not extended into the mesotympanum. A deliberate myringostapediopexy may be performed when the incus has been destroyed or must be removed, the surgeon depressing the upper edge of the intact pars tensa against the head of the mobile stapes.

### Extension of Cholesteatoma into the Mesotympanum Behind the Pars Tensa

This occasional occurrence requires excision of that portion of the pars tensa overlying the tympanic extension of cholesteatoma so as to exteriorize the latter, avoiding opening into the mucous membrane-lined portions of the tympanum.

In conclusion, the Bondy modification of the radical mastoidectomy is indicated in cases of cholesteatoma for which exteriorization of the involved areas is sought, this being the surest way of minimizing cholesteatoma residue or recurrence.

### Placement of the Meatal Flap and Packing of the Cavity

The plastic flap of meatal skin is turned back to cover the facial ridge, with care not to cover areas of remaining matrix or even areas that had been covered by matrix. A closed sleeve of surgical rayon or wide strips of surgical rayon are inserted to line the cavity, with cotton balls soaked in Gantrisin otic (or ophthalmic) solution placed firmly, but not tightly, to fill the cavity. At no point should cotton touch raw surface. One or two sutures partially close the endaural incision, but the final meatal opening must be packed wide open to three or four times the original size so that when healing is complete, the final meatus will be twice the former size and the healed exteriorized cavity can easily be inspected and kept clean (Fig. 10–1J).

### Skin Grafting the Radical or Bondy Cavity

Siebenmann[23] was the first to recommend skin grafting by the method of Thiersch to promote rapid healing of the radical cavity. Experience in nearly 100

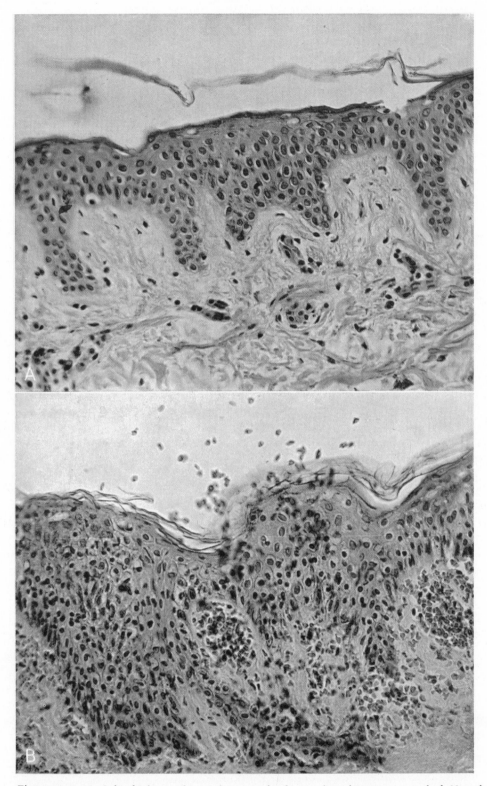

**Figure 10-5**   *A*, Split thickness skin graft removed 4 hours after placement on its bed. Note the intense spasm of the blood vessels, which are devoid of erythrocytes. *B*, Split thickness graft removed 24 hours after placement on its bed, showing beginning re-establishment of circulation with vessels filled with erythrocytes. (Courtesy of Dr. W. K. Wright.)

fenestration operations treated in this manner convinced the senior author[24] that primary split thickness skin grafting of the operative cavity is not desirable. When such a graft "took" by first intention, the epidermal lining of the healed cavity was closely applied to the bone without an intervening layer of connective tissue. Not only was the surface of the stratified squamous epithelium rough and uneven, but it continued to desquamate excessively, was very subject to localized areas of breakdown and granulations with discharge and there was a distinct tendency to invasion of crevices and cells requiring a later revision. With a thoroughly performed radical or Bondy operation with removal of matrix, the cavity will heal nearly always without troublesome granulations or suppuration provided careful sterile technique is observed in the operations and postoperative dressings.

Should the surgeon wish to shorten the time of final healing, he may apply a skin graft to the cavity two or three weeks postoperatively after it has become lined by a thin layer of healthy granulations that will then provide the desired subepithelial connective tissue layer[25] (Fig. 10–5).

## SECONDARY STAPES OPERATION, TYMPANOPLASTY OR FENESTRATION

The two requirements for effective sound conduction should be met by the Bondy operation. These requirements consist of an enclosed bubble of air against the round window, communicating with the eustachian tube, and sound transmission from the pars tensa of the tympanic membrane to the oval window via the intact ossicular chain, or via "nature's myringostapediopexy." After healing is complete and all inflammatory reaction within the tympanum has subsided, the patient should have little or no conductive hearing impairment as indicated by an audiometric air–bone gap. Should there be a persistent large air–bone gap, several possible problems exist:

1.   The round window may very rarely be occluded by bone.

2.   The incus, malleus or stapes may be immobilized by bone, tympanosclerosis or fibrous tissue.

3.   There may be an interruption of continuity between the pars tensa and mobile stapes.

4.   There may not be an air-containing cavity extending to the round window.

In the presence of an adequate cochlear reserve and a large air–bone gap, secondary exploration of the tympanic cavity by a stapes type of approach should be done. Depending upon the pathologic lesion found upon exposing the middle ear, a stapedectomy or tympanoplasty may be done as described in Chapters 18 and 16.

## POSTOPERATIVE CARE

The patient operated on under local anesthesia is encouraged to be out of bed the afternoon of surgery and may go home the next day in most cases. This early discharge and local rather than general anesthesia substantially reduce the costs of surgery, so important a consideration today.

The blood-stained outer dressing is changed before the patient returns home. The first postoperative treatment in the office is on the seventh or eighth day when the outer dressing is removed, the cotton ball packs and finally the surgical rayon sleeve are removed, and the one or two skin sutures are removed. The raw surface of the incision is painted with 2 per cent aqueous gentian violet to promote epidermization. Should there be a foul odor to the ear, Colymycin otic ear drops twice daily, half a dropperful, are prescribed. The ear should be seen and the endaural incision spread once or twice a week to prevent its edges from adhering, with resulting atresia. All postoperative dressing changes for the first several weeks should be performed with sterile technique so as not to introduce staphylococci or other fresh organisms. The application of 2 per cent aqueous gentian violet to the incision and any unhealed areas of the cavity promotes epidermization. When healing of the meatus is far enough along to prevent an atresia, the postoperative visits can be extended to several weeks. The occurrence of soft infected granulations requires that the patient place a dropperful of warmed 5 per cent boric acid in 70 per cent alcohol into his ear twice daily. This is an excellent promoter of epidermization of the cavity.

Once healed, the cavity should be inspected and cleaned every six to twelve months. The patient is instructed to place a medicine dropperful of Johnson's Baby Oil in his ear for three nights before these visits. This loosens and facilitates removal of crusts and epidermal debris.

## COMPLICATIONS OF THE RADICAL AND BONDY MODIFIED RADICAL OPERATIONS

The most serious complication and the cause of many malpractice suits is **facial nerve paralysis.** The patient must be examined and movement of the face on the operated side verified as soon as possible postoperatively. Sometimes a transient facial weakness occurs from the local anesthetic. This will recover within a few hours of surgery. If the face fails to move on the operated side on smiling, showing the teeth, wrinkling the forehead and closing the eye, the facial nerve should be explored and decompressed not later than the next day, with repair of any defect as described in detail in Chapter 20.

Due to aberrations in the course of the facial nerve, which in rare cases may be dehiscent and herniated into the oval window niche, or lie abnormally laterally at the posterior bend, or even run beneath the oval window, or emerge onto the lateral surface of the mastoid process, *surgical damage to the nerve may not be avoidable by the most experienced otologic surgeon.* Surgical damage to the nerve is especially unavoidable when previous surgery on that ear has resulted in distorted anatomy with loss of normal landmarks.

**Perichondritis** of the auricle, due to *Pseudomonas aeruginosa*, recognized by the red, tender thickening of the auricle and positive culture of pseudomonas, should be treated as described in Chapter 8 with ultraviolet irradiation and carbenicillin.

**Accidental tears of dura or sigmoid sinus** during a radical or Bondy operation should be treated as described in Chapter 9, with appropriate antibiotic coverage for predominant organisms.

**Chocolate or mucous cyst** in a healed radical cavity is the result of non-infected brownish serum collecting in a mucous membrane-lined pocket beneath the epidermal lining of a healed cavity. Simple puncture to evacuate the mucoid brownish serum reduces the cyst, but this does not prevent its recurrence. If such a cyst keeps recurring and is sufficiently troublesome, it should be exposed through an endaural incision, its mucoperiosteal lining curetted and a pedicle muscle-fascia graft used to obliterate this pocket.

**Cholesteatoma recurrence** in a healed radical or Bondy cavity occurs when a small island of matrix is covered by a muscle-fascia graft, or when healing of the cavity by epidermization covers over a tiny finger-like cholesteatoma extension. Since such recurrences (actually residues) of cholesteatoma are easily seen, they are easily uncapped, and they do not carry the risk of complication that follows residues and recurrences behind an intact canal wall, as described in Chapter 16.

**Granulation and discharge** from a once healed and dry radical or Bondy cavity arise when epidermal debris is allowed to accumulate and becomes infected. Thorough cleaning of the cavity and removal of granulations by a tiny cupped forceps or by wiping them off, followed by applying 2 per cent aqueous gentian violet, generally results in a dry ear.

Neglect of a radical mastoid or Bondy cavity that is allowed to fill with desquamated layers of keratinized epithelium brings back the original bone-eroding cholesteatoma with all its possible bone-eroding sequelae. The surgeon must impress upon his patient the inescapable necessity for periodic after-care of his radical cavity *at least once a year*, and oftener if accumulations of epidermal debris require such care. Periodic inspection of the ear is probably just as important, perhaps more so after an intact canal wall operation for cholesteatoma, to detect a hidden recurrence of cholesteatoma. Thus, all patients with cholesteatoma of the ear must continue under the care of an otologist for the rest of their lives, whether treated by attic irrigations (the rare case), by exteriorization of disease or by canal wall-up surgery.

## REFERENCES

1. von Tröltsch, A. F.: Lehrbuch der Ohrenheilkunde mit Einschluss der Anatomie des Ohres. Fogel, Leipzig, 1873.
2. von Bergmann, E.: Die chirurgische Behandlung von Hirnkrankheiten. Berlin, 1889.
3. Zaufal, E.: Technik der Trepanation des Proc. mastoid. nach Küster'schen Grundsätzen. Arch. Ohrenh., 30:291, 1890.
4. Stacke, L.: Stacke's Operationsmethode. Arch. Ohrenh., 35:145, 1893.
5. Körner, O.: Die eitrigen Erkrankungen des Schläfenbeins. Bergmann, Wiesbaden, 1899.
6. Bondy, G.: Totalaufmeisselung mit Erhaltung von Trommelfell und Gehörknöchelchen. Monatsschr. Ohrenheilk., 44:15, 1910.
7. Kopetsky, S. J.: Otologic Surgery, 2nd Ed. Paul B. Hoeber, Inc., New York, 1929.
8. Lempert, J.: Improvement of hearing in cases of otosclerosis: new one stage surgical technic. Arch. Otol., 28:42, 1938.
9. Baron, S.: Modified radical mastoidectomy. Arch. Otol., 49:280, 1949.
10. Zöllner, F.: Die Radikal-Operation mit besonderem Bezug auf die Hörfunktion. Ztschr. Laryng. Rhin. Otol., 30:104, 1951.
11. Wullstein, H.: Funktionelle Operationen im Mittelohr mit Hilfe des freien Spaltlappen-Transplantates. Arch. Ohren-, Nasen-u. Kehlkopfh., 161:422, 1952.
12. Cited by Babbitt, J. A.: The endaural surgery of chronic suppurations. In Kopetsky, S. J.: Loose-Leaf Surgery of the Ear. Thomas Nelson & Sons, New York, 1947.
13. Thies, F., Jr.: Die Radikaloperation durch den äusseren Gehörgang. Ztschr. Hals- Nasen-u. Ohrenh., 33:459, 1933.
14. Lempert, J.: Mastoidectomie sous-corticale. Ann. Mal. oreille, larynx., 48:111, 1929.
15. Passow, K. A.: Concerning closure of the bony defect after antrotomy. Pract. oto-rhino-laryng., 1:67, 1908.
16. Kisch, J.: Temporal muscle grafts in the radical mastoid operation. J. Laryng. & Otol., 43:735, 1928.
17. Meurman, Y., and Ojala, L.: Primary reduction of a large operation cavity in radical mastoidectomy with a muscle-periosteal flap. Acta Oto-laryng., 37:245, 1949.
18. Guilford, F. R.: Controlled cavity healing after mastoid and fenestration operations. Arch. Otol., 71:165, 1960.

19. Palva, T.: Surgery of chronic ear without cavity. Results in 130 cases with musculoperiosteal flap and fasciotympanoplasty. Arch. Otol. 77:570, 1963.

20. Adams, W. S.: The postoperative mastoid after fascial obliteration. J. Laryng. & Otol., 76:990, 1962.

21. Cody, D. T. R.: Mastoidectomy for acquired cholesteatoma: long-term results. Cholesteatoma First International Conference. Aesculapius Publ. Co., Birmingham, Alab., 1977.

22. Wright, W. K.: A concept for the management of attic cholesteatomas. Cholesteatoma First International Conference. Aesculapius Publ. Co., Birmingham, Alab., 1977.

23. Smythe, G. D. L.: Postoperative cholesteatoma. Cholesteatoma First International Conference. Aesculapius Publ. Co., Birmingham, Alab., 1977.

24. Siebenmann, F.: Die Radical-operation des Cholesteatoma mittelst Anlegung breiter permanenter Oeffnungen gleichzeitig gegen den Gehörgang und gegen die retroauriculare Region. Berl. klin. Wochnschr., 30:12, 1893.

25. Shambaugh, G. E., Jr., and Derlacki, E. L.: Primary skin grafting of the fenestra and fenestration cavity. Arch. Otol., 64:46, 1956.

26. Guilford, F. R., and Wright, W. K.: Secondary skin grafting in fenestration and mastoid cavities. Laryngoscope, 64:626, 1954.

## Gerhard Domagk

BORN 1895
DIED 1964

Demonstrated in 1932 the curative effects of prontosil, a red dye containing sulfanilamide, in streptococcic infection in mice, for which he received the Nobel Prize for Medicine.

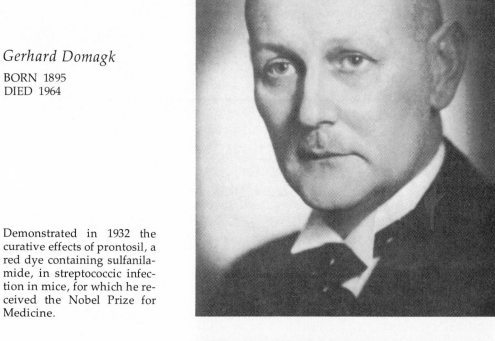

## Alexander Fleming

BORN 1881
DIED 1955

Alexander Fleming (on the left, demonstrating a bottle containing Penicillium notatum mold). Observed and recorded in 1928 lysis of staphylococcus colonies by Penicillium mold. The Nobel Prize, in 1945, was awarded Fleming, Florey and Chain "for the discovery of penicillin and its therapeutic effect for the cure of different infectious maladies."

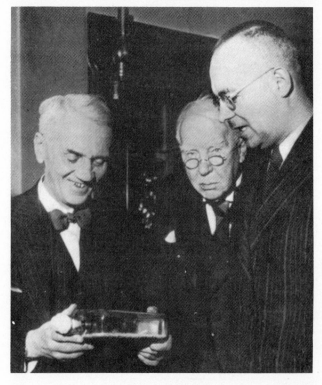

288

# Chapter 11

# Meningeal Complications of Otitis Media

HISTORICAL NOTES
FACTORS THAT INFLUENCE THE DEVELOPMENT OF
    COMPLICATIONS
PATHWAYS OF SPREAD IN THE PRODUCTION OF A
    COMPLICATION
EXTRADURAL AND PERISINUS ABSCESS
OTITIC MENINGITIS, LOCALIZED
OTITIC MENINGITIS, GENERALIZED
LATERAL SINUS THROMBOPHLEBITIS
OTITIC HYDROCEPHALUS
CEREBROSPINAL OTORRHEA

## HISTORICAL NOTES

Otitis media is a potentially serious disease chiefly because of its complications, which may threaten life and health. This has been recognized from antiquity when Hippocrates[1] about 460 B.C. noted that "acute pain of the ear with continued high fever is to be dreaded for the patient may become delirious and die." The Roman physician Celsus[2] mentioned around 25 A.D. that "inflammation and pains of the ear lead sometimes to insanity and death." The celebrated Arabian physician Avicenna,[3] who lived from 980 to 1037 A.D., related suppuration of the ear and of the brain, believing that the ear discharge was caused by the brain disease. It was Morgagni[2] (1682–1771) who first clearly recognized that the ear infection came first and brain abscess was secondary.

**Brain abscess** was the first complication of otitis media to be recognized, and it was the first one successfully treated by operation. In 1768 Morand[3] reported a successful operation for brain abscess, but nearly a century elapsed before Roux[4] reported the second successful operation. In 1856 Lebert[5] accurately described the pathology of brain abscess, confirming the fact that it follows infection of the ear, not the reverse. The surgical treatment of brain abscess then developed rapidly. In 1881 Macewen[6] reported the first of his remarkably successful series of 18 recoveries out of 19 operated cases of brain abscess, a record not to be surpassed until the advent of antibiotics. By 1908 Körner[7] was able to find 268 reported operations with 137 recoveries.

The surgery of brain abscess had reached its peak of otologic interest by the time of Eagleton's[8] text in 1922. The management of this relatively common complication of otitis media remained chiefly in the hands of the otologic surgeon until the sulfonamides began to be used for acute otitis media in 1935 and penicillin was introduced in 1942. Thereafter the incidence of brain abscess, which may already have begun to decline, decreased abruptly. Today few otologists see enough of these cases to remain familiar with the techniques of brain surgery, so that they frequently enlist the assistance of the neurosurgeon.

The relative success of surgery for brain abscess remained in sharp contrast for many years to the almost invariably fatal outcome of **purulent meningitis,** the most dreaded complication of otitis media and the most frequent cause of death. Since therapy of generalized otitic meningitis was rarely successful, the efforts of the otologic surgeon were directed toward prevention. Whenever possible, bone-invading types of acute and chronic otitis media were operated on before a complication had occurred. Careful clinical observation of patients with middle ear infections would not infrequently permit the detection of the earliest stages of beginning meningeal involvement. With prompt and thorough surgical drainage of the suppurative focus in the temporal bone considerable success was attained in arresting the meningeal invasion in many cases while it was still localized, preventing the development of the otherwise fatal generalized meningitis.[9] Despite these advances, meningitis remained the most frequent cause of death in otitis media, and otitis media was by far the most frequent cause for meningitis not due to the meningococcus.

The last of the three major intracranial complications of otitis media to be related to ear disease was infective **thrombosis of the lateral sinus,** first described by Hooper[7] in 1826. Thirty years later Lebert[10] accurately described the pathology of otitic sinus thrombosis. In 1880 Zaufal[11] proposed an operation for this complication and in 1884 he first attempted it, but the patient died.

The surgical treatment of sinus thrombosis was finally established by the publications of Lane[12] in 1889 and of Ballance[13] in 1890. However, a controversy over whether, as part of the surgical management, to ligate the jugular vein in all cases, in some cases or in none, continued for many years, only to be resolved by the introduction of effective antibacterial and anticoagulant medication in favor of non-ligation for most cases.

The two complications of otitis media due to extension **within** the temporal bone that often led to a fatal intracranial extension, namely **purulent labyrinthitis** and **petrositis,** were the last serious complications to be defined and effectively treated. A technique for draining the infected labyrinth was first described in 1895 by Jansen.[14] In 1904 Gradenigo[15] described a syndrome of continuing aural discharge and severe fifth nerve pain and sixth nerve paralysis due to infection of pneumatic cells in the petrous portion of the temporal bone with adjacent meningitis. In 1930 Kopetsky and Almour[16] and in 1931 Eagleton[17] described the first systematic attempts to drain an abscess of the petrous apex. Other methods for reaching this relatively inaccessible area were soon described by Frenckner,[18] Ramadier,[19] Lempert[20] and Farrior.[21] For a few years the literature contained numerous reports of successful operations for petrositis, many of them in patients with early meningitis. Just at the time that this frequent cause for otitic meningitis began to yield to surgical therapy, it virtually (but not quite) disappeared from the scene of otologic experience as the result of effective antibacterial medication for acute otitis media.

The most important single event in the history of complications of otitis media was unquestionably the introduction of sulfonamides and antibiotics. In the 5 year period immediately preceding their introduction, from 1928 to 1933, approximately 1 in every 40 deaths in a large general hospital was caused by an intracranial complication of otitis media, with meningitis heading the list, sinus thrombosis second and brain abscess last.[22] In a similar 5 year period from 1949 to 1954 only 1 in every 400 deaths was the result of ear disease, an amazing tenfold reduction in less than 20 years. The decrease in fatalities following acute otitis media was greatest, as this previously accounted for the majority of serious complications. Today the majority of fatal complications are the result of chronic suppurative otitis media, in which any decreased incidence has probably been due more to earlier recognition and better surgical treatment of cholesteatoma than to antibiotics, which are relatively ineffective against this bone-eroding disease.

Of the three major intracranial complications of otitis media the reduction in fatalities has been greatest for thrombophlebitis of the lateral sinus, which has nearly disappeared as a cause of death.[22] This is easily understood since infection of the blood stream was the usual mechanism of death from sinus thrombosis, and antibiotics act best in the blood stream. Brain abscess has been greatly reduced by antibiotics. Purulent otitic meningitis, though reduced, persists as by far the most frequent intracranial complication today of otitis media. However, it has been changed from a nearly 100 per cent fatal disease to one in which recovery can be expected in the majority of instances if it is diagnosed early and treated adequately.

The marvelous reduction in the frequency of otitic complications and the markedly improved prognosis of the intracranial complications have been accompanied, perhaps inevitably, by a less fortunate tendency to forget the importance of the middle ear in cases of brain abscess, sepsis and non-meningococcal meningitis. The family physician has come to rely more upon drugs to take care of ear infections than upon careful clinical study and early otologic consultation. The diagnostic acumen of the otologist has been blunted by his diminished experience and lessened familiarity with the symptomatology of otitic complications. The situation has been made more difficult by the masking effect of antibiotics on the symptoms of continued infection. These factors may be resulting in a recent increase in serious complications of otitis media, particularly in proportion to the number of cases of surgical mastoiditis.[23]

In a recent report of 50 intracranial complications of otitis media from 1961 to 1977,[24] more than half were due to brain abscess, with involvement of the temporal lobe 5 times more frequent than that of the cerebellum. Meningitis was second in frequency; lateral sinus thrombosis and cortical thrombophlebitis each caused two cases; there was one case of cerebral hernia and three of otitic hydrocephalus.

All but 3 of the 50 complications were in cases of chronic otorrhea with cholesteatoma or granulations or both. Three cases were unresolved acute otitis, two of which were due to pneumococcus.

The relatively high mortality of 36 per cent between 1939 and 1949 during early antibiotic therapy fell to 6 per cent between 1950 and 1960, and to no deaths between 1961 and 1971, owing to earlier diagnosis, the use of massive amounts of antibiotics, based on culture of the offending organism, and the use of steroids to reduce cerebral edema in cases of brain abscess and otitic hydrocephalus.

Today the neurosurgeon is often the first to be called in consultation for intracranial complications. While he should direct therapy of the complication, he must recognize the frequent otitic (sometimes nasal accessory sinus) origin and always request otolaryngologic consultation and help in the management, with surgical removal of the suppurative focus, which is usually in the ear. It is concluded that a quoted incidence of as high as 40 per cent postoperative cholesteatomas after intact canal wall techniques does not justify the use of this method for patients in the presence of an intracranial complication.

The patient with chronic suppurative otitis media who is not "doing well" may indicate trouble. Earache with chronic otitis means that something has gone wrong, and if pus is under pressure in the middle ear cleft, then an intracranial complication may be impending. Certainly, headache and drowsiness are danger signals. It must be stressed again that one of the earliest signs of brain abscess is a visual field defect, and this is almost invariably present if tested for carefully. A raised temperature suggests a meningitis or sinus thrombosis. Awareness of the significance of these symptoms and signs will result in earlier diagnosis, prompt treatment and a further reduction in mortality.

## FACTORS THAT INFLUENCE THE DEVELOPMENT OF COMPLICATIONS

The tendency of an acute middle ear infection to spread beyond the confines of the middle ear and its pneumatic spaces is influenced by the variety of infecting organism, its virulence in a particular epidemic, its susceptibility to available antibacterial medication, the adequacy of such medication, the resistance of the host and to a lesser degree the type of pneumatization and the history of previous otitis medias. Thus, certain strains of hemolytic streptococcus cause more complications than other strains of the same organism. The type III pneumococcus has a particular predilection for intracranial extension. The resistance of the host, especially to pneumococcus type III infection, is lowered in infancy, old age[21] and diabetes. Too small doses of an antibiotic, given for too brief a time, and the use of a less effective drug when a more effective one could have been selected by culture and sensitivity tests are important contributing causes to complications of otitis media. There is the increasingly important problem of bacteria that develop resistance to antibiotics, a resistance thus far definitely established only for staphylococcus infections.

Intracranial extension of acute otitis media occurs somewhat more often from poorly pneumatized than from well pneumatized temporal bones, and in ears with a history of previous attacks of otitis media.

The tendency of a chronic middle ear infection to produce a complication depends above all upon the pathologic lesion causing the chronic otorrhea. The benign type of chronic otorrhea with a mucoid discharge coming from a central perforation does not by itself invade bone and cause complications. There is, however, nothing to prevent a fresh virulent organism from entering such an ear, and causing an acute exacerbation and a complication by the same mechanism as in any acute otitis media. The bone-invading types of chronic otitis media that lead to complications are the relatively uncommon chronic osteomyelitis of the temporal bone and the much more common cholesteatoma of either the attic retraction or the secondary acquired variety (see Chapter 7), and the rare infected congenital cholesteatoma.

## PATHWAYS OF SPREAD IN THE PRODUCTION OF A COMPLICATION

Complications of otitis media occur when the normal defense barriers of the middle ear are overcome, permitting the infection to spread to an adjacent structure.

In Chapter 7 we saw how the mucoperiosteum of the middle ear is a continuation of the respiratory mucous membrane, possessing considerable ability to localize and overcome infection. When this first line of defense fails to halt the infection, the intact bony walls of the tympanic cavity and pneumatic cells afford a further effective barrier against extension of infection. Interruption of the bony barrier exposes the soft tissue of an adjacent structure to the infecting organism. If the adjacent structure is the periosteum of the outside of the skull, an easily diagnosed and relatively harmless subperiosteal abscess results; within the temporal bone a more serious facial nerve paralysis or labyrinthitis may occur; and inside the skull the infection may produce an extradural or perisinus abscess. In most cases, as the bony barrier is penetrated, a layer of protective granulations forms on the exposed structure as a third and last line of defense. In the case of an extradural abscess or perisinus abscess, this may localize the infection for a varying period of time before the development of a meningitis, lateral sinus thrombosis or brain abscess.

The pathway by which an infection may spread through the normal defense barriers is not always the same. In certain acute infections the spread is by **osteothrombophlebitis** through intact bone. In many acute and in most chronic infections the spread is by **bone erosion.** In certain cases the spread occurs along a **preformed pathway.** Each method of spread has certain characteristics by which it may be recognized. Since each requires a somewhat different therapeutic approach, it is necessary that the clinician attempt to ascertain the probable pathway of spread causing the complication in each particular case.

## Extension by Osteothrombophlebitis

Körner[7] in 1902 demonstrated by histopathologic studies that it is possible for infection to pass from the lining mucosa of the tympanum and mastoid cells **through intact bone** by means of a progressive thrombophlebitis of small venules. This manner of spread may occur in acute middle ear infections or in acute exacerbations of a chronic infection when a fresh virulent organism has entered the ear. In the preantibiotic era osteothrombophlebitis was a frequent pathway of spread in the virulent form of hemolytic streptococcus otitis media known as "acute hemorrhagic mastoiditis" (see Chapter 7). It also accounted for intracranial extensions from certain cases of pneumococcus type III otitis media so mild and transitory as almost to escape notice[25] (see Figs. 12–1 and 12–2).

A complication by osteothrombophlebitic spread may be recognized by these characteristics:

1.  The complication occurs **early** in the acute infection, sometimes within a day or two of the onset, usually within the first 10 days.

2.  In certain complications such as purulent meningitis there is lacking the prodromal period of beginning invasion with localized serous meningitis, such as is usually seen in extension by bone erosion.

3.  At operation the bony walls of the middle ear and mastoid cells are intact. The bone and mucoperiosteal lining of the mastoid cells may be inflamed and bleed excessively — hence the term "hemorrhagic mastoiditis" — but there is no coalescent abscess and the bone is not dehiscent.

The treatment of a complication by osteothrombophlebitic extension is directed toward the complication itself, as will be described, relying upon antibacterial medication to control the infection in the middle ear mucosa and thrombosed venules.

### Extension by Bone Erosion

This is the most frequent manner of spread leading to a complication in cases of acute otitis media in well pneumatized temporal bones, and it is nearly always the manner of spread in cases of chronic suppurative otitis media. In acute otitis media, bone erosion is the result of a coalescent mastoiditis, as described in Chapter 7. In chronic otitis media the bone erosion is usually due to a cholesteatoma; less often it is the result of a chronic osteomyelitis.

The bone-eroding process first exposes the soft tissue of a neighboring structure. Protective granulations form on the structure as a third and last line of defense. Then, after a period of time that varies with the virulence of the organism, the pus under pressure finally penetrates the wall of protective granulations by pressure necrosis.

Bone erosion as the pathway of spread may be recognized by these characteristics:

1. The complication occurs several weeks or more after the onset of an acute otitis media, or in a chronic otitis of long duration.

2. A prodromal period of partial or intermittent involvement of the structure frequently precedes the diffuse involvement. Thus a mild or intermittent facial weakness may precede complete facial paralysis; recurring mild vertigo often precedes diffuse purulent labyrinthitis; localized serous meningitis usually precedes diffuse purulent meningitis.

3. At operation a dehiscence of the bony barrier is found between the suppurative focus and the neighboring structure. The exposed soft tissue of the neighboring structure is covered by a layer of granulations.

The treatment of a complication by bone erosion is directed toward the complication **and always includes** surgical removal of the suppurative bone-eroding focus in the temporal bone. If the latter is neglected, the complication is likely to recur or to respond poorly to treatment.

### Extension by Preformed Pathway

This manner of spread may occur in acute exacerbations of chronic otitis media, but it can also occur in cases of acute and chronic otitis media. The preformed pathway may be a normal anatomic opening in the bony wall such as the oval or round window leading from the middle ear to the labyrinth, or the internal auditory meatus, perilymphatic duct or endolymphatic duct and sac leading from the labyrinth to the meninges. The pathway may be a developmental dehiscence, such as a patent petrosquamous suture in infants or a dehiscence of the floor of the hypotympanum over the jugular bulb. The preformed pathway may be the result of a skull fracture, or of previous aural surgery such as a fenestration, a stapes operation, a labyrinthotomy for Meniere's disease or a mastoidectomy with dural exposure. Perilymph fistula, which may be a congenital or an acquired rupture of the oval or round window, or which may follow partial or complete stapedectomy, establishes a wide-open pathway for infection to extend to the labyrinth and thence to the meninges from the first attack of otitis media to occur in such an ear. Occasionally a previous otitis media with a coalescent mastoiditis heals but leaves a scar tissue tract to a neighboring structure; this tract acts as a preformed pathway for a succeeding acute middle ear infection.

Extension by preformed pathway is not always easily diagnosed preoperatively. It is suggested by these characteristics:

1.   There is a history of repeated attacks of meningitis, skull fracture, operation on the temporal bone or previous healed otitis media.

2.   The complication occurs early in the acute infection, thus resembling extension by osteothrombophlebitis.

3.   At operation a dehiscence of the bony barrier not due to bone erosion is found.

4.   The patient has an intracranial complication following a suppurative labyrinthitis.

The treatment of a complication by preformed pathway is directed toward the complication along with closure of a fistula, and surgical evacuation of any collection of pus within the temporal bone. An example is a beginning meningitis via the internal auditory meatus from a suppurative labyrinthitis; the labyrinth should be drained at the same time that the meningitis is being treated by antibacterial medication.


## EXTRADURAL AND PERISINUS ABSCESS

If a coalescent mastoiditis is regarded as a stage in the development of an acute otitis media and not as a complication, then the **most frequent** complication of otitis media due to extension of infection beyond the bony barriers of the middle ear and pneumatic cells is an extradural collection of pus. If this lies against the dura of the middle fossa or of the posterior fossa medial to the sigmoid sinus, it is called an **extradural** or **epidural** abscess. If it lies against the split of posterior fossa dura enclosing the lateral sinus, it is called a **perisinus** abscess.

Extradural and perisinus abscesses are alike in their etiology, pathology, danger of extension through the dura and **usual dearth of symptoms.**


### Etiology

Extradural and perisinus abscess can develop by any of the three pathways of extension: rarely by breakdown of a thrombosed venule beneath an intact plate of bone, occasionally along a preformed fibrous tissue pathway and most often by bone erosion.


### Pathology

The bone erosion of coalescent mastoiditis frequently exposes the sigmoid portion of the lateral sinus to produce a perisinus abscess. The bone erosion of a cholesteatoma more often exposes the dura of the middle cranial fossa to produce an extradural abscess. In either case protective granulations always form between the pus and the dura. However, it is possible for an enlarging cholesteatoma, with a minimum of active infection of its debris, to expose dura with little or no granulation formation, the epidermal lining of the cholesteatoma lying directly on the dura. Even though there is no collection of pus or granulations against the dura, such a case is classified as an extradural abscess since the dura lies exposed to the infected area.

The clinical importance of extradural and perisinus abscesses is that, although frequently asymptomatic so that they are an incidental and often unexpected finding during a simple or radical mastoidectomy, they carry a grave risk of extension through the dura to produce a lateral sinus thrombophlebitis, a subdural abscess, meningitis or brain abscess. An extradural abscess may exist for a long time without symptoms to betray its presence, sometimes extending into months or even years in the case of cholesteatoma, until the protective granulations are finally penetrated or until a fresh virulent organism gains access to the ear, resulting, with little or no warning, in a rapid spread of infection to the meninges or brain.

## Symptoms

The majority of perisinus and extradural abscesses produce **no symptoms** and are a chance finding at operation. Their presence may be suspected when:
1.   There is a profuse or a markedly intermittent otorrhea.
2.   There are marked pulsations of the purulent discharge accentuated by compression of the internal jugular vein. The pulsations of the serosanguineous discharge of an early acute otitis media should not be confused with the pulsations of the thick, purulent aural discharge from an extradural abscess.
3.   There is a low grade fever of unknown origin following an acute otitis media.
4.   There is persistent headache on the side of the otitis media.
5.   There are symptoms and signs of localized protective meningitis.
6.   There are recurring attacks of non-meningococcal generalized meningitis.
7.   The x-ray shows an unusually large coalescent or cholesteatoma cavity.
8.   Occasionally a very large extradural abscess may cause symptoms of cerebral compression, with somnolence, projectile vomiting, papilledema and slowed pulse, resembling but without the localizing symptoms of a brain abscess.

## Treatment

The treatment of perisinus or extradural abscess is **surgical.** Antibacterial medication reaches pus under pressure in an abscess cavity only poorly and cannot be trusted to control the infection, especially in cases of chronic otitis media with cholesteatoma infected by more or less antibiotic-resistant organisms.

If the symptoms and findings suggest a possible extradural or perisinus abscess, the tegmen and sinus plates should be removed at operation and the dura exposed. If an abscess is found, the granulation-covered portion of the dura or lateral sinus should be uncovered until normal-appearing dura is reached in all directions, to be certain that there are no remaining areas of trapped extradural pus. The protective granulations on the dura or sinus wall should be disturbed as little as possible unless a necrotic lead to a subdural abscess or a brain abscess is found. Such a necrotic lead should be explored cautiously to avoid breaking through protective localizing meningeal adhesions. If a dural exposure by cholesteatoma is found covered by healthy-appearing epidermis, the latter need not be disturbed as long as the cholesteatoma is well exteriorized by means of a radical mastoidectomy.

In addition to the wide exposure of an extradural or perisinus abscess the causative coalescent or cholesteatomatous bone-eroding disease must be dealt with by the appropriate simple or radical mastoidectomy (see Chapters 9 and 10). At the same time, specific antibacterial medication for the particular infecting organism, as determined by culture and sensitivity tests, is indicated. This is done to prevent postoperative extension of infection through the protective granulations that are inevitably disturbed to some degree by surgery, an occurrence not infrequently observed in the presulfonamide and preantibiotic days.

## OTITIC MENINGITIS, LOCALIZED

The two most important complications, because they continue to be the most frequent cause of death in otitis media, are meningitis and brain abscess. The latter will be considered in the next chapter.

Two clinical types or degrees of meningitis should be distinguished: localized, circumscribed, serous or protective meningitis, sometimes called meningismus; and diffuse, purulent, generalized meningitis, also called leptomeningitis.

Localized meningitis may be defined as a localized inflammation of the dura and pia-arachnoid confined to the region adjacent to a suppurative focus or dural irritation, **without viable organisms in the spinal fluid.**

### Pathology

The usual suppurative focus causing a localized meningitis is an extradural abscess, most often secondary to an otitis media. If the extradural abscess exists long enough, there may be local dural necrosis and an adjacent but still localized intradural or subdural abscess. The process of localization involves both the dura itself, which becomes thickened by deposition of fibrin and proliferation of fibroblasts, and the arachnoid, which, when irritated, reacts with fibroblastic proliferation and accumulation of round cells, until the inflamed area is walled off by granulations and adhesions between the dura, the arachnoid and the cortex of the brain.

Besides an extradural abscess, other suppurative otogenic foci that may incite a localized meningitis are: a broken-down, infected thrombus in the lateral sinus (actually an intradural abscess); suppurative labyrinthitis; osteomyelitis of the temporal bone, especially of the petrous portion; and brain abscess. Laceration of the dura by surgical trauma causes a localized meningeal reaction that soon walls off and arrests the escape of cerebrospinal fluid. Electrocoagulation of the dura causes a similar meningeal reaction that may be utilized to wall off the cerebrospinal space preparatory to draining a brain abscess. In infants a localized meningeal inflammation known as "meningismus" may occur via the patent petrosquamous suture from an unperforated acute otitis media.

### Symptoms

The symptoms of localized meningitis range from those that are so minimal that they are detected only by the alert clinician who is watching for them in every otitis media, to those that are severe and resemble diffuse purulent meningitis. The two most constant symptoms are **headache** and **an increase in temperature.** Cerebral irritation may cause the patient to be **irritable or drowsy.** There may be non-projectile **vomiting.** Infants with meningismus may have **convulsions.**

### Signs

The most constant and the earliest sign of localized meningitis is slight to moderate **neck rigidity,** with resistance to flexing the neck, so that the chin does not touch the chest. With this there is often a positive **Kernig** sign — inability to extend the leg completely with the thigh flexed on the abdomen. Infants with meningismus may also have a true opisthotonos, with a positive Brudzinski sign — flexion of the hip and knee when the neck is bent; positive Babinski test — extension of the toes instead of flexion on stimulating the sole of the foot; and the ankle clonus reflex — pressure on the sole with flexion of the foot causes clonic contractions of the calf muscles.

## Diagnosis

The diagnosis of localized meningitis is conclusively established by the spinal fluid examination showing **increased numbers of cells but normal sugar and no organisms on culture.** The fluid may appear grossly clear, slightly opaque, or "ground glass," or cloudy, and the cells may be as few as 10 or 16 to as many as a thousand per cubic millimeter, but with lymphocytes predominating. The spinal fluid pressure may be normal or increased. The protein is increased in proportion to the cells. Localized otitic meningitis must be differentiated from tuberculous and non-bacterial meningitis (see Table 11–1).

## Treatment

The treatment of localized otitic meningitis is directed toward the suppurative focus in the temporal bone. In the case of infants with meningismus or children and adults with an **early** acute otitis media, a myringotomy with antibacterial medication for the causative organism may suffice. Whenever localized meningitis occurs

TABLE 11–1   SPINAL FLUID FINDINGS IN VARIOUS ETIOLOGIC
FORMS OF MENINGITIS

| Etiologic Form | Cells Number and Predominance | Sugar | Culture |
|---|---|---|---|
| Bacterial Often otitic { Streptococcus Pneumococcus Staphylococcus Pseudomonas aeruginosa Coliform organisms | 1000 + polymorphonuclear | low | positive |
| Meningococcus | 1000 + polymorphonuclear | low | positive |
| Tuberculous | fewer than 1000 lymphocytes | low | positive only by special media |
| Fungal Cryptococcus (torula) | fewer than 1000 lymphocytes | normal (or low) | positive only by special media |
| Syphilis | fewer than 1000 lymphocytes | normal | negative |
| Protozoal Malaria Toxoplasmosis | fewer than 1000 lymphocytes | normal | negative |
| Viral Poliomyelitis Mumps Lymphocytic choriomeningitis | fewer than 1000 lymphocytes | normal | negative |
| Localized Otitic Meningitis | fewer than 1000 lymphocytes | normal | negative |

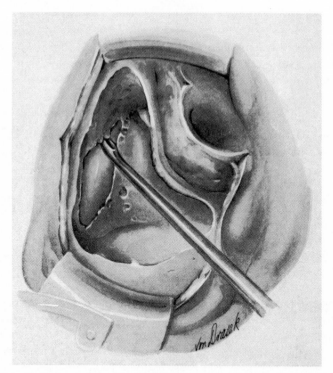

**Figure 11–1** Technique of exposing middle fossa dura in search for extradural abscess.

in a chronic otitis media or after the first week or two of an acute otitis media, **immediate surgical exploration** is indicated to search for and remove or drain the suppurative focus. This is a true otologic emergency for within a few hours of the earliest minimal symptoms of localized meningitis the infection may penetrate the inflammatory barriers to become the much more serious and difficult to control generalized meningitis.

Surgical exploration should include wide exposure of the dura of the middle and posterior cranial fossae in the search for an extradural abscess (Fig. 11–1). If insufficient pathologic change is found in the mastoid portion of the temporal bone, the perilabyrinthine area should be explored for a lead to the petrous portion. When a localized meningitis is secondary to a suppurative labyrinthitis, the labyrinth must be drained (see Chapter 12).

## OTITIC MENINGITIS, GENERALIZED

Generalized otitic meningitis may be defined as a pyogenic infection of the pia-arachnoid over the entire brain and spinal cord, **with viable organisms in the spinal fluid.** In the presulfonamide days disease of the ear was the most common cause of generalized meningitis not due to the meningococcus. Today ear disease still ranks as an important cause of non-meningococcal purulent meningitis.

### Pathology

It is important to remember that diffuse generalized otitic meningitis is **usually** preceded by a localized meningitis lasting several hours to a few days or longer. As the bacteria penetrate the barriers of localized meningitis they finally reach and begin to multiply rapidly in the cerebrospinal fluid itself, utilizing the sugar and spreading to infect the pia-arachnoid around the entire brain and spinal cord. At autopsy a plastic exudate is found over the entire brain and spinal cord, but the exudate is usually most marked and oldest over the base of the brain near the site of invasion from the ear. In patients autopsied after penicillin treatment, perivascular areas clear of exudate have been described,[22] showing that the penicillin acts through the blood stream rather than through the cerebrospinal fluid.

### Symptoms

The symptoms of generalized meningitis are similar to those of the localized variety but **greater in degree.** A **chill** may accompany the initial rise in temperature. The **pulse is rapid and fever is high** and in the terminal stages may be very high indeed (107 to 108° F.), perhaps owing to involvement of the temperature-regulating center. **Headache** is constant and may become excruciating; it may be temporarily lessened by lumbar puncture. The **neck is retracted and the spine stiff** so that the entire body can be lifted by elevating the head. The sensorium becomes clouded, with restlessness and delirium progressing to **coma.** Convulsions, ocular paralyses, hemiplegia and other paralyses may occur as the plastic exudate involves the cerebral cortex and cranial nerves. As the intracranial pressure rises in the terminal stages there may be slowed pulse, elevated blood pressure, Cheyne-Stokes respiration and projectile vomiting. Choked discs may appear toward the end.

### Diagnosis

The conclusive diagnosis of generalized meningitis is made by lumbar puncture revealing a **grossly cloudy fluid,** containing **more than a thousand cells** per cubic millimeter, **predominantly polymorphonuclear** with **reduced sugar** and **organisms on smear and culture.** Epidemic cerebrospinal meningitis due to the meningococcus will need to be differentiated from otitic meningitis by means of culture and stained smear.

### Treatment

The treatment of generalized otitic meningitis is twofold: evacuation of the suppurative focus in the temporal bone and specific antibacterial medication parenterally rather than intrathecally for the organism in the spinal fluid. The heroic and usually unsuccessful attempts to save the patient in the presulfonamide era by operations to provide continuous drainage from the cisterna magna are no longer indicated.

Since the prognosis of purulent meningitis is directly dependent upon the **earliest possible correct diagnosis** and the **prompt application of appropriate therapy,** the management of the patient with meningitis is worth describing in detail.

The first **invariable rule** is for the physician routinely to examine **every** patient with a fever for stiffness of the neck and a Kernig sign. If neither is present, it is unlikely that meningitis is present, the only exception being in infants when a bulging fontanelle or a low weak cry in the presence of fever may point to a meningitis.[26]

The second step is to perform a lumbar puncture **as soon as possible** if the neck is even slightly stiff on flexion or the Kernig sign is positive. The spinal fluid pressure should be noted, and its gross clarity or cloudiness, the total and differential cell count and the sugar, protein and chloride content determined. The fluid should be cultured and the centrifuged sediment stained with Gram's stain and acid-fast stain.

When the cells exceed 1000 and are predominantly polymorphonuclear with reduced sugar and a positive culture, the meningitis is bacterial, due either to a streptococcus, pneumococcus, staphylococcus, *Pseudomonas aeruginosa, Bacillus proteus* or colon bacillus, any of which may be of otitic origin, or to the meningococcus of non-otitic origin.

When the cells are fewer than 1000 and are predominantly lymphocytes, the meningitis is of fungal, viral, protozoal or spirochetal origin, or is due to the tubercle bacillus, or **it may be a localized meningitis of otitic origin.** The usual spinal fluid findings in the various etiologic forms of meningitis are given in Table 11–1.

The third step in the treatment of generalized bacterial meningitis is to administer adequate and appropriate antibacterial medication. Immediately after the diagnostic lumbar puncture the patient is started on massive doses of soluble (not long-acting) penicillin, 1 million units intramuscularly every 2 hours, or up to 150 million units intravenously every 24 hours. If the course is favorable and the spinal fluid becomes clear, with normal sugar and no more than 100 lymphocytes per cubic millimeter, this may be reduced on the third day to 600,000 units every 6 hours.

As soon as culture and sensitivity tests have revealed a more suitable agent, this should be added to, or substituted for, the penicillin. However, penicillin and Aureomycin should not be given concurrently, as they appear to be antagonistic.[26] Streptomycin should always be used rather than dihydrostreptomycin because of the delayed irreversible cochlear deafness that may follow the latter, even after a lapse of several months.[27] Chloromycetin (chloramphenicol) given orally, 0.6 Gm. for the first dose and 0.3 Gm. every 6 hours, passes readily into the cerebrospinal fluid and is effective against *Bacillus coli* and *Hemophilus influenzae*, a frequent cause of acute otitis in infants. *Pseudomonas aeruginosa* and staphylococcus meningitis present special problems. The former responds to carbenicillin and gentamycin. Staphylococcus may be resistant to all of the known antibiotics, but ampicillin should be given for this and for proteus infections. New antibiotics are constantly being discovered with added effectiveness against particular organisms. The reader will need to consult the recent literature in addition to utilizing sensitivity tests in order to treat resistant infections.

Intrathecal medication is considered detrimental because of the meningeal irritation and fibrosis, sometimes resulting in deafness and blindness.[28]

Excessive intracranial pressure may need to be relieved by lumbar or ventricular punctures. Frequent changes in the position of the patient may help to prevent accumulations of pus in dependent portions of the arachnoid.[29] Other suggestions for the treatment of meningitis are included in Chapter 23.

The fourth step in the treatment of generalized non-meningococcal bacterial meningitis is to search for a suppurative focus in the middle ear, accessory sinuses or lungs. If there is a history of otitis media in the preceding months, the possibility of a silent or masked mastoiditis must be considered even though there are no recent ear symptoms, only mild changes in the tympanic membrane and questionable x-ray mastoid changes. The only positive finding may be a slight loss of hearing or slight tenderness over the mastoid, and yet at operation a coalescent mastoiditis and an extradural abscess may be found as the primary focus for the meningitis. If there is doubt, an exploratory mastoidectomy may be indicated when no other source can be found to account for a non-meningococcal meningitis. If disease is found, the middle and posterior fossa dura should be exposed for a possible extradural abscess, and leads to the petrous portion of the temporal bone should be explored. For recurrent meningitis, surgical exploration for a perilymph fistula may be necessary.

The otologist should not overlook a tiny crust or polyp in the superior meatal wall above the short process of the malleus, concealing an asymptomatic attic cholesteatoma, as a possible source of otitic meningitis.

## LATERAL SINUS THROMBOPHLEBITIS

Phlebitis and thrombophlebitis of the sigmoid portion of the lateral sinus ranked second to meningitis in the presulfonamide era as the most frequent fatal complication of otitis media. Although rarely seen today, this complication does occur, and is very easily overlooked because of the masking effect of antibiotics on fever, the most constant symptom.

### Pathology

Lateral sinus thrombophlebitis is characteristically a hemolytic streptococcus complication; the majority of reported cases in the presulfonamide days were due to this organism. The type III pneumococcus and the staphylococcus are next in order of frequency.

The usual pathway to the sinus is by coalescent or cholesteatomatous bone erosion and formation of a perisinus abscess. After a period of time that varies with the virulence of the organism, the resistance of the host and the use of antibacterial medication, the pus under pressure in the perisinus abscess penetrates by pressure necrosis the protective granulations and the dural outer wall of the sinus. When the inflammatory process reaches the intima of the lateral sinus, fibrin, blood cells and platelets adhere to it, producing a **mural thrombus.** As the progressing infection begins to invade the mural thrombus, the latter propagates until an **obliterating thrombus** occludes the lumen of the sinus. Infection and purulent breakdown within the thrombus are accompanied by the formation of fresh thrombus in either direction, the thrombus thus tending to propagate downward toward the jugular bulb and internal jugular vein, backward toward the torcular Herophili, and into the mastoid emissary vein, superior petrosal sinus and inferior petrosal sinus. Meanwhile the broken-down purulent contents of the sinus, actually an intradural abscess, may incite a localized and later a generalized meningitis or brain abscess.

The lateral sinus may also become involved by osteothrombophlebitic extension through intact bone early in an acute otitis media. Sometimes the infected venules empty organisms directly into the bloodstream in the sinus, producing a septicemia without an occluding thrombosis, but more often the thrombi in the venules propagate into the lumen of the sinus. In either event the bony sinus plate will be found to be intact when exposed surgically, and the outer dural wall of the sinus may appear normal.

The formation of the thrombus within the lateral sinus is regarded as a protective mechanism attempting to localize the spreading infection. In some cases it is successful: the thrombus organizes, and recovery ensues. In such a patient an old, healed, obliterated lateral sinus may be noted months or years later at autopsy. These cases of spontaneous healing of an infected lateral sinus are rare. In most cases of untreated lateral sinus thrombosis the infection within the sinus cannot drain externally, and death is due to sepsis as infected material continues to escape into the systemic circulation, or to obstructed venous return from the brain, or to inward spread, producing a brain abscess or terminal meningitis.

### Symptoms

The most constant, characteristic and sometimes the **only symptom** of lateral sinus thrombophlebitis is the **fever.** Typically the fever is septic in type, with wide swings in the temperature curve producing a "picket-fence" temperature chart. Chills usually precede the sharp rises in temperature, and profuse sweats accompany the downward swings. Each rise in temperature corresponds to the escape of a fresh batch of organisms into the systemic circulation, occurring at irregular intervals but averaging once or twice in 24 hours. The temperature curve resembles that of malaria but lacks its regularity. Variations in the fever curve are seen, some cases having a high sustained fever and some having moderate elevations occurring only once every few days.

Between the bouts of fever the patient with lateral sinus thrombophlebitis is **alert with a sense of well-being** out of proportion to his serious illness and downhill course, in contrast to the apathy of brain abscess and the prostration of meningitis.

**Progressive anemia** is the third symptom of infection of the lateral sinus, and is especially rapid and pronounced in hemolytic streptococcus infections.

**Progressive emaciation** is the fourth symptom, especially noticeable to the consultant or relative who see the patient again after a lapse of several days, but not as rapid and pronounced as in cerebellar abscess.

**Obstruction of venous return** from the brain produces symptoms more often when the larger right lateral sinus is thrombosed than when the smaller left lateral sinus is diseased. The symptoms and signs resemble those of otitic hydrocephalus with **headache, increased cerebrospinal fluid pressure** and **eyeground changes.** The latter occur in 50 per cent of cases and consist of papilledema, especially on the affected side, as the most frequent finding, half with retinal hemorrhages, blurring of the disc margins and dilatation of retinal veins.[30]

Less common symptoms of lateral sinus thrombophlebitis are: edema over the posterior aspect of the mastoid process due to thrombosis of the mastoid emissary vein, known as **Greisinger's sign;** tender enlarged cervical glands along the internal jugular vein on the involved side; extension to the cavernous sinus via the superior or the inferior petrosal sinus, with the usual symptoms of cavernous sinus thrombosis, namely chemosis, proptosis, fixation of the eyeball and papilledema; and pain when there is dural inflammation.

### Diagnosis

There is no infallible diagnostic test for infective thrombosis of the lateral sinus, and the final diagnosis depends upon surgical exploration. The most helpful diagnostic aid is the blood culture.[31] This should be taken if possible at the time of a chill when a fresh batch of organisms has entered the systemic circulation. Several cultures may be necessary before a positive one is obtained. **A positive blood culture cannot be obtained while the patient is on effective antibacterial therapy.**

A positive blood culture is very strong evidence in favor of a lateral sinus thrombophlebitis. However, a negative blood culture on one or several occasions does not rule it out. If the culture is positive, lateral sinus thrombophlebitis should be differentiated from other causes for positive blood culture, such as the transient bacteremia after tonsillectomy or a tooth extraction, and bacterial endocarditis.

The second most helpful diagnostic test of lateral sinus thrombosis is the **Tobey-Ayer** or **Queckenstedt test.** This test is performed as follows:

A spinal needle is introduced into the lumbar canal, a manometer is attached and the resting spinal fluid pressure is recorded. The change in pressure produced by digital compression of first one internal jugular vein, then the other and then both at once, and the pressure changes occurring when compression of one jugular vein is released, then the other and then both, are all noted and recorded. When the spinal fluid pressure fails to rise after compression of the internal jugular vein on the side of the diseased ear, and fails to fall when this vein is released, with a prompt response from the opposite side, the test is positive. Like the blood culture, a positive Tobey-Ayer or Queckenstedt test is strong evidence in favor of an occlusion of the lateral sinus, but it is not infallible. A false positive test occurs when one lateral sinus is much smaller than the other and this is usually the left one. A false negative test occurs when there is unusually good collateral circulation around the obstructed lateral sinus via the mastoid emissary vein, inferior petrosal sinus and sinus of Englitsch (see Chapter 1).

The presumptive diagnosis of lateral sinus thrombophlebitis could be made in the presulfonamide era, even with a negative blood culture and a negative Tobey-Ayer-Queckenstedt test, from the characteristic chills and "picket-fence" fever curve. Today both the fever and the blood culture are masked by antibacterial medication, leaving only the Tobey-Ayer-Queckenstedt test for diagnosis. In case of doubt it may be advisable to discontinue antibacterial therapy for several days to unmask a suspected lateral sinus thrombophlebitis. The possibility of this complication should be kept in mind whenever a perisinus abscess is found at operation and when following evacuation of such an abscess the patient fails to do well. Surgical exploration of the sinus may then be indicated, as described in the following paragraphs.


*Treatment*

The accepted treatment of lateral sinus thrombophlebitis in the presulfonamide era was **always surgical.** The details of the surgical management varied among different authors, but certain principles were generally agreed upon.[32] These will be described first, followed by a description of today's treatment of these cases as modified by antibacterial and anticoagulant medication.

As noted before, the final diagnosis of lateral sinus thrombosis was made by surgical exploration. When the clinical symptoms, especially a high swinging "picket-fence" fever with chills, and the diagnostic blood culture and Tobey-Ayer-Queckenstedt tests pointed toward infection of the lateral sinus, exploration was carried out as follows:

A complete simple mastoidectomy (or a radical mastoidectomy if the patient

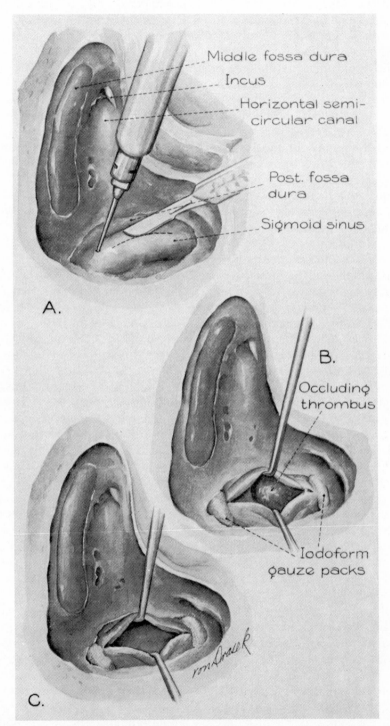

**Figure 11–2** Technique for exploring for sigmoid sinus thrombosis. *A*, Wall of the sinus and adjacent posterior fossa dura has been exposed by removal of sinus plate. The sinus may be aspirated with a short bevel, large bore needle. Most authors prefer to incise the sinus wall using the belly of the curved blade. *B*, Exposure of thrombus within the sinus. *C*, Thrombus evacuated from sinus lumen. (Note: The sinus lumen is usually occluded above and below by gauze packs, as shown in *B* and *C*, before exploratory incision but not for exploratory aspiration.)

had a chronic suppurative otitis with cholesteatoma) was performed, including removal of the bony sinus plate so as to expose the outer dural wall of the sigmoid portion of the lateral sinus (Fig. 11–2). The exposed wall of the sinus was inspected and palpated, but all authors agreed that its appearance could be deceptive, a broken-down purulent thrombus sometimes having a consistency similar to a normal blood-filled sinus, and a normal-appearing outer dural wall sometimes concealing a thrombus within. If a perisinus abscess was found, the exposure of the granulation-covered wall of the sinus was continued in all directions until normal-appearing wall and posterior fossa dura were reached. If the symptoms and signs of sepsis were not severe and the sinus appeared soft, nothing further was done at this time. If the temperature dropped and the patient proceeded to recovery, there was no way of knowing whether a thrombus was present or not.

If on the other hand the sinus wall looked and felt suspicious, and the symptoms and signs of sepsis were severe, or if following mastoidectomy and simple exposure of the sinus wall the septic symptoms continued, the lumen of the sinus was explored as follows:

A tampon of tightly rolled ½ inch iodoform gauze, a little wider than the sinus, was inserted between the sinus wall and the bony plate at the upper end of the exposed area, and a second plug was inserted between the bone and sinus wall at the lower end of the exposure, thus occluding the lumen at both ends (Fig. 11–2B). A vertical ½ inch incision was then made through the outer dural wall of the sinus, great care being taken not to wound the inner dural wall. The interior of the sinus was examined. If no clot was found, the upper plug was loosened; free bleeding indicated that there was no thrombus above the area of exposure, and the plug was replaced. The lower plug was then loosened and if there was free bleeding, the conclusion was that the jugular bulb was not thrombosed. When, on exploration, the sinus was not thrombosed but the septic symptoms and signs were severe and the exposed wall of the sinus was discolored, the plugs obliterating the lumen above and below the area of exposure were left in place to obliterate the sinus and prevent further infection of the systemic circulation from the localized phlebitis. In other cases when the sinus was found not thrombosed, the bleeding from the incision in its wall was controlled by holding iodoform gauze against it while the upper and lower plugs were slowly removed. This gauze was left in place 4 to 6 days until firm healing of the incision occurred.

If, when its wall was incised, a thrombus was found in the sigmoid sinus, the internal jugular vein was ligated in the neck just above the entrance of the common facial vein. This was done to prevent particles of infected thrombus from being broken off and carried to the lung, and to prevent air embolism. The incision in the sinus wall was then extended until the end of the thrombus was reached, with further removal of the bony sinus plate if necessary as far as the torcular Herophili posteriorly and the jugular bulb inferiorly if the thrombus was that extensive. The exposed thrombus was then lifed out of the lumen with forceps, with care to avoid trauma to the inner dural wall. Removal of thrombus was continued until free bleeding was encountered from both ends, and this bleeding was controlled by iodoform gauze plugs inserted between the bone and sinus wall as before. These plugs could be removed in 3 or 4 days, by which time the sinus lumen would have been obliterated by adhesions between its outer and inner walls. Following removal of the thrombus, the outer wall of the diseased sinus was sometimes excised with scissors, leaving an open trough.

Variations in the surgical procedure just described consisted of: simple aspiration of the sinus through a large needle instead of an exploratory incision (Fig.

11–2*A*) or removal of only the central, broken-down portion of the thrombus, leaving firm thrombus at either end as nature's method of localizing the infection. Some authors advised excision of the cervical portion of the internal jugular vein rather than simple ligation of the vein. The problem of when to perform jugular vein ligation in cases of suspected lateral sinus thrombophlebitis was a much debated one. Some otologists advised jugular ligation in every case of otogenic sepsis; others advised ligation only when a thrombus was found to be present; others reserved ligation for the cases of continuing sepsis after evacuation of a thrombus from the lateral sinus; a few advised against jugular ligation in any case. Numerous statistical studies were made to show the value or uselessness of jugular ligation, without solving the problem. The advent of effective antibacterial and anticoagulant therapy has finally settled the debate in favor of simple evacuation of the central broken-down portion of the thrombus from the lateral sinus without routine jugular ligation in every case, relying upon an anticoagulant such as heparin or Dicumarol to prevent further extension of the thrombus, and antibacterial medication selected according to culture and sensitivity tests to sterilize the blood stream.

In addition to surgical exploration and evacuation of the thrombus from the lateral sinus, with or without jugular ligation, subsequent supportive therapy for the septic patient in the presulfonamide era consisted of repeated blood transfusions and evacuation of any metastatic abscesses.

In the presulfonamide era the mortality rate of surgically treated lateral sinus thrombophlebitis varied greatly in different reports, probably depending more upon the virulence of the particular organism and the duration of septic symptoms before the patient was seen than upon the details of surgical management. An average mortality of around 20 per cent for surgically treated cases, and around 100 per cent for untreated cases, could be expected. Today the recognized and surgically and antibiotically treated patient with thrombosis of the sigmoid sinus should recover.

### Jugular Bulb Thrombosis

Propagation of a thrombus from the sigmoid portion of the lateral sinus to the jugular bulb was considered an indication for surgical exposure and evacuation of the bulb. Grunert[33] and Piffl[34] devised elaborate operations to expose and drain the bulb. The simpler methods described by Voss[35] and Whiting[36] consisted in following the sigmoid sinus to the bulb by removing the bony posterior wall of the bulb medial to the facial nerve and inferior to the posterior semicircular canal.

Primary jugular bulb thrombosis without involvement of the sigmoid sinus was sometimes seen in early acute middle ear infections, by osteothrombophlebitic spread from the hypotympanum. The diagnosis was made by surgical exploration of the mastoid, revealing absence of a thrombus in the sigmoid portion with no bleeding from the lower end when the occluding plug of iodoform gauze was removed, but free bleeding from the upper end.

### Treatment Today of Lateral Sinus Thrombophlebitis

Sinus thrombosis caused 0.3 per cent of deaths during the first quarter of this century, and only 0.01 per cent of deaths during the 5 years 1956 to 1960,[37] a three hundred fold decrease. Formerly due most often to acute otitis media and the hemolytic streptococcus, the majority of cases today occur in chronic otorrhea with cholesteatoma, and the invading organism is of the type found in infected cholestea-tomas, namely, *B. proteus, Pseudomonas aeruginosa, Bacillus coli* or staphylococ-cus. These organisms, unlike the hemolytic streptococcus, do not cause a septi-cemia, but may spread to the lungs by infected emboli, or more often directly through the inner wall of the sigmoid sinus, causing a brain abscess.

The rarity of sinus thrombosis today and the masking effect of antibiotics on fever, the most frequent and characteristic symptom of this complication, have made early diagnosis more difficult. As a result, although the total number of deaths from sinus thrombosis is exceedingly low today, the mortality rate continues to be high; it was 25 per cent in the 12 cases that occurred in 5 years in Denmark.[37] Each of these three deaths was due to brain abscess, two cerebellar and one temporal lobe.

The possibility of lateral sinus thrombosis should be considered in a patient with an acute suppurative otitis media who begins to run a high or septic type of fever, and in any patient with a chronic draining ear who begins to run even a slight or intermittent fever, for a chronic otitis media by itself, even when due to a very large infected cholesteatoma, rarely causes an elevation in temperature. Loss of weight, anemia, headache due to obstructed venous return, deterioration in general health and metastatic lung abscess suggest sinus thrombosis. A negative blood culture and a negative Tobey-Ayer-Queckenstedt test do not rule out the possibility of a thrombosed lateral sinus.

With the single exception of the patient with an early acute suppurative otitis media and sepsis due to the hemolytic streptococcus, in whom penicillin may be sufficient to control the infection within the sinus as well as blood stream, the treatment of suspected sinus thrombosis is surgical: an immediate radical mas-toidectomy (if there is a chronic otorrhea) with wide exposure of the wall of the sigmoid sinus. Should a perisinus abscess be found, the organism should be cultured with antibiotic sensitivity tests. If the patient does well, with no further fever or metastatic infection, nothing more need be done beyond treatment with the effective antibiotic. If the fever continues for 48 hours, and the patient's general condition does not improve, the mastoid wound should be reopened and the sinus wall incised by a vertical incision. If an infected thrombus is found, the exposure of sinus wall and incision should be extended in both directions until solid red thrombus or free bleeding is encountered. Ligation of the internal jugular vein may not be necessary except in patients with metastatic lung infection, or those who continue to do poorly after evacuation of the infected thrombus. In addition to full doses of the effective antibiotic, as determined by sensitivity tests, the patient should receive heparin or Dicumarol to prevent further propagation of the thrombus, and he should be watched for symptoms of cerebellar or temporal lobe brain abscess. Transfusions, formerly indicated in all cases to combat the septicemia and resulting anemia, should be withheld in most cases because of the increased risk today of serum hepatitis.

### Technique of Jugular Vein Ligation

The technique of internal jugular vein ligation (only rarely required today) is as follows: The patient should lie flat on his back, with the head turned to the side and a folded sheet beneath the shoulders to stretch the neck. A skin incision 5 to 7 cm.

long is made along the anterior border of the sternocleidomastoid muscle, beginning 2.5 cm. above the angle of the jaw and continuing to the level of the thyroid cartilage (Fig. 11–3). The incision is deepened by sharp dissection through the superficial fascia and platysma, with the external jugular vein retracted back out of the way. The deep fascia encloses the sternocleidomastoid muscle and the carotid sheath, and must be divided by sharp dissection along the anterior border of the muscle (Fig. 11–3). The latter can then be retracted posteriorly, exposing the carotid sheath enclosing the internal jugular vein, the bifurcation of the common carotid artery and the vagus nerve. The vein lies superficial and slightly posterior to the artery, with the vagus nerve behind and between the vein and artery. The jugular vein is easily recognized by its dark blue color and the fact that it empties with each inspiration and refills with each expiration. The common carotid artery is easily identified by palpation of its strong pulsations. By blunt dissection the internal jugular vein is carefully freed from the fascia and from the vagus nerve. The common facial vein should be identified. With a blunt curved aneurysm needle a double ligature of No. 1 chromic gut is passed around the internal jugular vein just above the common facial, and is tied (Fig. 11–3D).

In cases of jugular bulb thrombosis the internal jugular vein above the common facial may be found collapsed and empty of blood. Should the internal jugular vein contain a thrombus, it should be tied off lower in the neck below the thrombus. The internal jugular vein is a very large but very thin-walled structure. It must not be torn because of the risk of air embolism or massive hemorrhage.

The superficial fascia should be approximated with No. 00 plain gut and the skin closed with interrupted silk sutures. Unless the vein contains infected thrombus the wound may be closed without drainage.

Unnecessary ligation of the internal jugular vein should be avoided, as fatal consequences occasionally occur owing to impeded cerebral circulation when the lateral sinus in the opposite side is very small.[38, 39]

## OTITIC HYDROCEPHALUS

In 1927 Symonds[40, 41] described a syndrome of increased intracranial pressure without a brain abscess, following several weeks or more after an acute otitis media. He named the syndrome "otitic hydrocephalus." The condition occurs most often in children and adolescents. The most constant **symptom** is **headache,** often with **sixth nerve paralysis** on the same side, sometimes with vomiting. Otherwise the patient looks and feels quite well. The most constant **findings** are **papilledema,** which may reach 5 or 6 diopters, and a **spinal fluid pressure exceeding 300 mm. of water.** Unlike localized meningitis the spinal fluid is clear without increase in cells or protein. Unlike brain abscess there are no localizing neurologic changes, and ventriculography or CT scan does not show a space-occupying lesion.

The exact mechanism of the increased cerebrospinal fluid pressure is not known, but it is assumed to be due to increased production or decreased resorption of cerebrospinal fluid secondary to a previous mild nonpurulent or localized meningeal inflammation. In some cases there is a cystic accumulation of spinal fluid in the cerebellopontine angle. An occasional reported case followed lateral sinus thrombosis; but most patients with otitic hydrocephalus do not have evidence of this condition, and most patients with proved lateral sinus thrombosis do not develop otitic hydrocephalus. One reported case followed a subarachnoid-endolymphatic operation.

*Text continued on page 312*

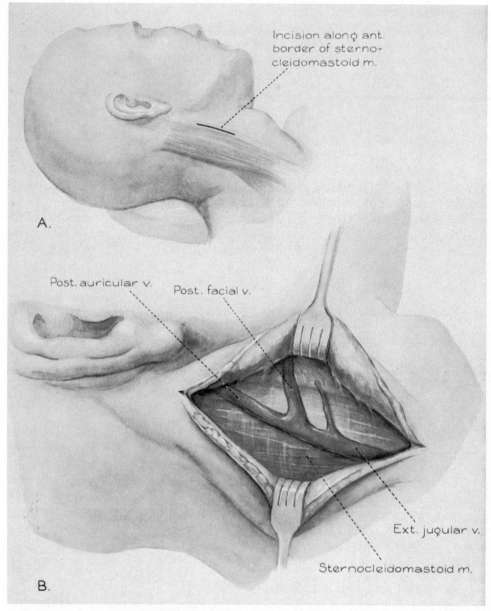

**Figure 11–3**  Technique of internal jugular vein ligation. *A*, Skin incision. *B*, Retraction of skin and platysma. (Continued on following page.)

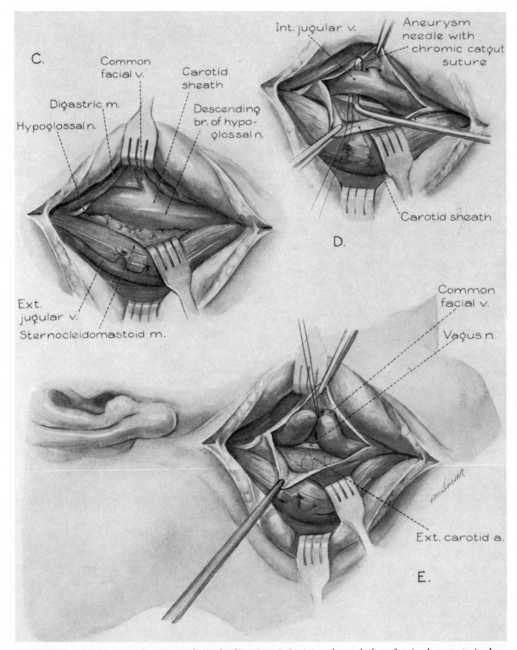

**Figure 11–3** (Continued)   Internal jugular ligation. C, Incision through deep fascia along anterior border of sternocleidomastoid muscle. D, Carotid sheath incised and internal jugular vein isolated above common facial vein. E, Internal jugular vein ligated.

The **diagnosis** of otitic hydrocephalus is made by lumbar puncture showing a normal spinal fluid under markedly increased pressure, in a patient who develops headache and papilledema with or without sixth nerve paralysis one to several weeks or more after an otitis media.

The **treatment** of otitic hydrocephalus is to reduce the increased intracranial pressure by repeated lumbar or ventricular punctures, diuretics and, if necessary, to perform a subtemporal decompression, until the condition subsides, so as to prevent optic atrophy from prolonged papilledema. After weeks or months the increased cerebrospinal fluid pressure slowly returns to normal.

## CEREBROSPINAL OTORRHEA

Drainage of spinal fluid from the ear may be a complication of chronic suppurative ear disease, or it may result from surgery on the ear. A frequent cause is fracture through the temporal bone. It may develop following irradiation of tumors involving the temporal bone;[42] in rare cases it begins spontaneously without previous ear disease, the result usually of a congenital malformation; or it may follow barotrauma or physical exertion, with rupture of the oval or round window. The symptoms, diagnosis and treatment of cerebrospinal otorrhea are the same, irrespective of the cause.

### Symptoms and Diagnosis

Clear, colorless, watery fluid draining from a mastoid cavity, or from the external auditory meatus, that reaccumulates immediately after removal by suction or cotton applicators, should be assumed to be spinal fluid. The conclusive diagnosis is made by a positive test for sugar on a specimen of the fluid. Occasionally there will be no external drainage from the ear but the patient will complain of fullness in the ear due to accumulation behind the intact tympanic membrane, and there may be a cerebrospinal rhinorrhea due to escape of this fluid down the eustachian tube. Obtaining clear watery fluid from the middle ear with a positive test for sugar after myringotomy establishes the fact that this is a cerebrospinal fluid leak and not the usual secretory otitis media.

### Technique of Surgical Repair

Cerebrospinal otorrhea carries the same grave risk of meningitis due to retrograde infection through the eustachian tube or from the external ear as does cerebrospinal rhinorrhea. Unless it ceases spontaneously (and this is rare) or is surgically corrected, the patient sooner or later develops meningitis.

When a spinal fluid leak occurs through a minute or gross dural tear during mastoid surgery, the dura should be exposed on all sides of the tear to ascertain that a spicule of bone does not project through it. If the leak is a slow seepage, it may cease if a small free graft of temporalis muscle is placed against it and held in place by compressed Gelfoam. The arachnoid mesh within and the muscle outside the dura effect an adequate fibrous tissue repair. If at the conclusion of the operation there is any evidence of continued drainage of clear fluid, the dura around the tear should be elevated from the bone in all directions, and a temporalis fascia graft applied and tucked between dura and bone on all sides, covered by compressed Gelfoam, surgical rayon and firm packing.

More troublesome and dramatic is the flow of spinal fluid from a dural tear in the posterior fossa near the superior petrosal sinus and medial to the sigmoid sinus. Here lies the lateral prolongation of the basal cistern, an area devoid of arachnoid mesh. The explosive and profuse flow of spinal fluid is difficult to control by a fascial graft, and may continue after operation, soaking pillow and mattress. A large graft of temporalis or leg muscle or abdominal fat filling the mastoid cavity snugly, as employed following transtemporal bone removal of acoustic neuroma, may suffice to stop the flow. The author has utilized the irritant effect of iodoform gauze packing to stimulate fibrosis at the site of the tear, and in one such case (a fenestration operation) the profuse flow of spinal fluid ceased after a week and the patient made an uneventful recovery. Blatt[43] has successfully used sterile peanut oil on gauze packing to produce a vigorous inflammatory response with fibrosis.

Special mention should be made of the profuse flow of clear fluid from the oval window, a "gusher," encountered occasionally during stapes surgery. Ward[44] suggests that a fracture or direct instrument trauma to the inner wall of the vestibule or through an otosclerotic focus might be the cause. More likely, however, is Schuknecht's[45] explanation that these patients have an abnormally patent cochlear aqueduct allowing a free flow of spinal fluid to the scala tympani, rather than the slow seepage that usually occurs. Elevation of the patient's head during and after surgery reduces the flow. A snug-fitting fat graft on wire, as described by Schuknecht,[46] is an effective method for stopping the flow after a stapedectomy.

More insidious and difficult to recognize is the development of a perilymph fistula months or years after a partial or complete stapedectomy. These cases carry the same risk of labyrinthine and then meningeal infection from an otitis media as do other cases of cerebrospinal otorrhea, and should be dealt with as described in Chapter 18. Rupture of the oval or round window from barotrauma or physical exertion is known to occur, with symptoms resembling sudden labyrinthine deafness or endolymphatic hydrops, the cochlear symptoms predominating.[47] Rest in bed with the head elevated 30 degrees may suffice to cause the perilymph leak to heal. If symptoms persist, surgical repair by application of a tissue graft is indicated. Recovery of hearing is more likely in cases of spontaneous repair than in those requiring surgical repair.

Cerebrospinal otorrhea following skull fracture, that occurring spontaneously without previous trauma or ear disease and that following irradiation for a tumor, can be repaired either by the neurosurgical approach through the middle cranial fossa (if this is the site of the dural defect) or by transtemporal bone exploration. The advantage of the latter is that the site of the defect can be ascertained without subjecting the patient to craniotomies of both the middle and posterior fossae when the site is uncertain, and any causative temporal bone lesion that might be encountered can be dealt with at the same time. The neurosurgeon generally utilizes fascia to repair the dural defect, sometimes reinforced by a bone graft.[48]

## REFERENCES

1. Quoted by Cawthorne, T.: The surgery of the temporal bone. J. Laryng. & Otol., 67:377, 1953.
2. Quoted by Heine, B., and Beck, J., in Denker, A., and Kahler, O.: Handbuch der Hals-Nasen-Ohrenheilkunde. Vol. 8. Berlin, 1927.

3. Morand, S. F.: Opuscules de chirurgie. Paris, 1768.

4. Roux, J.: Tableu des blessés reçus dans différens hopitaux de Paris. Union méd. Paris, 2:105, 1848.

5. Lebert: Ueber Gehirnabscesse. Virchows Arch. path. Anat., 10:78, 1856.

6. Macewen, W.: Pyogenic Infective Diseases of the Brain and Spinal Cord. Glasgow, 1893.

7. Körner, O.: Die otitischen Erkrankungen des Hirns, der Hirnhäute und der Blutleiter. Wiesbaden, 1908.

8. Eagleton, W. P.: Brain Abscess, Its Surgical Pathology and Operative Technic. The Macmillan Co., New York, 1922.

9. Shambaugh, G. E., Jr.: The surgical treatment of meningitis of otitic and nasal origin. J.A.M.A., 108:696, 1937.

10. Lebert: Ueber Entzündung der Hirn-Sinus. Virchows Arch. path. Anat., 9:381, 1856.

11. Zaufal, E.: Operation der Sinusthrombose und Versuche mit Cocaïn am Gehörorgane. Prag. med. Wchnschr., 9:474, 1884.

12. Lane, W. A.: Middle ear suppurations and their complications. Brit. M. J., 1:998, 1889.

13. Ballance, C. A.: Pyemic thrombosis of the lateral sinus. Lancet, 1:1057, 1114, 1890.

14. Jansen, A.: Referat die Operationsmethoden bei den verschiedenen otitischen Gehirnkomplikationen. Verhandl. deutsch. otol. Gesellsch., 4:96, 1895.

15. Gradenigo, G.: Sulla leptomeningite circoscritta e sulla paralisi dell' adducente di origine otitica. Gior. Accad. med. Torino, 10:59, 1904.

16. Kopetsky, S. J., and Almour, R.: Suppuration of the petrous pyramid. Ann. Otol. Rhin. & Laryng., 39:996, 1930; 40:157, 1931.

17. Eagleton, W. P.: Unlocking the petrous pyramid for localized bulbar meningitis secondary to suppuration of the petrous apex. Arch. Otol., 13:386, 1931.

18. Frenckner, P.: Some remarks on treatment of apicitis (petrositis) with or without Gradenigo's syndrome. Acta oto-laryng., 17:97, 1932.

19. Ramadier, J. A.: L'ostéite profonde du rocher. Paris, 1933.

20. Lempert, J.: Complete apicectomy; new technic for complete exenteration of apical carotid portion of petrous pyramid. Arch. Otol., 25:144, 1937.

21. Farrior, J. B.: The sublabyrinthine exenteration of the petrous apex. Ann. Otol. Rhin. & Laryng., 51:1007, 1942.

22. Courville, C. B.: Intracranial complications of otitis media and mastoiditis in the antibiotic era. Laryngoscope, 65:31, 1955.

23. Rosenwasser, H., and Adelman, N.: Otitic complications. Arch. Otol., 65:225, 1957.

24. Lund, W. S.: A review of 50 cases of intracranial complications from otogenic infection, between 1961 and 1977. Clinical Otolaryngology and Allied Sciences, Blackwell Scientific Publications, 1978.

25. Faunce, C. B., and Shambaugh, G. E. Jr.: Abscess of the brain following mild transitory otitis media. Arch. Otol., 17:673, 1933.

26. Lepper, M. H., and Dowling, H. F.: Management of the patient with meningitis. GP, 7:47, 1953.

27. Glorig, A.: The effect of dihydrostreptomycin on the auditory mechanism. Ann. Otol. Rhin & Laryng., 60:327, 1951.

28. Hoyne, A. L., and Riff, E. R.: Terramycin therapy for meningitis; a report of 14 recoveries without other medication. J. Pediat., 39:151, 1951.

29. Harpman, J. A.: On the management of otorrhinogenic intracranial infections. J. Laryng. & Otol., 69:180, 1955.

30. White, L. E.: Papilledema of otitic origin. Arch. Otol., 2:371, 1925.

31. Friesner, I., Druss, J. G., Goldman, J. L., and Rosenwasser, H.: Sinus thrombosis. Am. J. Surg., 42:116, 1938.

32. Braun, A.: Sinus Thrombophlebitis. Paul B. Hoeber, Inc., New York, 1928.

33. Grunert, K.: Die operative Auräumung des Bulbus venae jugularis, Bulbus operation, in Fällen otogener Pyömie. Vogel, Leipzig, 1904.

34. Piffl, O.: Zur operativen Freilegung des Bulbus der Vena jugularis interna. Arch. Ohrenh., 58:76, 1903.

35. Voss, O.: Zur operativen Freilegung des Bulbus venae jugularis. Ztschr. Ohrenh., 48:265, 1904.

36. Whiting, F.: Jugular bulb operation. Laryngoscope, 35:494, 1925.

37. Jensen, A. M.: Sinus thrombosis and otogenic sepsis. Acta Otol., 55:237, 1962.

38. Rohrbach, R.: Ueber Gehirnerweichung nach isolierter Unterbindung der Vena jugularis interna. Beitr. klin. Chir., 17:811, 1896.

39. Linser, P.: Ueber Cirkulationsstörungen im Gehirn nach Unterbindung der Vena jugularis interna. Beitr. klin. Chir., 28:642, 1900.

40. Symonds, C. P.: Some points in the diagnosis and localization of brain abscess. J. Laryng. & Otol., 42:444, 1927.

41. Symonds, C. P.: Otitic hydrocephalus. Brain, 54:55, 1931.

42. Alberti, P. W. R. M., and Dawes, J. D. K.: Cerebrospinal otorrhea in chronic ear disease. J. Laryng. & Otol., 75:123, 1961.

43. Blatt, I. M.: Surgical repair for cerebrospinal otorrhea due to middle ear and mastoid disease. Laryngoscope, 73:446, 1962.

44. Ward, P. H.: Cerebrospinal fluid otorrhea. Arch. Otol., 74:399, 1961.
45. Schuknecht, H. F., and Seifi, A. E.: Experimental observations on the fluid physiology of the inner ear. Ann. Otol. Rhin. & Laryng., 72:687, 1963.
46. Schuknecht, H. F., McGee, T. M., and Colman, B. H.: Stapedectomy. Ann. Otol. Rhin. & Laryng., 69:597, 1960.
47. Goodhill, V.: Sudden deafness and round window rupture, Laryngoscope 81:1462, 1971.
48. Lang, E. R., and Bucy, P. C.: Cerebrospinal fluid otorrhea. Arch. Otol., 75:415, 1962.

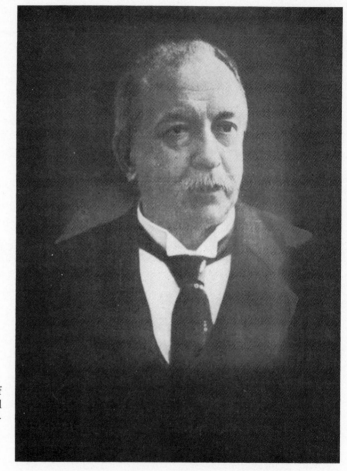

*Giuseppe Gradenigo*

BORN 1859
DIED 1926

Described the syndrome of
suppuration of the apical
portion of the petrous pyramid.

*Chapter 12*

# Non-meningeal Complications of Otitis Media

BRAIN ABSCESS
LABYRINTHITIS
PETROSITIS
FACIAL PARALYSIS

## BRAIN ABSCESS

Otitis media, despite the benefits of antibacterial therapy, continues to be a frequent cause of brain abscess.[1] Particularly since sulfonamide and antibiotic treatment of **acute** middle ear infections, the great majority of otitic brain abscesses encountered today are the result of **chronic** suppurative otitis media with cholesteatoma.

Otitic brain abscess occurs in the temporal lobe twice as often as in the cerebellum. Although cerebellar abscess is virtually always from the ear, temporal lobe abscess may be secondary to pulmonary infection or a staphylococcus bacteremia, although many cases are from the ear.

As a rule otitic brain abscess is single. In rare cases it may be multiple, it may become multilocular and involve the parietal and occipital lobe and it sometimes occurs primarily in the parietal lobe rather than the temporal lobe or cerebellum.

### Pathways of Extension to the Brain

The pathways of extension are the same for brain abscess as for other complications of otitis media. The most frequent pathway of spread to the brain is by means of coalescent or cholesteatomatous **bone erosion and an extradural abscess.**

Extension by **preformed pathway** is a common cause of cerebellar abscess from a suppurative labyrinthitis. In these cases the infection may extend through the internal auditory meatus, producing first a localized meningitis and then a cerebellar abscess; it may produce an empyema of the endolymphatic sac, actually an intradural abscess, and then a brain abscess; or it may produce a necrosis of the posterior osseous semicircular canal and an extradural abscess, and thence a cerebellar abscess. A broken-down thrombus in the lateral sinus is a common cause of cerebellar abscess.

**317**

**Osteothrombophlebitic extension** to the brain through intact bone from an early acute suppurative otitis media was not uncommon in the preantibiotic era, but is rare today.

### Pathology of Brain Abscess

The actual pathology of penetration of infection into the brain substance explains the fact that a brain abscess always begins subcortically in the white matter. This penetration begins as a periphlebitis or a thrombophlebitis of dural veins adjacent to an extradural or intradural abscess, and proceeds as a perivascular inflammation along veins connecting the dura with the rich venous network over the surface of the brain and thence extending into the sulci of the brain (Fig. 12–1). A localized meningitis probably always accompanies the perivascular spread of infection from the dura to the brain. On and in the cerebral cortex with its good blood supply the infection remains confined to the connective tissue surrounding the veins (Fig. 12–2), but when the perivascular infection reaches the avascular zone of white matter it spreads into the brain tissue. The actual formation of an abscess in the white matter proceeds in **three stages** or steps. In many cases each stage can be recognized by its clinical symptoms, but in some cases the stages blend and are indistinguishable.

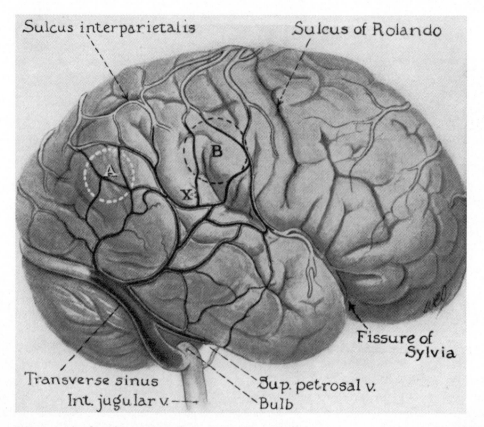

**Figure 12–1**    Thrombosis of lateral sinus and pial veins leading to cerebral brain abscesses, *A* and *B*, in a child of 10 following a brief otitis media with aural discharge for 2 to 3 days. *X* indicates the area from which tissue was taken for the microscopic section shown in Figure 12–2.

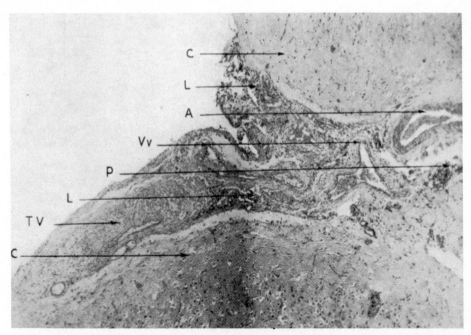

**Figure 12–2**  Photomicrograph, from same patient as in Figure 12–1, taken from area X, showing retrograde thrombophlebitis which produced subcortical abscess. *TV*, Thrombosed vein; *L*, Perivascular lymphocytes; *P*, Perivascular polymorphonuclear leucocytes; *Vv*, Normal veins; *A*, Normal artery; *C*, Cerebral cortex.

The first stage is the **initial encephalitis** in the white matter surrounding an infected vein, with edema and sometimes bacteria demonstrable in the tissue by microscopic study, and local softening of the brain tissue on gross examination. With vigorous antibacterial therapy the infection may be arrested at the stage of encephalitis, and may resolve without abscess formation. Even before the advent of sulfonamides and antibiotics, cases of nonpurulent otogenic encephalitis that did not proceed to a brain abscess were sometimes observed.

The second stage in the development of a brain abscess is a beginning **localization** of the area of encephalitis by a surrounding zone of dilated capillaries and round cell infiltration (Fig. 12–3). As this occurs the symptoms of initial encephalitis subside and the patient enters a symptom-free **latent or quiescent stage.**

The third stage is that of a walled-off but actively **enlarging abscess.** By this time the area of initial encephalitis has broken down into pus and necrotic debris. Around the pus a wall of granulation tissue has formed, and on the outer surface of the granulation tissue a wall of fibrous tissue has begun to form (Fig. 12–4). The central cavity filled with pus proceeds to enlarge like any undrained abscess, at the expense of its walls, by pressure necrosis and proteolytic digestion by enzymes liberated by the polymorphonuclear leucocytes; new areas of edema and encephalitis precede the new formation of granulation and fibrous tissue as the abscess advances. The pressure on adjacent centers produced by the expanding abscess and **even more by the surrounding edema and encephalitis** produces localizing symptoms and signs. Accordingly this is known as the **manifest stage of cerebral compression.**

A temporal lobe abscess generally expands away from the cortex toward the ventricle, producing a pear-shaped cavity narrower at the point of origin beneath the

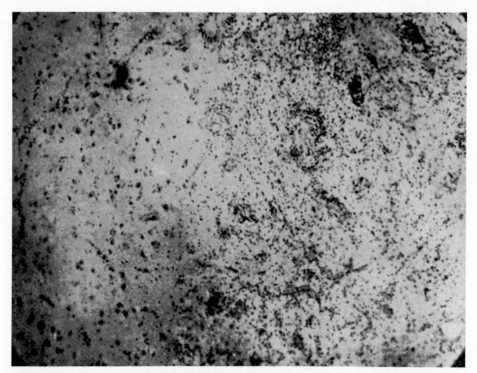

**Figure 12–3** Photomicrograph of edge of brain abscess 14 days old. To the left, normal brain tissue. To the right, perivascular infiltration and new connective tissue. (From Eagleton, W. P.: Brain Abscess, New York, Macmillan Co., 1922.)

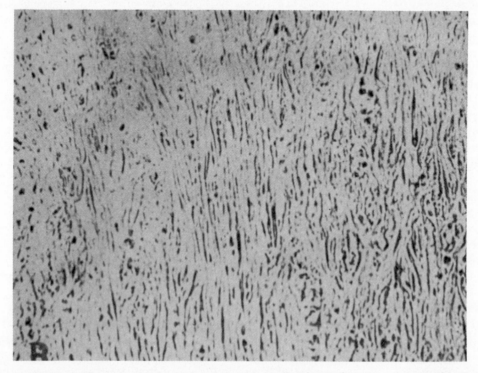

**Figure 12–4** Photomicrograph of connective tissue wall of brain abscess 3½ months old. (From Eagleton, W. P.: Brain Abscess. New York, Macmillan Co., 1922.)

cortex and wider toward the ventricle. If expansion is rapid, the walling-off process is less effective, the advancing encephalitis is more severe and a multilocular abscess may develop.

A cerebellar abscess is usually ovoid or irregular in shape, and it rarely becomes very large since pressure on the respiratory center occurs relatively early in the restricted space of the posterior fossa.

The further course of a brain abscess varies with the type and virulence of the infecting organism, the location of the abscess, the effectiveness of antibacterial medication and the success of surgical therapy. The anaerobic and putrefactive bacteria found in cholesteatoma are less easily localized and eradicated by antibacterial medication than the pneumococcus or streptococcus of an acute otitis media.

A temporal lobe abscess, if not drained, in most cases eventually ruptures into the lateral ventricle, either by means of a slow intermittent leak permitting effective therapy, or by a sudden and catastrophic rupture with an overwhelming meningitis and rapid death. Rupture onto the surface of the brain is less common; when it occurs a localized meningitis may wall off the infection with the establishment of a fistulous tract from the abscess to the ear. Such a tract is nearly always due to outward extension of an abscess from within, rather than the reverse. In some cases temporal lobe abscess causes herniation of the brain through the tentorium, with respiratory death.

Cerebellar abscess, unless treated surgically, usually ends with respiratory paralysis due to herniation of the brain stem into the foramen magnum with a pressure cone, but it too may rupture superficially producing a basilar meningitis or a fistulous tract to the ear.

In rare cases a brain abscess may become so well encapsulated that the surrounding encephalitis subsides and with it the symptoms disappear, only to recur months or years later when for some reason such a "silent" abscess becomes reactivated.

### Symptoms and Signs

The symptoms of the first stage of **initial encephalitis** rarely last more than a few days and are generally so mild and evanescent as to escape notice except in retrospect, but they are sufficiently characteristic to alert the keen clinician to the possibility of beginning brain involvement in a patient with otitis media. A **chill** or chilly sensation, followed by a slight or moderate **rise in temperature** lasting several days, frequently heralds the invasion of the brain. **Headache** and **nausea,** sometimes with non-projectile **vomiting,** are often present. If observed closely, the patient may appear **apathetic, drowsy** or **irritable.** In children a **convulsion** may be the first evidence of cerebral involvement.

As a rule there are no localizing neurologic changes in the stage of initial encephalitis. Should there be a localized meningeal reaction there may be **slight stiffness of the neck** and the spinal fluid will show a slight to moderate increase in cells and protein, but without organisms and with a normal sugar content.

The symptoms of the second **latent or quiescent stage,** as its name implies, are minimal or absent in many cases. In others malaise, poor appetite, intermittent headache and a slight temperature elevation may persist, with listlessness, drowsiness, slowed cerebration and fretfulness or irritability due to continued encephalitis. The latent or quiescent stage lasts from 10 days to several weeks or, rarely, several months. As a rule there are no neurologic signs, and the number of cells in the spinal fluid diminishes or returns to normal.

The symptoms and signs of the third stage of **manifest expanding abscess** are due to cerebral compression caused **more by edema and encephalitis around the abscess than by the space-occupying abscess itself.** As the encephalitis and edema fluctuate from hour to hour and day to day, so the symptoms and signs may come and go. Therefore repeated frequent examination of the patient is often necessary to make the diagnosis of a brain abscess.

The **symptoms and signs** of an expanding brain abscess are of two types: those due to **generalized increased intracranial pressure** and those due to **localized pressure on brain centers.**

The most constant generalized symptom of brain abscess is severe and usually continuous **headache. Projectile vomiting** is common and characteristic. Intermittent **slowing of the pulse** due to pressure on the vagus center in the brain stem is more common than **Cheyne-Stokes respiration** due to pressure on the respiratory center. The **temperature** may be **slightly elevated, normal** or **subnormal. Apathy** and **drowsiness** may be accompanied by **disorientation.** Jacksonian **convulsions** and **ocular paralyses** with **pupillary changes** may occur.

The most constant **signs** of increased intracranial pressure are in the eyegrounds, occurring in about half the cases, with **blurring of the disc margins, hyperemia or papilledema.** The **spinal fluid** is rarely normal in brain abscess and **usually shows a slight increase in cells and protein.** If the abscess is beginning to leak into the ventricle or onto the surface of the brain, the spinal fluid will show the changes of meningitis, localized or generalized. Spinal fluid should be withdrawn by lumbar puncture cautiously and in small amounts in cases of suspected temporal lobe abscess, and only by ventricular puncture in case of a suspected cerebellar abscess, to avoid herniation of the brain stem into the foramen magnum.

Symptoms and signs of increased intracranial pressure are more constant and definite in cerebellar than in temporal lobe abscess, because of the restricted space of the posterior fossa and its proximity to the brain stem. In addition to the slowed pulse and Cheyne-Stokes respiration there may be elevation of blood pressure due to pressure on the brain stem.

The **localizing or focal** symptoms and signs of brain abscess occur late and are less constant than the general symptoms. As a rule the general symptoms are sufficient to make the presence of a brain abscess likely before focal symptoms occur. Like the general symptoms the focal symptoms are due more to pressure on adjacent centers by the encephalitis around an abscess than by the abscess itself, and so the focal symptoms and signs are often **evanescent** and **intermittent,** being detected only by daily observation of the patient. Localizing and focal symptoms and signs occur earlier and are more constant in cerebellar than in temporal lobe abscess, and if the latter is on the right side in a right-handed person, there may be no localizing findings.

The most constant symptom of a left temporal lobe abscess in a right handed patient is **aphasia,** usually of the naming variety, so that the patient cannot remember the name of a familiar object like a pencil or pen, although he knows perfectly well its purpose and quickly recognizes the correct name when he hears it. The next most common focal symptom is **paresis** of the face and mouth on the opposite side, later of the arm and hand, due to pressure on the motor cortex. This paresis is of the central type. It may be most apparent with emotional facial movements of laughing or crying, and it does not affect the frontalis muscle. **Visual field defects** may be found, though these are not easy to demonstrate in a confused or lethargic patient.

The most constant symptom and sign of a cerebellar abscess is **ataxia** on the same side, most easily demonstrated for the hand and arm. The patient does poorly on the finger-to-nose test, there is decreased ability to alternate movements rapidly (adiadochokinesia) and there may be a coarse intention tremor. Muscular **hypotonia** and **weakness** on the involved side are present without paralysis. The **gait is ataxic,** with a tendency to fall toward the diseased side. Especially characteristic is a **spontaneous nystagmus** that fluctuates in degree and direction, and is often vertical or oblique. A striking symptom of cerebellar abscess is **rapid emaciation** of the patient despite a fair appetite, probably due to pressure on vegetative centers in the brain stem.

*Diagnosis*

The suspicion of brain abscess or lateral sinus thrombosis arises in any patient with a chronic suppurative otitis media with cholesteatoma who has a chill followed by a low grade fever and headache. If after a latent period symptoms and signs of increased intracranial pressure develop, the probability is that there is a brain abscess. When localizing symptoms and signs occur, there is almost the certainty of an abscess. In some cases a latent brain abscess becomes manifest soon after a radical mastoidectomy, with severe headache and fever followed by localizing symptoms.[2]

Difficulties in diagnosis are frequent and are due to the dearth of definite symptoms and signs in the early stages, even with a well encapsulated abscess. It is necessary to remember that encephalitis without abscess formation will simulate a brain abscess, and, indeed, always precedes the formation of a discrete abscess. Otitic hydrocephalus will show the same symptoms and signs of increased intracranial pressure, but without the fever or localizing symptoms of an abscess. A very large extradural or intradural abscess may simulate a brain abscess. Other conditions that must be differentiated from brain abscess are brain tumor, vascular intracranial accidents, lateral sinus thrombosis with choked disc, and suppurative labyrinthitis with localized meningitis. The points used in differentiation of suppurative labyrinthitis from cerebellar abscess are given in Table 12–1.

TABLE 12–1   DIFFERENTIATION OF SUPPURATIVE LABYRINTHITIS FROM CEREBELLAR ABSCESS

| | *Cerebellar Abscess* | *Suppurative Labyrinthitis* |
|---|---|---|
| *Spontaneous nystagmus* | Irregular and variable in direction and degree. May be vertical or oblique. | Horizontal-rotary, regular and constant. Rarely vertical or oblique. Slow component toward disease. |
| *Spontaneous past-pointing* | May be present without nystagmus or vice versa; may be variable and affect only the hand and arm on the diseased side. | Proportional to the nystagmus, bilateral and always toward the slow component of the nystagmus. |
| *Falling* | Not affected by the position of the head; usually toward the diseased side. | Depends on the position of the head and proportional to the nystagmus. |
| *Gait* | Deviates toward the diseased side, and is independent of the direction of nystagmus. | Deviates toward the slow component of the nystagmus. |
| *Caloric reaction* | Deranged (abnormal) response. | Absent response. |

Additional diagnostic aids are:

**Pneumoventriculography** will show a displacement and distortion of the lateral ventricles away from the side of a temporal lobe abscess, but encephalitis without abscess can show the same change. In a cerebellar abscess both lateral ventricles will be dilated and the ventricular puncture will improve headache and coma.

**Electroencephalography** is more helpful in localizing a temporal lobe than a cerebellar abscess. A negative electroencephalogram is evidence against the presence of a brain abscess.

**Intracranial angiography** by injection of Thorotrast into the carotid artery may be helpful in diagnosis and localization of an abscess by demonstrating displacement of the larger cerebral arteries.

**Brain scanning** is used for the detection of space-occupying lesions. A radioactive solution is injected intravenously, and 3 or 4 hours later a Geiger counter is used to scan the brain. The radioactive material is detected in vascular channels. In the case of an abscess, there is likely to be a void in the center corresponding to the purulent contents, with increased uptake around it corresponding to the capsule.

Computerized axial tomography (CAT scan) is the most recent and one of the most valuable diagnostic aids for the detection of space-occupying lesions.

The final diagnosis of brain abscess depends upon diagnostic brain puncture. However, indiscriminate exploratory punctures of the uninfected brain through a contaminated field may induce an encephalitis, and exploratory puncture of an encephalitis without abscess probably aggravates the encephalitis.

*Treatment*

The question of whether a brain abscess is best drained by the otologic surgeon through the area of invasion or by the neurosurgeon through a clean area is still debatable, although with the latter method there is not as much risk of producing meningitis today as in the preantibiotic era. The increasing rarity of otitic brain abscess is causing many otologic surgeons to defer the management of the occasional case to the neurologic surgeon. However, when a mastoidectomy reveals a dural fistula with pus coming from the brain, it is logical to proceed to utilize this route to drain the abscess.

Certain principles have been established by experience in the treatment of brain abscess. The most important to remember is that the edema and encephalitis around an abscess are the major causes of symptoms and the major sources of difficulty once the abscess has been located and drained. Encephalitis responds to appropriate antibacterial therapy for the causative organism, whereas encapsulated pus needs to be drained. The best results of surgical drainage will occur when judicious delay combined with antibacterial medication has allowed the abscess to become well localized and the surrounding encephalitis to subside. The less the brain is traumatized in the search for and draining of the abscess, the less the ensuing flare-up in encephalitis, which is always increased by any manipulation. The optimum time for draining a brain abscess is in the manifest stage of a localized encapsulated abscess. Since this is the time that definite focal symptoms and signs first appear, **in general an abscess should be drained as soon as the diagnosis is made.** However, if the clinical history indicates that the process is in the stage of initial encephalitis, antibacterial medication should be given and operation deferred unless increasing pressure on vital centers makes surgical intervention imperative. Not infrequently an otitic encephalitis will resolve under antibacterial therapy without proceeding to abscess formation. Probing an encephalitis in the search for a possible abscess aggravates the edema and inflammation. On the other hand, unnecessary delay in draining an expanding abscess that is causing increasing intracranial pressure can have disastrous consequences.

A well encapsulated abscess may be removed intact by the neurosurgeon just as he would remove an encapsulated tumor. This method of treatment is preferred today by many neurosurgeons, since with antibiotic protection the dangers of contamination of normal brain tissue and meninges by leakage are lessened.

The **technique of draining** a brain abscess is tending toward conservatism with as little trauma to the brain as possible. With the help of antibacterial medication to combat encephalitis and any concomitant meningitis, and to take care of small remnants of pus, it is probably better to rely upon simple tapping of the abscess, repeated once or several times if necessary, than to try to marsupialize the abscess by extirpating the overlying cerebral cortex, or to provide continuous drainage by means of a large tube.

If a dural fistula is found at mastoidectomy, the exploring blunt brain needle should be gently introduced through this tract directly inward to a depth of 3 or 4 cm. and if pus is not encountered, at several angles. The needle is allowed to slide in almost of its own weight, and any lateral movements that would tear the brain tissue are avoided. Frequently a slight or definite resistance is encountered when the wall of the capsule is reached, and added force is required to penetrate the wall. In the case of encephalitis without abscess there will be no resistance (less than normal) and no pus will be encountered. If clear fluid is obtained the lateral ventricle has been tapped. As the brain needle is introduced the cannula should be removed intermittently to allow pus to escape, should the abscess have been reached. Pus should be allowed to flow out by itself without aspiration or irrigation. The pressure of the surrounding encephalitis will be sufficient to evacuate the major part of the pus. When pus no longer escapes, the needle should be withdrawn, with the surgeon carefully recording the exact depth and direction in case a repeat tap is required.

If it is decided to explore for abscess through intact dura, a small incision should be made, exposing the surface of the brain so that the exploring needle can avoid any large vessels. A cerebellar abscess should be searched for and drained through an incision of the dura just medial to the sigmoid sinus, between this sinus and the posterior semicircular canal. A temporal lobe abscess should be searched for directly above the lesion in the attic or antrum by first removing the tegmen plate. A cerebellar abscess is more likely to be reached within 1 or 2 cm. of the cortex whereas a temporal lobe abscess may be deeper, and the exploring needle may have to be introduced repeatedly in various directions before pus is encountered.

The greatest problem after the abscess has been drained is the edema and encephalitis of the surrounding brain. A wide **subtemporal decompression** is helpful for a temporal lobe abscess, as the dura has some elasticity and "give." This may be accomplished simply by extending the endaural or postaural mastoid incision upward, elevating the periosteum and temporal muscle from the temporal fossa and removing the squama superiorly, anteriorly and posteriorly. Decompression of the posterior fossa is accomplished by exposing the posterior fossa dura from the labyrinth to well behind the sigmoid sinus.

**Wide incision of the dura** to permit the underlying brain to expand may be necessary but should be avoided if possible, for a herniation of the brain tends to start a vicious circle: As the hernia increases, the circulation of that part of the brain is impaired, with more edema and encephalitis and more herniation. Eventually a large **fungus cerebri** results, large portions of which may slough before the mass begins to recede, unless the patient meanwhile succumbs to the spreading encephalitis.

**Dehydration of the brain** by intravenous hypertonic glucose, sorbitol, urea or mannitol will temporarily ease the pressure on vital centers and improve the circulation to the inflamed brain tissue. **Concentrated plasma** has a similar but a somewhat more lasting effect, and has the further advantage of supplying protein for nutrition. **Steroids** may be administered pre- and postoperatively to prevent cerebral or cerebellar edema. The possible disadvantage of reduced inflammatory response from steroids is probably outweighed by the reduced edema.

Whenever the patient with a brain abscess begins to "go bad," the surgeon must decide quickly whether the worsening of symptoms is due to reaccumulation of pus in the abscess or spreading encephalitis. The latter will be aggravated by unnecessary probing of the brain, but the former must be drained to save the patient.

### Prognosis

The prognosis of brain abscess varies greatly in published reports of cases, from the extraordinary series of 18 recoveries in 19 surgically treated abscesses reported by Macewen, to 80 per cent or 90 per cent mortality reported by others. Recent reports indicate an average mortality of 28 per cent[3] to 66 per cent.[4] Untreated manifest brain abscess usually ends fatally, although in rare cases one may encapsulate and become quiescent for months or years. The prognosis is better with abscesses due to antibiotic-sensitive organisms than in abscesses due to anaerobic or mixed infections such as occur in cholesteatoma. The prognosis is better for older, well localized abscesses than for early, poorly encapsulated lesions.

Residual neurologic defects following surgical treatment of brain abscesses are surprisingly few when the conservative method of drainage by repeated tapping is employed, proving that the focal signs and symptoms are more the result of reversible surrounding encephalitis than of actual necrosis of tissue within the abscess.

## LABYRINTHITIS

Labyrinthitis is the most frequent complication of otitis media due to extension of infection **within** the temporal bone. Like meningitis, labyrinthitis has two clinically distinguishable types or degrees: localized, circumscribed or **serous labyrinthitis** without total and permanent loss of function, and diffuse, purulent or **suppurative labyrinthitis** with permanent total destruction of the sensory elements within the labyrinth. In addition to these two degrees of inflammatory involvement of the labyrinthine contents, there may be a **fistula of the labyrinth,** with or without simultaneous inflammatory labyrinthitis; there may be a **dead labyrinth** with total loss of function long after an acute suppurative process has healed, or following some other destructive event such as a massive hemorrhage, skull fracture or operative destruction of the labyrinth; and there may be a **sequestrum of the osseous labyrinth.**

### Fistula of the Labyrinth

#### Pathology and Etiology

Fistula of the labyrinth may be **surgically produced,** or it may occur **spontaneously** in the course of suppurative or neoplastic ear disease or the result of physical exertion or barotrauma[5]

**Spontaneous fistula** of the labyrinth is in the **majority of cases** due to bone erosion by **cholesteatoma.** In fact the development of a spontaneous labyrinthine fistula is so characteristic of cholesteatoma that it immediately suggests the presence of the latter in a case of chronic suppurative otitis media, or in a patient with a dry attic perforation, despite the absence of the usual symptoms and findings of cholesteatoma, namely a foul discharge coming from a marginal perforation, x-ray enlargement of the attic and antrum and masses of epidermal debris retrieved from the attic by instrumentation or irrigation through an attic cannula. Rarely a spontaneous fistula of the labyrinth may arise in a gummatous syphilitic osteitis of the labyrinthine capsule, in a tubercular otitis media, in a chronic perilabyrinthine osteomyelitis or in a neoplasm such as carcinoma or glomus jugulare tumor. In non-cholesteatomatous infection the erosion of the bony labyrinthine capsule to produce a fistula is accompanied by simultaneous localized or diffuse inflammation of the labyrinthine contents. In the case of cholesteatoma, however, the epidermal lining of the advancing cholesteatoma sac covers the fistula and in at least some cases protects the labyrinthine contents from inflammatory involvement. For this reason the term "circumscribed labyrinthitis," which implies that there is always an inflammatory change within the labyrinth, is not as suitable for labyrinthine fistulas as the simpler term "fistula of the labyrinth."

**Surgically produced fistula of the labyrinth** may be **accidental** during a simple or radical mastoidectomy, in which case an inflammatory labyrinthitis usually results. **Purposeful** fistula of the labyrinth is produced by the fenestration operation and by horizontal canal labyrinthotomy for intractable Meniere's disease, and it may follow stapedectomy.

The surgically produced fistula of the fenestration operation resembles the fistula produced by cholesteatoma in many respects: It is covered by a thin layer of epidermis; the labyrinthine contents may remain free from inflammation, or may be involved in a serous and, sometimes (very rarely after fenestration), in a suppurative labyrinthitis; the fistula is usually on the convex surface of the horizontal semicircular canal; and, in part owing to the osteogenic-inhibiting effect of the epidermal covering (see Chapter 19), the fistula tends to remain open permanently.

The fistula produced by horizontal canal labyrinthotomy for Meniere's disease should be filled with bone dust at the time of operation in order to induce osteogenic closure. The fistula that may follow stapedectomy, especially with the use of Gelfoam or a polyethylene tube prosthesis, is characterized by a minute leak of perilymph, unsteadiness and fluctuation in hearing.

### Symptom and Diagnosis

The only symptom, and the means of diagnosis, of uncomplicated fistula of a semicircular canal is the **fistula test.** This consists of **nystagmus and vertigo** when positive or negative pressure is applied to the soft tissue covering the fistula. The nystagmus is produced by a movement of endolymph toward the ampulla with inward pressure displacement, with the quick component toward the affected ear. With negative pressure there is outward displacement and a movement of endolymph away from the ampulla, with the quick component of nystagmus toward the normal ear.

The fistula test is elicited by means of a pneumatic Siegel type of speculum with a short piece of soft rubber tubing around the narrow end of the speculum to produce an airtight meatal closure (Fig. 12–5). With a very active fistula test each slight increase in pressure causes nystagmus toward the affected ear, and each slight

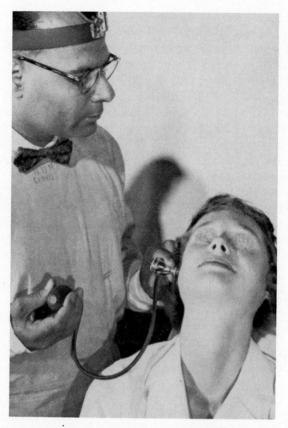

**Figure 12–5** Technique of eliciting a positive labyrinthine fistula test. The patient's eyes are watched for nystagmus, while intrameatal pressure is slowly increased and decreased.

decrease in pressure causes nystagmus in the reverse direction. With a fistula of the horizontal semicircular canal the nystagmus is always horizontal. With a fistula of either vertical canal the nystagmus is vertical. With a large fistula far forward exposing at the same time the ampulla of the horizontal canal and that of the superior vertical canal the nystagmus is rotary.

The fistula test obviously can be elicited only when there is retained function of that semicircular canal. Thus a **falsely negative** fistula test will be present when the fistula is accompanied by a localized loss of function of the ampulla of the involved canal or by a generalized loss of labyrinthine response. A **falsely positive** fistula test may be elicited by eustachian tube inflation or pneumatic massage of the tympanic membrane in rare cases of abnormally mobile stapes without other ear disease. These cases are not only rare, but the fistula test is weakly, not strongly, positive.

The patient with an active fistula of the labyrinth often complains of dizziness if he presses against the tragus or manipulates the auricle, or if he turns the head quickly. Rarely he may experience momentary vertigo when exposed to a loud noise — the Tullio phenomenon.

*Treatment*

Fistula of the labyrinth due to cholesteatoma is a positive indication for the radical or modified radical mastoidectomy to exteriorize the cholesteatoma sac and prevent the retention of infected debris. In a few patients who refused surgery the cholesteatoma has been kept relatively inactive by the author for many years by periodic attic irrigations. However, this type of conservative management is accompanied by a definite and unwarranted risk: In two such patients, despite the oft-repeated admonition to **return at once** if the ear began to drain, a recurrence of otorrhea was ignored, or the patient found it "inconvenient" to return, and a suppurative labyrinthitis ensued. Both patients then returned with acute labyrinthine symptoms and a dead labyrinth, and both showed evidence of beginning meningitis. Fortunately appropriate therapy resulted in recovery from the localized meningitis, though not of labyrinthine function.

Fistula of the labyrinth occurring in a chronic perilabyrinthine osteomyelitis will be accompanied by symptoms of serous or suppurative labyrinthitis calling for surgical intervention to remove the diseased bone. Syphilitic or tubercular fistulas of the labyrinth require specific antisyphilitic or antitubercular medication.

Fistula due to oval or, less often, round window membrane rupture occurs in divers or after sudden physical exertion where rapid change in intracranial and intralabyrinthine pressure causes a rupture by implosion or explosion. Bed rest with the head kept elevated 30 degrees to reduce intracranial and intralabyrinthine pressure will allow spontaneous healing of the fistula in many cases. If the impaired hearing with rest in bed persists, and the history of onset after barotrauma or physical exertion suggests rupture of the oval or round window membrane, surgical exploration should be considered after 10 or 12 days, and repair performed with perichondrial or fascial grafts held in place by compressed gelfoam.[5]

## Inflammatory Labyrinthitis, Serous

### Etiology

Inflammation of the labyrinthine contents is rarely hematogenous and is nearly always the result of an osteitis of the labyrinthine capsule or of extension by preformed pathway. Diffuse suppurative inflammatory labyrinthitis is usually preceded by a localized serous labyrinthitis.

Extension of inflammation to the labyrinth by a preformed pathway may occur rarely in early acute suppurative otitis media via the annular ligament of the oval window or the secondary tympanic membrane of the round window. It frequently occurs from a generalized purulent meningitis via the internal auditory meatus and acoustic nerve fibers, and less often via the cochlear aqueduct or the endolymphatic sac and duct. Serous labyrinthitis of varying degree is frequent following surgical fenestration and stapedectomy.

Serous labyrinthitis is frequent (but not invariable) with cholesteatomatous fistula of the labyrinth. It is sometimes seen in acute coalescent mastoiditis, in petrositis and in chronic perilabyrinthine osteomyelitis. It is the usual mechanism of the deafness of congenital syphilis, and it may occur in tuberculosis of the middle ear.

Serous (or suppurative) labyrinthitis by the hematogenous route occurs very rarely indeed. Conceivably an infected embolus in a patient with subacute bacterial endocarditis might lodge in an end-artery of the labyrinth. Possibly a distant focus of infection such as an abscessed tooth or infected tonsil can produce a hematogenous serous labyrinthitis with symptoms of Meniere's disease, as described by Wright.[6]

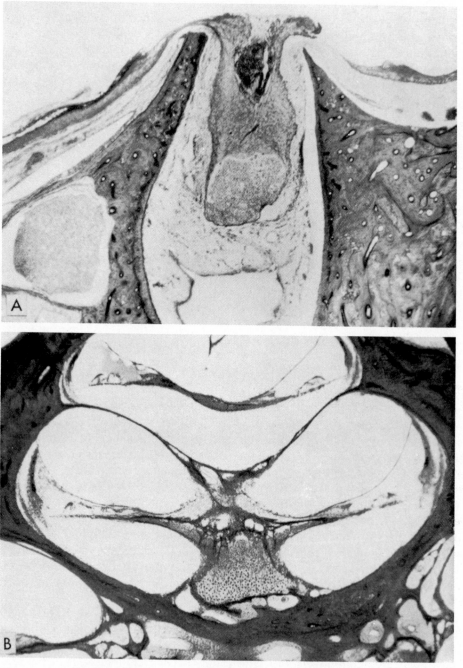

**Figure 12–6**   Serous labyrinthitis one week following fenestration in rhesus monkey. *A*, Cellular infiltration of arachnoid mesh of perilymphatic space surrounding invaginated meatal flap. *B*, Serous exudate in cochlear duct, in the same ear as in *A*.

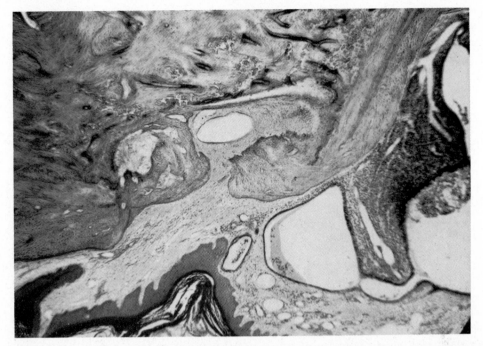

**Figure 12–7**  Late effects of serous labyrinthitis one year after fenestration in rhesus monkey. Note dense fibrosis of perilymphatic space with secondary osteogenic replacement surrounding endolymphatic semicircular duct.

## Pathology

The earliest pathologic change of serous labyrinthitis is capillary dilatation and increased permeability in the vessels of the delicate arachnoid mesh of the perilymphatic space, with a serous or serofibrinous exudate both in the perilymphatic and in the endolymphatic space near the site of extension to the labyrinth. The loose wide spaces of the arachnoid mesh soon fill with round cells and fibroblasts. These changes may remain fairly well localized to the area of invasion, but often there is a diffuse labyrinthine involvement with more or less serous exudate or albuminous material in all portions of the endolymphatic and perilymphatic labyrinth (Fig. 12–6A and B).

The inflammatory changes of serous labyrinthitis may resorb leaving no trace, but more often a varying degree of perilymphatic fibrosis remains at the site of invasion. There is a great tendency toward later invasion of such perilymphatic fibrous tissue by endosteal bone (Fig. 12–7). This constitutes a frequent mechanism of osseous closure of the fenestra when it occurs later than one year after a fenestration operation.

## Symptoms and Diagnosis

The **symptoms** of serous labyrinthitis are the result of disturbed vestibular and cochlear function, nearly always with a **depression** of sensory response.

The **vestibular symptoms** precede the cochlear symptoms by a few hours to several days when the site of invasion is a semicircular canal, as after a fenestration operation. They consist of **spontaneous nystagmus toward the opposite ear** (very rarely toward the involved ear), nausea and vomiting, vertigo and ataxia with past-pointing. The symptoms are proportionate to each other and constant, as contrasted with cerebellar disease in which the vestibular symptoms are disproportionate (nystagmus without vertigo, for example) and variable (nystagmus varies in direction and degree from time to time).

A peculiar variety of pendulous nystagmus with a to-and-fro movement of the eyes synchronous with the pulse is sometimes seen after surgical fenestration, especially following release of pressure on the tympanomeatal flap. This is due to movements of the endolymph produced by the pulsation of dilated arterioles in the inflamed flap.

The **cochlear symptoms** of serous labyrinthitis consist of an impairment of hearing of the sensorineural type greater for tones of high pitch, frequently with **distortion of hearing and diplacusis.** The diplacusis is usually binaural dysharmonic: A pure tone is heard at a different pitch in the two ears, usually higher pitched in the diseased ear. Rarely there is a monaural diplacusis: A pure tone is heard as two tones of different pitch in the affected ear. Or there may be an echo diplacusis: A pure tone is heard a fraction of a second later in the ear with serous labyrinthitis.[7]

In cases of serous labyrinthitis of mild to moderate degrees of severity, **definite retention of labyrinthine function** can be demonstrated by either the caloric test or the masked hearing tests. In cases of severe serous labyrinthitis there may be temporary suppression of all labyrinthine response. **It is impossible to differentiate such a severe serous labyrinthitis during the acute stage from a diffuse suppurative labyrinthitis.** This differentiation can be made only by tests made some weeks later when definite recovery of response indicates that the patient has had a serous involvement of the labyrinth, whereas failure to recover a caloric or cochlear response indicates that the patient had a suppurative involvement.

### Treatment

As long as the labyrinthitis is of the serous type, as indicated by definite labyrinthine responses, there is no danger of intracranial invasion. Treatment of the serous labyrinthine inflammation is directed toward the etiologic factor. If it is an early acute suppurative otitis media, myringotomy and antibacterial therapy will suffice. If it is a perilabyrinthine osteitis or a cholesteatoma, mastoidectomy with removal of diseased bone should be combined with antibacterial medication. Acute serous labyrinthitis, immediately after fenestration or occurring months or years after fenestration, due to infection of the cavity, should be treated by antibacterial medication and local cleanliness but with care to avoid unnecessary trauma or manipulation of the flap over the fenestra.

Every patient with serous labyrinthitis should be watched for evidence of beginning diffuse suppurative involvement, heralded by an abrupt increase in vestibular symptoms and sudden loss of all hearing.

### Inflammatory Labyrinthitis, Suppurative

### Etiology and Pathology

The same etiologic factors and pathways of invasion apply to diffuse suppurative labyrinthitis as to serous labyrinthitis, a stage of localized serous inflammation

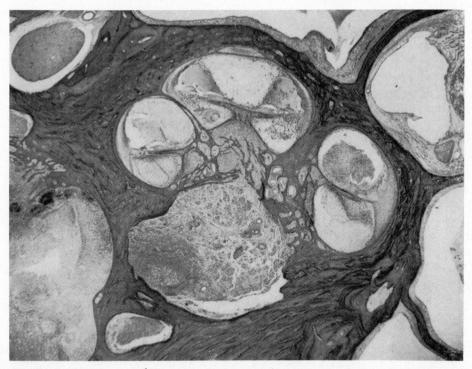

**Figure 12–8**   Diffuse suppurative labyrinthitis 7 days following fenestration in rhesus monkey. Note purulent exudate in cochlea and internal acoustic meatus with beginning meningitis.

generally preceding the stage of diffuse purulent involvement. An exception to this rule is involvement of the labyrinth secondary to a generalized meningitis, in which case a purulent labyrinthitis usually occurs without a prodromal period of serous labyrinthitis.

In suppurative labyrinthitis pus is found in all parts of the labyrinth, more in some areas than others, but without any effective localization (Fig. 12–8). The sensory elements in the cochlear duct, ampullas of the semicircular canals and maculas of the utricle and saccule degenerate and disappear. If the patient does not die of a cerebellar abscess or meningitis due to intracranial extension, or if the labyrinth is not operated on, healing eventually occurs by fibrosis followed by an obliterative osteitis. In untreated suppurative labyrinthitis pus may remain trapped in the bony labyrinth for weeks or even months before it finally makes its way intracranially or is replaced by fibrous tissue. Such a "latent" labyrinthitis may exist with no symptoms to betray its presence until the patient suddenly develops meningitis.

*Symptoms*

The symptoms of suppurative labyrinthitis are vestibular and cochlear, without fever, just as are the symptoms of serous labyrinthitis, but with these differences:

1.   The onset of severe vertigo, nystagmus and vomiting is more abrupt in the suppurative form. The more rapid the destruction of the end-organs within the labyrinth, the more violent the vestibular disturbances. In some cases of gradual progression from a serous to a suppurative labyrinthitis there may be no more than a

slight sense of unsteadiness.[8] The labyrinthine symptoms of suppurative labyrinthitis are believed to be due to sudden loss of the normal tonic impulses from one labyrinth, with nothing to balance the tonic impulses that continue to come from the opposite intact labyrinth. Thus when both labyrinths are destroyed simultaneously, there is no nystagmus and vertigo; and when one labyrinth is destroyed slowly, compensation keeps pace with the gradual loss of function, with mild or even absent vestibular symptoms.

2.   The onset of severe vestibular symptoms is accompanied by a complete loss of cochlear response. This can be ascertained only by the use of maximum narrow-band masking of the normal ear while testing the hearing in the diseased ear.

3.   The vestibular symptoms are most intense at the onset of suppurative invasion, with a gradual lessening during the following days, requiring usually 3 to 5 weeks for compensation to occur with complete recovery from nystagmus and vertigo. Compensation occurs more rapidly in the young than in the aged.

4.   The caloric reaction is absent from the diseased ear.

5.   With subsidence of the acute vestibular symptoms there is no recovery of cochlear or vestibular response in the diseased ear.

It should be emphasized that in uncomplicated suppurative labyrinthitis there are **no symptoms other than those due to sudden loss of sensory function.** Headache, pain, malaise or fever **does not** occur from a labyrinth filled with pus. The explanation is that the total amount of pus contained in the labyrinth is small, and the opportunity for systemic absorption of toxic products is extremely limited from the bony walls of the intact labyrinthine capsule.

### Treatment

The most important treatment of suppurative labyrinthitis is to keep the patient in bed under **close and continuous observation for symptoms and signs of beginning intracranial extension.** Antibacterial medication should be given, more to aid in preventing intracranial extension than in the expectation that the drug will enter the infected labyrinth in therapeutic concentration. The symptoms and signs that are watched for **hourly** are: headache, usually occipital; stiffness of the neck, even very slight; Kernig sign (rarely present without stiffness of the neck); elevation of temperature above normal even though slight; and facial paralysis. At the **first appearance of any of these symptoms a spinal fluid examination should be made.** If there are increased numbers of cells, beginning spread of the infection intracranially is certain and the labyrinth should be drained surgically as an emergency operation. With the help of antibacterial medication drainage of the labyrinth should arrest the further advance of infection to the meninges or cerebellum.

### Prognosis

Before the advent of sulfonamide and antibiotic therapy the mortality rate of suppurative labyrinthitis was particularly high in the cases occurring postoperatively due to accidental opening of the labyrinth or luxation of the stapes into the vestibule. Some authors recommended immediate operation to open the labyrinth as soon as the diagnosis of suppurative labyrinthitis was established, but others advised surgical intervention only when there was evidence of beginning meningitis. Even with operation on all patients with suppurative labyrinthitis as soon as the diagnosis was established, Ruttin[9] reported 40 per cent mortality in a series of 20

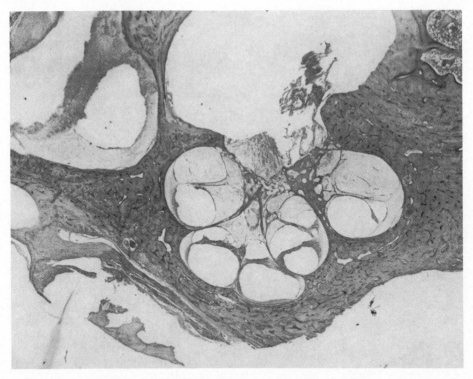

**Figure 12–9** Labyrinthitis secondary to meningococcal meningitis in child age 3. (Courtesy of Dr. Elmer W. Hagens.)

cases. Today, with careful observation of the patient to detect the earliest evidence of meningeal invasion permitting prompt drainage of the labyrinth, combined with antibacterial medication, the relatively high mortality rate of suppurative labyrinthitis should be greatly reduced, and with few exceptions the patient should recover good health, but of course he cannot recover labyrinthine function. Suppurative labyrinthitis secondary to meningitis does not require drainage of the labyrinth (Fig. 12–9)

### Technique of Labyrinth Drainage

Operations for opening the labyrinth for suppurative labyrinthitis have been described by Jansen,[10] Hinsberg[11] and Richards.[12] In all of these procedures all three semicircular canals were opened above the horizontal portion of the facial canal, and the vestibule and cochlea were opened below the bony facial canal by removing the promontory. In addition, Neumann advised exposing the posterior fossa dura as far as the internal auditory canal, which was then opened to expose the auditory and facial nerves. All of these labyrinthine operations involved great risk of injury to the facial nerve, especially in its horizontal portion, and all were time-consuming and difficult to perform with the mallet and gouge and without the help of magnification.

With the added protection of antibacterial medication, and the use of magnification and the dental-type drill, drainage of the labyrinth can be accomplished today easily, quickly and with safety to the facial nerve, as follows:

After a preliminary radical mastoidectomy, using a small diamond burr and the operating microscope, the prominence of the horizontal semicircular canal is taken

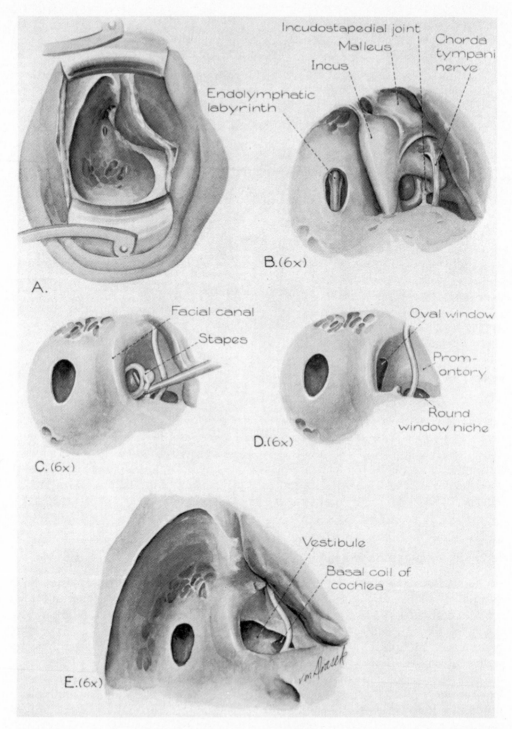

**Figure 12–10**  Technique of labyrinthectomy. *A*, Fenestra in horizontal semicircular canal without enchondralization. *B*, Same, under operating microscope. (In most cases the incus lies partly over the ampulla.) *C*, Endolymphatic labyrinth extracted; incus and head of malleus removed. *D*, Stapes and footplate extracted. *E*, Oval and round windows connected.

down exactly as in the fenestration operation, with a fenestra created far forward into the ampulla (Fig. 12–10B). The vestibule is easily entered from above, and the endolymphatic duct is extracted with a small hook. The cochlea and vestibule are then opened from below by extracting the stapes and burring away the promontory until the oval and round windows are connected. A small probe or hook may then be passed into the vestibule under the bony bridge of the facial canal from above or below.

### Dead Labyrinth

Following subsidence of the acute vestibular symptoms of suppurative labyrinthitis, usually after 3 to 5 weeks, the patient is symptom-free, showing only continued absence of caloric response and of cochlear response from the diseased ear. For varying periods of time such a labyrinth may continue to harbor viable microorganisms. The term "latent labyrinthitis" has been applied to such an asymptomatic persisting infection. Unfortunately there are no symptoms or tests to differentiate a dangerous latent labyrinthitis from a harmless healed labyrinth following a suppurative labyrinthitis. Because of the possibility that a radical mastoid operation might light up a latent labyrinthine infection by the repeated shock of mallet on gouge and thus cause a fatal meningitis, the former teaching was that a labyrinthectomy must always accompany the radical operation on a patient with a dead labyrinth. Today with the use of the rotary dental drill instead of the mallet and gouge and with antibiotic protection it is safe to reserve opening of the labyrinth for those cases of dead labyrinth with spinal fluid evidence of beginning meningeal invasion.

### Sequestrum of the Labyrinth

Sequestration of part or all of the bony labyrinth may occur in extensive perilabyrinthine osteitis, usually associated with a dead labyrinth. The senior author, however, removed a sequestrum of the bony semicircular canals of **both** ears of a child following a scarlet fever necrotizing otitis, who had total loss of vestibular response but definite retained hearing in one ear.

The presence of a sequestrum of the bony labyrinth should be suspected when a patient, following a suppurative labyrinthitis, develops a facial paralysis. In most cases a sequestrum of the labyrinth is an unexpected finding in the course of a radical mastoidectomy in a patient with a dead labyrinth and chronic otorrhea.

The treatment of sequestrum of the labyrinth is simply to lift out the loose necrotic bone from the bed of granulations in which it lies, with great care not to injure the facial nerve. If necessary the sequestrum should be broken into several pieces to permit its removal without facial nerve injury. Remnants of bone of the labyrinthine capsule that are not loose or obviously osteitic should not be disturbed.

## PETROSITIS

### Definition and Pathology

Petrositis is an inflammation of the petrous portion of the temporal bone. Except for the rather rare acute fulminating osteomyelitis of the petrosa in infants, petrositis occurs only in temporal bones with pneumatic cells in the petrous pyramid.[13] Just as there is an inflammation of the mucsoal lining of mastoid air cells in every acute suppurative otitis media of any degree of severity, so there is a similar inflammation of any air cells that have developed in the petrosa. As in the mastoid, this inflammation recedes, in the great majority of cases, as the otitis media subsides, without producing any symptoms referrable to the petrous involvement and without producing bony changes in the cell walls. Such cases are not clinically diagnosed as petrositis. The diagnosis of petrositis is reserved for infected petrous cells with inadequate drainage causing bony changes of coalescence in the cell walls, and resulting often in symptoms referrable to the petrosa.

In these respects petrositis behaves exactly like mastoiditis in an acute middle ear infection, and the involvement of air cells in the petrous portion might simply be considered as part of the pneumatic cell involvement of acute otitis media that includes cells in the mastoid process, squama and petrosa. In certain respects, however, petrositis differs from mastoiditis, justifying its consideration as a separate entity. These differences are:

1.   The petrous pyramid is pneumatized[14] in only a third of temporal bones past the age of 3 years, whereas the great majority of mastoid processes after the first year are pneumatized to some degree. Moreover, the petrous pyramid is never completely pneumatized, areas of bone marrow remaining adjacent to pneumatic cells, so that osteomyelitis frequently accompanies a coalescent petrositis.

2.   The bony labyrinth that nearly fills the base of the petrous pyramid interposes a "bottleneck" between the middle ear and any petrous air cells, increasing the tendency toward impaired drainage from these cells.

3.   The petrous pyramid is situated so that pus cannot find its way outward to produce a relatively harmless and easily diagnosed and drained subperiosteal abscess as in the case of the mastoid and squama, but has a greater tendency toward intracranial extension. In the immediate preantibiotic era it became evident that the majority of cases of fatal otitic meningitis were the result of inward extension from a petrositis.

### Etiology

Acute coalescent petrositis is usually associated with an acute coalescent mastoiditis, and, like the latter, is due most often to the beta hemolytic streptococcus or pneumococcus. Chronic petrositis may be due to one of these organisms in a trapped abscess, or it may be due to a staphylococcus with a chronic osteomyelitis of the petrosa or, in the case of a cholesteatoma, to pseudomonas or other gram-negative organism.

### Symptoms

The symptoms of petrositis depend upon the area of the petrous pyramid affected. Air cells extend into the petrous pyramid in two main groups:[14] a **posterior group** of air cells from the epitympanum and antrum that finds its way around the semicircular canals into the base of the pyramid, not infrequently extending to the apex, and an **anterior group** of cells from the tympanum, hypotympanum and eustachian tube that finds its way around the cochlea into the apex of the pyramid. The posterior group of cells is present in about 30 per cent of temporal bones, whereas the anterior group of cells is present in about 15 per cent of temporal bones.

The two most constant symptoms of petrositis are **pain** and **persistent aural discharge** following a simple mastoidectomy. In the case of a posterior petrositis the pain is occipital, parietal or temporal, and the persistent discharge is from the mastoid wound. In the case of an anterior petrositis the pain is frontal or behind the eye, and the persistent discharge is from the tympanum. **Diplopia** due to sixth nerve paralysis may occur when the apex is involved, the nerve being compressed by edema where it passes through Dorello's canal beneath the petrosphenoid ligament at the tip of the petrous apex. The three symptoms, diplopia, pain around the eye and persistent otorrhea, constitute **Gradenigo's syndrome.**[15]

Additional symptoms of petrositis, less constant than the preceding, are: **transient facial paresis, mild recurrent vertigo** and **fever** that is usually low grade and intermittent. If the suppuration begins to extend beyond the petrosa, there may be added the symptoms of **localized,** then of **generalized meningitis,** or of a **cerebellar or a temporal lobe abscess,** or of **thrombophlebitis** of the inferior petrosal sinus and jugular bulb, or of a **lateral pharyngeal, retropharyngeal or deep neck abscess.**

### Diagnosis

Effective antibiotic therapy has virtually eliminated cases of acute coalescent petrositis following an acute suppurative otitis media. The few cases that are seen today are associated with a chronic otorrhea, rarely with a cholesteatoma, more often with a chronic osteomyelitis of the petrosa or a chronic coalescent abscess cavity in the apex.[16]

Suppuration in the petrous portion of the temporal bone should be suspected whenever there is a persistent purulent discharge following a well done simple or radical mastoidectomy, for after thorough exenteration of all mastoid cell tracts, the usual source for continued purulent drainage is from perilabyrinthine peritubal or apical petrous cells. The addition of pain around or deep to the eye, diplopia due to sixth nerve paresis, facial weakness or vertigo, often with fever, is almost certain evidence of petrositis. The occurrence of meningitis during an otitis media with an insufficient pathologic lesion in the mastoid to account for it, and the occurrence of repeated attacks of meningitis,[17] always suggest the possibility of a petrositis, even without the other symptoms. X-ray studies are helpful to demonstrate a large abscess of the petrous apex[16] or differences in pneumatization and density of the two sides.

### Treatment

Acute coalescent petrositis in the preantibiotic era sometimes cleared following a complete simple mastoidectomy. Today most cases of acute petrositis can be cured by antibacterial medication in sufficient dosage. Cases of acute petrositis requiring surgery have almost disappeared, but chronic cases due to organisms resistant to the usual antibiotics still require operation.[18]

In some of these chronic cases a low grade osteomyelitis is present in marrow-containing perilabyrinthine and apical bone. Surgical intervention becomes necessary when the chronic otorrhea is accompanied by pain behind the eye, intermittent vertigo, facial weakness, transient diplopia and intermittent low grade fever. Since it is difficult to remove every vestige of infected marrow-containing bone, operation should be followed by antibacterial medication selected by culture taken at operation with sensitivity tests.

**Choice of Surgical Approach.** The objective of surgery is to provide adequate drainage from the suppurative focus in the petrosa without damage to the facial nerve and to the labyrinth if this is still functional. Although the symptomatology and x-ray studies may point toward one particular group of cells as the site of the disease, a systematic surgical routine should be employed.

A **preliminary complete simple mastoidectomy** should always be performed, if it has not already been done. If there are not urgent indications of threatened meningitis and considerable disease was found in the mastoid, further surgery may be delayed for a week or 10 days while the patient is kept under close observation. If the symptoms and signs of petrositis persist, the petrosa should be explored as follows:

The **easiest and safest** surgical approach to infected petrous cells is along the route by which the cells invaded the petrosa. Accordingly, the areas where cell tracts commonly extend into the petrous pyramid should be explored systematically. This is best done with very small curets, No, 000, 0000 or 00000 in size, with which any softened bone can be removed and a cell tract followed inward. It is easier to distinguish between cellular osteitic bone and the ivory-like healthy labyrinthine capsule with a curet than with a rotating burr.

Exploration of posterior cell tracts into the petrosa can be accomplished without destroying hearing. It begins by **skeletonizing** the bony semicircular canals, and **defining** the tegmen plate of the middle cranial fossa and the dural plate of the posterior cranial fossa by carefully clearing them of any cellular bone. These bony plates should then be removed, exposing the dura of the middle fossa above and posterior fossa behind the osseous semicircular canals (Fig. 12–11). The following areas are then examined and explored for cell tracts leading inward:

1.   Above the superior vertical semicircular canal, posterior to the geniculate ganglion, a cell tract frequently exists (Fig. 12–11 B,1). This may lead directly inward to the upper part of the apex, but since the facial nerve usually runs very close to the middle fossa dura from the internal auditory meatus to the geniculate ganglion, this particular cell tract should be explored very cautiously.

2.   A cell tract above the horizontal semicircular canal and behind the superior vertical canal frequently leads inward, paralleling the superior petrosal sinus toward the internal auditory meatus and sometimes to the apex (Fig. 12–11B,3). This tract can be explored more thoroughly with safety than the previously described tract.

3.   A cell tract sometimes extends through the arch of the superior semicircular canal to the apex (Fig. 12–11B,2). This is the approach described by Frenckner.[19]

4.   Beneath the posterior semicircular canal and above the jugular bulb, but posterior to the vertical mastoid portion of the facial nerve, a cell tract not infrequently leads to the apex beneath the internal auditory meatus (Fig. 12–11B,4). This is the approach described by Dearmin,[20] Farrior[21] and others.

5.   An additional method of reaching the apex without destroying hearing should be mentioned. This is to elevate the middle fossa dura medially over the arcuate eminence from the attic to open into an extradural abscess lying on the anterior middle fossa surface of the apex. If there is not an extradural middle fossa abscess and if the roof is thinned by disease, it is sometimes possible to break through the cortex with a curet into an apical abscess, as described by Eagleton.[22]

*Text continued on page 344.*

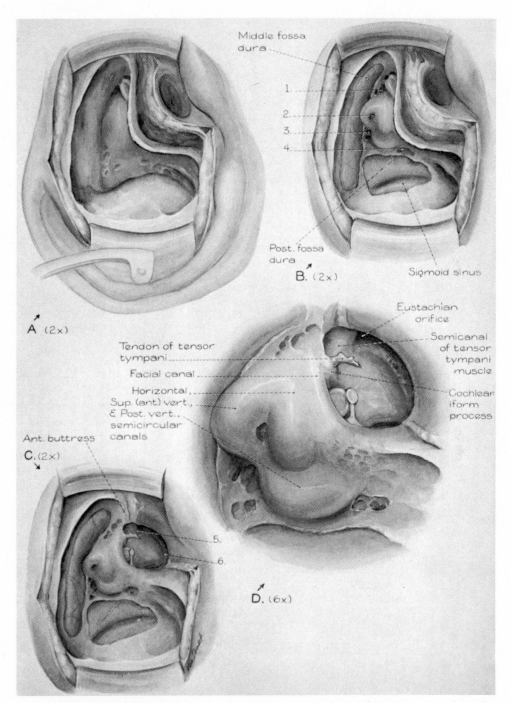

**Figure 12–11** Surgical approach for suppuration of petrosa. *A,* Initial simple mastoidectomy. *B,* Exposure of dura of middle and posterior fossae and exploration of perilabyrinthine cell tracts. *1,* Cells between superior semicircular canal and geniculate ganglion. *2,* Arch of superior semicircular canal. *3,* Cells between superior and posterior semicircular canals. *4,* Cells beneath posterior semicircular canal. *C,* Conversion to radical mastoidectomy and exploration of *5,* peritubal cells and *6,* hypotympanic cells. *D,* Same, under operating microscope. (Continued on following page.)

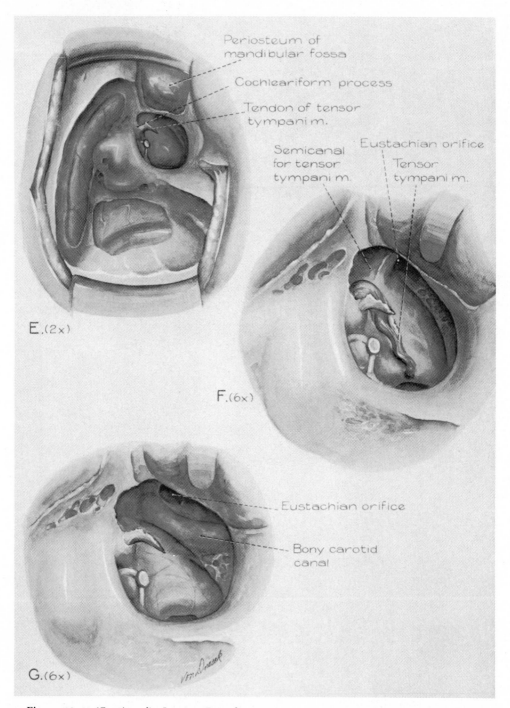

**Figure 12–11** *(Continued)*   Lempert-Ramadier petrosectomy. *E,* Anterior osseous meatal wall removed to gain access to eustachian orifice. *F,* Tensor tympani muscle removed from its semicanal. *G,* Outer rim of eustachian orifice removed; bulge of carotid canal exposed. (Continued on following page.)

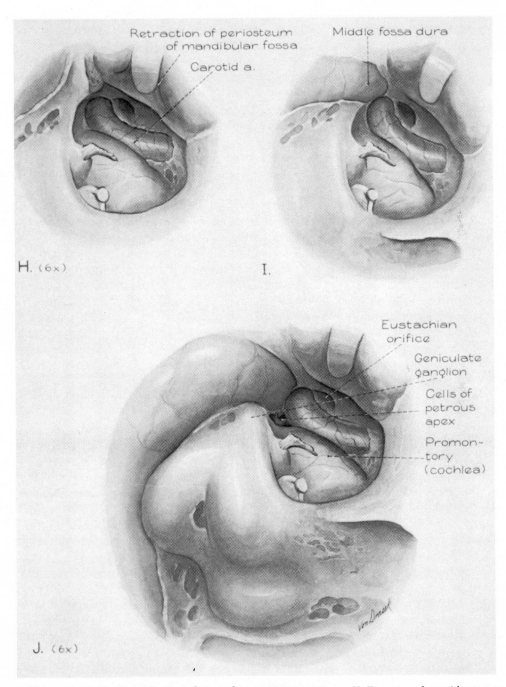

**Figure 12–11** *(Continued)* Completion of Lempert petrosectomy. *H,* Exposure of carotid artery to the apex. *I,* Exposure of middle fossa dura to the apex. *J,* Petrous apex excavated between carotid artery, middle fossa dura, geniculate ganglion and cochlea.

Copious removal of cerebrospinal fluid by lumbar puncture preliminary to the dural elevation facilitates the procedure. With the posterosuperior border or crest of the petrous pyramid kept in view, the dura and temporal lobe are elevated in an anteromedial direction; four landmarks are used: the elevation of the arcuate eminence, the depression between the arcuate eminence and the internal auditory meatus, the elevation of the internal auditory meatus and the depression of the trigeminal ganglion[23] fossa. The latter lies exactly 1 inch or 2.5 cm. beyond the arcuate eminence, and is the usual site for a middle fossa extradural apical abscess. This approach is not recommended as it has the serious disadvantages of being relatively blind and of not providing continuous drainage since the dura falls back onto the arcuate eminence as soon as the elevation is terminated; moreover, elevation of the dura from the arcuate eminence may be difficult, causing an accidental dural tear.

When thorough exploration of **posterior cell tracts** around the semicircular canals fails to open into diseased bone or an abscess cavity, it is necessary to proceed to explore the **anterior group of cells** that may lead to the apex in front of or beneath the cochlea. This requires sacrifice of hearing with a **radical mastoidectomy,** including removal of the tympanic membrane, malleus and incus (Fig. 12–11C and D). The hypotympanum and the mouth of the eustachian tube are then explored for a cell tract leading inward between the cochlea and the jugular bulb or between the cochlea and the carotid artery. If no lead can be found, it is then necessary to follow the carotid artery to the apex according to the method of Ramadier[24] and Lempert.[25] Ramadier exposed the carotid artery at the mouth of the eustachian tube, retracted it anteriorly and entered the apex through the medial wall of the carotid canal. Lempert added to this the removal of a wedge of bone between the carotid canal, the cochlea and the middle fossa to establish a permanently open drainage tract. The operation as described by Lempert is done as follows:

To the usual endaural incision with a radical mastoidectomy is added an incision in the skin of the anterior meatal wall from the root of the zygoma extending downward to the floor of the meatus at the junction of the osseous and cartilaginous meatus. The skin of the anterior osseous meatal wall is elevated as a flap attached to the floor of the meatus.

The anterior osseous meatal wall is removed, exposing the periosteum of the mandibular fossa as far as the mouth of the eustachian tube (Fig. 12–11E and F). Since this is the non-articular portion of the temporomandibular fossa, there is no risk of injuring this joint. The jaw is held open by means of a bite-block, thus retracting forward the soft tissue of the mandibular fossa with improved visualization of the eustachian orifice.

The dura of the middle cranial fossa is exposed by removal of the tegmen plate and root of the zygoma to the level of the geniculate ganglion, just above the cochleariform process (Fig. 12–11E). The tensor tympani muscle is lifted from its semicanal and removed. The mouth of the eustachian tube now lies fully exposed. A smooth rounded eminence in the medial wall of the eustachian tube just in front of the promontory identifies the bony carotid canal (Fig. 12–11G).

The outer bony wall of the carotid canal is carefully removed with a small sharp curet, exposing the vertical portion of the carotid artery (Fig. 12–11H). The carotid artery is enclosed by a venous plexus which may be wounded, with profuse **venous** bleeding easily controlled by a Gelfoam pack. A much more serious laceration of the artery itself has been described.[26]

The triangle of bone between the middle fossa, carotid artery and cochlea is now entered with a small curet, and as this bone is removed the horizontal apical portion of the carotid artery is exposed, with the cup of the curet kept against the carotid and the sharp cutting edge directed away from the carotid. As the apex is entered the tegmen plate is removed (Fig. 12–11I and J). By this approach it is possible to exenterate all cellular and cancellous bone from the petrous apex, exposing the middle and posterior fossae dura of the apex.

In addition to the risk of lacerating the carotid artery, the facial nerve may be injured at the geniculate ganglion or in its petrosal course to the internal auditory meatus, the cavernous sinus may be injured at the tip of the apex, the superior petrosal sinus may be injured, the dura may be torn or the cochlea may be entered when the vertical portion of the carotid lies close to the promontory. Before attempting this approach to the apex, the surgeon should refresh his memory of the anatomic relationships by one or several cadaver dissections.

The Ramadier-Lempert approach to the petrous apex is the most satisfactory method for thorough exploration of the apex, and the one most often employed today for chronic petrositis. It resembles, but is preferable to, the relatively blind approach with a burr previously described by Kopetsky and Almour.[27]

## FACIAL PARALYSIS

The facial nerve is more frequently paralyzed than any other motor nerve in the body, and it has the longest course in a bony canal of any nerve. In a series of 347 cases of peripheral facial paralysis observed by Cawthorne[28] over 90 per cent were due to lesions within the temporal bone. Two thirds of these (69 per cent) were cases of Bell's palsy; surgical injury to the nerve within the temporal bone accounted for 15 per cent; and 8 per cent were the result of otitis media. It is the latter group that will be considered in this chapter.

Facial paralysis may be a complication of either acute or chronic otitis media. When it occurs in the first week or 10 days of an acute otitis media it is not due to bone erosion of the facial canal, but to an edema of the nerve within its bony canal, similar to a Bell's palsy (see Chapter 20).[29] In these cases complete recovery from the facial paralysis may be expected with conservative treatment of the otitis media.

Facial paralysis that comes on in the stage of coalescent bone erosion of an acute suppurative otitis media, that is, after 2 weeks or more of the infection, should be assumed to be the result of erosion of the osseous facial canal with exposure of the nerve to the advancing suppuration. Immediate surgical intervention is indicated to arrest the coalescent process and protect the nerve from partial destruction. A complete simple mastoidectomy should be done without an attempt to identify or further to expose and decompress the nerve if the paralysis is incomplete. Should such a patient show complete paralysis with loss of electrical excitability, indicating a severe lesion, decompression of the nerve in its vertical mastoid segment should be done as described in Chapter 20. Such cases are rare.[30]

Facial paralysis occurring in a chronic otitis media is the result of bone erosion affecting the bony facial canal. Formerly it was a frequent symptom of tubercular otitis media. When it occurs after a suppurative labyrinthitis it suggests a sequestrum of the bony labyrinth. It may be a symptom of a chronic osteomyelitis of the petrous pyramid, in which case the facial nerve involvement is more likely to be partial and transient. It may occur by cholesteatomatous bone erosion. However, exposure of the facial nerve by cholesteatoma without paralysis is more common than exposure with paralysis. The explanation is that the epidermal lining of the advancing cholesteatoma acts as a protective covering for the nerve as its bony canal

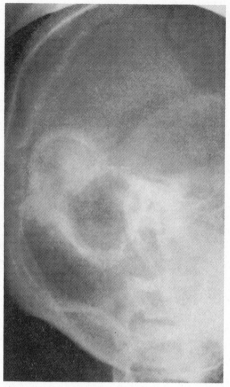

**Figure 12–12**   Cholesteatoma that had exposed the entire vertical mastoid portion of the facial nerve, without paralysis.

is eroded away. In one case observed by the senior author the entire vertical mastoid portion of the facial nerve was found to have been exposed by a huge cholesteatoma (Fig. 12–12), without any evidence of facial weakness before or after surgery. Progressive facial paralysis in a patient with long-standing severe deafness and without otorrhea suggests a congenital cholesteatoma of the petrosa (see Chapter 23).

Facial paralysis occurring in a chronic otitis media is an indication for immediate operation. Careful removal of the diseased structures should be done and the exposed portion of the nerve should be carefully examined. Decompression of the nerve above and below the area of disease should be carried out until normal healthy nerve is reached, to make certain that no granulation tissue or cholesteatoma has infiltrated the bony facial canal. Should a dehiscence of the nerve trunk be found, repair should be carried out by nerve graft or rerouting and end-to-end anastomosis.

For the details of medical and surgical management of facial paralysis, including electrodiagnosis, decompression and repair, see Chapter 20.

## REFERENCES

1. Stuart, E. A., O'Brien, F. H., and McNally, W. J.: Some observations on brain abscess. Arch. Otol., 61:212, 1955.
2. Williams, H. L.: Latent brain abscesses which manifest themselves after mastoidectomy in chronic suppurative otitis media. Laryngoscope, 74:346, 1964.
3. Jeanes, A.: Otogenic intracranial suppuration. J. Laryng. & Otol., 76:388, 1962.

4. Tarkkanen, J. V.: Otogenic brain abscess. Acta oto-laryng., Suppl. 185, 1963.
5. Goodhill, V.: Labyrinthine membrane ruptures in sudden sensorineural hearing loss. Pro. Royal Soc. Med. 69:565, 1976.
6. Wright, A. J.: Further clinical observations on the nature and treatment of Meniere's disease. J. Laryng. & Otol., 55:388, 1940.
7. Shambaugh, G. E., Jr.: Diplacusis: a localizing symptom of disease of the organ of Corti. Arch. Otol., 31:160, 1940.
8. Braun, A., and Friesner, I.: The Labyrinth. Rebman & Co., New York, 1913.
9. Ruttin, E.: Klinik der serösen und eitrigen Labyrinth-Entzündungen. Safár, Wien, 1912.
10. Jansen, A.: Referat über die Operationsmethoden bei den verschiedenen otitischen Gehirnkomplikationen. Verhandl. deutsch. otol. Gesellsch., Jena, 1895, p. 96.
11. Hinsberg, V.: Über Labyrinth-eiterungen. Verhandl. deutsch. otol. Gesellsch., Jena, 1906, p. 30.
12. Richards, J. D.: Surgery of the labyrinth. Laryngoscope, 17:741, 1907.
13. Lindsay, J. R.: Suppuration in the petrous pyramid. Ann. Otol. Rhin. & Laryng., 47:3, 1938.
14. Rainer, A.: Development and construction of pyramidal cells. Arch. Ohren- Nasen- u. Kehlkopfh., 145:3, 1938.
15. Gradenigo, G.: Sulla leptomeningite circoscritta e sulla paralisi dell' abducente di origine otitica. Gior. Accad. med. Torino, 10:59, 1904.
16. Pulec, J. L., and Williams, H. L.: Chronic abscess of the petrous apex. Arch. Otol., 75:419, 1962.
17. Eby, L. G.: Petrositis and lateral sinus thrombosis due to antibiotic-resistant infections. Laryngoscope, 71:1165, 1961.
18. Rambo, J. H. T., and Petti, G. H.: Petrous apicitis. Arch. Otol., 65:523, 1957.
19. Frenckner, P.: Some remarks on treatment of apicitis with and without Gradenigo's syndrome. Acta oto-laryng., 17:97, 1932.
20. Dearmin, R. M.: Logical surgical approach to tip cells of petrous pyramid. Arch. Otol., 26:314, 1937.
21. Farrior, J. B.: The sublabyrinthine exenteration of the petrous apex. Ann. Otol. Rhin. & Laryng., 51:1007, 1942.
22. Eagleton, W. P.: Unlocking of petrous pyramid for localized bulbar meningitis secondary to suppuration of petrous apex. Arch. Otol., 13:386, 1931.
23. Myerson, M. C.: Suppuration of petrous pyramid. Arch. Otol., 26:42, 1937.
24. Ramadier, J.: Les ostéites pétreuses profondes (pétrsites). Oto-rhino-laryng. internat., 17:816, 1933.
25. Lempert, J.: Complete apicectomy (mastoidotympano-apicectomy), new technic for complete apical exenteration of apical carotid portion of petrous pyramid. Arch. Otol., 25:144, 1937.
26. Podesta, R., and Tato, J. M.: Histopathologic report on case of petrositis (Ramadier's operation); tear and hemorrhage of internal carotid, suppurating meningitis. Acta oto-laryng., 25:254, 1937.
27. Kopetsky, S. J., and Almour, R.: Suppuration of petrous pyramid: pathology, symptomatology and surgical treatment. Ann. Otol. Rhin. & Laryng., 39:996, 1930; 40:157, 396, 922, 1931.
28. Cawthorne, T.: The surgery of the temporal bone. J. Laryng. & Otol., 57:437, 1953.
29. Kettel, K.: Facial palsy of ototic origins. Arch. Otol., 37:303, 1943.
30. Farrier, J. B.: Facial paralysis in otology. South. M. J., 41:348, 1948.

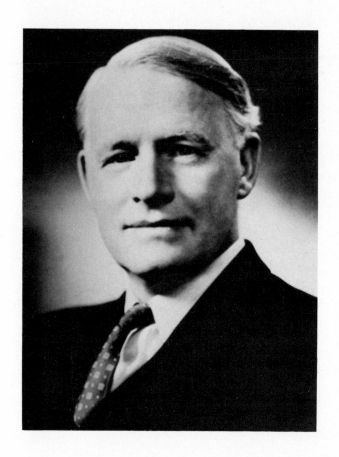

*Carl Olaf Nylén*

BORN 1892
DIED 1978

Initiated in 1921 the otomicroscope for ear surgery.

# Part Three

*"Fenestration does not pretend to cure the lesion of oto-sclerosis in the region of the oval window but it can and does cure clinical otosclerosis by rendering it symptom free. . . ."*

LEMPERT

# Surgery of Deafness

## Hermann von Helmholtz

BORN 1821
DIED 1894

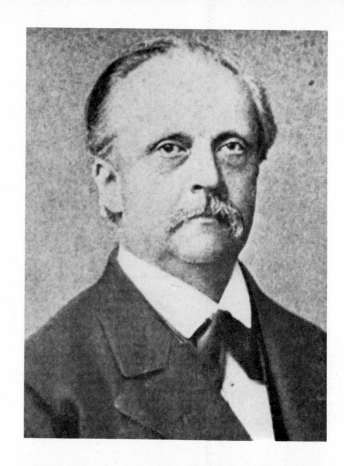

Foremost physiologist of the nineteenth century, who developed the theory of the mechanics of the middle ear transformer.

## Georg von Békésy

BORN 1899
DIED 1972

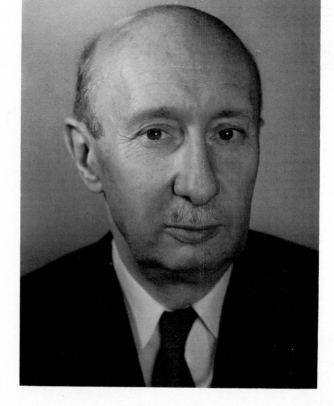

Awarded the Nobel Prize in 1961 for his fundamental studies of the physiology of the middle and inner ear.

# Chapter 13

# Mechanics of Hearing

HISTORIAL ASPECTS
NATURE OF SOUND AND SENSITIVITY OF THE EAR
PHYLOGENETIC EVOLUTION OF THE MIDDLE EAR
   TRANSFORMER
LEVER EFFECT OF THE OSSICULAR CHAIN
HYDRAULIC EFFECT OF THE MIDDLE EAR
   TRANSFORMER
FUNCTION OF THE ROUND WINDOW
PHASE DIFFERENCE BETWEEN THE OVAL AND ROUND
   WINDOWS
RESONANCE AND EFFICIENCY OF THE OUTER AND
   MIDDLE EAR
BONE CONDUCTION HEARING
FUNCTION OF THE INTRATYMPANIC MUSCLES
THE COCHLEAR RESPONSE AND FREQUENCY ANALYSIS
SUMMARY OI MECHANICS OF NORMAL HEARING
BONE CONDUCTION IN THE DISEASED EAR
MECHANICS OF AIR CONDUCTION IN THE DISEASED
   EAR
      OCCLUSION OF THE MEATUS
      PERFORATION OF THE TYMPANIC MEMBRANE
      INTERRUPTION OF THE OSSICULAR CHAIN
      OCCLUSION OF THE EUSTACHIAN TUBE
      THE COLUMELLA EFFECT
      ABSENCE OF THE TYMPANIC MEMBRANE AND
         OSSICLES
      CLOSURE OF THE ROUND WINDOW
      STAPES FIXATION
      MECHANICS OF THE FENESTRATED EAR

## HISTORICAL ASPECTS

Accurate information regarding the mechanics of hearing has been available for a little over a century. The mechanics of hearing have begun to be explored in considerable detail only in the last 50 years, and this information has been applied deliberately and systematically to the surgical reconstruction of the sound-conducting mechanism for only 30 years.

The early Greek physicians, like Empedocles who lived from 500 to 428 B.C., knew of the tympanic membrane and tympanic cavity and believed the seat of the hearing resided in the latter.[1] To this rudimentary concept Galen,[2] who lived from

A.D. 131 to 201, added the auditory nerve, which he thought ended in the middle ear cavity, but meanwhile he forgot about the tympanic membrane.

No further progress was made in the physiology of hearing until the sixteenth century when the great anatomists of the Renaissance made their monumental contributions. The greatest of the anatomists was the Belgian Vesalius,[3] who in 1543 named the malleus and incus and described them in detail. Three years later, in 1546, the Italian anatomist Ingrassia[4] discovered the stapes and the oval and round windows, and in 1561 Fallopius,[5] another Italian anatomist, described and named the cochlea, labyrinth and canal for the facial nerve. Shortly thereafter, in 1564, still another Italian anatomist, Eustachius,[6] discovered the auditory tube that is generally referred to by his name.

These anatomic discoveries enabled Coiter[7] in 1566 to trace for the first time the path of sound vibrations from the external auditory meatus through the tympanic membrane to the labyrinth and cochlea. Neither Coiter nor Duverney,[8] who a century later further elaborated on the conduction of sound to the inner ear, suspected the important **transformer** action of the middle ear for the purpose of overcoming the sound barrier between air and water since they, like their predecessors, believed that the labyrinth contained air. That the labyrinth is filled with fluid was first maintained by Cotugno[9] in 1760, and conclusively proved when Meckel[10] placed fresh temporal bones outside in freezing weather and found the labyrinths always filled with ice. The description in 1851 by Corti[11] of the tectorial membrane, basilar membrane, hair cells and supporting cells was followed some time later by the demonstration by Retzius[12] that the hair cells are the ultimate receptors, innervated by the auditory nerve fibers.

The final steps toward appreciation of the transformer function of the middle ear were taken by Müller[13] in 1837 and by Helmholtz in 1863. These celebrated German physiologists noted the difference in the acoustic properties of air and water, and the need for a mechanism to convert air vibrations of large amplitude and low pressure to fluid vibrations of small amplitude and higher pressure. Helmholtz suggested that this was accomplished by a combination of three processes: a lever action of the drum membrane itself, a lever effect of the ossicular chain and the hydraulic action of a large tympanic membrane acting upon the small stapes footplate.[14]

Helmholtz' explanations met with immediate favor. They were so advanced for his time and so well documented by his detailed experimental investigations that for a long time they were accepted with scant question. Except for some original work by Bezold, little more was added to the physiology of hearing until about 1922 when the details of the hearing mechanism began to be restudied by an increasing number of investigators. Among them were: Pohlman,[15] Frank,[16] Herzog[17] and Dahmann,[18] who re-examined the mechanics of sound conduction by the tympanic membrane and ossicles; Wever, Lawrence and Davis,[19] who included in their studies the mechanism of the cochlear response; and Lüscher[20] and Kobrak,[21] who investigated especially the function of the intratympanic muscles. Probably the foremost of the recent contributors to the physiology of hearing was Békésy, whose ingenious and detailed studies have helped to confirm certain of the principles of sound conduction proposed by Helmholtz, but at the same time have demonstrated errors and deficiencies in the earlier work. Even today our knowledge of the mechanical properties of the outer and middle ear is sketchy, and our understanding of the translation of mechanical movements within the cochlea to nerve impulses is even more fragmentary.[22] Further research into the details of the hearing mechanism is continuing and is very much needed to elucidate the function of the normal and, even more, of the diseased ear.

The final chapter in our understanding of the mechanics of hearing is only beginning to be written. This is the application of the principles of the middle ear transformer to the diagnosis and therapy of conductive losses. It is perhaps not too surprising that this clinical application has been so slow and late in arriving, in view of the incompleteness and gaps in our knowledge. For example, Bezold[23] was well acquainted with the work of Helmholtz, yet he failed to see that the construction of a skin-lined meatus to the antrum for congenital meatal atresia must include contact with the mobile stapes to reconstruct a transformer action. Neither Holmgren nor Sourdille understood the mechanics of hearing after fenestration. Actually, a clear comprehension of the pathway of sound in the fenestrated ear did not begin until 10 years after this procedure had been firmly established by Lempert and his followers. In 1947 Békésy[24] and in 1948 Juers[25] made preliminary studies of the mechanics of the fenestrated ear. In 1950 Davis and Walsh[26] made their important definition of the residue of unrestored conductive loss following successful fenestration; this was followed shortly by the significant studies by Nilsson[27] and Skoog[28] on the transmission of sound in the fenestrated ear.

Meanwhile in 1948 Johansen[29] applied the impedance formula to the middle ear transformer to explain audiometric configurations, and Campbell's[30] study followed in 1950.

It remained for Zöllner[31] in 1951 and Wullstein[32] in 1952 to finally apply the mechanical principles of the middle ear transformer to the surgical reconstruction of the middle ear following destructive suppurative disease. For the first time the mechanical principles first defined by Helmholtz nearly a century before began to be applied systematically to the therapy of conductive losses.

## NATURE OF SOUND AND SENSITIVITY OF THE EAR

Sound is a vibratory motion with a frequency within the human audible range, namely between 10 cycles per second and 24,000 cycles per second. Each sound wave consists of a compressional phase followed by a rarefaction phase, these phases following one another at different distances according to the frequency of the tone. From the sound source the alternate waves of compression and rarefaction travel at a fixed speed in air of 344 meters (1129 feet) per second at 20° C. at sea level. In water sound travels more than four times as fast, at a speed of 1437 meters (4714 feet) per second; in ivory (not unlike the petrous bone) the speed of sound is even more rapid, 3013 meters (9886 feet) per second.

A pure tone is a simple wave form termed "sinusoidal." A complex tone consists of a fundamental pure tone combined with various overtones generally of lesser intensity.

The **frequency** of a tone determines its pitch and is the number of cycles per second, each cycle consisting of a compression phase and a rarefaction phase. The wavelength of a tone is easily calculated by dividing the speed of sound by the frequency. For example, the wavelength of the frequency of 1000 cycles per second is the speed of sound of 344 meters, or 34400 centimeters, divided by 1000, or 34.4 cm. In very cold air the molecules are closer together and sound travels more rapidly without changing direction, as occurs when layers of air of different temperatures are encountered. This and the lack of fog or smoke account for the unusual clarity and sharpness of hearing of distant sounds on a very cold, clear night.

The **intensity** of a tone determines its loudness as heard by the ear, and is the amplitude of displacement of molecules in the sound waves. For clinical purposes

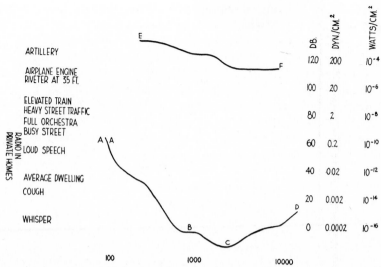

**Figure 13–1**   Range of sensitivity of the human ear from threshold to pain. Curve *ABCD* represents the threshold of hearing in a normal young adult. *B* is the threshold at 1000 cycles, chosen as the reference level for human hearing with a sound pressure of $2 \times 10^{-4}$ dynes per square centimeter. *EF* represents the threshold for pain. (From Lindsay, J., et al. *In* Coates, G. M., et al. (Eds.): Otolaryngology. Vol. 1. Hagerstown, Md., W. F. Prior Co., 1955.)

the intensity of a tone is expressed in decibels, and the **threshold** of hearing for a healthy young adult is taken as 0 decibels of loudness. For the tone of 1000 cycles this amounts to a pressure of approximately 0.0002 dyne per sq. cm. The sensitivity of the human ear is greatest for the frequencies of 1000 to 3000 cycles; it is a little less for higher frequencies and considerably less for lower frequencies (Fig. 13–1). For example, the sensitivity of the normal human ear for 100 cycles is 1000 times less than for 1000 cycles, representing a decrease of 30 decibels. The audiometer is constructed to correct for these differences in sensitivity between frequencies so that whatever the frequency, the threshold will be 0 decibels of intensity for the normal ear. Clinical audiometers are actually set so that their 0 decibels is approximately 5 decibels louder than the true threshold, as measured in a completely noise-free room. This is to compensate for the masking effect of the usual ambient noise found in the average sound-treated (but not truly soundproof) testing room.

Normal ears of different people vary slightly in their threshold of sensitivity, so that audiograms within 20 decibels of 0 are considered to be within the range of normal hearing (A.N.S.I., American National Standards Institute).

The enormous range of intensities over which the ear operates is one of the most amazing attributes of the human organism. At the threshold of hearing in the range of greatest sensitivity the amplitude of vibration of the tympanic membrane is about one tenth the diameter of a hydrogen molecule and the corresponding movement of the basilar membrane in the cochlea is one hundredth as large as this. At the other end of the scale the ear responds to sound vibrations with a sound intensity one trillion times the intensity at threshold! Such extremely loud sounds cause a tickling or pain in the ear and are termed the threshold of feeling (Fig. 13–1, curve *EF*). At the threshold of feeling for 10 cycles the movements of the tympanic membrane are so large (0.2 to 0.4 mm. of excursion[33]) that they are visible to the naked eye, especially if aided by stroboscopic illumination. It should be noted that at these high intensities the sensory structure of the cochlea may be permanently damaged.

Because of the extraordinary range of intensities of normal hearing it is convenient to employ a condensed scale for intensity measurements. This is accomplished by expressing intensities in terms of the logarithm of the numbers. For example, a sound intensity 10 times above threshold is termed 10 decibels, a hundred times above threshold is 20 decibels and a thousand times above threshold is 30 decibels. An intensity of 120 decibels, at the threshold of feeling for 1000 cycles, is one trillion times above the threshold of hearing and, as already mentioned, can permanently damage the neurosensory structure in the cochlea. The intensity of 100 decibels, or 10 billion times the intensity of barely audible sound, is generally considered the limit of non-damaging sound, so that clinical audiometers are not constructed to produce sound of more than 100 or 110 decibels. Some ears will be damaged even at 100 decibels above threshold if they are exposed long enough.

The marvels of hearing do not end here.[34] The normal human ear at a cocktail party is able to suppress a large amount of noise and babble of voices and concentrate on one speaker. Exactly how this is done is not known except that **binaural hearing** becomes important for this refined function. The monitoring of one's own voice occurs by a feedback system which continually adjusts and corrects the voice as we speak. The feedback is partly by air-conducted sounds, but also by bone-conducted sounds, especially from the mandible to the external meatus. The result is that our own voice sounds different to us than to others who hear it only by air conduction. This accounts for the amazing, embarrassing and disappointing experience of listening to a high-fidelity tape recording of one's own voice, which sounds thinner, less resonant, decidedly less impressive and hardly recognizable to the speaker, but quite natural to his friends.

The unconscious monitoring of one's own voice by air- and bone-conducted hearing accounts for the voice alterations produced by long-standing severe hearing losses. In otosclerosis, bone-conducted hearing is enhanced compared to air-conducted hearing, and the victim fails to increase the intensity of his voice in the presence of noise and speaks too softly. In high-frequency sensorineural hearing loss the quality of the voice is altered by the failure to hear the higher frequencies in speech. In total binaural deafness the quality and loudness of the voice soon become markedly altered, flat and disagreeable if not corrected by a voice teacher.

The localization of the direction of sound is another attribute of normal hearing, requiring two ears with nearly equal "balanced" sensitivity. This localization is accomplished by a slight time delay in the arrival of sound to one of the ears, as well as by differences in loudness. In attempting to locate the source of a sound one unconsciously turns the head to bring one ear a little closer, accentuating the time and loudness differences.

Finally, the ability of the ear to discriminate pitch and to analyze complex sounds so as to separate one tone from many others has mystified and amazed physiologists for many years.

In this *Surgery of the Ear* it is neither possible nor necessary to present a complete discussion of the mechanism of hearing. We shall concern ourselves mainly with the mechanics of sound conduction from the outside air to the cochlea, with only a brief mention of the transformation of vibratory motion in the cochlea to nerve impulses.


## PHYLOGENETIC EVOLUTION OF THE MIDDLE EAR TRANSFORMER

Far back in the process of evolution when the world was young our distant ancestors lived in the sea. Their hearing organ, like that of many of today's crustaceans and fishes, consisted of a simple sac filled with fluid (at first sea water) and contained sensory cells in contact with a dense but mobile membrane (Fig. 13–2A). Its chief function, like the macula of the human vestibule, which it resembled, was equilibratory, but it could also respond to coarse vibrations. Since the acoustic properties of soft tissues with their high water content are very nearly the same as those of water, sound vibrations from the sea passed easily through the skin and soft tissues to the fluid within the primitive ear. There was no need for a complicated mechanical apparatus to transmit sound to the inner ear. Thus fish respond quickly to splashing or similarly produced sound in the water. On the other hand, fish are not disturbed by any but the loudest sounds produced in the air **above** water, for because of the different acoustic properties of air and water, often referred to as the difference in sound impedance between air and water, 99.9 per cent of the energy of air-borne sound is reflected away from the surface of water, and only 0.1 per cent enters the water.[1] The existence of this very great air-water **sound barrier** is easily demonstrated by the swimmer who, with his head under water, clearly hears faint sounds originating under water, such as two stones clicked together, but fails to hear a loud noise above the water (Fig. 13–3).

As the face of the world began to wrinkle with age our restless and enterprising ancestor about 260 million years ago crept out of the sea onto dry land. To breathe air he developed lungs, but at first he was comparatively deaf, for only 0.1 per cent of sound energy reached the fluid of his inner ear, 99.9 per cent being reflected away by the air-water sound barrier. This proved to be a great disadvantage in the struggle for existence, for survival often depended upon timely flight. For better hearing an apparatus was needed to transform air-borne sounds of large amplitude but small force to fluid vibrations of small amplitude but large force. This was accomplished by a marvelous salvage-adaptation of the gills, no longer needed for respiration, one of the most remarkable transformations of evolution. The first gill cleft became the external auditory meatus and tympanic cavity with an intervening tympanic membrane acquired by a simple arrest of the usual process of embryologic develop-ment in which the first branchial groove grew toward and finally joined the first pharyngeal pouch. The cartilages of the first and second branchial arches on either side of the first gill cleft were modified to form a lever-like ossicular chain leading from the large tympanic membrane to the small oval window. The middle

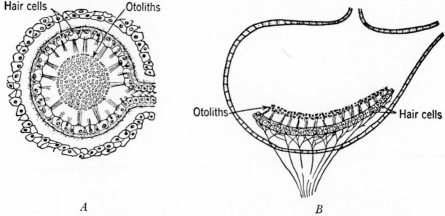

*A*                                        *B*

**Figure 13–2** *A*, Otolithic organ of a mollusc *(Pectus inflexus)*, after Butschli. *B*, The saccule of man. (From Wever, E. G., and Lawrence, M.: Physiological Acoustics. Princeton, Princeton University Press, 1954.)

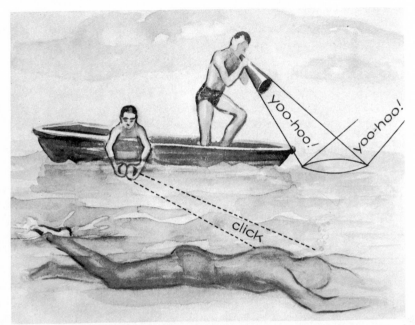

**Figure 13–3** Swimmer with head immersed clearly hears click of stones under water but not the voice above water.

ear pressure transformer thus evolved is often referred to as the impedance-matching mechanism of the ear, since it overcomes or matches the difference in acoustic impedance between air and water.

## LEVER EFFECT OF THE OSSICULAR CHAIN

Helmholtz attributed the pressure transformation of the middle ear to three factors: a mechanical amplification of force by the tympanic membrane itself, a lever effect of the ossicular chain and the hydraulic action of the much larger size of the tympanic membrane (90 sq. mm.) acting upon the smaller stapes footplate (3 sq. mm.).

Recent studies of Dahmann,[17] Békésy[22] and Wever and Lawrence[1] indicate that Helmholtz was mistaken about the first factor, namely that the tympanic membrane by virtue of its conical shape amplifies the force exerted upon the manubrium. Actually the membrane moves as a solid plate on an axis that runs through the short process of the malleus and body of the incus, and the handle of the malleus merely follows its excursions without any increase in force (Fig. 13–4).

The second factor described by Helmholtz is the lever effect of the ossicular chain. After studying the shape of the ossicles, their articulations and the tensions of their ligaments, with visual observations of their movements, Helmholtz arrived at a rather complicated concept of ossicular motion. This began with piston-like movements of the manubrium, a twisting motion of the head of the malleus and a rocking motion of the incus imparted to the stapes. He concluded that there was an increase of force of 1.5 times from the manubrium to the stapes.

Certain discrepancies in Helmholtz' measurements and reasoning are pointed out by Dahmann and Wever and Lawrence. Actually the incus and malleus move as a unit pivoted on an axis that runs through the posterior process and ligament of the

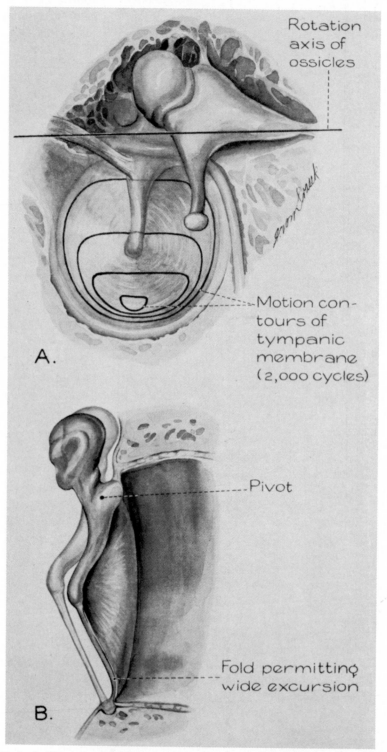

**Figure 13–4** *A*, Movements of the tympanic membrane for 2000 cycle tone (Békésy). *B*, Axis of rotation of tympanic membrane and ossicles.

incus and the anterior process and ligament of the malleus (Fig. 13–4A). The lever effect of the ossicular chain is simply the length of the malleus handle compared to the length of the long process of the incus, which in the human ear is 1.3 to 1, representing an increase of force at the oval window of 1.3 times rather than the 1.5 times described by Helmholtz. In the cat this ratio is 2.5 to 1.[1]

## HYDRAULIC EFFECT OF THE MIDDLE EAR TRANSFORMER

The third factor contributing to the pressure transformation of the middle ear according to Helmholtz is the difference in size between the tympanic membrane and stapes footplate. The recent studies of Békésy[22] indicate that the effective vibrating area of the tympanic membrane is somewhat smaller than Helmholtz thought, about 55 sq. mm. rather than 85 to 90 sq. mm. The ratio of this effective area to the average size of the footplate (3.2 sq. mm.) is 17 to 1. This represents the **hydraulic ratio** of the tympanic membrane and stapes footplate, producing an increase of force at the oval window of 17 times for the human ear. This compares with an effective tympanic membrane–oval window ratio of 24.3 for the cat.[1]

The final transformer ratio of the human tympanic membrane and ossicular chain is the product of the lever ratio of 1.3 times the hydraulic ratio of 17, or **22**, according to Békésy.[22] This is considerably less than for the cat, in which the ossicular chain ratio of 2.5 times the 24.5 ratio gives a transformer ratio of **61 to 1**.[1]

## FUNCTION OF THE ROUND WINDOW

The function of the round window has been the subject of much speculation and debate. This structure lies at the opposite end of the cochlear duct from the oval window. It is closed by a thin membrane having an area of 2 sq. mm., a little smaller than the oval window, which is slightly larger than 3 sq. mm. in the human ear. (In the cat the oval window averages 1.2 sq. mm. compared to 3.01 sq. mm. for the round window.[1]) The membrane of the round window in man is usually concealed from view by the overhang of the niche of the round window, but occasionally part or all of the round window membrane is clearly seen during the operation of stapedectomy, when it can be observed to lie approximately at right angles to the oval window and to have a somewhat convex surface toward the middle ear.

Recent authors agree that in the normal ear the round window acts merely as a relief opening in the bony labyrinth at the opposite end of the cochlear perilymphatic duct from the stapes footplate to permit maximum movement of the cochlear column of fluid. The increase of force of **22 times** at the oval window imparted by the middle ear transformer far exceeds any force exerted by sound on the round window. Moreover the intact tympanic membrane acts to shield the round window from the direct impact of sound and probably alters the phase, further minimizing any canceling effect produced by sound reaching both windows at the same time. It is interesting that in the frog the round window membrane lies against the lymph sac and in some birds' ears it lies against the jugular vein. In these animals it can act only as a relief opening to permit maximum movement of the cochlear fluid column and cannot be the portal of entry for sound.[15]

Although the round window as a competitive portal of entry for sound is relatively unimportant in the normal ear, in the **diseased middle ear** it may be very important, both for the canceling effect on sound entering the oval window without the advantage of a pressure transformer and because in certain conditions the round window may actually become the portal of entry for sound.[35]

## PHASE DIFFERENCE BETWEEN THE OVAL AND ROUND WINDOWS

Each sound vibration consists of a compression phase followed by a rarefaction phase. If a sound reaches the oval and round windows at the height of the compression phase (Fig. 13–5A), there will be a tendency toward less displacement of the fluid column in the cochlea than if the sound reaches one window at the compression phase and the other window at the rarefaction phase. A phase difference between the two windows can arise when one window lies closer to the sound source than the other. This is the situation when there is a total loss of tympanic membrane and malleus and incus, and the sound wave reaches the head of the stapes a little sooner than it reaches the round window because of the protrusion of the stapes compared to the recessed round window membrane (Fig. 13–5B). A phase difference can also arise from the presence of an intact tympanic membrane

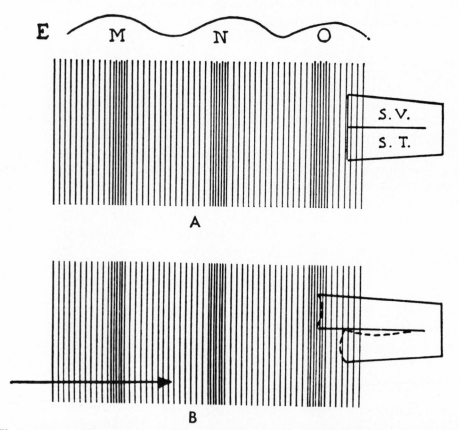

**Figure 13–5**   *A*, Effect of sound reaching oval and round windows in the same phase and with equal force: no movement of the cochlear partition. *B*, Sound pressure reaching both windows with equal force but in different phase: movement of cochlear column and partition. (From Juers, A. L.: Observations on bone conduction in fenestrated cases. Ann. Otol. Rhin. & Laryng., 57:28, 1948.)

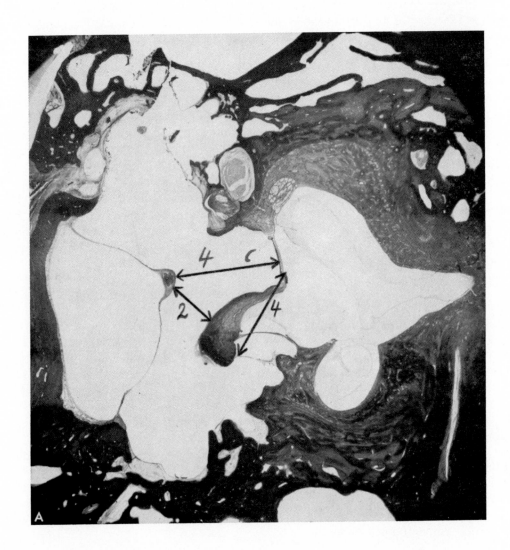

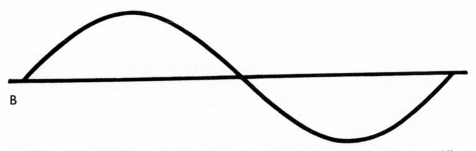

**Figure 13–6** Comparison of wavelength of 1000 cycles *(B)* and dimensions of human middle ear in millimeters *(A)*. (From Lindsay, J., et al. *In* Coates, G. M., et al. (Eds.): Otolaryngology. Vol. 1. Hagerstown, Md., W. P. Prior Co., 1955.)

acting on the enclosed tympanic bubble of air. Because of its mass and elasticity the tympanic membrane movements lag slightly behind the waves of alternate compression and rarefaction in the external meatus. The inward movement of the tympanic membrane reaches its maximum, with maximum compression of the elastic bubble of air, at the moment that the sound vibration in the meatus has begun to enter its rarefaction phase. Then as the tympanic membrane begins to move outward, pulling the stapes footplate with it, the round window is still being pushed inward by the compressed bubble of air, providing the phase difference at the two windows necessary for optimum hearing. A large perforation of the tympanic membrane eliminates this phase-changing action by allowing the sound to reach the round window without having its phase delayed or reversed, and as a result the phase relationship between the two windows becomes unfavorable.

It should be noted that phase differences between the two windows have a very minor effect on hearing acuity of the **normal ear,** because of the 22 times increase of force at the oval window compared to the round window by virtue of the hydraulic and lever effects of the tympanic membrane and ossicular chain. Thus Wever and Lawrence[1] report for the normal ear only a 3.5 decibel difference in the hearing acuity for 100 cycles between no phase difference and maximum phase difference at the two windows.

In contrast to the minor effect of phase differences on hearing acuity in the normal ear, these differences begin to play a critical though variable role when the ear is deprived of the middle ear transformer. These variations are due to the particular pathologic lesion and to the anatomic dimensions of the particular ear in relation to the wavelength of sound (Fig. 13–6). Thus a sound vibration of 8000 cycles, measuring less than 0.5 cm. from peak of compression phase to peak of rarefaction phase, may reach the head of the stapes and the round window of an ear without a tympanic membrane at opposite phases, with enhanced hearing for this frequency, but at a little higher frequency the sound may reach both windows in the same phase, with poorer hearing for this higher frequency.

How much the intact tympanic membrane dampens or shields the round window from sound, in addition to altering the phase at the round window, has not been clarified. For practical clinical purposes it may be asssumed that for optimum hearing the round window must be **maximally free to move,** lying against an elastic air cushion, and it must be **maximally shielded** from the direct impact of sound by an intact tympanic membrane.


## RESONANCE AND EFFICIENCY OF THE OUTER AND MIDDLE EAR

The ear is not a high-fidelity instrument, but because of its anatomic size and structure it responds better to certain frequencies than to others. In the human external auditory meatus the natural resonance frequency is near 3000 cycles, explained by the fact that the meatus is 2.7 cm. long, and a tube closed at one end resonates best to a frequency four times its length, or 10.8 cm.; the wavelength of 3000 cycles is 11.4 cm. This natural resonance increases the sound pressure at the tympanic membrane for tones around 3000 cycles by about 10 decibels.[22] In addition to this resonating amplification of the meatus itself there is in many animals, but not in man, a large, funnel-shaped auricle, which further concentrates sound at the tympanic membrane. This concentration amounts to an additional 8 decibels in the deer as compared to the human — a valuable survival advantage for the deer versus the hunter. The natural resonance frequency of the tympanic membrane and ossicular chain is around 800 cycles.[36]

The efficiency of the tympanic membrane in receiving and transmitting sound energy to the manubrium is relatively poor for low frequencies below 500 and is greatest between 800 and 1600 cycles.[1] The pressure transformation between tympanic membrane and stapes is greatest between 500 and 2000 cycles. Thus both the natural resonances and the efficiency of the outer and middle ear mechanism for the human ear are greatest in the speech range, so that the greatest sensitivity lies between 1000 and 3000 cycles (Fig. 13–1).

## BONE CONDUCTION HEARING

Hearing by bone conduction is the result of sound vibrations that reach the cochlear fluid column through the skull. Vibrations may be communicated from the skull to the cochlear fluid in several ways. One way is a to-and-fro shaking movement of the entire skull, as one would shake the fluid in a cocktail shaker, termed **translatory bone conduction** (Fig. 13–7A). For optimum translatory bone conduction two windows of equal mobility at either end of the cochlear duct are needed.

Another form of bone conduction to the cochlea is by intermittent compression and expansion of the skull bones, rhythmically reducing and increasing the size of the cochlear space. This is termed **compressional bone conduction** (Fig. 13–7B) and is greater when one window is more movable than the other. If both windows are equally movable, or if both windows are immobile, bone conduction is diminished somewhat but not eliminated, since alternating distortion of the cochlear wall will alter the relative sizes of the scala vestibuli and scala tympani, with resultant movement of the basilar membrane.[37]

Below 200 cycles bone-conducted sound is conducted to the cochlea entirely by

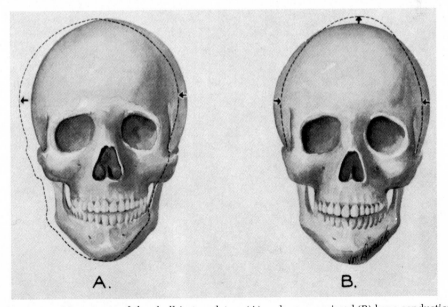

A.                                          B.

**Figure 13–7**   Movements of the skull in translatory (A) and compressional (B) bone conduction.

the translatory method. Near 800 cycles compressional bone conduction becomes more important, whereas above 1500 cycles the skull continues to vibrate by the compressional method, but in several sections like a bell rather than as a whole.[22]

Bone conduction can also occur by the vibrations of the skull being communicated to the air column in the meatus and to the bubble of air in the tympanum, and thence to the tympanic membrane and via the ossicular chain to the oval window. Moreover, the ossicles themselves, owing to their mass and inertia, will fail to follow translatory movements of the skull, thus vibrating relative to the skull. The resulting movements of the tympanic membrane and ossicular chain are then transmitted to the cochlea in the usual manner. This is termed **transmitted bone conduction,** or the middle ear contribution to bone conduction.

In the normal ear, bone conduction has very little influence on the hearing of air-conducted sound, since the middle ear transformer is much more effective than the small amount of sound energy absorbed by the skull from air, since most of this energy is reflected. As we have seen, bone-conducted hearing is much more important in hearing one's own voice, the vibrations of the larynx being communicated to the mandible and thence to the air of the meatus.[34] In the diseased ear deprived of a pressure transformer, bone-conducted sound becomes much more important in its contribution to hearing by air, and because bone-conducted sound is slightly out of phase with air-conducted sound, the result may be unfavorable.[36]

## FUNCTION OF THE INTRATYMPANIC MUSCLES

A discussion of the mechanics of sound conduction should include a consideration of the tensor tympani and stapedius muscles. As long ago as 1837 Müller[13] proposed that these muscles act to muffle or decrease the transmission of sound to the cochlea. Extensive studies by Lüscher and Kobrak confirm the protective role of these muscles in preventing excessively loud sounds from reaching the cochlea by dampening them. Kobrak[38] noted that these muscles do not respond to faint or moderate intensities but contract reflexly in response to loud sounds. As the loudness of a sound increases, the stapedius muscle contracts first, and with a further increase in loudness the tensor tympani also contracts. The stapedius contraction inhibits the movements of the stapes footplate; the tensor tympani acts at the opposite end of the chain by lessening the movements of the manubrium. The louder the tone, the stronger the contraction of these muscles. Although the amount of sound protection is not large, around 10 decibels for most sounds, it can be the difference between no damage and irreversible cochlear damage for sounds near the threshold of feeling. Since there is a brief latent period in the reflex contraction of these muscles, they do not protect the cochlea from sudden, sharp or explosive sounds such as gunfire.

An incidental function of these muscles is simply to increase the rigidity of the ossicular chain and thus protect it against dislocation. Recently Wever[39] has demonstrated an additional function in the cat in which very faint sounds cause a weak contraction that appreciably increases the acuity of hearing. A similar sharpening of the hearing for faint sounds in the human ear has yet to be demonstrated.

## THE COCHLEAR RESPONSE AND FREQUENCY ANALYSIS

The theory of Helmholtz that the basilar membrane consists of a series of resonators of different length and under different tension, each tuned to a different frequency, like a piano, has had to be modified as further information has accumulated. Békésy in particular studied the movements of the cochlear structures in response to sound. He found that the basilar membrane is not under tension. The movements of the cochlear partition, consisting of the basilar membrane, hair cells, tectorial membrane, endolymph of the scala media and Reissner's membrane, occur as a traveling wave that begins at the oval window in the normal ear. For frequencies below 60 cycles the whole partition vibrates, and the auditory nerve is stimulated with each vibration according to the frequency. Above 60 cycles the basilar membrane begins to vibrate unevenly, with a point of maximum vibration that varies with each tone. Gradually as the frequency increases this takes the place of the periodicity of stimulation of the nerve in determining pitch, until above 4000 cycles pitch is determined entirely by the site of maximum stimulation. Apparently an inhibiting mechanism suppresses the weaker stimuli from adjacent areas of less amplitude of vibration. The basilar membrane makes a rough frequency analysis, and the central auditory nervous system sharpens the analysis in ways not yet understood.[34]

## SUMMARY OF MECHANICS OF NORMAL HEARING

Before considering the mechanics of hearing in the diseased middle ear, we should summarize the principal factors that contribute to the conduction of sound in the normal ear.

By far the most important single factor in sound conduction is the **hydraulic ratio** of the middle ear, because of the large area of the tympanic membrane acting on the small area of the stapes footplate. This great hydraulic advantage of 17 to 1 is enhanced by a small and relatively unimportant **lever factor** of 1.3 to 1, due to the difference in length of the manubrium and long process of the incus, to give a total **transformer ratio** of 22 to 1 for the human ear.

The mechanical lever advantage of the human ossicular chain is so small that one wonders why we do not have a single ossicle like the columella of the frog and bird instead of a chain of three ossicles. The chief reason for our more complicated chain appears to be protection for the cochlea. It affords opportunity for two muscles instead of one to dampen loud sounds, and in addition the movements of the ossicles in response to very loud sounds change so as to diminish the corresponding movements of the cochlear fluid column.[22] As we shall see, the human ear deprived of an incus but with contact between the tympanic membrane and stapes operates like the bird's ear, with only slight loss of efficiency.

Additional mechanical factors that contribute to normal hearing acuity are the greater efficiency, due to their natural resonances, of the outer and middle ear structures for the speech range than for lower frequencies, and the phase-reverser and shielding action of the intact tympanic membrane and enclosed bubble of air on the round window. Bone-conducted sound is unimportant for normal hearing except for one's own voice.

## BONE CONDUCTION IN THE DISEASED EAR

Audiometers today are constructed and calibrated so that the air and bone curves interweave or superimpose at or within 20 decibels of 0 (A.N.S.I.) for the normal ear. Audiometric bone-conducted hearing is considered the measure of sensorineural function in the cochlea or eighth nerve or central auditory pathways. When

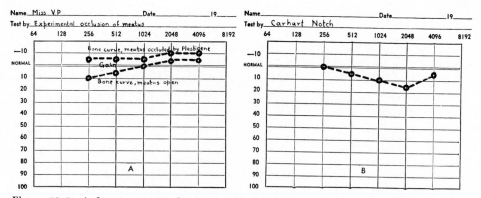

**Figure 13–8**  *A*, Improvement in bone conduction produced by occlusion of the outer end of the meatus, in a normal-hearing young adult in a quiet testing room. *B*, Carhart notch. This is the average bone conduction curve in patients with otosclerotic stapes fixation without cochlear deterioration.

the hearing by air is impaired more than hearing by bone, the resulting air-bone gap is considered the measure of hearing impairment due to a conductive lesion of the outer or middle ear. Although bone-conducted hearing is our most useful measure of sensorineural function, it is not always a precise measure. Thus more than a century ago Schwabach[40] and Weber[41] noted that in lesions of the outer and middle ear, hearing by bone conduction was better than that in the normal ear. In 1926 Pohlman and Kranz[42] showed that improved bone conduction was no longer evident when most patients with middle ear lesions were tested in a soundproof room. They and Knudsen and Jones[43] in 1931 showed that the greater masking effect of noise on the normal ear is responsible for the apparent discrepancy in bone conduction between normal patients and those with middle ear lesions tested in noise. Later studies have shown that there **can** be an absolute increase in bone conduction in a few conditions, such as occlusion of the external auditory meatus at its outer end (Fig. 13–8A)*, but in **most** middle ear lesions bone conduction is actually impaired for certain frequencies. In 1950 Carhart[44] described a notching in the bone conduction audiogram in patients with stapedial fixation otospongiosis. (Fig. 13–8B). This is now known to be due to loss of transmitted bone conduction to the inner ear imparted by the skull vibrations to the ossicles.[45] Unexplained are the rather marked variations in the shape and size of Carhart's "otosclerotic" notch as revealed by improvement in bone conduction following fully successful stapes surgery (Fig. 13–9). When the partially fixed stapes footplate is the site of a large otospongiotic thickening that increases its mass, the bone conduction loss is especially great so that the air and bone hearing tests resemble those of a sensorineural more than of a conductive lesion.[37]

Thus the bone curve must not be accepted as a completely accurate measure of inner ear function, but it must be interpreted in the light of other tests, including speech discrimination.

## MECHANICS OF AIR CONDUCTION IN THE DISEASED EAR

We have already seen how complicated are the factors that contribute to sound conduction in the normal ear. When we try to define the mechanical effects on

*Note: all audiograms in this chapter A.S.A., the former American Standards Association.

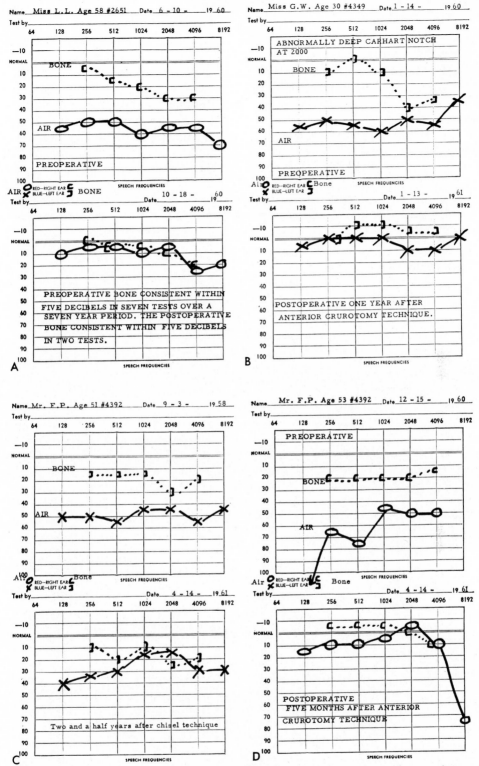

**Figure 13–9** Otosclerotic (Carhart) notches as revealed by improved bone conduction after stapes surgery. *A,* Improvement in bone conduction after stapedectomy with fat graft and wire. *B,* Improved bone conduction after anterior crurotomy mobilization of stapes. *C,* Bone conduction unchanged by stapes mobilization with partial closure of air-bone gap. *D,* Same patient as in *C.* Top: Stapes refixed. Bottom: Partial stapedectomy with complete closure of air-bone gap and improved bone conduction. (From Shambaugh, G. E., Jr., and Adamson, M.: Bone conduction changes following stapes surgery as related to indications for surgery. Laryngoscope, 74:513, 1964.)

hearing of different lesions of the outer and middle ear we find ourselves in an area of conjecture still largely unexplored by exact measurements. Nevertheless, as otologic diagnosticians and surgeons we must attempt to fit what is known concerning the mechanics of normal hearing to the pathologic situation, with the acknowledgment that we will doubtless be guilty of oversimplification and that our interpretations must be subject to revision as further research is done. The practical results that are being achieved by applying the principles of sound conduction to the surgical reconstruction of the outer and middle ear (Chapter 16) are sufficient justification for the clinician's attempt to interpret where the acoustic physiologist has not yet fully explored.

The impedance formula for an acoustic system as proposed by Johansen[29] helps to explain the varieties of hearing curve encountered in different conductive lesions. This formula states that impedance equals the square root of friction² plus

$$\left(\text{mass times frequency minus }\frac{\text{stiffness}^2}{\text{frequency}}\right)$$

or

$$I = \sqrt{\text{friction}^2 + m \times f - \frac{s^2}{f}}$$

In this formula impedance is defined as the resistance to being set into vibration of an acoustic system. When the mass of such a system is increased, the hearing threshold for high frequencies is impaired; when stiffness is increased, the threshold for low frequencies is impaired; and when friction is increased, the threshold for all frequencies is impaired, especially for those near the resonance of the middle ear between 800 and 1600 cycles (Fig. 13–10). Examples of increase of mass are moist

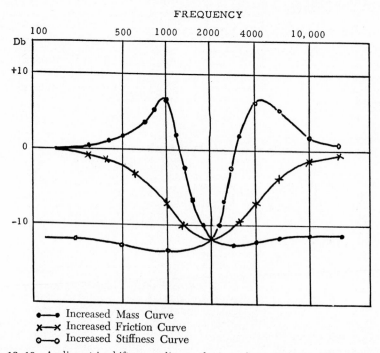

●——● Increased Mass Curve
✕——✕ Increased Friction Curve
○——○ Increased Stiffness Curve

**Figure 13–10**   Audiometric shifts according to the impedance formula. (After Johansen.[29])

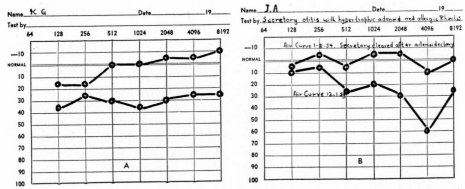

**Figure 13–11** *A*, Lower curve is loss produced by moist cotton resting on the tympanic membrane of a normal young adult. *B*, Lower curve is "mass tilt" produced by fluid in the tympanic cavity.

debris in the external auditory meatus resting upon the tympanic membrane (Fig. 13–11A) or fluid in the tympanic cavity resting upon the inner surface of the tympanic membrane (Fig. 13–11B). Examples of increase of stiffness are increased presssure in the meatus (Fig. 13–12A) or negative intratympanic pressure due to recent eustachian tube occlusion (Fig. 13–12B) or an early beginning otospongiotic

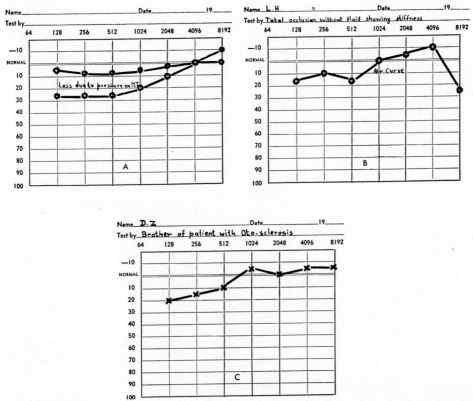

**Figure 13–12** *A*, Lower curve is loss produced by increased air pressure in the meatus. (After Dishoect and DeWit, Acta Oto-laryng., *32*:99, 1944.) *B*, Air curve produced by increased stiffness due to eustachian tube occlusion without fluid. *C*, Air curve showing stiffness tilt in a patient with suspected otosclerosis, indicating the earliest stage of stapes fixation.

stapes fixation (Fig. 13–12C). Changes in friction in the middle ear transformer are less obvious. Although the impedance formula helps to explain some of the different audiometric curves encountered by the clinician in pure conductive lesions, its strict application to the ear is probably an oversimplification.[46]

The traditional concept that the low frequencies are impaired more than the high frequencies in all lesions of the sound-conducting system, whereas the high frequencies are impaired more in lesions of the sensorineural apparatus, must be discarded, for in certain pure conductive lesions the loss is entirely or predominantly for high tones (see Fig. 13–11B), whereas in the pure inner ear lesion of endolymphatic hydrops the loss may be confined to, or be greater for, the tones of low pitch.

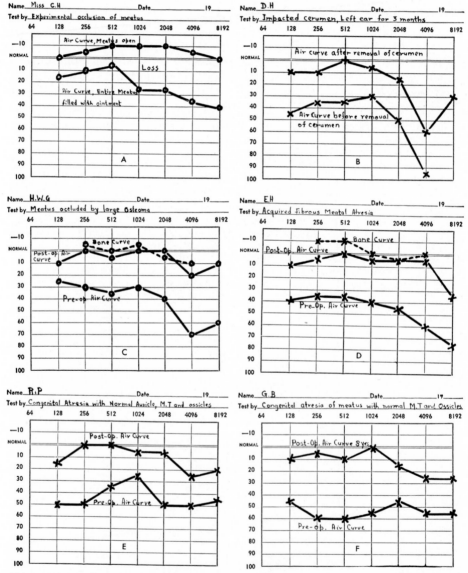

**Figure 13–13**  Clinical varieties of occlusion of the meatus. *A*, Loss due to ointment occluding the meatus. *B*, Loss due to impacted cerumen. *C*, Loss due to osteoma occluding the meatus. *D*, Loss due to acquired fibrous atresia of the meatus. *E*, Loss due to congenital meatal atresia. *F*, Loss due to congenital meatal atresia.

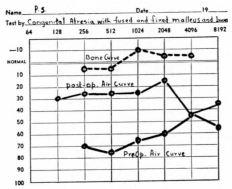

**Figure 13–14** Maximum air-bone gap due to congenital osseous meatal atresia with fused and fixed (ankylosed) malleus and incus.

In studying the hearing effects on the air-conduction audiogram of different kinds of conductive pathology it is best to consider uncomplicated isolated pathologic lesions rather than combinations of several types of lesions, and "pure" conductive lesions rather than combined conductive and sensorineural lesions. The fact that a hearing loss is eliminated by removing or correcting the lesion indicates that the loss was due to that particular isolated lesion.

## Occlusion of the Meatus

At first glance the simplest form of conductive hearing impairment appears to be that produced by putting the finger in the external meatus, yet when we examine the various audiometric curves encountered in clinical practice produced by occlusions of the meatus we find that there are several factors that contribute to the hearing results. One factor is that air-borne sound is simply excluded from the ear, from which we might expect a uniform loss for all frequencies. Even this factor will vary with the solidity and acoustic resistance of the occluding material or tissue, as is seen in the examples in Figure 13–13 of various types of clinical occlusion of the meatus. When in addition to a bony atresia the incus and malleus are fused and fixed, there is an even greater loss due to the addition of the ossicular fixation to the meatal occlusion (Fig. 13–14). When occlusion of the meatus is confined to its outer end, the trapped column of air vibrates with a somewhat different type of curve, probably owing to resonance in the region of 1000 cycles (Fig. 13–15). When

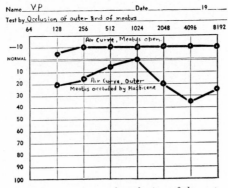

**Figure 13–15** Loss produced by experimental occlusion of the outer end of the meatus by plasticene.

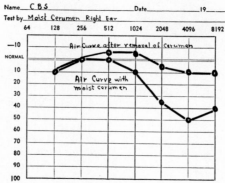

**Figure 13–16**  Loss due to moist cerumen resting against the tympanic membrane, producing "mass tilt."

occlusion is confined to the inner end of the meatus with moist debris weighting the tympanic membrane, a still different audiometric curve is seen with a loss confined to the high frequencies (Fig. 13–16).

## Perforation of the Tympanic Membrane

Another seemingly simple lesion of the conducting mechanism is a perforation of the tympanic membrane. Békésy[47] compared the movements of the ossicles in response to sound in fresh cadavers when the tympanic membrane was intact and when it had a small central perforation 1 mm. in size. He found no impairment of ossicular motion above 400 cycles, with a loss of 12 decibels for 100 and 200 cycles, of 29 decibels for 50 cycles and of 48 decibels for 10 cycles. However, a tympanic membrane perforation clinically causes a loss of hearing for all frequencies, so that obviously the impairment of ossicular motion is not the only factor. Thus Payne and Githler[48] found increasing hearing losses for all frequencies as the size of the

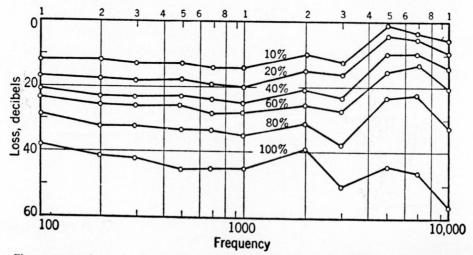

**Figure 13–17**  Increasing hearing impairment with increasing size of tympanic membrane perforation in a cat; the percentages refer to the proportion of membrane involved in the perforation. (From Payne, M. C., and Githler, F. J.: Effects of perforations of the tympanic membrane on cochlear potentials. Arch. Otol., 54:666, 1951.)

perforation in the cat's ear was increased (Fig. 13–17). In patients with tympanic membrane perforations there is in general a greater loss of hearing with larger than with smaller perforations, but this relationship is not constant, as may be seen in the examples (Fig. 13–18).

The mechanism of the hearing impairment in simple perforation of the tympanic membrane is twofold:[1] a primary effect due simply to a reduced surface on which the sound pressure is exerted, with a reduced effective hydraulic ratio; and a secondary effect due to sound reaching the round window directly, tending to cancel the movements of the stapes footplate. A larger perforation admits sound more easily with less friction from the edges of the perforation. The size of the perforation is more important in determining the hearing loss than its location.

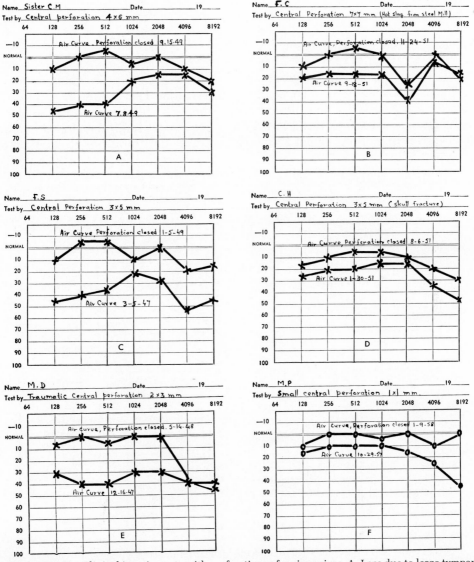

**Figure 13–18** Clinical impairments with perforations of various sizes. A, Loss due to large tympanic membrane perforation measuring 4 × 6 mm. B, Loss due to very large tympanic membrane perforation measuring 7 × 7 mm. C, Loss due to medium perforation measuring 3 × 5 mm. D, Loss due to medium perforation measuring 3 × 5 mm. E, Loss due to small perforation measuring 2 × 3 mm. F, Loss due to tiny perforation measuring 1 × 1 mm.

### Interruption of the Ossicular Chain

Experimental interruption of the incudostapedial joint in the cat produces a particularly great loss of around 60 decibels (Fig. 13–19A).[1, 49] Clinically the incus and stapes may be separated as a congenital ossicular anomaly (Fig. 13–19B), as the result of surgical or head trauma (Fig. 13–19C and D) or as the result of necrosis of the tip of the long process of the incus. As in the cat, the loss from interruption of the human ossicular chain is particularly great, for now both movable windows are shielded from sound, whereas whatever sound that does reach them does so with nearly equal force and in nearly the same phase, with a canceling effect. These observations point to the futility of mobilizing the stapes footplate without maintaining a communication between the tympanic membrane and the mobilized area of footplate (Fig. 13–20A and B).

### Occlusion of the Eustachian Tube

The first hearing change produced by eustachian tube occlusion is due to absorption of oxygen and then of nitrogen from the dead air by the middle ear mucosa, producing a negative intratympanic pressure with increased stiffness of the conducting system and a greater loss for low frequencies (Fig. 13–12B). After a time the negative pressure pulls fluid from the mucosa until fluid fills the middle ear,

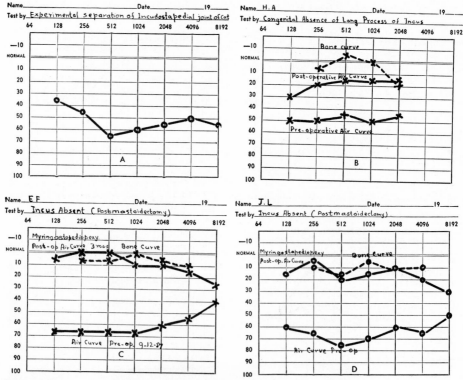

**Figure 13–19** *A,* Loss due to separation of the incus from the stapes of a cat. (From Wever, E. G., Lawrence, M., and Smith, K. R.: The middle ear in sound conduction. Arch Otol., 48:19, 1948.) *B,* Air-bone gap due to congenital interruption of the ossicular chain. *C,* Loss due to traumatic interruption of the ossicular chain. *D,* Loss due to traumatic interruption of the ossicular chain. Note gain in *C* and *D* after surgical correction, proving that the large conductive loss was due to interruption of the ossicular chain.

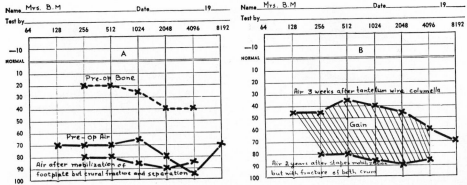

**Figure 13–20** *A*, Further loss produced by interruption of ossicular continuity during stapes mobilization. *B*, Gain produced by simple restoration of ossicular continuity.

adding mass to stiffness, with a flattened curve and a loss for all frequencies (Fig. 13–21*A* and *B*). Diminution in the negative pressure and stiffness factor leaves a greater loss for high frequencies (Fig. 13–11*B*). Thus as simple a lesion as eustachian tube obstruction can produce three variations in the audiometric curve.

### The Columella Effect

We have seen that the lever effect contributed by the incus and malleus is relatively unimportant in the middle ear transformer. We should expect that a movable stapes connected directly to a mobile tympanic membrane might function almost as well as the normal ear, and indeed this is the case, as shown in patients with a Bondy type of modified radical mastoidectomy without an incus but with a "nature's" myringostapediopexy (Fig. 13–22*B*, *C* and *D*). The same near-normal hearing may be obtained by a deliberate myringostapediopexy in patients without an incus (Fig. 13–22*A*).

### Absence of the Tympanic Membrane and Ossicles

Total loss of the tympanic membrane and ossicular chain affects the hearing in two ways: The middle ear transformer with its 22 to 1 increase of force at the oval

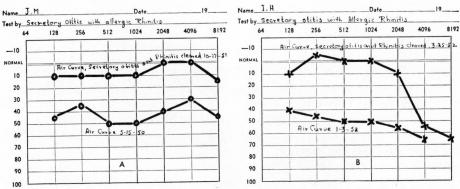

**Figure 13–21** *A* and *B*, Stiffness plus mass in secretory otitis, producing loss for all frequencies.

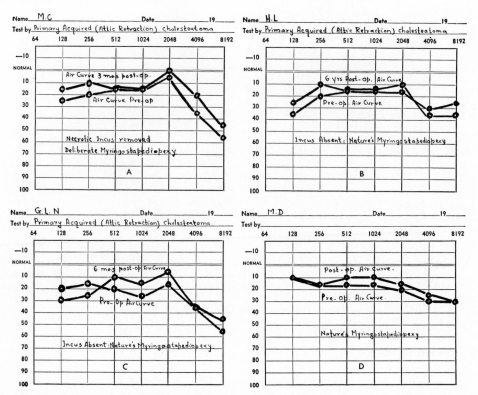

**Figure 13–22**  *A*, Bondy modified radical mastoidectomy with deliberate myringostapediopexy. *B*, *C* and *D*, Bondy operations with "nature's" myringostapediopexy.

window is gone, and sound now reaches both windows at nearly the same time and with the same force, with a marked canceling effect. If the stapes is present, sound will reach its head before it reaches the round window, providing a phase difference for certain frequencies of appropriate wavelength and a little better hearing than if the crura are absent. In such an ear the restoration of hearing must aim to shield one of the windows from direct exposure to sound by construction of an intact membrane enclosing an air bubble, and if possible the hydraulic ratio of large tympanic membrane and small oval window must be restored by construction of a large movable membrane in contact with the stapes. These two principles form the basis for the various tympanoplasty operations of Zöllner and Wullstein (see Chapter 16).

### Closure of the Round Window

The hearing effects of round window closure are similar to the effects of oval window closure, on both air and bone conduction.[50] The closure of the round window must be by bone and it must be complete, for displacement of the round window membrane by only a third of a cubic millimeter is sufficient for normal hearing.[1] Marked bony narrowing of the round window niche and scar tissue closure have had no effect on the hearing.

Simultaneous bony closure of both windows occurs rarely in advanced otospongiosis. This might be expected to cause a profound loss of hearing by bone as well as by air, with a spectacular improvement in hearing if two new windows are

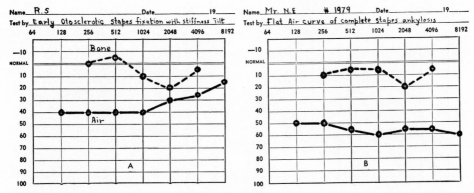

**Figure 13–23** *A*, Loss due to early otosclerotic stapes fixation, with fairly typical otosclerotic notch by bone and stiffness tilt by air. *B*, Loss due to advanced stapes ankylosis, with fairly typical otosclerotic notch by bone, equal loss for all frequencies by air.

constructed. This hope has not been realized; the addition to stapes ankylosis of round window closure appears to add only a little greater impairment of hearing by air and by bone, because the canals for the cochlear aqueduct and for the inferior cochlear vein offer auxiliary outlets for the scala tympani.[37, 51]

## Stapes Fixation

Fixation of the stapes as an isolated lesion occurs typically in otospongiosis (otosclerosis). It can also be the result of a congenital ossicular anomaly involving the stapes alone, or it may result from scar tissue adhesions or tympanosclerosis following a middle ear infection.

The earliest stage in otospongiotic stapes fixation is often (but not always) manifested by a greater loss for low frequencies, due presumably to increased stiffness of the stapediovestibular joint (Fig. 13–23*A*). Occasionally the imminent onset of hearing impairment may be predicted when a tilt develops in the air curve of a patient with normal hearing but with a family history of otospongiosis (Fig. 13–12*C*). As the fixation of the footplate increases, the mass of the labyrinthine capsule begins to be added to the stiffness factor, and the audiogram assumes a horizontal curve (Fig. 13–23*B*).

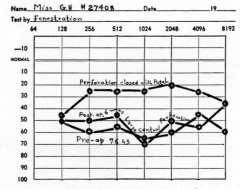

**Figure 13–24** Gain achieved by closing a large tympanic membrane perforation following fenestration.

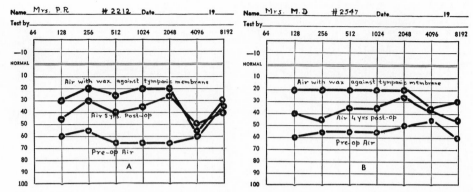

**Figure 13–25**  *A* and *B*, Improvement achieved by blocking tympanic membrane after fenestration.

## Mechanics of the Fenestrated Ear

The fenestration operation obviously does not restore a normal sound-conducting system, for such an ear lacks a middle ear transformer. The residual conductive loss after successful fenestration due to this lack was first defined by Davis and Walsh[26] as a loss of at least 20 decibels. A later study by Shambaugh[52] indicated that the average residual conductive loss after fenestration is 25 decibels for the speech frequencies.

The question of whether sound enters the fenestrated ear through the new fenestra or through the round window was studied by Nilsson[27] and Skoog[28] with the conclusion that the predominant stimulus reaches the inner ear via the new fenestra. The importance of an intact tympanic membrane to enclose an elastic bubble of air against the round window while shielding it from sound is shown by the clinical observation that a perforation markedly impairs the hearing after successful fenestration (Fig. 13–24).

In successfully fenestrated ears a significant sharpening of the hearing occurs if sound transmission to the round window is further dampened by ointment or other material placed against the tympanic membrane (Fig. 13–25*A* and *B*).[53]

## REFERENCES

1. Wever, E. G., and Lawrence, M.: Physiological Acoustics. Princeton, Princeton University Press, 1954.
2. Galen, C.: Opera omnia. Edited by D. C. G. Kuhn. Lipsiae, 1822.
3. Vesalius, A.: De humani corporis fabrica. Basileae, 1543.
4. Ingrassia. Quoted by Schelhammer, G. C.: De auditu, 1684.
5. Fallopio, G.: Observationes anatomicae ad Petrum Mannam. Venetiis, 1561.
6. Eustachius, B.: Opuscula anatomica. Venetiis, 1564.
7. Coiter, V.: De auditus instrumento. Noribergae, 1573.
8. Duverney, J. G.: Traité de l'organe de l'ouïe. Paris, 1683.
9. Cotugno, D.: De aquaeductibus auris humanae internae. Vienna, 1760.
10. Meckel, P. F.: De labyrinthi auris contentis. Argentorati, 1777.
11. Corti, A.: Recherches sur l'organe de l'omie des mammifères. Ztschr. wiss. Zool., 3:109, 1851.
12. Retzius, G.: Die Endigungsweise des Gehörnerven. Biol. Untersuch., 3:29, 1892.
13. Müller, J.: Handbuch der Physiologie des Menschen. 1837.
14. Helmholtz, H. L. F.: Die Mechanik der Gehörknöchelchen und des Trommelfells. Pflügers Arch. ges. Physiol., 1:1, 1868.
15. Pohlman, A. C.: The problem of middle ear mechanics. Ann. Otol. Rhin. & Laryng., 31:1, 430, 1922.

16. Frank, O.: Die Leitung des Schalles im Ohr. Sitzungs. Akad. Wiss., München. Vol. 11. 1923.
17. Herzog, H.: Das Knochenleitungsproblem. Theoretische Erwägungen. Ztschr. Hals-,Nasen- u. Ohrenh., 15:300, 1926.
18. Dahmann, H.: Zur Physiologie des Hörens. Ztschr. Hals-, Nasen- u. Ohrenh., 24:462, 1929.
19. Davis, H., et al.: Electrical response of cochlea. Am. J. Physiol., 107:311, 1934.
20. Lüscher, E.: Die Funktion des Musculus stapedius beim Menschen. Ztschr. Hals-, Nasen- u. Ohrenh., 23:105, 1929.
21. Kobrak, H.: Zur Physiologie der Binnenmuskeln des Ohres. Beitr. Anat., Physiol., Path. u. Therap. Ohres, 28:138, 1930.
22. Békésy, G. von, and Rosenblith, W. A.: The mechanical properties of the ear. In Stevens, S. S. (Ed.): Handbook of Experimental Psychology. New York, J. Wiley and Sons, 1951.
23. Bezold, F.: Textbook of Otology. Translated by J. Holinger. Chicago, E. H. Colgrove Co., 1908, p. 102.
24. Békésy, G. von: The sound pressure difference between the round and oval window and the artificial window of the labyrinth fenestration. Acta oto-laryng., 35:301, 1947.
25. Juers, A. L.: Observations on bone conduction in fenestrated cases. Ann. Otol. Rhin. & Laryng., 57:28, 1948.
26. Davis, H., and Walsh, T. E.: The limits of improvement of hearing following the fenestration operation. Laryngoscope, 60:273, 1950.
27. Nilsson, G.: The immediate improvement of hearing following the fenestration operation. Acta oto-laryng., Suppl. 98, 1952.
28. Skoog, T.: On the transmission of air borne sounds in the fenestrated ear in clinical otosclerosis. Acta oto-laryng., Suppl. 100, 1952.
29. Johansen, H.: Relation of audiograms to the impedance formula. Acta oto-laryng., Suppl. 74, 1948.
30. Campbell, P. A.: The importance of the impedance formula in the interpretation of audiograms. Tr. Am. Acad. Ophth., 54:245, 1950.
31. Zöllner, F.: Die Radikal-Operation mit besonderem Bezug auf die Hörfunktion. Ztschr. Laryng. Rhin. Otol., 30:104, 1951.
32. Wullstein, H.: Die Eingriffe zur Gehörverbesserung. In Uffenorde, W.: Anzeige und Ausführung der Eingriffe an Ohr. Nase und Hals. 2nd Ed. Revised by H. Uffenorde. Stuttgart, Georg Thieme, 1952.
33. Békésy, G. von: Über die Messung der Schwingungsamplitude der Gehörknöchelchen mittels einer kapazitiven Sonde. Akust. Ztschr., 6:1, 1941.
34. Békésy, G. von: The ear. Scient. Am., 197:66, 1957.
35. Békésy, G. von: Zur Physik des Mittelohres und über das Hören bei fehlerhaftem Trommelfell. Akust. Ztschr., 1:13, 1936.
36. Kobrak, H. G.: Physiology of the ear. In Coates, G. M., et al. (Eds.): Otolaryngology. Vol. 1. Hagerstown, Md., W. F. Prior Co., 1955.
37. Tonndorf, J.: Animal experiments in bone conduction: clinical conclusions. Ann. Otol. Rhin. & Laryng., 73:659, 1964.
38. Kobrak, H.: The physiology of sound conduction. Ann. Otol. Rhin. & Laryng., 47:166, 1938.
39. Wever, E. G., and Vernon, J. A.: The control of sound transmission by the middle ear muscles. Ann. Otol. Rhin. & Laryng., 65:5, 1956.
40. Schwabach, D.: Über den Wert des Rinnéschen Versuches für die Diagnostik der Gehörkrankheiten. Ztsch. Ohrenh., 14:61, 1885.
41. Weber, E. H.: De pulsu, resorptione, auditu et tactu. Lipsiae, 1834.
42. Pohlman, A. G., and Kranz, F. W.: Quantitative tests on bone and air acuity in paracusis Willisi. Arch. Otol., 3:136, 1926.
43. Knudsen, V., and Jones, I. H.: Bone conduction. Arch. Otol., 13:489, 1931.
44. Carhart, R.: The clinical application of bone conduction audiometry. Arch. Otol., 51:798, 1950.
45. Huizing, E. H.: Bone conduction: the influence of the middle ear. Acta oto-laryng., Suppl. 155, 1960.
46. Reger, S.: Discussion of paper by P. A. Campbell. Tr. Am. Acad. Ophth. and Otolary., 54:245, 1950.
47. Békésy, G. von: Über die mechanisch-akustischen Vorgänge beim Hören. Acta otolaryng., 27:281, 388, 1939.
48. Payne, M. C., and Githler, F. J.: Effects of perforations of the tympanic membrane on cochlear potentials. Arch. Otol., 54:666, 1951.
49. Wever, E. G., Lawrence, M., and Smith, K. R.: The middle ear in sound conduction. Arch. Otolaryng., 48:19, 1948.
50. Harrison, W. H., et al.: Congenital absence of the round window. Laryngoscope, 74:967, 1964.
51. Groen, J. J., and Hoogland, G. A.: Bone conduction and otosclerosis of the round window. Acta oto-laryng., 49:206, 1958.
52. Shambaugh, G. E., Jr.: Correlation of the predicted with the actual result of fenestration in 164 consecutive cases. Laryngoscope, 62:461, 1952.
53. Shambaugh, G. E., Jr.: Technic for increasing sound pressure differential between fenestra and round window to enhance hearing improvement following successful fenestration. Tr. Am. Acad. Ophth. and Otolary., 58:454, 1954.

# Chapter 14

# Surgical Correction of Congenital Malformations of the Sound-Conducting System

HISTORICAL ASPECTS
EMBRYOLOGIC CONSIDERATIONS
DIAGNOSIS
INDICATIONS FOR SURGICAL CORRECTION
AGE OF PATIENT AT OPERATION
SURGICAL TECHNIQUE
    RECONSTRUCTION OF A MICROTIC OR ABSENT
      AURICLE
    CONSTRUCTION OF AN OSSEOUS MEATUS
    THE MANAGEMENT OF OSSICULAR
      MALFORMATIONS
    CONSTRUCTION OF A SUBSTITUTE TYMPANIC
      MEMBRANE AND SKIN GRAFTING THE MEATUS
    THE PROBLEM OF POSTOPERATIVE OSSICULAR
      FIXATION BY FIBROSIS
POSTOPERATIVE CARE
HEARING RESULTS OF SURGICAL CORRECTION OF
  MEATAL ATRESIA
HEARING RESULTS IN ISOLATED OSSICULAR
  MALFORMATIONS

## HISTORICAL ASPECTS

The first reported operation for congenital meatal atresia was by Kiesselbach[1] in 1883; it resulted in facial paralysis. Perhaps influenced by this, operations to improve hearing in patients with congenital atresia were opposed for many years as being useless, irrational and dangerous, by most of the leaders in otology, including Schwartze,[2] Trautmann[3] and Politzer.[4] Although sporadic reports of improved hearing following construction of a substitute meatus did appear from time to time, including those of Scheibe,[5] Alexander,[6] Page[7] and Dean,[8] the prevailing attitude continued to be pessimistic. This was clearly expressed in Kopetsky's text, *Otologic Surgery*, in 1929:[9] "Operative procedures in congenital atresia of osseous character, whereby the auditory apparatus is involved, give poor results at best."

It was not until the climate of otologic opinion had begun to change, as the result of the proved success and increasing use of fenestration surgery for otosclerosis, that operations to correct congenital malformations of the sound-conducting apparatus began to be looked upon more favorably. The change in attitude may be dated from 1947 when Ombrédanne[10] in Paris and Pattee[11] in America each reported a series of cases of atresia successfully treated by surgery to improve the hearing. In the next few years a succession of reports appeared of increasing numbers of cases successfully operated on. The reports of Siirala,[12] Shambaugh,[13] House,[14] Rüedi[15] and Meurman[16] have helped to establish surgical correction of congenital malformations of the sound-conducting mechanism as desirable and useful.

## EMBRYOLOGIC CONSIDERATIONS

The embryologic development of the hearing mechanism was described in detail in Chapter 1, and need not be repeated except to emphasize certain facts that apply to the surgical correction of malformations.

Particularly important is the observation, first made many years ago by Alexander,[6] that in the majority of cases of hearing impairment due to congenital malformations only the sound-conducting system, or only the sensorineural apparatus is involved, with simultaneous involvement of both parts of the hearing mechanism being the exception rather than the rule. This is accounted for by the entirely different embryonic origin of the two parts of the hearing organ; the sensory labyrinth is derived from the ectodermal **otocyst** whereas the sound-conducting system comes from the **branchial or gill apparatus.**

The particular malformation present in each case depends upon the age in embryonic life at which normal development was arrested, as well as upon the portion of the branchial apparatus affected (Table 14–1).[13]

The first evidence of the outer ear is seen in the 4 week old human embryo as a funnel-shaped cleft on either side of the head, the first branchial groove (Figs. 14–1 and 14–2). This is the "primitive meatus" destined to become the outer part of the external auditory meatus; the inner portion is not formed until much later, in the seventh fetal month.

The auricle begins to form in the sixth week of embryonic life (Figs. 14–3 and 14–4) as knob-like hillocks from the first and second branchial arches, on either side of the primitive meatus. By the third month the hillocks have fused to form the auricle, the tragus coming from the first branchial arch and the remainder of the auricle from the second arch. Where the hillocks from these two arches join, just

*Text continued on page 385.*

**TABLE 14–1   TIMETABLE OF EMBRYOLOGIC DEVELOPMENT OF THE EAR\***

| *Time* | *Branchial Apparatus—Outer and Middle Ear* | *Membranous Labyrinth Otocyst* |
|---|---|---|
| 3 weeks | First pharyngeal pouch appears. | Otic placode appears. |
| 4 weeks | Primitive funnel-shaped meatus from first branchial groove. | Otocyst formed. |
| 6 weeks | Knoblike hillocks from first and second branchial arches appear. | Endolymphatic sac and duct, semicircular canals and cochlea begin to form in that order from otocyst. |
| 8 weeks | Solid epithelial cord grows from primitive meatus toward tympanum. Ossicles begin to form from cartilages of first and second branchial arches. | Cartilaginous otic capsule appears. |
| 12 weeks | Hillocks fuse to form auricle. Ossicles differentiating. Tympanic ring begins to ossify. | Endolymphatic labyrinth fully differentiated except for part of the organ of Corti in apical turn. Fissula ante fenestram appears. |
| 16 weeks | Ossicles fully formed in cartilage. They begin to ossify. | Ossification of labyrinthine capsule begins as endolymphatic labyrinth reaches adult form. |
| 23 weeks | Pneumatization of upper half of tympanum and epitympanum. Antrum appears. | Ossification of labyrinthine capsule nearly complete. |
| 28 weeks | Solid epithelial cord canalizes and fuses with primitive meatus to form tympanic membrane and external auditory meatus. | Periosteal layer of capsule continues to thicken, but endochondral layer of capsule and labyrinth remain unchanged for remainder of life except for possible occurrence of new bone or cartilage in the fissula ante fenestram, and cochlear degeneration of senescence. Endolymphatic sac continues to grow in size until puberty. |
| 35 weeks | Pneumatic cells begin around antrum. Ossicles reach adult form. | |
| Birth | Resorption of embryonic subepithelial connective tissue in tympanum, antrum and pneumatic cells. Pneumatization accelerates. | |
| Age 1 | Osseous meatus deepens. Mastoid process appears. | |
| Puberty | Osseous meatus complete. Pneumatization complete except in petrous pyramid. | |

\*From Bast, T. H., and Anson, B. *In* Coates, G. M., et al. (Eds.): Otolaryngology. Vol. 1. Hagerstown, Md., W. F. Prior Co., 1955.

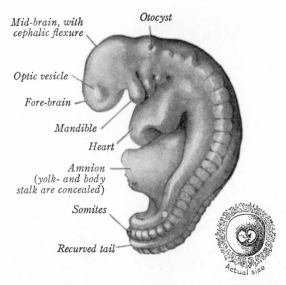

*Mid-brain, with*
*cephalic flexure*

*Otocyst*

*Optic vesicle*

*Fore-brain*

*Mandible*

*Heart*

*Amnion*
*(yolk- and body*
*stalk are concealed)*

*Somites*

*Recurved tail*

*Actual size*

**Figure 14–1**   Human embryo of 26 days, showing first and second branchial grooves and the otic pit preliminary to formation of otocyst. (From Arey, L. B.: Developmental Anatomy, 7th ed. Philadelphia, W. B. Saunders Co., 1965.)

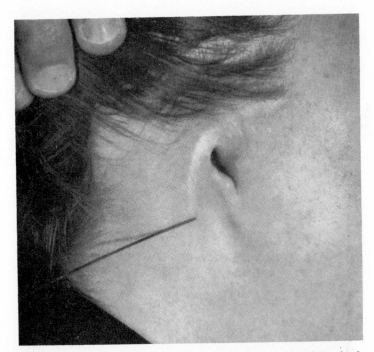

**Figure 14–2**   Malformation due to arrested development about the fourth week of embryonic life. Compare with Figure 14–1. Cleftlike opening of the first branchial groove led to a cholesteatoma sac, exteriorized at surgery. Note the curved scar of incision. Tiny fistula of the second branchial groove at the tip of the pointer.

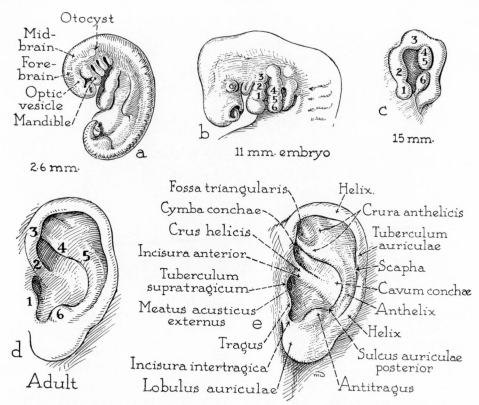

**Figure 14–3**   Developmental and adult anatomy of the auricle. *a*, The primordial elevations on the first (mandibular) and second (hyoid) arches *(b)* which fuse *(c)* to form the adult auricle *(d)*, marked with numerals to indicate the derived parts. *e*, Adult form of the auricle with the parts identified. (From Anson, B. J.: Morris' Human Anatomy, 12th ed. New York, McGraw-Hill Book Co., 1966.)

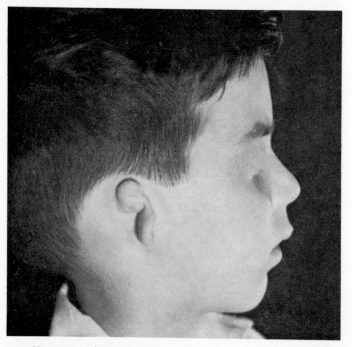

**Figure 14–4**   Malformation of auricle with atresia due to arrested development at 6 weeks of embryonic life.

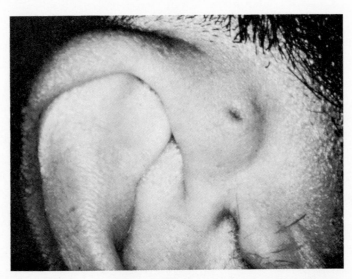

**Figure 14–5**    Preauricular cyst due to defective fusion of auricular knobs from the first and second branchial arches.

above and in front of the meatus, an epithelial-lined pit (Fig. 14–5) may persist into adult life (see Chapter 8, Congenital Preauricular Cyst and Fistula).

Toward the close of the second fetal month a solid cord of epithelial cells grows inward from the primitive funnel-shaped meatus, ending in a disc-like expansion that lies close to the epithelium of the tympanic cavity, separated from it only by a thin seam of connective tissue destined to become the circular and radial fibers of the tympanic membrane. This epithelial cord remains solid until it begins to canalize in the seventh fetal month, first at its inner end, forming the outer surface of the tympanic membrane, and then proceeding outward to fuse with the primitive meatus. It is thus possible, though not common, for arrest of development late in fetal life to result in an atresia near the isthmus but with a well formed tympanic membrane and ossicles, and a pouch-like meatus adjacent to the tympanic membrane filled with cerumen or cholesteatomatous epidermal debris.

Meanwhile, as the outer ear is formed from the first branchial groove and first and second arches, the middle ear and eustachian tube have been developing from the first pharyngeal pouch, which appears in the 3 week old embryo. At 2 months the tympanic cavity occupies only the lower half of the future middle ear cavity; the upper half is filled with connective tissue containing the early cartilaginous stapes, incus and malleus. Extension of the tympanic cavity into the attic to surround the ossicles and to enwrap them and their ligaments with epithelium is completed relatively late, in the seventh and eighth fetal months.

The malleus and incus are derived from Meckel's cartilage of the first branchial arch, which also forms the mandible. Malformation of the auricle, bony meatal atresia and malformation of the incus and malleus occur very often in the same person together with a poorly developed mandible, owing to arrest of development of the first branchial groove and first branchial arch in the second month of fetal life. If the maxilla is also malformed, the patient then presents the Franceschetti-Zwahlen[17] or Treacher-Collins syndrome of mandibular-facial dysostosis, marked by outward-downward slanted eyes termed anti-Mongoloid, notched lower lid, short mandible, bony meatal atresia and malformed incus and malleus (Fig. 14–6).

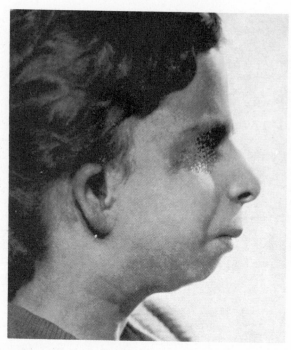

**Figure 14–6**   Mandibular-facial dysostosis with meatal atresia; Treacher-Collins syndrome.

The facial nerve not infrequently has an abnormal course through the temporal bone in severe malformations of the outer and middle ear.[18] It may lie free in the tympanic cavity; it may emerge onto the lateral surface of the skull, as in the infant; and it may be small and poorly developed, with a facial paresis. These abnormal relationships render surgical intervention for congenital atresia difficult and hazardous.

Malformations of the stapes, derived from Reichert's cartilage of the second branchial arch and cleft, may accompany malformations of the incus and malleus with meatal atresia from involvement of the first branchial arch, but more often they occur independently. Thus cases of **isolated congenital stapes ankylosis** are not uncommon, and may be erroneously diagnosed as otosclerosis.[13] In the majority of patients with meatal atresia with deformed and fused incus and malleus, the stapes is well developed and mobile. Therefore fenestration of the labyrinth or oval window surgery is not required for the surgical reconstruction of an effective sound-conducting system in the majority of patients with meatal atresia.[16]

The surgeon should remember that the ossicles reach full adult size by the end of the fourth fetal month, when ossification occurs. The incus and malleus thereafter remain constant in form and size, whereas after ossification the stapes undergoes a process of variable emaciation resulting in a loss of bulk with marked variations in the eventual size, shape and strength of its crura, head and neck.[19] These very great differences in the adult stapes should be regarded as normal variants rather than true anomalies, as long as there are two crura, a stapedius tendon, a head and neck attached to the lenticular process of the incus and a movable footplate.

As we saw in Chapter 1, pneumatization of the temporal bone begins to extend out from the antrum toward the end of fetal life. The entrance of air into the tympanic cavity at birth permits the resorption of the embryonic subepithelial connective tissue, whereupon pneumatization proceeds rapidly into the mastoid process, into the hypotympanum and peritubal area, and lastly into the petrous pyramid. Although there is a slight tendency toward poor pneumatization in patients with marked malformation and aplasia of the outer and middle ear, this is not at all constant. Thus, in a series of 74 cases of congenital meatal atresia Meurman[16] observed absent or scant pneumatization in 38 per cent as compared to 25 per cent for normal ears. On the whole the ears with the greater deformity had a somewhat higher incidence of scant or absent pneumatization. In the senior author's series of 25 cases of congenital meatal atresia in which the degree of pneumatization was recorded, this was fairly good or normal in 20 (80 per cent) and poor or absent in 5 (20 per cent).

The **mechanism** of congenital malformations of the branchial apparatus is not known in most cases.[20] Only rarely does the family history in such malformations indicate an hereditary tendency. Rubella[21, 22] toward the end of the first trimester of pregnancy has been implicated. A sharp increase in multiple congenital malformations in Germany during 1959 to 1962 was traced to the administration of thalidomide, a tranquilizer, to pregnant women. Between 6500 and 7000 babies were born with defective limbs during the thalidomide era; another 3000 had minor defects of the fingers and hand. About 10 per cent of the affected babies, or close to 1000, were born with malformations of the ear (Fig. 14–7).

Thalidomide-induced defects of the ear are of all degrees, but they tend to be severe, with simultaneous involvement of the inner ear and microtia and atresia, and often with facial paresis on the side with the greater involvement.[23] Of particular interest is the correlation of the embryologic development as shown in Table 14–1 with the time of administration. Thalidomide taken between the 35th and 38th day of pregnancy caused absence of the auricle with facial paresis and damage to the eye

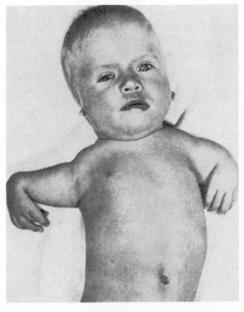
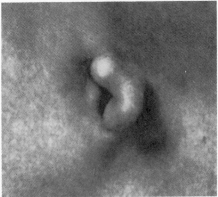

**Figure 14–7**  *A*, Typical malformations following thalidomide administration during pregnancy. Marked aplasia of outer, middle and inner ears, bilateral abducens paralysis, right-sided facial paralysis and defective arms. *B*, Left side of same infant showing microtia with meatal atresia and retroauricular fistula. (From Mündnich, K.: Hearing improvement and plastic operations for malformations of the ear. Hals- Nasen- Ohrenh., *3*:668, 1965.)

muscle nuclei; between the 38th and 46th day of pregnancy, less severe microtia; between the 39th and 44th day, absence or near absence of the arms; between the 41st and 44th day, absence of legs; and around the 50th day, stenosis of the rectum or anal atresia.[24]

Unilateral atresia is somewhat more common than bilateral, but in a unilateral case it is not uncommon to observe a less marked malformation on the opposite side with a small meatus and tympanic membrane or an anomaly of one or more of the ossicles. Many authors have commented upon the greater frequency of congenital atresia in males than in females, in the proportion of 2 to 1, and the more frequent involvement of the right ear than the left, in the proportion of 3 to 2.[16] The reasons for these differences are not known.

## DIAGNOSIS

The diagnosis of congenital malformation of the auricle and meatus is self-evident and offers no difficulty, but the presence or absence of a tympanic membrane beyond a meatal atresia and the condition of the ossicles cannot be determined preoperatively and can only be surmised. Tomographic and conventional x-ray examination may demonstrate the presence of a malleus and incus but does not prove that they are functionally mobile, nor does their absence from the usual mastoid film always mean that they are not present.[16] As noted before, the degree of pneumatization by radiologic examination does not show any constant relationship to malformations of the auricle, meatus, tympanic membrane or ossicles.

The best indication of the probable degree of middle ear malformation in cases of congenital atresia is the condition of the auricle. Remembering that the auricle is well formed by the third month of fetal life, a microtic or absent auricle indicates arrest of development of the branchial apparatus earlier in embryonic life with the probability of absence of the tympanic membrane and malformation of the malleus and incus. Thus in the senior author's series of 18 cases of congenital meatal atresia with an absent or microtic auricle there was a rudimentary tympanic membrane only twice (11 per cent), with normal incus and malleus in only one patient (5.5 per cent). By contrast, in 9 cases of meatal atresia with a well formed auricle, a mobile tympanic membrane was found in 4 (44 per cent) and a fairly well formed mobile incus and malleus in every case.

**Ossicular malformations without atresia** are more common than they were once thought to be. These patients resemble those with otosclerotic stapes fixation in having a severe conductive hearing loss without a history of preceding otitis media and with an essentially normal meatus, tympanic membrane and eustachian tube. They may be distinguished from those with otosclerosis by these differences:[13]

1. Otosclerosis rarely causes a hearing loss before the age of 12, whereas congenital ossicular malformation produces a hearing impairment from birth, although it is rarely detected by the parents before the child is 4 or 5.

2. The hearing impairment of otosclerosis comes on insidiously and progresses gradually, whereas the loss due to congenital malformation remains constant. As the demands on the child's hearing increase with age there may **seem** to be an increase in the impairment in patients with congenital ossicular malformation, but repeat hearing tests will show that the loss is a stable one.

3. A family history of progressive hearing impairment is found in half of cases of otosclerosis. Rarely is there a positive family history in congenital malformations of the outer and middle ear.

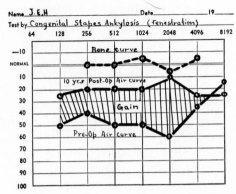

**Figure 14-8**   Audiogram in a patient with congenital stapes fixation without atresia.

4. Ossicular malformation with a conductive hearing loss and a patent meatus is rather frequently found in one ear when there is congenital meatal atresia of the opposite ear. Minor abnormalities of the derivatives of the branchial apparatus, such as a very narrow, though patent, meatus, a small tympanic membrane or a small mandible, in the presence of a conductive loss dating from early childhood, suggest an ossicular anomaly rather than otosclerosis (Fig. 14-8).

The final diagnosis of congenital ossicular malformation without atresia can be made only by surgical exploration. A number of these cases have been encountered during fenestration or stapes mobilization operations for supposed clinical otosclerosis.[26] Fixation of the stapes, absence of the long process of the incus and ankylosis of the malleus head to the attic wall are among the congenital malformations encountered. A careful review of the history in these patients will usually indicate that a hearing loss was probably present in early childhood.

## INDICATIONS FOR SURGICAL CORRECTION

Operation to improve the hearing in cases of congenital meatal atresia or some other malformation of the sound-conducting apparatus was formerly advised only in bilateral cases with good cochlear function. With improved understanding of the mechanics of sound conduction and with the improved results achieved by modern technique, patients with unilateral malformation with hearing loss may be operated on provided the cochlear function is sufficient to anticipate a hearing level within 20 or 25 decibels of the normal ear. With this improvement in hearing the patient will begin to benefit from binaural hearing, with improved ability to localize sound, to understand speech in the presence of noise and to understand speech from the affected side. Moreover, the improved cosmetic appearance of a patent meatus is of some value to the patient.

The hearing result from surgery will depend upon the particular malformation found at operation as well as upon the surgical technique employed. In patients with a functioning tympanic membrane and ossicular chain the construction of a patent meatus should eliminate the air–bone gap. The same result can be achieved with a substitute tympanic membrane against a mobile incus and malleus. In patients with a mobile stapes the construction of a substitute meatus and tympanic membrane in contact with the stapes should produce a hearing level only slightly poorer than the cochlear reserve, provided secondary fibrotic ossicular fixation does not occur. In patients with a fixed stapes a stapedectomy by the usual technique (see Chapter 18) should eliminate the air–bone gap.[27]

## AGE OF PATIENT AT OPERATION

As soon as the diagnosis of bilateral atresia has been made, it is extremely important to place a bone conduction hearing aid on the infant. This can be done between the ages of six weeks to six months. Only if the hearing aid is instituted before two years of age will the youngster develop normal speech. Failure to institute amplification prior to the two-year age limit most often results in poor, if any, speech development.

Surgical correction of a unilateral malformation of the sound-conducting apparatus may well be deferred until the patient is 15 to 17 years old, at which time the operation can be done under local anesthesia with adequate sedation and by which time the growth of the temporal bone will have provided easier access to the structures.

Operation on at least one ear between the ages of 5 and 7 is advisable in cases of bilateral malformation of the outer and middle ear. This will allow the child to start school without the stigma of a hearing aid.

In rare cases of congenital atresia combined with a moderate cochlear involvement, operation on one ear may be contemplated as early as age 4. Two such patients with bilateral meatal atresia seen by the senior author had not acquired speech by the age of 4, and would not tolerate a hearing aid. By means of noise makers and tuning forks it was possible to demonstrate fairly good, though not normal, cochlear function. Within 2 weeks of the construction of a substitute meatus and tympanic membrane in contact with the stapes both of these children began to talk, rapidly acquiring normal speech for their age. While these two cases were dramatic, they must be considered unusual. Therefore, the authors would like to re-emphasize the need for early amplification.

## SURGICAL TECHNIQUE

The earliest operations for congenital meatal atresia sought to construct a skin-lined opening to the antrum (Fig. 14–9), without particular attention to the reconstruction of an effective impedance-matching mechanism to overcome the air-water sound barrier. Recent authors[13, 16] recognize that for the best hearing results the operation must be designed to reconstruct a middle ear air cavity closed by a movable membrane in contact with a mobile ossicular chain or stapes. **No single technique is appropriate for all cases;** rather the technique in each operation must be modified to fit the particular lesion that is found so as to construct the most effective impedance-matching mechanism. The surgeon must be prepared to modify his plan of attack as he proceeds; he must have a clear comprehension of the mechanics of sound conduction; and he must have familiarity and experience with tympanoplasty and fenestration operations. Because the distortions of anatomy and possible misplacements of the facial nerve make these operations particularly difficult and hazardous, they should not be attempted by the novice.

The surgical correction of congenital malformations of the outer and middle ear comprises four types of problem: the reconstruction of an absent or microtic auricle, the construction of a new osseous skin-lined meatus, the management of ossicular

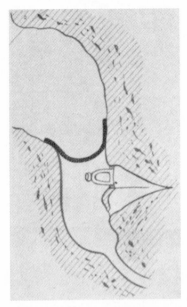

**Figure 14–9**  Skin-lined opening to the antrum with the poor hearing result of an ossicular interruption. (From Mündnich, K.: Hearing improvement and plastic operations for malformations of the ear. Hals-Nasen-Ohrenh., 3:668, 1965.)

malformations and the construction of a substitute tympanic membrane. The first problem, that of reconstructing the auricle, is primarily cosmetic and belongs more to the plastic surgeon. The last three problems are auditory and should be attacked only by the otologic surgeon who is thoroughly familiar with the mechanics of hearing and the complicated surgical anatomy of the temporal bone.

## Reconstruction of a Microtic or Absent Auricle

The auricle is without doubt the most difficult feature to restore, partly because of its intricately shaped cartilage and partly because of its thin delicate skin, which cannot be duplicated in a skin graft.[27] The construction of an entirely new auricle by means of tube grafts, scalp flaps and bone or cartilage implants is often disappointing, and the result is less acceptable than a well made prosthesis. Technical advances in plastics and the increased use of prostheses in head and neck surgery have greatly improved the quality of these devices. The longer hair styles tend to camoflauge the area more readily for men and women alike, thus making the artificial prosthesis more acceptable.

Until a satisfactory and dependable surgical technique is evolved, construction of a new auricle should be regarded as an experimental procedure for those with considerable familiarity and experience with this unique problem. Among the techniques that have been experimented with are the implantation of an homologous cartilage graft from the auricle of the mother[28] and the construction of an auricular cartilage by means of diced autogenous rib cartilage placed in a Vitallium ear mold that is buried beneath abdominal skin for 5 or 6 months.[29]

Auricular rudiments can be utilized and appreciably improved in their cosmetic appearance by relatively simple operations to unroll a curled-up auricular cartilage and to transplant a misplaced rudiment to a more normal position.[16, 27] The microtic

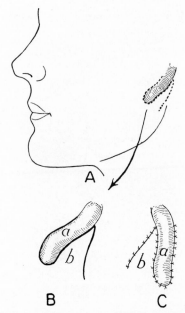

**Figure 14–10**   Z-plasty to move auricular remnant. *A*, Abnormally placed auricular rudiment with line of incision dotted. *B*, Auricular rudiment *a* and flap *b* mobilized by incisions. *C*, Auricular rudiment moved posteriorly to more normal position, with incisions sutured. (From Barsky, A. J.: Principles and Practice of Plastic Surgery. Baltimore, Williams and Wilkins Co., 1950.)

auricle is sometimes found abnormally far forward and inferiorly. It may be transplanted by means of a Z-plasty as shown in Figure 14–10. An elongated rudiment may be given a curve suggesting the helix of the normal auricle by transplanting its middle portion posteriorly, as shown in Figure 14–11. Further operations may be contemplated at a future date to improve the appearance of the rudiment by elevating the tissue and skin-grafting its posterior aspect, or by placing a curved tube graft around its upper and posterior border to simulate the

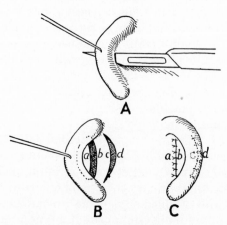

**Figure 14–11**   Creating a curve in an auricular remnant. *A*, Incision to free the midportion of the auricular remnant. *B*, Remnant retracted from its bed *ab*, with incisions *cd* for the new bed. *C*, Remnant sutured to the new bed, with the old bed sutured after flap *bc* has been mobilized. (From Barsky, M. J.: Principles and Practice of Plastic Surgery. Baltimore, Williams and Wilkins Co., 1950.)

normal helix. Extensive reconstruction of a microtic auricle, like the construction of an entirely new auricle, is better left to the plastic surgeon who has had previous experience with this particular problem.

## Construction of an Osseous Meatus

Although reconstruction of a deformed or absent auricle may be left to the plastic surgeon who has had previous experience with this difficult problem, the construction of a patent meatus should be undertaken only by an otologic surgeon who has had previous experience with tympanoplasty operations and clearly comprehends the mechanics of the normal sound-conducting system.

### Incision

When there is a primitive funnel-shaped meatus at the normal site, the usual endaural type of incision extending upward from the meatus is employed. If there is absence of a meatus, a 3 cm. vertical incision with a 1 cm. cross incision is used; the four corners of these incisions will be undermined to produce a rounded meatus (Fig. 14–12A). The correct position of these incisions is determined by palpation of the root of the zygoma, the anterior wall of the mastoid process and the head of the mandible.

### Periosteal Retraction and Exposure

The incisions are deepened to the bone of the zygomatic root and mastoid process. Retraction of periosteum exposes these structures and allows inspection of the usual site of the osseous meatus (Fig. 14–12B). As a rule the normal landmarks, including the suprameatal spine of Henle, are absent or obscured by an irregular mass of bone and fibrous tissue. When the auricle is well formed there is a possibility that a tympanic membrane may be present beyond the atresia. In such cases, if the head of the mandible is seen to occupy its normal position, with an irregular mass of fibrous tissue, cartilage and bone filling the space normally occupied by the osseous meatus, an attempt should be made to explore the meatus without doing a preliminary attico-antrotomy. On the other hand, when the auricle is microtic, the chance of finding a functionally mobile tympanic membrane is remote; and also when the head of the mandible is found to lie against the anterior wall of the mastoid process, an attico-antrotomy must be used.

### Exploration of the Osseous Meatus

The problem is to discover and expose a tympanic membrane without destroying it and without opening the attic or antrum. This may be accomplished in some cases by cautiously removing the atretic mass of irregular bone, cartilage and fibrous tissue between the root of the zygoma above, the head of the mandible in front and the anterior wall of the mastoid process behind. It may thus be possible to reach the notch of Rivinus where the posterior-superior edge of the tympanic membrane, if present, can be elevated, permitting inspection and palpation for mobility of the

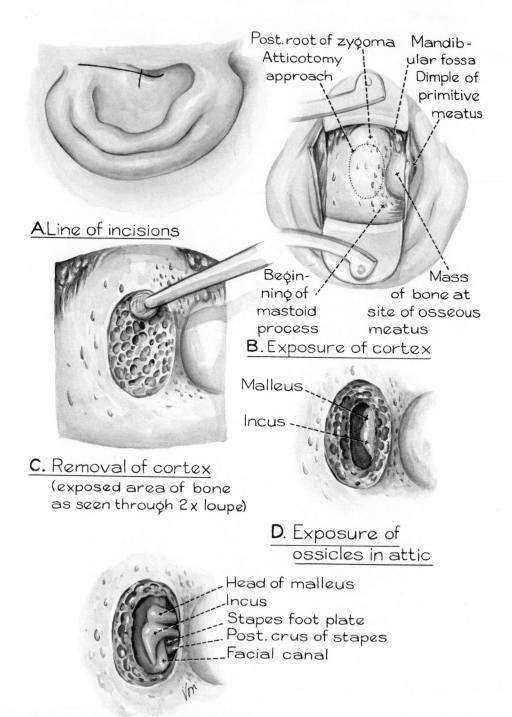

A. Line of incisions

Post. root of zygoma    Mandib-
Atticotomy               ular fossa
   approach              Dimple of
                         primitive
                         meatus

Begin-                                  Mass
ning of                              of bone at
mastoid                             site of osseous
process                                meatus

B. Exposure of cortex

C. Removal of cortex
(exposed area of bone
as seen through 2 x loupe)

Malleus
Incus

D. Exposure of
   ossicles in attic

Head of malleus
Incus
Stapes foot plate
Post. crus of stapes
Facial canal

E. Completion of cavity,
   tympanum exposed from above

**Figure 14–12**   Surgical correction of congenital meatal atresia. *A,* Crucial incisions. *B,* Exposure of cortex. *C,* Atticotomy approach. *D,* Atticotomy. *E,* Bone removal completed. (Continued in Figures 14–13 and 14–17.)

ossicular chain, as in a stapes operation. The outer surface of the tympanic membrane (if one is found) is cleared of any fibrous tissue, and the osseous meatus is enlarged to the adult size and then lined by split thickness skin grafts.

## Attico-antrotomy

The easiest and safest approach to the tympanum, and the one used by the senior author for the majority of cases of congenital meatal atresia, is by endaural attico-antrotomy. This method should be employed when the head of the mandible lies against the mastoid process and when preliminary exploration of the osseous meatus fails to disclose a tympanic membrane.

An oval-shaped area of cortex is removed with the dental-type cutting burr, just above and behind the site of atresia (Fig. 14–12C). The tegmen plate is defined and followed inward to the attic and antrum; sufficient cellular, diploic or solid bone is removed to create a bony meatus about twice the size of the adult meatus. This part of the operation is the most difficult and the most dangerous to the facial nerve, and it must be accomplished slowly and carefully; avoid working in a narrow hole and watch at all times for a misplaced facial nerve. When the tegmen plate lies close to the superior meatal wall, it may be necessary to expose the middle fossa dura and to follow it inward. When neither the antrum nor the attic is encountered at the usual depth in a very constricted and poorly pneumatized bone, it may be wiser to terminate the operation (as in one of the author's series) than to risk injury to the facial nerve or labyrinth.

The attic and antrum are opened wide enough to expose the malleus and incus (Fig. 14–12D); take care not to dislocate these ossicles when they are normally mobile. The tympanic facial canal is identified. A bony atresia plate usually occupies the site of the tympanic membrane. This plate is removed from above downward until the stapes and oval window are brought into view (Fig. 14–12E). It is often impossible to visualize the round window niche.[16]

A complete mastoidectomy is to be avoided; it is not necessary and results in an unduly large postoperative cavity that will be more difficult to care for.

## The Management of Ossicular Malformations

Congenital ossicular malformations may occur independently as isolated lesions, or they may be part of a more widespread arrest of development of the branchial apparatus.

In the great majority of cases of congenital meatal atresia with microtia, indicating arrest of development before the third fetal month, the malleus and incus are deformed and usually fused and immobile (Fig. 14–13). In most of these the stapes, however, is fairly well formed and mobile. If the incus is well formed it may be mobilized by being separated from the head of the malleus, with amputation of the latter (Fig. 14–14). Markedly deformed, fused and fixed ossicles should be removed and the substitute tympanic membrane placed against the mobile stapes to produce a myringostapediopexy (Fig. 14–15).

In cases of atresia with a well formed auricle, indicating arrest of development **after** the third fetal month, the incus and malleus are usually well formed and mobile, though there may not be a tympanic membrane. Routine removal of these ossicles, even when they are functionally mobile, has been advised by some because

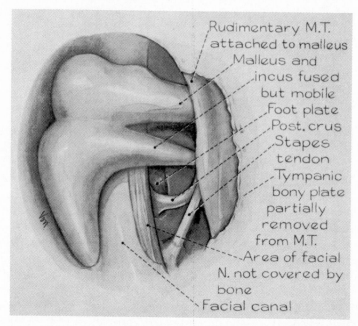

**Figure 14–13**  Malformed fused incus and malleus as seen through the operating microscope, magnified 16 times. Same patient as in Figure 14–12.

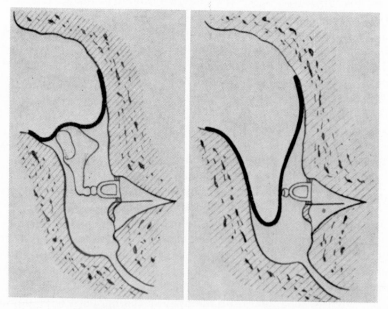

Figure 14–14                                               Figure 14–15

**Figure 14–14**  Incus mobilized by amputation of ankylosed head of malleus, with substitute tympanic membrane resting against it. (From Mündnich, K.: Hearing improvement and plastic operations for malformations of the ear. Hals- Nasen- Ohrenh., 3:668, 1965.)

**Figure 14–15**  Substitute tympanic membrane placed against mobile stapes. (From Mündnich, K.: Hearing improvement and plastic operations for malformations of the ear. Hals- Nasen- Ohrenh., 3:668, 1965.)

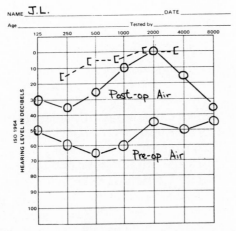

**Figure 14–16** Hearing result in a patient with meatal atresia with substitute tympanic membrane against a mobile malleus and incus.

of the possibility of secondary fibrous fixation. Recent authors[13, 16] believe that a more nearly normal impedance-matching mechanism will result when the lever advantage of the malleus and incus is added to the hydraulic ratio of a large tympanic membrane and small stapes footplate by placement of the substitute tympanic membrane against the mobile incus and malleus (Fig. 14–16). Should these ossicles become fixed by secondary postoperative fibrosis, they may be removed at a second operation and the substitute tympanic membrane placed against the stapes.

When the stapes is fixed, the surgeon must choose between fenestration of the horizontal semicircular canal or stapedectomy. The latter is preferred when there is a mobile malleus handle or incus to which the wire of a prosthesis may be attached; the former is better for more severe malformations in which the middle ear is very constricted, with inadequate access to the stapes, or when there is no mobile ossicle to which a substitute stapes can be attached.

An alternate method of incision and exposure preferred by the junior author has been described by Crabtree.[32] This technique creates a flap that is used to partially line the new meatus and approaches the exposure of the middle ear and ossicles via a post-aural mastoidectomy using a dental-type drill and irrigation-suction. The facial recess[33] is employed to identify the facial nerve and to expose the incudostapedial joint. This joint is separated before the bony atresia is drilled away, to avoid sensorineural hearing loss due to vibrations transmitted through the fixed malleus to the stapes. Ossicular reconstruction is aimed at building upon the superstructure of the stapes to increase the middle ear space. This may require a transposed autogenous or homograft incus or cartilage. Should a stapedectomy be performed for a fixed stapes when the malleus and incus are fixed, it may be necessary to place the incus or cartilage against a connective tissue graft (perichondrium, fascia, vein) over the open oval window. The T.O.R.P. (total ossicular replacement prosthesis) may have some role in this type of reconstruction.

The Crabtree grafting procedure, which involves rebuilding the drum head and creating a skin-lined external auditory canal, is described in the next chapter.

In the occasional patient with atresia but a mobile tympanic membrane and ossicular chain, these structures should be disturbed as little as possible, and the operation should be confined to construction of a skin-lined osseous meatus.

Isolated ossicular malformations without atresia should be dealt with according to the particular lesion.

## Construction of a Substitute Tympanic Membrane and Skin Grafting the Meatus

When a mobile tympanic membrane and ossicular chain are found beyond the atresia, it is necessary only to line the enlarged bony meatus with skin grafts. Unlike skin grafts against soft tissue, which may be very thin, the grafts placed against bare bone should be thicker: either thin full thickness or thick split thickness. Otherwise the resulting epidermis will lack a layer of subepithelial connective tissue, and it will be unhealthy, will desquamate excessively and will be subject to frequent localized infection and breakdown.[30]

In most cases of congenital meatal atresia the tympanic membrane is absent or is so rudimentary as to be non-functional. It is then necessary to construct a substitute tympanic membrane in contact with a mobile incus and malleus or with a mobile stapes. The substitute tympanic membrane consists of a fascial graft[34] with split thickness skin to cover it and to line the meatus (Fig. 14–17B).

Because of a tendency for a skin graft that lines the meatus to contract during healing, there may be an advantage in using a separate graft against the substitute tympanic membrane from that used to line the meatus.[16] The edges of the grafts should be approximated without overlapping. To insure good approximation with the skin of the outer meatal opening, the graft should be sutured to it.

Pedicle grafts to line the meatus and to form a substitute tympanic membrane can be used, but they are more difficult to construct and to fit to the meatus than free grafts and they add to the scarring about the ear. They appear to have no advantages over free grafts.[16]

The skin grafts lining the meatus and closing the tympanic cavity are held in place snugly, but **without pressure,** by means of small cotton balls or sponge packs moistened with Gantrisin or other antibiotic otic solution (Fig. 14–17C). To prevent the packs from becoming adherent, strips of cigarette paper or surgical rayon are first placed against the floor and walls of the new meatus.

Because of a certain amount of scar tissue contraction that always occurs with healing, the new skin-lined meatus should be of large adult size, and the outer meatal opening should be at least twice the size eventually desired (Fig. 14–17D).

## The Problem of Postoperative Ossicular Fixation by Fibrosis

One of the major problems of surgery for congenital meatal atresia has been postoperative fibrosis causing fixation of the malleus and incus when these have been left in, or of the stapes when they have been removed.[15] Because of this, every effort should be made to minimize fibrosis, by these means:

1. Local anesthesia should be used if possible because it **lessens bleeding.** The preoperative use of Premarin by intramuscular injection and during the operation by intravenous injection helps to further diminish bleeding.

2. A meticulously perfect **aseptic technique** in the operating room and postoperative dressings is essential.

3. **Unnecessary trauma** to the mucoperiosteum of the tympanic cavity and epitympanum, including that around the ossicles, must be avoided with the help of

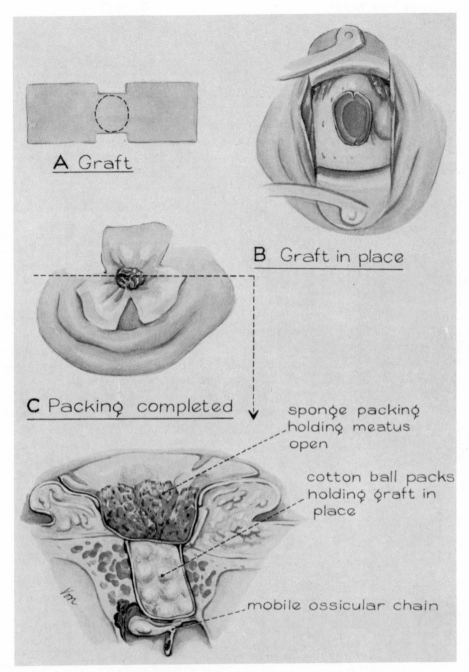

**A** Graft

**B** Graft in place

**C** Packing completed

sponge packing
holding meatus
open

cotton ball packs
holding graft in
place

mobile ossicular chain

**Figure 14-17**  Placement of a thick split thickness graft against a mobile though fused incus and malleus. Same patient as in Figures 14–12 and 14–13.)

operating microscope magnification. Bone dust should be thoroughly removed by irrigation with Tis-U-Sol or Ringer's solution.

4. Gelfoam thoroughly soaked in cortisone or one of its derivatives, such as Hydeltrasol, should be placed in the middle ear and around the ossicles beneath the substitute tympanic membrane. In the senior author's experience this effectively reduces postoperative fibrosis after operations on the stapes and following various tympanoplastic procedures.

## POSTOPERATIVE CARE

The cotton ball packs and surgical rayon strips are removed on the fourteenth postoperative day. Except for the application of 2 per cent aqueous gentian violet to any unhealed area or granulation, little more need be done except to keep the ear and meatus clean. It is most important to observe complete sterile technique for all postoperative dressings for the first 6 weeks.

The use of a rubber tube or other prosthesis to hold the meatus open should not be necessary and should **not** be used since it actually promotes the formation of a cicatricial ring that rapidly closes the meatus once the prosthesis is removed. A properly constructed large meatus should remain open by itself.

Beginning 2 weeks after operation an occasional inflation of the eustachian tube will help to establish an air-containing tympanic cavity, as well as demonstrate any dehiscence in the substitute tympanic membrane that may require repair.

## HEARING RESULTS OF SURGICAL CORRECTION OF MEATAL ATRESIA

The hearing results of operations for congenital atresia and other malformations vary with the degree of deformity, the preoperative cochlear function and the occurrence of secondary fibrosis. Patients with a moderate preoperative loss usually have less extensive malformations, and chances are more favorable for a high level of hearing after operation than in those with a profound preoperative loss.

Of the 34 operations for congenital meatal atresia performed by the senior author one was not completed because of failure to find the attic at the usual depth and four were on children aged 4 whose hearing could not be tested audiometrically before operation.

Of the remaining 28 patients, 6 were operated on again because of loss or partial loss of the hearing improvement. At the end of 1 to 16 years following operation, no patient had a further hearing loss, 3 patients had hearing within 10 decibels of the preoperative level, one had lost an initial improvement and 24 had maintained improvement of 12 to 48 decibels for the speech frequencies. The average gain was 26.5 decibels at an average time after operation of 6½ years. The permanence of the

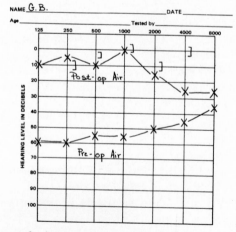

**Figure 14-18**  Hearing result after construction of a patent meatus in a patient with meatal atresia with a well formed tympanic membrane and normal ossicles.

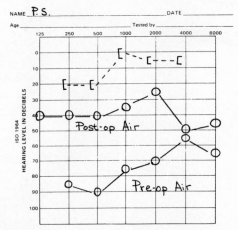

**Figure 14–19** Hearing result in a patient with meatal atresia after removal of the incus and malleus. Substitute tympanic membrane in contact with the stapes (myringostapediopexy).

hearing improvements achieved in these cases of congenital meatal atresia was as good as the results of classic fenestration for otosclerosis.

In this series the two best hearing results (3 decibel level and 0 decibel level) occurred when the substitute tympanic membrane was placed against a mobile incus and malleus (Fig. 14–18). Nearly as good results were obtained in three patients in whom a mobile tympanic membrane and ossicular chain were found beyond the atresia and were preserved. Myringostapediopexy after removal of the incus and malleus gave generally good results (Fig. 14–19). Fenestration also gave good results, but no better than myringostapediopexy except in the one patient in whom the stapes became fixed. With the local use in the ear of a cortisone preparation to prevent secondary fibrosis and ossicular fixation, the hearing results after myringostapediopexy, and especially when the substitute tympanic membrane is placed on a movable malleus and incus, should be excellent and should exceed those of classic fenestration.

## HEARING RESULTS IN ISOLATED OSSICULAR MALFORMATION

Congenital ossicular malformations without atresia are not uncommon (Fig. 14–20),[26] and may be confused preoperatively with stapedial otosclerosis. The congenital origin of the ossicular fixation should be suspected whenever a severe conductive hearing loss dates from early childhood without a history of previous otitis media, when the loss is not progressive, when other malformation of the outer or middle ear is present, and when a severe conductive loss is unilateral. Conventional x-ray and tomographic studies may be helpful in establishing the preoperative diagnosis.

Impedance studies with special attention to stapedial reflexes may be helpful as well. There is a wide variety of congenital combinations that will produce a conductive hearing loss with a normal tympanic membrane and external auditory canal.

Malleus head fixation[35] is much more common than once realized and may be managed in several ways. One way is by placing the tympanic membrane on the

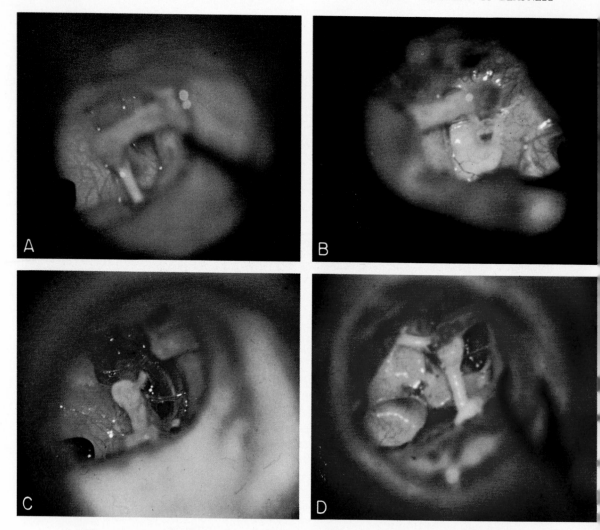

**Figure 14–20** Congenital ossicular malformations. *A*, Congenital fixation of the stapes. *B*, Solid stapes without crural arch or tendon. *C*, Congenital absence of lenticular process of incus. *D*, Congenital malformation with bony bridge from malleus to stapes. (From Hough, J. V. D.: Congenital malformations of the middle ear. Arch. Otol., 78:335, 1963.)

head of the stapes after amputation of the malleus head, as in Case 9 (Figs. 14–21 and 14–22). This gives a satisfactory result, as one can see from the postoperative audiogram, but has the disadvantage of lowering the eardrum into the middle ear cavity, thus creating a retraction pocket. This pocket will sometimes cause the ear to drain if water is not kept from the external canal. In addition, with time, the drum may pull away from the stapes, allowing the conductive loss to recur.

A newer and more reliable method of handling the problem is to disarticulate the incus and extract it along with the head of the malleus. The incus is then sculptured[35] into a fitted prosthesis that can be placed between the handle of the malleus and the capitulum of the stapes. This allows the drum head to remain at its normal level and consistently results in a satisfactory hearing result.

Stapes fixation alone is managed in the same manner as one would a case of otospongiosis. When malleus head fixation is present as well, an alternate method must be employed. The technique of Sheehy[36] works well in this situation. The malleus head is amputated after the incus has been removed. An I.R.P. (incus replacement prosthesis) is then attached to the malleus handle and brought into contact with a connective tissue graft over the opened oval window.

Besides the Sheehy technique, another method of dealing with this problem is to use cartilage or a T.O.R.P. (total ossicular replacement prosthesis) from the oval window directly to cartilage placed against the tympanic membrane.

In the rare case of absence of the stapes arch or long process of the incus, similar techniques are used to reconnect the ossicular chain.

Illustrative case reports follow.

## Case 1

Miss M. St. J., age 12. Hearing impairment noted at age 4. Preoperative clinical diagnosis: otosclerosis with stapes fixation. Fenestration of R. ear: stapes immobile. Hearing gain of plus 23 decibels after 12 years, to 27 decibel level. Fenestration L. ear: absence of mastoid process with abnormal position of facial nerve which emerged into soft tissue at the posterior end of its tympanic portion, and was accidentally severed. Nerve ends approximated and fenestration with a gain of plus 39 decibels after 4 years, to a 15 decibel level, with moderately good recovery of facial nerve function.

Postoperative diagnosis: congenital malformation with stapes fixation in both ears, absence of mastoid process and abnormal course of facial nerve L. ear.

## Case 2

Miss J. E. H., age 7. Hearing impairment noted since early childhood. Preoperative clinical diagnosis: otosclerosis with stapes fixation. Fenestration R. ear: stapes immobile without visible otosclerotic focus. Hearing gain of plus 35 decibels to 17 decibel level, after 10 years. Fenestration L. ear: stapes immobile; footplate free of otosclerotic changes. Hearing gain of plus 31 decibels to 27 decibel level, after 7 years.

Postoperative diagnosis: congenital stapes fixation with small mandible.

## Case 3

Miss M. R. D., age 5. Congenital absence of R. auricle and meatus with narrow but patent L. meatus and bilateral conductive hearing loss.

Fenestration L. ear: incus and stapes deformed; distortion of anatomy of tympanum and epitympanum. Hearing gain of plus 44 decibels to 15 decibel level, after 8 years.

## Case 4

Mr. L. I., age 4. Microtia and atresia R. ear; bilateral conductive hearing loss. Fenestration of L. ear: stapes footplate ankylosed and continuous with promontory. No hearing improvement: plus 2 decibels to 62 decibel level, after 3 years. Failure probably due to profuse bleeding at operation with serous labyrinthitis and probable intralabyrinthine fibrosis.

*Case 5*

Miss S. T., age 5. Hearing loss noted at age 3. Conductive loss established by air and bone audiometry and tuning fork tests. Diagnosis: congenital ossicular malformation without atresia. Stapes mobilization R. ear footplate with pneumatic hammer resulted in insignificant gain of plus 10 decibels to 50 decibel level, after 2 years. Stapes mobilization L. ear: deformed stapes lacking a head and neck, and the incus attached directly to the crura. Footplate immobile, anterior end being continuous with the promontory. Chisel fracture around margins of footplate with fracture of anterior crus but posterior crus remained intact. Hearing gain of plus 21 decibels to 30 decibel level, after one year.

*Case 6*

Miss H. A., age 8. Hearing loss noted at age 5. Did not speak until age 3. Is in school for hearing handicapped. Clinical diagnosis: congenital ossicular malformation without atresia. Operation: fused ankylosed incus and head of malleus removed. Stapes normally mobile but without a head and neck and with no connection with the incus. Myringostapediopexy with gain of plus 30 decibels to 20 decibel level, after one year.

*Case 7*

Mr. W. W., age 42. Hearing loss noted for 4 years. Clinical diagnosis: otosclerosis. Stapes mobilization approach to R. ear: mass of solid bone replaced incus and stapes, preventing access to footplate.

Postoperative diagnosis: congenital malformation and fixation of incus and stapes.

*Case 8*

Mrs. R. D. Bilateral conductive hearing loss of 26 years' duration. Large perforation R. tympanic membrane. L. tympanic membrane normal. Clinical diagnosis: otosclerosis L. ear. Stapes mobilization approach to L. ear: stapes footplate covered only by an extremely thin transparent membrane through which the utricle could be clearly seen. Attempt to mobilize footplate unsuccessful.

Postoperative diagnosis: congenital stapes fixation with congenital fenestra of footplate.

*Case 9*

Miss J. H. (Figs. 14–21 and 14–22). Unilateral conductive hearing loss of 2 years' duration. R. tympanic membrane normal. L. tympanic membrane retracted. Clinical diagnosis: unilateral otosclerosis L. ear. Stapes mobilization approach to L. ear: stapes and footplate normal and very movable. Long process of incus not seen. Soft

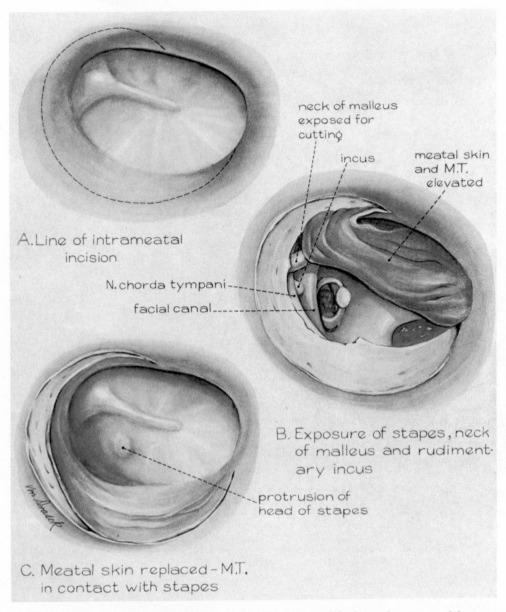

A. Line of intrameatal incision

neck of malleus exposed for cutting

incus

meatal skin and M.T. elevated

N. chorda tympani

facial canal

B. Exposure of stapes, neck of malleus and rudiment-ary incus

protrusion of head of stapes

C. Meatal skin replaced - M.T. in contact with stapes

**Figure 14–21**  Myringostapediopexy for congenital absence of the lenticular process of the incus. Same patient as in Figure 14–22.

fibrous adhesion between the head of the stapes and the upper edge of the bony meatus. Round window niche open. Flap replaced. Six months later, through an endaural incision, the skin of the osseous meatus, posteriorly, superiorly and anteriorly, elevated as a cuff resembling a mobilization cuff, exposing the middle ear cavity. Many loose filmy adhesions present, obscuring the stapes and the area of oval window, were removed. The stump of the incus seen projecting from the upper meatal wall. The head of the malleus amputated to get good contact between tympanic membrane and the head of the stapes (myringostapediopexy). Hearing gain of plus 33 decibels to 7 decibels, after one year (Fig. 14–22). Postoperative diagnosis: congenital absence of lenticular process of incus.

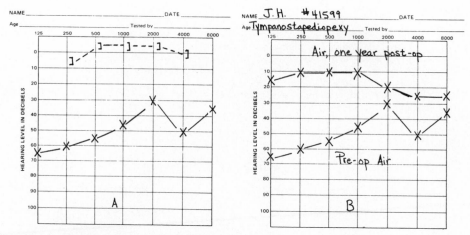

**Figure 14–22** Hearing tests of a patient with congenital absence of the lenticular process in the incus (same patient as in Figure 14–21). *A*, Preoperative audiograms, air and bone, *B*, Result one year after myringostapediopexy.

# REFERENCES

1. Kiesselbach, W.: Versuch zur Anlegung eines äusseren Gehörganges bei angeborener Missbildung beider Ohrmuscheln mit Fehlen der äusseren Gehörgänge. Arch. Ohrenh., *19*:127, 1882.
2. Schwartze, H.: Ueber erworbene Atresie und Strictur des Gehörganges und deren Behandlung. Arch. Ohrenh., *47*:71, 1899.
3. Trautmann, F.: Die persistente retroauriculär Oeffnung nach Radicaloperation und plastischer Verschloss derselben. Arch. Ohrenh., *48*:1, 1900.
4. Politzer, A.: Diseases of the Ear. Philadelphia, Lea & Febiger, 1908.
5. Scheibe, A.: Doppelseitige kongenitale Atresie des Gehörgangs. München. med. Wchnschr., *51*:88, 1904.
6. Alexander, G.: Zur chirurgischen Behandlung der kongenitalen Atresie. Ztschr. Ohrenh., *55*:144, 1908.
7. Page, J. R.: Congenital bilateral microtia with total osseous atresia of the external auditory canals, operation and report of cases. Tr. Am. Otol. Soc., *13*:376, 1914.
8. Dean, L. W., and Gittins, T. R.: Report of a case of bilateral congenital osseous atresia of external auditory canal with exceptionally good functional result following operation. Tr. Am. Laryng. Rhin. & Otol. Soc., 1917.
9. Kopetsky, S. J.: Otologic Surgery. New York, Paul B. Hoeber, 1929, p. 47.
10. Ombrédanne, M.: Surgery of deafness: fenestration in cases of congenital atresia of the external auditory canal. Oto-rhino-laryng. internat., *31*:229, 1947.
11. Pattee, G. L.: An operation to improve hearing in cases of congenital atresia of the external auditory meatus. Arch. Otol., *45*:568, 1947.
12. Siirala, U.: Plastic correction of congenital atresia of the external auditory meatus combined with fenestration to improve hearing. Acta oto-laryng., *37*:307, 1949.
13. Shambaugh, G. E., Jr.: Developmental anomalies of the sound conducting apparatus and their surgical correction. Ann. Otol. Rhin. & Laryng., *61*:873, 1952.
14. House, H. P.: Management of congenital ear canal atresia. Laryngoscope, 64:916, 1953.
15. Rüedi, L.: The surgical treatment of the atresia auris congenita. Laryngoscope, 64:666, 1954.
16. Meurman, Y.: Congenital microtia and meatal atresia. Arch. Otol., 66:443, 1957.
17. Franceschetti, A., and Zwahlen, P.: Un syndrome nouveau: le dysostose mandibulofaciale. Bull. schweiz. Akad. med. Wissensch., 1:60, 1944.
18. Fraser, J. S.: Malformations of the auricle, external meatus and middle ear. Arch. Otol., *13*:1, 1931.
19. Anson, B. J., and Bast, T. H.: The surgical significance of the stapedial and labyrinthine anatomy. Quart. Bull. Northwestern Univ. Med. School, *32*:307, 1958.
20. Altmann, F.: The ear in severe malformations of the head. Arch. Otol., 66:7, 1957.
21. Richards, C. S.: Middle ear changes in rubella deafness. J. Otol. Soc. Australia, 1:173, 1963.
22. Leicher, H.: Deaf-mutism, vestibular pathology and malformation of the outer ear as a symptom of rubella-embryopathy. Ztschr. Laryng. Rhin. Otol., *31*:128, 1952.
23. Mündnich, K.: Hearing improvement and plastic operations for malformations of the ear. Hals-Nasen-Ohrenh., *3*:668, 1965.
24. Lenz, W.: The thalidomide syndrome. Fortschr. Med., *81*:148, 1963.

25. House, H. P., House, W. F., and Hildyard, V. H.: Congenital stapes footplate fixation. Laryngoscope, 68:1387, 1958.
26. Hough, J. V. D.: Malformations and anatomical variations seen in the middle ear during the operation for mobilization of the stapes. Laryngoscope, 68:1337, 1958.
27. Barsky, A. J.: Principles and Practice of Plastic Surgery. Baltimore, Williams & Wilkins Co., 1950.
28. Gillies, Sir H., and Millard, D. R., Jr.: The Principles and Art of Plastic Surgery. Boston, Little, Brown & Co., 1957.
29. Peer, L. A.: Reconstruction of the auricle with diced cartilage grafts in a vitallium ear mold. Plast. & Reconstruct. Surg., 3:653, 1948.
30. Shambaugh, G. E., Jr., and Derlacki, E. L.: Primary skin grafting of the fenestra and fenestration cavity. Arch. Otolaryng., 64:46, 1956.
31. Dubs, R.: A new method for attaching an auricle prosthesis. Pract. oto-rhino-laryng., 27:172, 1965.
32. Crabtree, J. A.: Tympanoplastic techniques in congenital atresia. Arch. Otol., 88:89, 1968.
33. Sheehy, J. L., and Patterson, M. E.: Intact canal wall tympanoplasty with mastoidectomy. Laryngoscope, 77:1502, 1967.
34. Glasscock, M. E.: Tympanic membrane grafting: overlay vs undersurface technique. Laryngoscope, 83:754, 1973.
35. Pennington, C. L.: Incus interposition techniques. Ann. Otol., Rhinol. & Laryngol., 82:518, 1973.
36. Sheehy, J. L.: Stapedectomy in the fenestrated ear. Ann. Otol. Rhinol. & Laryngol., 71:1027, 1962.

# Chapter 15

# Closure of Tympanic Membrane Perforations

HISTORICAL ASPECTS
ETIOLOGY AND PATHOLOGY OF PERMANENT CENTRAL
    PERFORATIONS
EFFECTS ON THE HEARING OF PERFORATIONS OF THE
    TYMPANIC MEMBRANE
INDICATIONS FOR AND ADVANTAGES OF CLOSURE
CONTRAINDICATIONS TO CLOSURE OF A PERFORATION
CLOSURE OF PERFORATIONS BY A PROSTHESIS
SPLINTING OF TRAUMATIC PERFORATIONS
TECHNIQUE OF CLOSURE BY PROMOTION OF HEALING
        RESULTS OF CLOSURE BY PROMOTION OF
            HEALING
CLOSURE BY MYRINGOPLASTY
        THE OVERLAY TECHNIQUE OF MYRINGOPLASTY
        THE UNDERSURFACE TECHNIQUE OF
            MYRINGOPLASTY

## HISTORICAL ASPECTS

The closure of tympanic membrane perforations to improve the hearing was confined at first to the use of **prostheses.** In 1640 Banzer[1] recommended pig's bladder membrane stretched over an ivory tube. In 1841 Yearsley[2] applied a simple ball of moist cotton against the perforation, a method still used occasionally today. Toynbee[3] in 1853 devised as an "artificial membrana tympani" a thin rubber disc with a silver wire stem to assist in its placement (Fig. 15–1), and in 1887 Blake[4] introduced the still widely used paper patch. Various other sheets, membranes and tubes closed at one end have been described to occlude a perforation of the tympanic membrane or to substitute for it when it is absent. A useful and practical prosthesis introduced by Pohlman[5] is the "Korogel insert," consisting of a tube closed at one end and made of flexible plastic material in different sizes and shapes to fit the individual ear.

**Promotion of healing** as a method for closing a tympanic membrane perforation

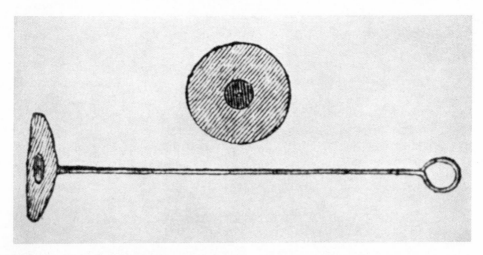

**Figure 15–1**  Toynbee's artificial membrani tympani made of rubber with a silver wire stem. (From original illustration by Toynbee.)

by cautery destruction of its rim was first mentioned by Roosa[6] in 1876; he used a silver nitrate bead. Trichloracetic acid, the cauterizing agent generally used today, was introduced by Okuneff[7] in 1895. In 1919 Joynt[8] observed that a patch on the perforation after cautery gave a higher percentage of closures, and Linn[9] found a patch of moist cotton with repeated cautery at weekly intervals very effective. This last method with a few minor changes was utilized by Derlacki[10] and Wright[11] and is the one described in this text.

The **surgical repair** of permanent perforations of the tympanic membrane was first described as a "myringoplasty" by Berthold[12] in 1878. He placed a court plaster against the tympanic membrane for 3 days to remove the epithelium, and then applied a thick skin graft. Despite success reported in two cases, little more was heard of myringoplasty until Schulhof and Valdez[13] mentioned it in 1944, and then not again until 1952 when Wullstein[14] published a method of closing perforations with a split thickness skin graft. Only a year later Zöllner[15] described his experiences with a similar graft; Wullstein and House[16] then advised a full thickness graft taken from behind the ear. The remarkable rebirth of interest in surgical closure of perforations has continued with a veritable flood of articles describing different methods. The operating microscope, first applied to these operations by Wullstein and Zöllner, has become indispensable for this type of surgery.

For several years the grafting material consisted of skin, generally in the form of free grafts, taken from the arm or from behind the ear. Soon the disadvantages of this material became evident: excessive desquamation into the meatus required frequent cleaning and a number of apparently well healed perforations reopened because of ingrowth of stratified squamous epithelium from hair follicles, sweat and sebaceous glands that had been cut across when the graft was prepared.

In 1956 Zöllner,[17] following the suggestion of Unterberger, first used fascia lata to close a perforation. In 1958 Heermann[18] began to use temporal fascia; in 1960 Shea[19] and Tabb[20] independently described the closure of tympanic membrane perforations using a vein graft. The advantages of connective tissue over skin as a transplant soon became evident in the higher percentage of successful closures and fewer late reopenings of the perforation.

Meanwhile meatal skin, sometimes used as a pedicle graft,[21-23] more often as a free graft,[24, 25] proved to be better than skin from other areas. The skin of the bony meatus is nearly free of glands and hair follicles, and since it is elevated with its periosteum, the danger of cutting across one of these epithelium-lined tubules is minimized. Equally important are the facts that the skin of the bony meatus is accustomed to and thus remains healthier in the moisture-retaining confines of the meatus, it normally desquamates much more slowly than skin elsewhere,[25] and it cleans itself by outward migration of the cornified layer.

In the late 1960's, homograft tympanic membranes were used sporadically but never gained universal acceptance. The best take rates were reported to be about 70 to 90 per cent.[26] To date the most widely used grafting material is temporalis fascia. Regardless of the technique employed, take rates are commonly reported at 96 to 97 per cent.[27]

## ETIOLOGY AND PATHOLOGY OF PERMANENT CENTRAL PERFORATIONS

Permanent central perforations of the tympanic membrane may be of **traumatic origin,** but more often result from an **acute suppurative otitis media of the necrotic type.** In Chapter 7 the usual type of acute suppurative otitis media, with a tiny tympanic membrane perforation and with a self-limiting course leading to a restoration of the structures to normal, was contrasted with the necrotizing form of acute suppurative otitis media that occurs especially in children suffering from measles or scarlet fever. In this disease large portions of the tympanic membrane where the blood supply is poorest become necrotic and slough, usually leaving intact the better nourished annular rim, the area near the handle of the malleus and the pars flaccida. Such a typical kidney-shaped perforation is termed "central" because of the marginal rim that remains. After the acute necrotic otitis media has subsided, the perforation may heal spontaneously by means of a thin atrophic scar, or it may remain permanently open (see Fig. 7–1). In such a middle ear the mucous membrane is exposed to repeated reinfection, both via the meatus and through the eustachian tube, with a chronic continuous discharge or with recurring episodes of suppurative otitis media. Allergic sensitization of the exposed middle ear mucosa occurs frequently.[28, 29]

**Trauma** leading to a permanent perforation of the tympanic membrane may be the result of sudden or explosive alterations in air pressure in the external meatus, or of hot water, slag or acid entering the meatus; or it may follow a lightning stroke or skull fracture. Surgical trauma, especially during the operation of stapes mobilization, and prolonged use of ventilation tubes are additional causes. Traumatic perforations more often become permanent when accompanied or followed by an acute suppurative otitis media.

The very great tendency toward spontaneous healing of even very large perforations of the tympanic membrane was noted as long ago as 1876 when Roosa[6] stated: "Yet the tympanic membrane has a regenerative power second to that of no other membrane in the body. I have repeatedly seen it entirely restored after all but a narrow rim had been entirely swept away. That even occurred in cases of long standing. The prompt healing of the drum-head after operative perforation and in acute inflammations is a matter of common experience."

In the experimental animal[30] proliferation of stratified squamous epithelium at the edges of a perforation begins within 12 hours and granulation tissue begins at 36 hours; regeneration of the pavement epithelium on the inner mucosal surface is more sluggish and begins only after several days. As long as there is a suitable flat surface, stratified squamous epithelium grows at the rate of 1 mm. a day.

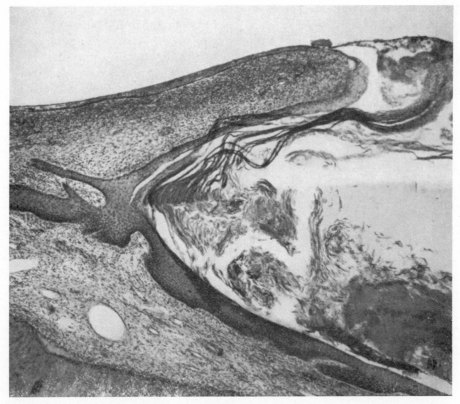

**Figure 15–2** Old central perforation of tympanic membrane showing stratified squamous epithelium of meatus and outer surface (below) extending over the rim to meet the tympanic epithelium (above). (Courtesy of Dr. H. F. Schuknecht.)

The question arises as to why most small and some large perforations of the tympanic membrane heal spontaneously, but others do not. The answer, which gives the clue to stimulating closure of such perforations, was provided by Dunlap and Schuknecht[31] in 1947. By histologic examination of permanent perforations they found that the stratified squamous epithelium of the outer surface had grown inward over the edges of the perforation to meet the tympanic epithelium within (Fig. 15–2). It is a familiar clinical observation that fistulous openings onto the surface of the body tend toward spontaneous closure except when stratified squamous epithelium has extended inward to line the opening, and that closure in these cases requires complete removal or destruction of this epithelium. Fortunately, stratified squamous epithelium does not grow easily over the sharp edge of a skin incision; otherwise, permanent fistulas would follow many surgical procedures, and permanent perforations of the tympanic membrane would be far more common than they actually are.

## EFFECTS ON THE HEARING OF PERFORATIONS OF THE TYMPANIC MEMBRANE

As we have seen in Chapter 13, a simple perforation of the tympanic membrane without other lesion of the middle ear transformer has two different effects on the hearing. First, there is the diminished surface of tympanic membrane on which sound pressure is exerted, causing diminished excursions of the ossicular chain. For a small perforation 1 mm. in size Békésy[32] found that the loss of ossicular motion is confined to sounds below 400 cycles; it is 12 decibels for 100 and 200 cycles, 29 decibels for 50 cycles and 48 decibels for the lowest audible frequency of 10 cycles. The larger the perforation, the greater the loss of surface on which sound pressure can act, with the additional factor that sound pressure entering the middle ear through the perforation acts on the posterior surface of the tympanic membrane against the sound pressure on the outer surface.

The second effect on the hearing of a simple perforation results from sound reaching the round window directly without the dampening and phase-changing effect of the intact tympanic membrane. Because of friction on the margins of a perforation this effect becomes greater with a larger perforation. Moreover, as the size of the remnant of tympanic membrane decreases, the hydraulic advantage produced by a large tympanic membrane on a small oval window disappears, so that sound reaches both windows with more nearly equal force and at nearly the same time. The resultant cancellation of vibratory movement of the cochlear fluid column produces the maximum hearing loss observed in simple perforation, as much as 42 decibels for the speech frequencies.[10, 33]

When healing of a perforation of the tympanic membrane results in the elimination of the air–bone audiometric gap, with the restoration of normal hearing, it is reasonable to assume that the hearing loss was solely the result of the perforation and not due in part to other lesions of the ossicles or cochlea. In general, the larger the perforation, the greater the hearing impairment,[33] but this relationship is not constant and consistent in clinical practice; seemingly identical perforations in size and location produce different degrees of hearing loss (see Fig. 13–18). The reasons for the variations in the hearing effects of simple perforations are not easily defined.

## INDICATIONS FOR AND ADVANTAGES OF CLOSURE

Closure of a tympanic membrane perforation restores the vibratory area of the membrane and affords round window protection, thus improving hearing and lessening tinnitus. It also lessens the susceptibility of the middle ear mucosa to infection via the eustachian tube and external auditory meatus.

An approximate estimate of the improvement in hearing and tinnitus that may be expected from permanent closure of a perforation is obtained by temporary patching with cigarette paper or cellophane. If a carefully applied airtight patch does not eliminate the conductive loss, one may assume that an additional ossicular lesion is present, either fixation or interruption. In such cases simple myringoplasty will not suffice: closure must be accompanied or followed by correction of the ossicular problem by tympanoplasty, as described in Chapter 16.

## CONTRAINDICATIONS TO CLOSURE OF A PERFORATION

Simple closure (office cautery method or surgical patching) should be performed only for a central type of perforation when no skin underlies the tympanic membrane or involves the middle ear. Preferably the eustachian tube should be functional; however, this state cannot be readily determined prior to repair.

Contributing factors such as allergic rhinitis and sinusitis should be brought under control prior to any attempt at closure. A full discussion of contraindications to "closure" of an ear is presented in the following chapter.

## CLOSURE OF PERFORATIONS BY A PROSTHESIS

In the early days of myringoplasty, it was a common practice to patch the perforation of the tympanic membrane with cigarette paper or thin onionskin paper to demonstrate to the patient and physician the improvement in hearing as well as the reduction in tinnitus that could be achieved by permanent closure. This is still useful when a patient hesitates to undergo myringoplasty.

The paper disc, moistened on one side with a solution of 1 per cent phenol in glycerin to make it adhere, is introduced with a small alligator-type forceps and teased into place with a tiny blunt ear hook or ring. Since it rarely remains in place more than a week or two (it is carried backward and outward onto the posterior meatal wall by the normal migration of the outer layers of stratified squamous epithelium), it is not satisfactory for long-time use. A prosthesis such as the Korogel insert[5] may be applied to perforations unsuitable for permanent closure or when closure has failed: the patient is instructed in removing it at night and reinserting it the next morning.

## SPLINTING OF TRAUMATIC PERFORATIONS

A paper patch applied as a splint to a fresh traumatic perforation helps to keep the edges approximated and prevents them from curling under. Oppenheimer[34] treated successfully within 4 days of occurrence 12 traumatic perforations under the operating microscope with local infiltration anesthesia as for a stapes operation (see Chapter 6). The torn edges were carefully everted and held in this position by Gelfoam thoroughly soaked in Neo-Hydeltrasol placed in the middle ear beneath the tear, with a strip of surgical rayon left against the outer surface of the tympanic membrane for 10 days. Occasionally, small tears can be splinted with a piece of Steri-Strip tape applied to the outer surface of the drumhead.

## TECHNIQUE OF CLOSURE BY PROMOTION OF HEALING

In 1851 Toynbee demonstrated five distinct layers of the pars tensa of the tympanic membrane that could be separated by dissection:

1. An outermost **epidermis** of stratified squamous epithelium that is continuous with that of the meatus.

2. A thin **dermis** of fibrous tissue, blood vessels and nerves, which is also continuous with that of the meatus. Unlike dermis elsewhere, that of the tympanic membrane and adjacent osseous meatus lacks glands and hair follicles and the rete pegs that help to anchor the epidermis elsewhere. Therefore the epidermis may be stripped with relative ease from the dermis of the tympanic membrane and osseous meatal wall.

3. An outer **radiate fibrous layer,** which inserts into the fibrocartilaginous annulus and the handle of the malleus.

4.   An inner **circular fibrous layer,** which is better developed peripherally than centrally.

5.   An innermost thin **mucous layer** with a single row of cuboidal epithelial cells on a thin layer of subepithelial connective tissue.

When a large perforation of the tympanic membrane heals spontaneously, it often results in a very thin atrophic scar that lacks the dense fibrous layers of the pars tensa and consists only of an outer epidermis resting on an inner mucous layer. Such a thin scar does as well, or nearly as well, as the normal tympanic membrane as far as hearing is concerned, but it is ruptured easily by external trauma or by forcible inflation of the eustachian tube, and it melts away rapidly in acute otitis media. By contrast a perforation closure induced by repeated acid cautery of its rim often results in a perfectly normal-appearing tympanic membrane possessing all five layers.

Three guiding principles should be kept in mind in attempts to promote healing of perforations by acid cautery of the rim. The first is that the outer stratified squamous epithelium that has grown inward across the edges, preventing spontaneous closure, must be destroyed not just once but repeatedly, to permit fibroblastic proliferation of the fibrous layer. The second is that the rim of the perforation should be kept moist, for drying immediately kills the young fibroblasts and permits the more hardy stratified squamous epithelium to extend under the dry crust to meet the tympanic epithelium. The third is that hyperemia stimulates fibroblastic proliferation, and should be induced by mild irritation.

**Topical anesthesia** of the perforation margins may be achieved by a small cotton ball moistened in 10 per cent cocaine in freshly prepared aniline left against the perforation for 5 or 10 minutes, or by Bonaine's solution (equal parts of menthol, phenol and cocaine) applied to the outer surface and rim of the perforation with a small cotton-tipped applicator. In most cases no anesthetic agent is necessary.

**Cautery of the perforation margin** is carried out with a saturated solution of trichloracetic acid made by adding a drop or two of water to a bottle with some acid crystals to permit them to dissolve slowly. A small "bead" of cotton is wound tightly to the end of a fine metal applicator, moistened with trichloracetic acid and touched to paper tissue to remove the excess. The applicator is stroked over the edge of the perforation in an inward-to-outward direction to break the epithelial barrier, producing a white cauterized margin 0.5 mm. wide. Care is taken not to cauterize the promontory. Juers[35] further fragments and everts the edges of the perforation under the operating microscope with tiny curets, angled knives and hooks: Derlacki,[10] who has the largest reported series, uses cautery alone to destroy the epidermis of the perforation margin.

**Repetition of the cautery** at weekly intervals is required until a new, pink, actively growing margin is seen around the entire perforation. The intervals may then be lengthened to 2 weeks as long as the margins continue to be active.

**Patching** by a flat disc of cotton kept moist by ear drops twice daily of 5 per cent urea in isotonic sodium chloride,[31] or 5 per cent neomycin in isotonic sodium chloride,[11] is necessary to keep the cauterized edge from drying. Juers[35] places equal parts of finely pulverized urea crystals and 5 per cent boric acid in lanolin ointment into the middle ear and on a paper disc placed against the perforation, for the same purpose.

### Results of Closure by Promotion of Healing

Closures occur more readily when the perforation is small or medium in size and involves no more than 65 per cent of the pars tensa. Juers[35] reports 88 per cent success with an average number of 3.7 treatments in perforations of this size using his marginal eversion method. Wright[11] obtained a similar rate of closure by marginal cautery; and Derlacki[10] closed 75 per cent of 131 perforations, some as large as four fifths of the pars tensa: 9 reopened spontaneously and 8 of these were successfully closed again. The quickest closure in his series was by two treatments, and the longest required 64 treatments. All authors emphasize the need for persistence on the part of both patient and physician if a high percentage of closures is to be achieved.

An adequate trial of closure by acid cautery, with or without marginal eversion,[35] is advised for small and medium-sized central perforations before myringoplasty is resorted to. Immediate myringoplasty is recommended for large perforations involving more than 65 per cent of the pars tensa, for narrow or curved external auditory canals preventing a view of the anterior edge of the perforation and for patients who come from afar or who refuse to return for a series of weekly treatments. When ingrowth of epidermis is suspected of forming an incipient or active cholesteatoma, tympanoplasty should be done.

## CLOSURE BY MYRINGOPLASTY

The term myringoplasty is reserved for the simple repair of a tympanic membrane perforation when no ossicular reconstruction is involved.

As we have seen, fascia has become the standard graft because it produces the most satisfactory eardrums, and the take rates are good.

Over the years, two basic grafting techniques have emerged; these are referred to as the overlay and undersurface procedures. Until recent years, the overlay method has been the most popular; however, in the last five years, the undersurface technique has been used more frequently.

### The Overlay Technique of Myringoplasty

The overlay procedure may be performed through a transcanal or postauricular approach. In either case, the initial steps require a set of incisions in the external auditory canal. In Figure 15–3 an outline of this technique using a transcanal approach is presented. Once the ear canal and postauricular area have been injected, an incision is made above and posterior to the auricle to obtain temporalis fascia (Fig. 15–3A and C). A vascular strip is then created in the external auditory canal by making incisions at the tympanosquamosal and tympanomastoid suture lines. These converge near the annulus, and then a circumferential incision is made anteriorly at the level of the bony cartilaginous junction (Fig. 15–3D).

The skin of the anterior ear canal is dissected and removed as a free graft (Fig. 15–3E and F); the malleus is denuded of stratified squamous epithelium, as is the drum remnant (Fig. 15–3G); and the fascia graft is prepared for insertion (Fig. 15–3H). The graft itself may be kept moist with Tis-U-Sol or dried to a parchment-like consistency. A slit is placed into the graft so that it can be positioned medially to the handle of the malleus (Fig. 15–3I). Next, the canal skin is replaced into the ear, either totally over the fascia (Fig. 15–3K) or back into its original position (Fig. 15–3L). There is no need to fill the middle ear with Gelfoam, as the graft is supported by the drum remnant. The vascular strip is replaced, and the ear canal is packed with Gelfoam pledgets soaked either in Tis-U-Sol or in an antibiotic ear drop solution.

A mastoid dressing is applied for the first 24 hours postoperatively, and the patient is allowed to leave the hospital the day following surgery. Three weeks later,

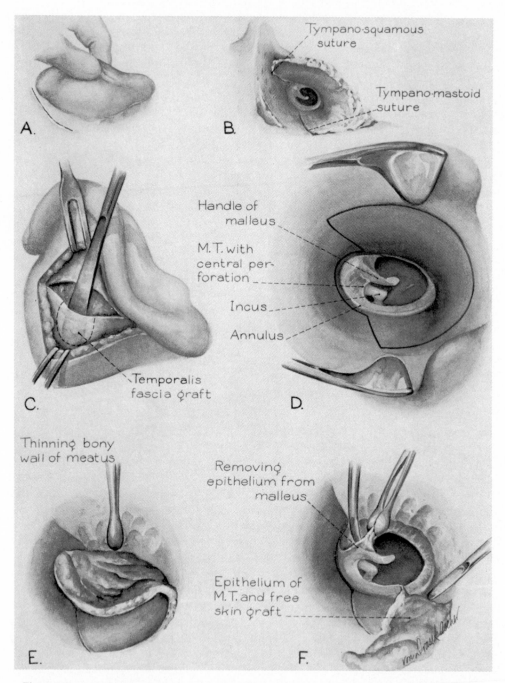

**Figure 15–3** *A,* Incision for temporal fascia graft. *B* and *D,* Incisions for meatal skin graft. *C,* Area of temporalis fascia removed for graft. *E,* Meatal skin elevated; anterior bony meatal wall thinned to expose anterior edge of tympanic membrane. *F,* Completion of removal of meatal skin graft; removal of epidermis from pars flaccida and malleus. (Continued on following page.)

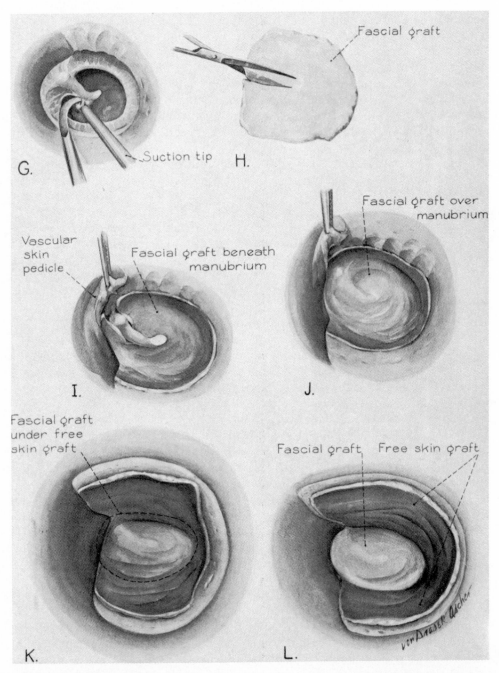

**Figure 15–3** *(Continued)* G, H and I, Method of applying fascial graft under malleus handle. J, Method of applying fascial graft on top of malleus handle. K, Meatal skin graft placed on top of fascial graft. L, Meatal skin graft replaced in meatus overlapping edges of fascial graft.

the patient instills into his ear half a dropperful of Johnson's Baby Oil to soften the Gelfoam. He is then seen at the office in four to six weeks for follow-up examination. Complete epithelialization may not take place for six to eight weeks.

There are several postoperative complications that may occur with the overlay procedure. The most common and bothersome of these is blunting of the anterior sulcus, which can be so excessive as to fix the malleus handle and produce a conductive hearing loss. Another difficulty with the overlay technique is the inability of the surgeon to completely remove all of the squamous epithelium in denuding of the drum remnant. Epithelial pearls can, therefore, arise anywhere in the new drumhead. Lateral migration of the tympanic membrane away from the malleus handle resulting in a conductive hearing loss may occur later on and is most frequently seen when the graft is placed lateral to the malleus handle rather than medial to it.

One other problem commonly associated with this operation is the relatively long duration of the healing process. Because the canal skin is completely removed and replaced as a free graft, there is a tendency for the ear to epithelialize slowly. It may easily take six weeks for the ear to completely heal.

If the blunting and lateralization are kept to a minimum, the hearing results of the overlay procedure can be quite good. Take rates are excellent[27] and account for the popularity of this procedure early in the historical course of myringoplasty surgery.

### The Undersurface Technique of Myringoplasty

Connective tissue grafts (fascia, vein and perichondrium) first began to appear in the late 1950's and early 1960's. With these tissues it became possible to place the grafting material under the drum remnant rather than on top of it. In contrast, the overlay technique had its origin in the early days of myringoplasty when skin of various types was used to close the perforation.

The concept of placing the graft under the drum remnant was set forth by Shea[19] and Tabb.[20] Their procedures were identical and employed vein as the grafting material. The procedure was initially described as an endomeatal approach and for many years was performed in the following classic manner.

Working through a standard ear speculum, the surgeon makes a meatal flap just as one would create to perform a stapedectomy. The edges of the perforation must be excised and the undersurface of the drum remnant denuded. The middle ear is then packed with Gelfoam, and the grafting material is placed under the perforation. The Gelfoam holds the graft against the undersurface while epithelialization is taking place. The new drum is usually healed in one to three weeks.

There are several problems associated with the undersurface technique. First, unless the surgeon is experienced with stapedectomies, he will not work well through a speculum. Second, if the external auditory canal is small and tortuous, it is extremely difficult to prepare the drum remnant or annulus, and graft placement is not as exacting as it should be. For these reasons, the take rate for endomeatal undersurface grafting has never been as good as that obtained by the average surgeon using the overlay procedure, thus accounting for the latter procedure's popularity.

The postoperative problems associated with overlay grafting, however, stimulated the junior author[36] to design an underlay technique that would encompass the advantages of both procedures. By routinely approaching the ear through a postauricular incision, it is possible to work transmeatally without the necessity of a speculum. Exposure is improved, graft placement is therefore more exact and the resulting take rates are significantly better.

The procedure is performed in the following manner. The ear canal and postauricular area are injected with 2 per cent Xylocaine with 1:100,000 Adrenalin. Working endomeatally through a speculum, a vascular strip incision is then made at the bony cartilaginous junction in the inferior part of the ear canal (Fig. 15–4A). This will create a small inferior flap. A postauricular incision is made about 3 mm. behind the fold, and a self-retaining retractor is used to expose the temporalis fascia. More injection solution is placed into the areolar tissue above the fascia, and a large piece of this loose connective tissue is removed. The "graft" is then placed on a Teflon block, teased out to a thin uniform layer, and set on the back table under a gooseneck lamp to dry to the consistency of parchment paper.

Meanwhile, the retractor is removed, and a T-shaped incision is made through the subcutaneous tissue and periosteum (Fig. 15–4B). The vascular strip is elevated from the ear canal, and the incision is held open with a self-retaining retractor (Fig. 15–4C). The surgeon can now work with both hands, free of the constraints of the ear speculum. A small knife is used to elevate the posterior annulus and attached lower flap (Fig. 15–4D). The ossicular chain is then inspected, and the undersurface of the drum remnant or annulus is denuded (Fig. 15–4E). Once the ear has been prepared for grafting, the middle ear space is filled with Gelfoam soaked in Tis-U-Sol (Fig. 15–4F). One common cause for failure with the undersurface technique is seen at the anterior annulus. If the Gelfoam should fall into the eustachian tube orifice during the immediate postoperative period, the graft will fall away from the undersurface of the annulus, resulting in a postoperative perforation in this area. To prevent this occurrence, the surgeon merely needs to start packing the middle ear cavity by first placing the Gelfoam into the eustachian tube and then working back into the tympanic cavity. Using this method, there is no potential space into which the Gelfoam can migrate.

Working through the posterior approach, the surgeon can obtain an excellent view of the anterior annulus simply by tilting the patient away from him. Even with a prominent anterior canal wall bulge, it is seldom necessary to remove bone in this area to see the annulus.

Once the middle ear has been packed, the fascia (or areolar tissue) graft is trimmed to size and placed into the ear. A slit is made for the malleus so the graft can be placed medially and brought up along the sides of the malleus onto the lateral attic wall (Fig. 15–4G). Under direct vision the edges of the graft can be tucked under the drum remnant or annulus, and there will be no question in the surgeon's mind that the graft is in good position (Fig. 15–4H).

Next, Polysporin ointment is placed into the anterior sulcus (Fig. 15–4I), and the vascular strip replaced into the ear canal. The postauricular incision is approximated with Dexon using a subcuticular closure. A small rubber band drain is left in place for 24 hours.

Finally, working through the speculum again, the final position of the vascular strip is adjusted, and the remainder of the ear canal is filled with Polysporin. A mastoid dressing is applied, and the patient is discharged from the hospital the following morning.

By using this procedure, the junior author has been able to solve the problems of blunting, lateralization, pearls and delayed healing associated with the overlay technique while at the same time obtaining a consistent take rate of 96 to 97 per cent.

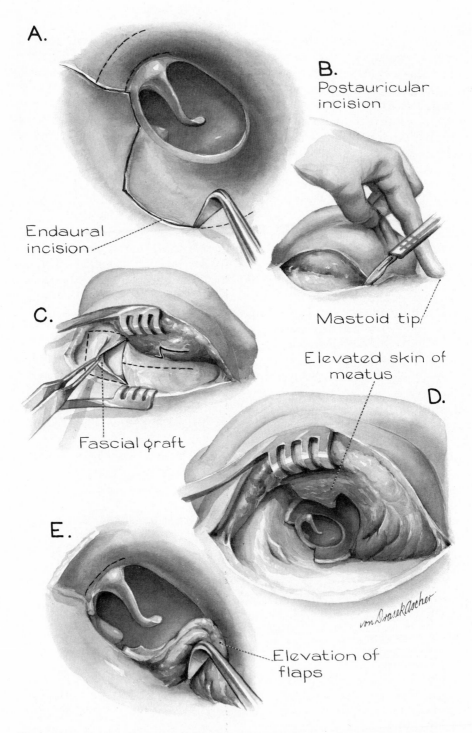

Endaural incision

B.
Postauricular incision

Mastoid tip

Elevated skin of meatus

C.

D.

Fascial graft

E.

Elevation of flaps

**Figure 15–4** *A*, Vascular strip incision. *B*, "T" shaped incision for elevating the auricle. *C*, Self-retaining retractor frees hands. *D*, Number 2 knife being used to elevate lower flap. (Continued on following page.)

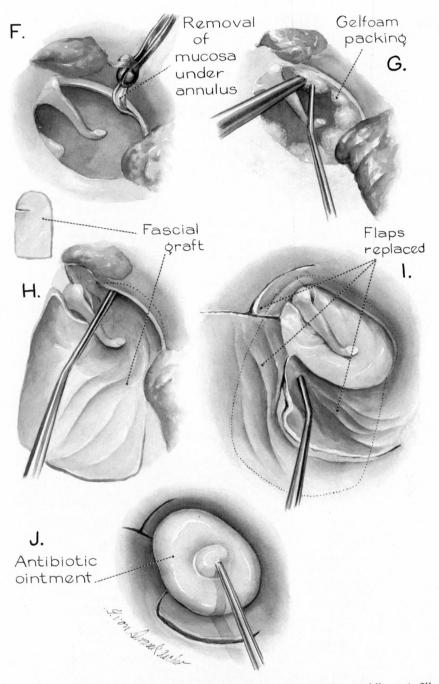

**Figure 15–4** *(Continued)* E, The under surface of annulus is denuded. F, Middle ear is filled with Gelfoam to support graft. G, The fascia is placed under the handle of the malleus. H, The graft is placed under the annulus. I, The external auditory canal being filled with Polysporin ointment to hold graft and vascular strip in place.

In the hands of the average surgeon, this postauricular undersurface myringoplasty will yield fewer complications as well as superior functional results.

# REFERENCES

1. Banzer, M.: Disputatio de auditione laesa. 1640.
2. Yearsley, J.: Deafness, Practically Illustrated. 6th ed. London, J. Churchill & Sons, 1863.
3. Toynbee, J.: On the Use of an Artificial Membrana Tympani in Cases of Deafness Dependent upon Perforations or Destruction of the Natural Organ. London, J. Churchill & Sons, 1853.
4. Blake, C. J.: Transactions of the First Congress of the International Otological Society. New York, D. Appleton & Co., 1887, p. 125.
5. Pohlman, M. E.: The artificial ear drum. Ann. Otol. Rhin. & Laryng., 60:118, 1951.
6. Roosa, D. B. St. J.: Diseases of the Ear. 3rd ed. New York, William Wood & Co., 1876.
7. Okuneff, W. N.: Ueber die Anwendung des Acidum trichloraceticum bei chronischen eitrigen Entzündungen des Mittelohres. Monatsschr. Ohrenh., 29:1, 1895.
8. Joynt, J. A.: Repair of drum. J. Iowa M. Soc., 9:51, 1919.
9. Linn, E. G.: Closure of tympanic membrane perforations. Eye Ear Nose & Throat Month., 23:185, 1944.
10. Derlacki, E. L.: Repair of central perforations of tympanic membrane. Arch. Otolaryng., 58:405, 1953.
11. Wright, W. K.: Repair of chronic central perforations of the tympanic membrane: by repeated acid cautery; by skin grafting. Laryngoscope, 66:1464, 1956.
12. Berthold, E.: Ueber Myringoplastik. Wien. med. Bl., 1:627, 1878.
13. Schulhof, E., and Valdez, G.: Pathology and therapeutics of the perforated ear drum. Franco-American Med. Assoc., Aug. 3, 1944.
14. Wullstein, H.: Funktionelle Operationen im Mittelohr mit Hilfe des freien Spalt-lappen-Transplantates. Arch. Ohren- Nasen- u. Kehlkopfh., 161:422, 1952.
15. Zöllner, F.: The principles of plastic surgery of the sound-conducting apparatus. J. Laryng. & Otol., 69:637, 1955.
16. House, H. P.: Surgical repair of the perforated ear drum. Ann. Otol. Rhin. & Laryng., 62:1072, 1953.
17. Zöllner, F.: Panel on myringoplasty. Second workshop on reconstructive middle ear surgery. Arch. Otol., 78:301, 1963.
18. Heermann, H.: Tympanic membrane plastic with temporal fascia. Hals- Nasen-Ohrenh., 9:136, 1960.
19. Shea, J. J.: Vein graft closure of eardrum perforations. J. Laryng. & Otol., 74:358, 1960.
20. Tabb, H. G.: Closure of perforations of the tympanic membrane by vein grafts. Laryngoscope, 73:699, 1960.
21. Bell, H. L.: Technique of tympanoplasty. Arch. Otolaryng., 66:554, 1957.
22. Bell, H. L.: The new meatal pedicle graft for restoration of the eardrum. Laryngoscope, 71:319, 1961.
23. Sooy, F. A.: A clinical and laboratory evaluation of tympanoplasty utilizing canal wall pedicle skin grafts. Laryngoscope, 74:979, 1964.
24. House, W. F., and Sheehy, J. L.: Myringoplasty. Arch. Otol., 73:407, 1961.
25. Plester, D.: Myringoplasty methods. Arch. Otol., 78:310, 1963.
26. Glasscock, M. E., House, W. F., and Graham, M.: Homograft transplants to the middle ear. A follow-up report. Laryngoscope, 82:868, 1972.
27. Sheehy, J. L., and Glasscock, M. E.: Tympanic membrane grafting with temporalis fascia. Arch Otol., 86:391, 1967.
28. Koch, H.: Allergical investigations of chronic otitis. Acta oto-laryng., Suppl., 62:1, 1947.
29. Derlacki, E. L., and Shambaugh, G. E., Jr.: Allergic management of some common ear conditions. Tr. Am. Acad. Ophth. and Otolary., 57:304, 1953.
30. Taylor, M., and McMinn, R. M. H.: Healing of experimental perforations of the tympanic membrane. J. Laryng. & Otol., 79:148, 1965.
31. Dunlap, A. M., and Schuknecht, H. F.: Closure of perforations of tympanic membrane. Laryngoscope, 57:479, 1947.
32. Békésy, G. von: Über die mechanisch-akustischen Vorgänge beim Hören. Acta oto-laryng., 27:281, 388, 1939.
33. Payne, M. C. and Githler, F. J.: Effects of perforations of the tympanic membrane on cochlear potentials. Arch. Otolaryng., 54:666, 1951.
34. Oppenheimer, P., Kaplan, J., Harrison, W., and Gandhi, K: Repair of traumatic myringorupture. Arch. Otol., 73:328, 1961.
35. Juers, A. L.: Perforation closure by marginal eversion. Arch. Otol., 77:76, 1963.
36. Glasscock, M. E.: Tympanic membrane grafting: Overlay vs. undersurface technique. Laryngoscope, 83:754, 1973.

## SUGGESTED ADDITIONAL READING

Wright, W. K.: Tissues for tympanic grafting. Arch. Otol., *78*:291, 1963.
Kley, W.: Progress in tympanoplasty. Monatsschr. Ohrenh. Laryngo-Rinol., *98*:385, 1964.
McLaughlin, C. R.: Composite ear grafts and their blood supply. Brit. J. Plast. Surg., *7*:274, 1954.
Sheehy, J. L.: Tympanic membrane grafting. Laryngoscope, *74*:985, 1964.
Tabor, J. R.: Repair of complete tympanic membrane perforations. Arch. Otol., *82*:14, 1965.

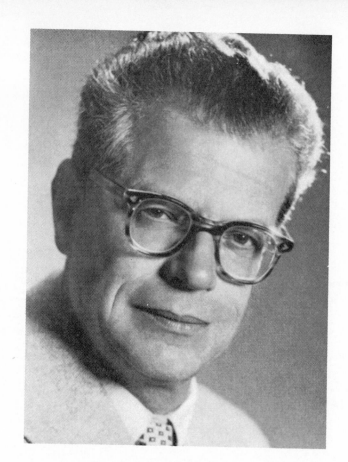

*Fritz Zöllner*

BORN 1901

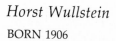

*Horst Wullstein*

BORN 1906

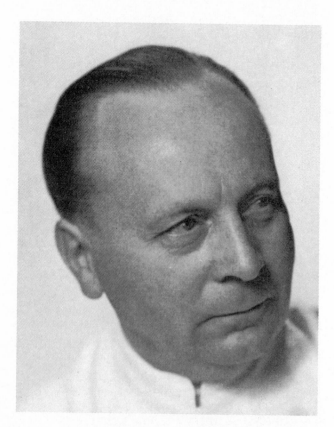

Eminent otologic surgeons
who developed the concepts
and techniques of tympanoplasty.

# Chapter 16

# Tympanoplasty

HISTORICAL ASPECTS
PHYSIOLOGIC PRINCIPLES OF TYMPANOPLASTY
DEFINITION OF TYMPANOPLASTY
INDICATIONS AND CONTRAINDICATIONS FOR
    TYMPANOPLASTY
PREOPERATIVE TESTS AND EVALUATION
ANESTHESIA FOR TYMPANOPLASTY
TECHNIQUES OF TYMPANOPLASTY
    TYMPANOPLASTY WITH INTACT TYMPANIC
        MEMBRANE
    TYMPANOPLASTY FOR CHOLESTEATOMA
    STAGING
    CANAL WALL DOWN TYMPANOPLASTY
    INTACT CANAL WALL TYMPANOPLASTY
COMPLICATIONS
RESULTS

## HISTORICAL ASPECTS

The term **tympanoplasty** was first used in 1953 by Wullstein[1] to describe surgical reconstructions of the middle ear hearing mechanism that had been impaired or destroyed by suppurative disease. These operations are designed to improve hearing in various types and degree of middle ear lesions and are largely replacing the old classic radical mastoidectomy described in Chapter 10.

Tympanoplasty is the final step in the surgical conquest of conductive hearing losses, and is the culmination of nearly 100 years of development of surgical procedures on the middle ear to improve hearing. The first of these was the stapes mobilization of Kessel[2] in 1878, soon followed by Berthold's[3] plastic repair of a perforated tympanic membrane in the same year and Kiesselbach's[4] attempt in 1883 to correct a congenital meatal atresia. These seven eventful years might well have been the beginning of a fruitful development of operations for conductive hearing losses, for the mechanics of the middle ear had been defined clearly by Helmholtz[5] shortly before, in 1868. In fact, however, despite the successes with stapes mobilization reported by Boucheron[6] in 1888 and Miot[7] in 1890, the new surgery of deafness declined and almost died out for reasons that are not entirely clear. By the end of the century a determined opposition by the leaders in otology had arisen toward all attempts to improve hearing by operations on the middle ear.

The completeness of the rejection of surgery for deafness was reflected in the standard texts of otology and otologic surgery, which scarcely mentioned, or mentioned only to condemn, such operations. For example, Kerrison's[8] 627 page *Diseases of the Ear* in 1930 devoted less than a single page to "Surgical Measures for the Relief of Deafness," concluding that: "These operations, mentioned for their

**425**

place in otological history, are quite obsolete today." It is even more surprising that Sir Charles Ballance[9] in his two volume *Surgery of the Temporal Bone* fails to mention any sort of operation to improve hearing.

Reasons for the opposition toward reconstructive surgery of the middle ear were no doubt the imperfect development of sterile technique and the absence of protective antibiotic preparations, with the danger and fear of infecting a clean field in the mastoid and labyrinth. There were few reports of serious infections following the early operations, but one can surmise that some unfortunate unreported results contributed to the opposition. An additional reason for the skepticism toward operations to improve hearing may have been the lack of audiometers for quantitative measurements of hearing before and after surgery.

Probably the greatest reason for the lack of interest in reconstructive operations on the ear was the intense preoccupation of the otologists of those days with infections of the ear and their complications. It is interesting that Schwartze[10] described the simple mastoid operation just three years before Kessel mobilized the stapes, and Küster,[11] Zaufal[12] and Stacke[13] described the radical mastoidectomy at exactly the time that Boucheron and Miot were reporting successes with stapes mobilization. It is evident that the **climate of otologic thought** was favorable toward procedures to control infection, and quite unfavorable toward operations on the ear to improve hearing.

The revival of interest in the surgery of deafness came about gradually. It began when Holmgren,[14] with considerable courage in the face of the concerted opposition, began his long series of operations on the labyrinth for otosclerosis, demonstrating that with modern methods of aseptic technique the non-infected mastoid and labyrinth could, after all, be opened safely. The development of the operating microscope, first by Nylén[15] in 1921, who used a monocular instrument and then by Holmgren, who introduced the binocular operating microscope in 1922, was an important advance destined to play an increasing role in the perfection of fenestration, stapes operations and tympanoplastic surgery. Sourdille's[16] ingenious and successful tympanolabyrinthopexy for otosclerosis added to the reviving interest in surgery for deafness.

The real turning point in the reorientation of otologic surgery away from operations for infection toward reconstruction of the hearing mechanism occurred when Lempert[17] combined Sourdille's several-stage operation into a more practical one-stage fenestration operation. At this time sulfonamide therapy of acute otitis media and otitic complications had begun to lessen the urgency and frequency of operations for acute mastoiditis. Lempert emphasized careful aseptic technique in the after-care as well as during the fenestration operation, and with the later addition to sulfonamides of prophylactic penicillin, postoperative infections lost much of their threat. Most important of all, Lempert taught his operation to otologists from all parts of the world. It was inevitable, as the number of patients successfully treated by Lempert and his pupils increased to hundreds and then thousands that the traditional and often bitter opposition should begin to decline. Thanks to Lempert the **climate of otologic thought** finally became favorable toward surgery for deafness. This led first to the successful operations for congenital meatal atresia in 1947 by Pattee[18] and Ombrédanne[19] and finally to the revival of stapes mobilization by Rosen[20] in 1953.

It is a remarkable fact, already noted in Chapter 13, that during all these years clinicians and surgeons failed to see clearly the applications to surgical techniques of the principles of the middle ear sound-pressure transformer as described by Helmholtz. Neither Holmgren, Sourdille, nor Lempert had a clear idea of how the fenestrated ear functions and why it cannot restore hearing to normal. Likewise,

Pattee and Ombrédanne failed to appreciate the need to restore sound-pressure transformation by placing the substitute tympanic membrane in contact with the mobile stapes.

The mechanics of the fenestrated ear remained obscure until Békésy and Juers began to study the problem. Juers[21] in 1948 noted that the drum membrane of the fenestrated ear must be intact "to protect the round window somewhat from sound pressure." Two years later, Davis and Walsh[22] defined the residue of unrestored conductive loss after successful fenestration as being "due to loss of the impedance-matching mechanism of the drum membrane, ossicular chain and oval window." The two basic principles of tympanoplasty had now been defined, namely, **sound protection for the round window** and **sound-pressure transformation for the oval window**.

It is interesting and surprising that the application of these principles to surgical reconstruction of the middle ear after chronic suppurative otitis media should have begun in Germany rather than in America, where fenestration surgery had reached a high degree of maturity and perfection.

In 1950 Moritz[23] first described the use of pedicle flaps to construct a closed middle ear cavity in cases of chronic suppuration, to provide sound shielding or protection for the round window preparatory to a later fenestration of the horizontal semicircular canal.

The logic of Moritz's procedure was immediately apparent. Zöllner[24] in 1951 and Wullstein[25] in 1952 began to write of similar operations to **provide sound protection for the round window** and to **reconstruct sound-pressure transformation for the oval window**. From the first Wullstein advocated free skin transplants rather than the pedicle grafts of Moritz, and Zöllner soon changed from pedicle to free grafts.

The subsequent development of tympanoplastic techniques has gone through major changes. Transplantation of skin from other parts of the body has been replaced by meatal skin removed as a free full thickness graft as first described by Zöllner. Vein, first used by Shea, is employed today less often than temporal fascia, as proposed by Heermann. Plastic prostheses for reconstruction of an ossicular chain were tried early and abandoned by Zöllner and Wullstein, but they continued to enjoy considerable vogue in America both for tympanoplasty and for connecting the incus to the oval window in stapedectomy. Soon the tendency toward rejection and extrusion of the plastic prosthesis when used in tympanoplasties became evident, and later the polyethylene tube "strut" in stapedectomy began to cause trouble. A wire prosthesis of stainless steel, platinum, or tantalum appears to be better tolerated in the middle ear. Ossicular repositioning, first used at about the same time by Wullstein and Zöllner[26] and described by Hall and Rytzner,[27] is a method of ossicular reconstruction favored today by many operators; wire or teflon from malleus to stapes or malleus to oval window is often utilized when the incus is absent. Homograft ossicles[28] have been popular since the early 1960's for reconstructing the chain in tympanoplasty. Recently there have been renewed attempts to use plastic struts[29]: total ossicular replacement prosthesis (T.O.R.P.) to produce a columella from the tympanic membrane to the oval window, and partial ossicular replacement prosthesis (P.O.R.P.) from stapes head to tympanic membrane.


## PHYSIOLOGIC PRINCIPLES OF TYMPANOPLASTY

In Chapter 13 we saw how, when animals emerged from the sea onto dry land, a mechanical device was needed to overcome the air-water sound barrier. The middle ear mechanism, developed from the discarded branchial apparatus no longer needed for breathing, was the answer. By means of a rather large hydraulic ratio of large tympanic membrane acting on small stapes footplate, combined with a rather small lever ratio of longer handle of the malleus acting on the slightly shorter long process of the incus, airborne sound vibrations of large amplitude but small force are transformed to fluid-borne sound vibrations of small amplitude but large force. Today Békésy's calculations of effective vibrating surface of tympanic membrane area compared to stapes footplate area of 17 to 1, and lever effect of ossicular chain of 1.3 to 1, are generally accepted, rather than the somewhat larger ratios calculated by Helmholtz (see Chapter 13). The 17 to 1 hydraulic ratio times the 1.3 lever ratio yields a total increase of pressure at the oval window of 22 times. This is termed the **sound-pressure transformer ratio** of the normal human ear. The 22 times increase of pressure equals 26.8 decibels.[30]

In Chapter 13 we also saw that the round window in the normal ear acts as a relief opening at the opposite end of the cochlear duct from the stapes footplate to permit maximum to-and-fro vibratory movements of the relatively non-compressible cochlear fluid column in the rigid bony cochlea. In the intact ear the round window membrane movements are largely passive in response to the stapes footplate movements. This is partly because the 22 times pressure increase at the oval window far exceeds any competitive pressure exerted on the round window from the tympanic cavity side. It is also because the intact tympanic membrane "protects" the round window from competitive sound, partly by damping and partly by a phase lag, so that what little sound does reach the round window may actually strengthen rather than cancel the movements of the cochlear fluid column. The relative importance of damping and phase shifting in the sound protection afforded the round window by the intact tympanic membrane remains to be determined.

In the diseased ear impaired by suppuration, the round window begins to play a more active and disturbing role in the mechanics of hearing. A perforation of the tympanic membrane removes sound protection from the round window, with a tendency for sound to reach both windows at nearly the same moment, thus cancelling the resultant movements of the cochlear fluid column. As long as the transformer ratio of the middle ear is larger, as in the case of a small tympanic membrane perforation with an intact ossicular chain, the cancelling effect of sound reaching the round window is small. As the perforation enlarges and the transformer ratio diminishes, the cancelling effect of sound on the unprotected round window rises rapidly until with a total perforation there is a loss of 40 to 45 decibels, or a loss of sound energy transmission of 10,000 times or more. An interruption of the ossicular chain does not add much to the loss of a large perforation, but behind an **intact** tympanic membrane an interrupted ossicular chain produces an enormous and maximum loss of hearing of the conductive type, because now both windows lie behind sound protection and there is no sound-pressure transformation for the oval window. This is one situation in which the 60 to 65 decibel loss, representing a loss of sound energy transmission of a **million times or more,** may be improved to a 40 decibel loss simply by removal of the tympanic membrane.

The ideal tympanoplasty restores sound protection for the round window by constructing a closed, air-containing middle ear against the round window membrane, and restores sound-pressure transformation for the oval window by connecting a large tympanic membrane or substitute membrane with the stapes footplate via either an intact or a reconstructed ossicular chain.

To accomplish the two physiologic principles of tympanoplasty, **sound protection** for the round window must first be provided by means of a tissue graft to repair the tympanic membrane defect, and the middle ear must be **lined with mucosa** and must **contain air** to the protected window. Then sound-pressure transformation for the oval window must be provided by **mobile ossicular continuity** between the large tympanic membrane and small oval window.

## DEFINITION OF TYMPANOPLASTY

Over the years, definitions and classifications of tympanoplasty have been proposed by various authors. It soon became apparent that some standardization was needed for reporting the type of disease present, the surgical procedure employed and the results obtained. In the *Transactions of the American Academy of Ophthalmology and Otolaryngology* of February 1965, a report of the Subcommittee of the Committe on Conservation of Hearing[31] set forth a standard classification for surgery of chronic ear infection, which has been adopted by most authors when reporting their tympanoplasty results:

1. *Myringoplasty*: An operation in which the reconstructive procedure is limited to repair of a tympanic membrane perforation.

2. *Tympanoplasty without mastoidectomy*: An operation to eradicate disease in the middle ear and to reconstruct the hearing mechanism without mastoid surgery, with or without tympanic membrane grafting.

3. *Tympanoplasty with mastoidectomy*: An operation to eradicate disease in both the mastoid process and middle ear cavity and to reconstruct the middle ear conduction mechanism, with or without tympanic membrane grafting.

In this classification, types of tympanoplasty according to the method of ossicular reconstruction are included. In other words, an author is expected to describe what was done. This new system replaced the original classification of Wullstein represented in Figure 16–1.

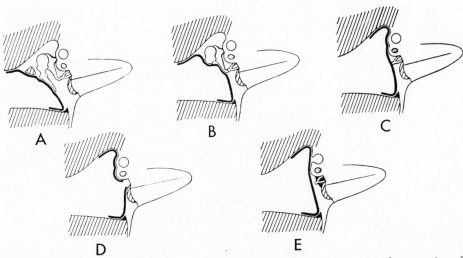

**Figure 16–1** Types of tympanoplasty according to Wullstein. *A,* Type I with restoration of the normal middle ear. *B,* Type II. Ossicular chain partially destroyed but preserved and continuity restored. Skin graft laid against the ossicles after removal of the bridge. *C,* Type III. Myringostapediopexy producing a shallow middle ear and a columella effect. *D,* Type IV. Round window protection with a small middle ear; mobile footplate left exposed. *E,* Type V. Closed middle ear with round window protection; fenestra in the horizontal semicircular canal covered by a skin graft.

The Subcommittee's classification also enumerates a set of rules for describing the gross pathology present at the time of surgery for chronic suppurative otitis media. These rules have to do with the type and location of a perforation of the tympanic membrane, the status of the ossicular chain, whether otorrhea is present and the status of the mucosa and eustachian tube. In addition, guidelines have been set forth for reporting results. In the past, most authors described success in terms of hearing improvement only, when, in fact, elimination of infection and preservation or restoration of anatomy are of equal importance. Therefore, results today are reported in relation to control of pathology, anatomical status, hearing improvement and postoperative complications. For a more detailed discussion of the subject, the reader is referred to the original report as it appears in the *Transactions of the American Academy of Ophthalmology and Otolaryngology*, February 1965.

## INDICATIONS AND CONTRAINDICATIONS FOR TYMPANOPLASTY

Tympanoplastic reconstruction of the conductive hearing mechanism is clearly useless in a functionally "dead ear" or in an ear without useful residual cochlear function. It is contraindicated in malignant neoplasms of the outer or middle ear, where eradication of the tumor must take precedence (see Chapter 22), in invasive life-threatening pseudomonas infection of the outer or middle ear in diabetics (see Chapter 10), and in threatened or actual intracranial complication of ear disease (see Chapters 11 and 12).

Relative contraindications to tympanoplasty include an acute exacerbation of chronic otitis media, which must first be brought under control by appropriate antibiotic therapy and an allergic type of chronic tubotympanitis with profuse mucoid discharge associated with an allergic rhinosinusitis, in which allergic factors must first be controlled by Rinkel's methods of optimum-dosage dust and mold therapy according to skin titration, plus elimination of food intolerance as determined by cytotoxic and provocative testing. A chronic external otitis due to *Pseudomonas, Aspergillus* or *Staphylococcus* should be controlled by appropriate local cleaning and antibiotics, and by allergic management in cases of allergic origin. Eustachian tube non-functioning is a relative contraindication to tympanoplasty, but as noted below, this is not always easily determined preoperatively.

Tympanoplasty is contraindicated on an only or much better hearing ear, for **any surgical procedure on the middle ear may result in an irreversible sensorineural hearing loss.** Only when the patient can use a hearing aid in the opposite ear with satisfactory results should tympanoplasty be considered on the better hearing ear.

The elderly patient in relatively good health without diabetes can be operated on quite safely under local anesthesia, so that age is not a contraindication. A child under three is a poor candidate for tympanoplasty because of its predilection for acute otitis media, as well as difficulties in postoperative care. Unless there is an actively infected cholesteatoma, tympanoplasty in children is best delayed until the teens when the demands on hearing increase, local anesthesia can be utilized and postoperative cooperation is better.

Repeated surgical failures with extensive middle ear fibrosis, a non-functioning eustachian tube, recurrent perforation or extrusion of a prosthesis are better left alone, and the patient advised to use a hearing aid, provided there is not recurrent or residual cholesteatoma.

Mention should be made of the uncooperative patient who does not keep appointments, fails to follow instructions or carries a "chip on the shoulder," ready to seek legal redress for failure to achieve the hoped for result. The surgeon should try to spot such a patient ahead of time and to advise a hearing aid instead of surgery.

## PREOPERATIVE TESTS AND EVALUATION

A complete history and otolaryngologic examination should be performed on all patients with a chronic draining ear. The otoscopic evaluation is best accomplished with a magnifying speculum or with the aid of an office or operating microscope. An audiogram is essential and should consist of pure-tone air and bone conduction curves with adequate narrow-band masking as well as of speech discrimination scores. All hearing tests should be confirmed with tuning forks with narrow-band masking. Mastoid x-rays are important for the preoperative evaluation of the patient. They will supply information about the ear that cannot be determined by careful otoscopic examination, such as whether or not the mastoid is pneumatic or sclerotic in nature, whether the sigmoid sinus is anteriorly placed and the middle fossa dura unusually low, whether the labyrinth has been fistulized by cholesteatoma or whether there is other pathology involved in the temporal bone, such as an acoustic tumor. Polytome x-rays may help to indicate ossicular defects and cholesteatoma size and extension.

If the individual's ear is actively draining at the time of the first office visit, the external auditory canal and tympanic cavity should be cleared of purulent material. This is most easily accomplished by using a small Barron suction tip with the aid of the operating microscope. The patient is then instructed to keep water out of the ear and to irrigate the ear copiously three times a day with a solution of 1.5 per cent acetic acid. The patient is asked to buy a 1 oz. rubber-ball syringe, and while holding the involved ear down, squeeze the bulb so that the clear liquid is forced into the ear to wash out the purulent material. After the irrigation, the ear should be allowed to dry. The head is then turned up and antibiotic solution is placed into the ear canal. This is followed by antibiotic steroid otic drops. Within a few days (usually four to seven) the otorrhea subsides. Ears with cholesteatoma may be refractory to local treatment and continue to drain up to the time of surgery. While most surgeons would prefer to operate on a "dry" ear, there is no contraindication to performing tympanoplasty in an actively draining one. Many times cholesteatoma disease must be removed surgically before the ear will become dry.

In addition to the above measures, an effort should be made to control any contributing factors, such as allergic rhinitis and sinusitis. The status of the upper respiratory tract directly influences eustachian tube function and therefore the outcome of any surgery in the tympanic cavity.

The patency of the eustachian tube is established by having the patient perform a Valsalva inflation (holding his nose and mouth closed while forcibly exhaling) or by using a Politzer inflation as described in Chapter 3. If the tube cannot be inflated in repeated attempts, the prognosis for satisfactory hearing after tympanoplasty is poor. However, removal of middle ear polyps, probing of the tube with a lachrymal probe from the middle ear, or insertion of a silastic film from eustachian orifice to round window, with closure of a perforation, sometimes results in improvement in eustachian tube function and a satisfactory hearing result. A Wright [32] eustachian tube prosthesis may restore function.

## ANESTHESIA FOR TYMPANOPLASTY

The senior author continues to prefer local anesthesia with adequate preoperative sedation as described in Chapter 6 for all types of mastoidectomy and tympanoplasty. These patients are ambulatory the afternoon of surgery and may return home the next day. The junior author prefers general anesthesia for prolonged procedures and whenever mastoidectomy is included. For children and excessively apprehensive patients, general anesthesia is best.

## TECHNIQUES OF TYMPANOPLASTY

### Tympanoplasty With Intact Tympanic Membrane

A conductive hearing loss behind an intact tympanic membrane is usually due to fixation of one or several ossicles or to interruption of the ossicular chain, most often at the incudostapedial articulation. Unless the meatus is unusually narrow, these cases can be approached by a stapes type meatal flap (see Chapters 6 and 18), modified by extending the incision outward superiorly so that should superior bony rim need to be removed to correct incus or malleus defects, the meatal skin flap will close the middle ear when replaced.

**Four basic types of ossicular interruption** are described by Austin:[33] malleus handle present (M+) or absent (M−) and stapes arch present (S+) or absent (S−). The usual defect is of the long process of the incus, most often with intact malleus handle (M+) and intact stapes arch (S+), accounting for 59.2 per cent of non-otosclerotic conductive losses. Next in frequency is intact malleus handle (M+) and absent stapes arch (S−) in 23.2 per cent of cases, while absent malleus handle (M−) and intact stapes arch (S+) accounts for 7.8 per cent of ossicular defects, and absent malleus handle and stapes arch (M−S−) accounts for 8.2 per cent of ossicular defects.

For simple ossicular interruption at the incudostapedial joint, the most common ossicular defect (M+S+), two methods are currently utilized:

**A. Incus transposition,** first described by Guilford,[34] is the method utilized by the senior author. The incus is separated from the malleus head with a long right-angled hook and extracted from the attic. This may require removal of some of the bony rim superiorly. The extracted incus is firmly held by the Sheehy clamp, and a hole of sufficient size to receive the head of the stapes is drilled through the body.

The incus is maneuvered into position so that the intact short process rests on the promontory or under the handle of the malleus, the head of the stapes being visible through the hole in the body.

The most frequent cause for failure after incus transposition is postoperative ankylosis to the facial ridge, promontory or posterior meatal wall. Thorough removal of osteogenic bone dust and insertion of silastic film between incus and adjacent bone help to avoid postoperative ankylosis. Displacement of the transposed incus from the head of the stapes is the next most common cause for failure. Careful inspection through the hole in the incus will verify its correct position on the head of the stapes, and packing the middle ear with Gelfoam soaked in Hydeltrasol helps to prevent its displacement.

**B. A fitted incus** sculptured with a drill to make a groove in its articular surface and an acetabulum on the short process, a technique described by Pennington[35] and

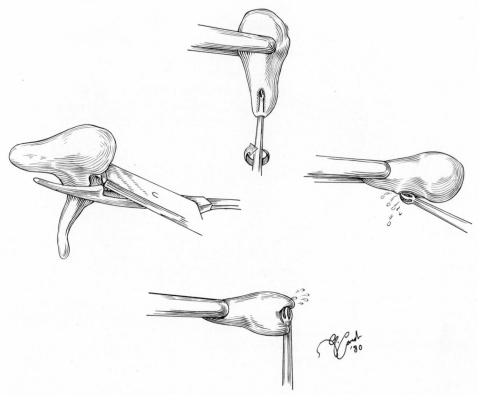

**Figure 16–2**  Sheehy clamp being used to hold incus while it is sculptured with a small cutting burr.

Austin,[33] is the method preferred by the junior author (Fig. 16–2). Again, the incus must be held securely by the Sheehy clamp while sculpturing with the drill. When properly fitted (Figs. 16–3 and 16–4), there should be just enough pressure to hold the incus firmly in place between malleus handle and stapes head with no need to pack the middle ear with Gelfoam. The sculptured incus must not be too long to fix the footplate by pressure nor too short to fit firmly between malleus handle and stapes footplate. When the malleus handle lies far anteriorly, preventing vertical placement of the sculptured incus between malleus handle and stapes head, this method is not suitable. In such cases, incus transposition as described previously should be employed.

Recently, the partial ossicular replacement prosthesis (P.O.R.P., Fig. 16–5) has been recommended for use from head of stapes to the tympanic membrane when an incus is not available. A thin slice of cartilage between prosthesis and tympanic membrane lessens the frequency of prosthesis extrusion. This method is too recent for evaluation of long-term results, so that transposed or sculptured autogenous or homograft incus is preferred by the authors.

When malleus handle is absent and stapes arch intact (M−S+), the incus is transposed if available, or tragal cartilage to connect the stapes head with the tympanic membrane may be used. The partial ossicular replacement prosthesis (P.O.R.P.) with a slice of tragal cartilage between it and tympanic membrane is an alternative but less proven technique.

When malleus handle is intact but stapes crura absent (M+S−), a sculptured incus from malleus handle to mobile footplate, held in place by Gelfoam, is the

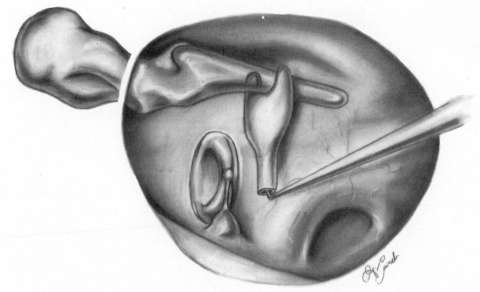

**Figure 16–3**   Fitted incus prosthesis being put into position with a right angle hook.

method of choice, while a total ossicular replacement prosthesis (T.O.R.P., Fig. 16–5) with a slice of cartilage between it and tympanic membrane is an alternative, less proven method.

The ossicular defect most difficult to correct is absence of malleus handle and stapes arch (M−S−). One may use an autogenous or homograft incus from mobile footplate to tympanic membrane or a T.O.R.P. prosthesis with slice of cartilage between it and tympanic membrane, either one held in place with Gelfoam.

All four techniques described here assume a mobile stapes footplate. When the footplate is fixed by otosclerosis or tympanosclerosis, a stapedectomy must be performed, the oval window being covered with vein or fascia to support the

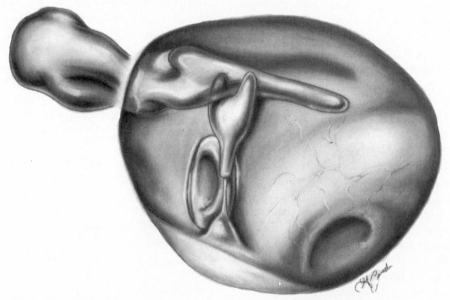

**Figure 16–4**   Fitted incus prosthesis in position between malleus and capitulum of stapes.

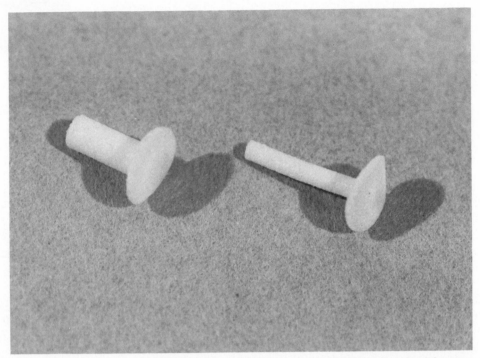

**Figure 16–5**  Total ossicular replacement prosthesis (T.O.R.P.) is on the right side of this picture. Partial ossicular replacement prosthesis (P.O.R.P.) is on the left side of this picture.

transposed incus or plastic columella. Behind an intact preoperative tympanic membrane, stapedectomy can be done safely at the first stage, but in the presence of a perforation, wet or dry, stapedectomy is likely to result in a permanent sensorineural hearing loss and must be delayed to a second stage.

**Ossicular fixation** of the incus only, due to tympanosclerosis or to ankylosis to the scutum, is an unusual problem requiring removal of sufficient superior canal wall rim to inspect and correct the fixation without displacing the incus. Much more frequent is ankylosis of the malleus head by a bridge of bone to the anterior or superior attic wall or by tympanosclerosis in the attic. This may be corrected by removal of tympanosclerosis or by drilling away the bridge of bone. It is essential that a drill never touch the ossicular chain until the incudostapedial joint is first severed, to prevent noise-induced cochlear hearing loss! After freeing the ankylosed malleus head, the joint should heal satisfactorily as long as the lenticular process of the incus is in contact with the stapes head. A sling made of a long thin fascial strip between the arch of stapes and around the long process of incus will help to maintain contact between stapes and incus.

An alternative method for correction of malleus ankylosis is simply to amputate the head of the malleus with the drill or the House malleus nipper, relying upon contact between incus and tympanic membrane to maintain ossicular sound transmission.

Combinations of malleus ankylosis and other ossicular defects can be corrected by combining the previous techniques.

Homograft ossicles are often successful when autogenous ossicles are not available. The homograft may be removed from a fresh cadaver or from patients operated on for acoustic neuroma by the translabyrinthine approach, the incus or malleus being preserved in 50 per cent alcohol and kept in an ordinary refrigerator until ready to use. A few surgeons utilize a homograft assembly of tympanic membrane and ossicular chain after preparation of the homograft by scrupulous removal of stratified squamous epithelium from the outer surface and mucous membrane from the inner surface of the tympanic membrane, thus removing tissues prone to immuno-rejection, leaving connective tissue and bone that do not incite rejection.

While great strides have been made in ossicular reconstruction since the first and second editions of *Surgery of the Ear*, the functional results are still poorer than in stapedectomy for otosclerosis, and revisions are more often indicated for failure to correct conductive defects.

**Aeration of a mucosa-lined tympanic cavity** is essential for a functioning middle ear. When there is mucosal pathology with a perforation or an intact but atelectatic tympanic membrane that fails to move on inflation, measures need to be taken to establish a functional eustachian tube with a mucosa-lined middle ear. An atelectatic tympanic membrane may be approached endomeatally by a stapes type flap, the atrophic tympanic membrane elevated from the promontory, intact if possible, and then reinforced with a fascial graft. A silastic film implant from eustachian orifice to round window will prevent postoperative adhesions and promote regeneration of normal mucosa. Insertion of a Wright eustachian tube prosthesis (Fig. 16–6) may be helpful for poorly functioning eustachian tubes, or a collar button type ventilation tube may be required to prevent recurrence of atelectasis.

Large polyps that fill the ear canal might be attached to the stapes, facial nerve or a fistula of a semicircular canal, and should not be avulsed. By-passing the external meatus, they are safely removed by an endaural atticotomy (method of senior author) or by a simple mastoidectomy and enlarged facial recess approach (method of junior author). By either approach, the base of the polyp can be visualized and the polyp safely removed.

Markedly thickened polypoid mucosa and granulations should be removed completely from the middle ear, along with scrupulous removal of every vestige of stratified squamous epithelium. Mild mucosal involvement generally reverts to normal once the perforation is closed and all cholesteatoma has been removed.

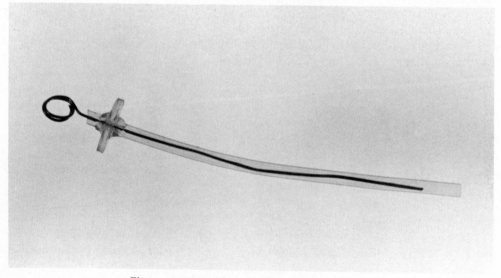

Figure 16–6    Wright eustachian tube prosthesis.

## Tympanoplasty for Cholesteatoma

When a cholesteatoma has been demonstrated preoperatively or when it is unexpectedly encountered at surgery, as may occur with a benign appearing central perforation, a simple stapes type of endomeatal approach is rarely sufficient. An exception is a small attic retraction cholesteatoma sac lying lateral to the incus and malleus, which can be brought into view, dissected and removed intact endomeatally by first removing some of the superior bony rim, as described by Linthicum (Fig. 16–7). Another exception is a small cholesteatoma confined to the mesotympanum, such as the congenital type so well described by Derlacki.[36]

For all other cholesteatomas involving the attic and antrum, and sometimes the mastoid, the surgeon has three choices: the traditional open cavity method by endaural approach, as described in Chapter 6; a postaural incision, as described below (see Fig. 16–8) for the intact canal wall technique by the enlarged facial recess approach; or the osteoplastic atticotomy of Guilford[37] and S. Wullstein.[38]

The open cavity method is preferred by the senior author and by certain well-known tympanoplasty surgeons, such as Gordon Smythe[39] of Belfast, Ireland; Thane Cody[40] of the Mayo Clinic; David Austin[41] of Chicago; and Tauno Palva[42] of Finland. A Bondy type of operation is performed, preserving, if possible, remnants of tympanic membrane and ossicles to be utilized in reconstructing sound conduction. The open cavity technique is rarely followed by cholesteatoma residues or recurrences, and it is as likely to improve hearing as the intact canal wall technique.

The size of the final healed postoperative Bondy type open cavity is often quite small when an attic retraction cholesteatoma occurs in a sclerotic non-pneumatized mastoid. The surgeon should avoid an extensive mastoidectomy, confining the bone removal to the superior and posterior wall of the attic, just sufficient to exteriorize the cholesteatoma, removing all matrix and constructing a cavity easily kept clean in future years. Remember that the seat of disease in this case is the attic, not the mastoid.

The size of the postoperative cavity can be reduced considerably by obliterative techniques, the method of Palva being most often used. Care must be exercised not to introduce muscular-fascial pedicle flaps on top of cholesteatoma matrix. If there is any question of tiny remnants of matrix extending deeply into bone, the obliterating flap should cover only that part of the mastoid bowl not involved in cholesteatoma.

The use of proplast to obliterate part of the mastoid cavity in the open technique has been recommended, but it is less satisfactory than living flaps, there being a tendency after a time for the plastic material to extrude.

Some authors have proposed rebuilding the canal wall months or years after an open Bondy type operation, using grafts of bone or cartilage, or implants of proplast. These techniques are difficult, and their results are not sufficiently encouraging to be recommended. When there is a large air–bone gap, a functioning eustachian tube and mucosa-lined mesotympanum in an old open cavity, reconstruction should be confined to closure of the perforation and ossicular reconstruction according to the existing defect, as described previously.

Other equally well-known tympanoplasty surgeons, such as Jansen[43] of Germany; Sheehy[44] of Los Angeles, California; William Wright[45] of Houston, Texas; and the junior author[46] of this text, prefer for most cases the intact canal wall technique, removing cholesteatoma through an enlarged facial recess. This method is techni-

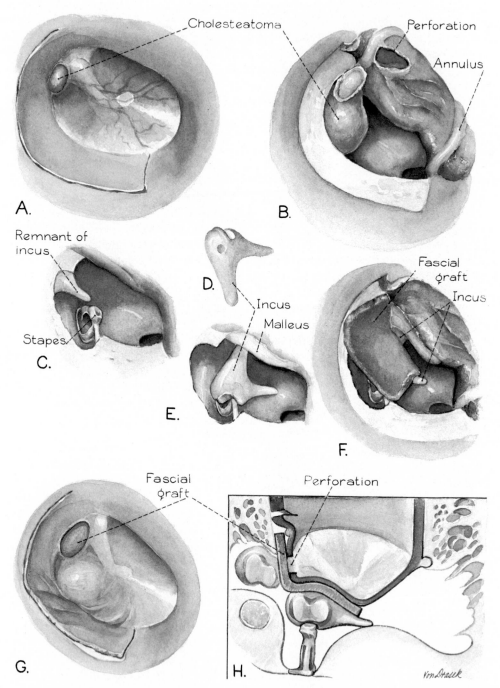

**Figure 16–7**  *A*, Meatal skin incisions for Linthicum endomeatal tympanoplasty Type II. *B*, Middle ear exposed. *C*, Medial attic wall removed; cholesteatoma sac lifted out in toto. *D*, Removed incus drilled to fit over stapes head. *E*, Transposed incus. *F*, Fascial graft to close attic perforation. *G*, Skin flap replaced after excising margin of attic perforation. *H*, Diagram of reconstructed ossicular chain.

cally more difficult, and cholesteatoma residues and recurrences are more frequent, so that a "second look" six months to two years later is advised. The advantages of the intact canal wall–facial recess technique include a normal external meatus that does not require periodic cleaning or preclude swimming.

A middle position is the osteoplastic atticotomy originated by Guilford[37] and practiced by Sabina Wullstein.[38] This method is technically more difficult than the open cavity operation and probably reduces the incidence of cholesteatoma residues and recurrences as compared to the facial recess intact canal wall operation.

Whatever the surgical approach, it is necessary that **all cholesteatoma matrix** be removed from the attic, antrum and mastoid. In some cases, the wall of the cholesteatoma sac can be dissected out, and the sac and its contents removed more or less intact. In other cases, there are finger-like extensions of cholesteatoma into small mastoid cells around the antrum and semicircular canals that must be followed to their end under the operating microscope. Cholesteatoma that extends under the malleus head and incus requires extraction of these ossicles, since complete removal of matrix from their undersurface is impossible. Cholesteatoma extending under the tympanic membrane into the mesotympanum must be exposed by a stapes type of meatal flap, and every vestige of stratified squamous epithelium must be removed before repairing the perforation. When skin lines the undersurface of the tympanic membrane remnant, it will be necessary to excise this portion of the tympanic membrane.

In a few situations, remnants of cholesteatoma matrix may be left in place at the initial operation. A fistula of the horizontal semicircular canal of a better hearing ear should not be disturbed, and in this case, an open cavity operation is indicated. Similarly, skin attached to an exposed facial nerve may be left in place in an open cavity. When skin covers a mobile stapes footplate, the surgeon may elect to stage the operation by first closing the perforation, then six months later, reopening the middle ear by a stapes type approach to remove remnants of cholesteatoma and proceeding with ossicular chain reconstruction.

## Staging

In a staged procedure, the disease (usually cholesteatoma) is removed from the ear and the tympanic membrane perforation repaired at the first operation. Three to eight months later ossicular defects are repaired. The junior author stages all cases of cholesteatoma operated by postaural mastoidectomy–facial recess–intact canal wall technique, so as to detect and remove any cholesteatoma residue or recurrence at the time of ossicular reconstruction.

The senior author, using an endaural atticotomy–open cavity technique as described in Chapter 10, includes removal of cholesteatoma matrix, tympanic membrane repair and ossicular reconstruction in one stage, but the patient is informed that a revision may be needed for a persistent conductive deficit of sufficient magnitude. Cholesteatoma residues behind the reconstructed tympanic membrane do not carry the risk of intracranial complications from residues in the attic and mastoid after intact canal wall operations. Otoscopic inspection fails to detect the latter, whereas mesotympanic residues are usually visible otoscopically.

Examples of a postaural Bondy type open cavity operation, of an osteoplastic atticotomy and of an intact canal wall facial recess operation are described below.

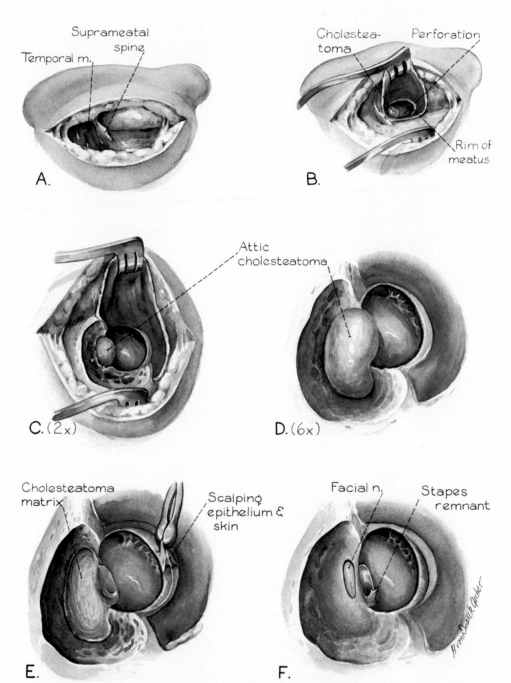

**Figure 16–8**   *A*, Postaural incision tympanoplasty, Type III. *B*, U-flap to expose meatus and tympanic membrane. *C*, Medial attic wall (bridge) removed to expose attic. *D*, Small attic cholesteatoma isolated. *E*, Cholesteatoma sac evacuated. Tympanic membrane and adjacent meatal skin removal. *F*, Cholesteatoma matrix removed. (Continued on following page.)

## Canal Wall Down Tympanoplasty

The canal wall down tympanoplasty procedure is essentially the classic modified radical mastoidectomy of Bondy, in which the tympanic membrane and ossicles are not disturbed and the attic cholesteatoma is exteriorized by removing the lateral attic wall and posterior canal wall. The canal wall down tympanoplasty involves repair of the tympanic membrane and ossicular chain after removal of cholesteatoma from the middle ear, attic and mastoid. The advocates of this technique feel that they can obtain better exposure of the middle ear and attic by removing the posterior-superior ear canal. An example of this procedure can be seen in Figure 16–8. A postauricular incision is performed in the routine manner, and temporalis fascia is removed (*A*). A self-retaining retractor is then inserted to expose the external auditory canal and middle ear (*B*). The mastoid is opened, and the lateral attic wall removed to expose the attic and middle ear (*C*). In *D* an attic cholesteatoma is uncapped. This is dissected free of the attic and middle ear. In this example the malleus, incus and stapes arch have been destroyed by the cholesteatoma (*E*). Once the cholesteatoma has been removed, the drum remnant is denuded (if an overlay grafting procedure is to be employed) and the anterior canal wall skin is removed. If an underlay technique is to be used, the annulus and the canal wall skin are left intact, and the undersurface of the annular rim is denuded of mucous membrane. At this time the ossicular chain can be reconstructed by using a homograft ossicle to the footplate or a T.O.R.P. with cartilage interposed between

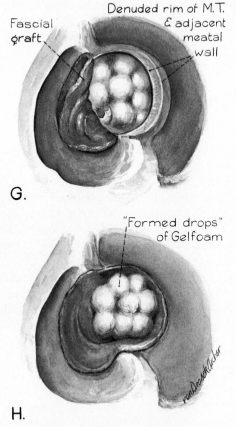

**Figure 16–8** *(Continued)*  *G*, Middle ear filled with soaked Gelfoam; fascial graft being applied. *H*, Fascial graft held in place by soaked Gelfoam, against homograft incus on stapes remnant.

the new drum and the prosthesis. The middle ear is filled with Gelfoam and the fascial graft inserted (G). The fascia is brought over the facial ridge to line the mastoid bowl, and Gelfoam is placed on top of the graft to stabilize it (H).

As in all canal wall down procedures, it is extremely important to create a large external auditory meatus. This is accomplished by fashioning a large flap of meatal skin and by removing a rim of conchal cartilage. This flap is sutured back to the subcutaneous tissue behind the mastoid cavity, which not only creates a large meatus but more rapidly re-epithelializes the bowl by means of the flap of skin. Suturing this flap into place negates the need for external packing of the ear canal and cavity with gauze. The postauricular incision is closed in the usual manner with subcuticular suture, and a mastoid dressing is applied for about 24 hours.

There are some definite advantages to this procedure that should be mentioned. First, it is in keeping with the classic techniques of modified mastoidectomy as taught in most residency programs; therefore, the surgeon will probably feel more comfortable with this type of procedure. Second, the less experienced surgeon can obtain better access to the anterior attic and middle ear in sclerotic and contracted mastoids. Third, the procedure eliminates the problem of residual disease in the mastoid (providing the meatus is large and the cavity can be readily visualized postoperatively). The fourth advantage concerns the nature of the disease present; attic and posterior superior quadrant cholesteatomas lend themselves to this type of procedure where the drum membrane has a tendency to retract toward the medial wall of the middle ear and attic.

However, this technique has no advantage concerning middle ear residual cholesteatoma. With a grafted tympanic membrane, the middle ear is closed to the environment, although the mastoid cavity is exteriorized. Middle ear disease may present as much of a problem with wall down tympanoplasty as with the intact technique.

## Intact Canal Wall Tympanoplasty

The advocates of the intact canal wall tympanoplasty[43-46] contend that in the majority of cases cholesteatoma can be satisfactorily removed from the mastoid and middle ear with the posterior ear canal wall in place. They also feel that with exposure of the facial recess[43] (a triangular area bounded by the fossa incudus, facial and chorda tympani nerves) and attic from behind, the middle ear is accessible for removal of cholesteatoma. The postoperative result is a more normal ear anatomically and functionally, with an intact ear canal and tympanic membrane. With this type of functional result the patient can participate in active water sports and does not need to keep water from the ear.

Admittedly there are some disadvantages to this procedure. First, the technique itself is difficult to perform and requires special training; in addition, it is not routinely taught in most residency programs but is available through a number of temporal bone dissection courses offered several times a year in different parts of the country. Without proper training and careful selection of cases, the postoperative results will be poor.

The second disadvantage is the continual risk of residual disease in the mastoid and attic. One must remember that residual disease is likewise a hazard with canal wall down tympanoplasty, though less frequent.

Third, recurrent attic and posterior-superior quadrant retraction cholesteatomas are more frequent with this technique. However, when properly performed in the hands of a surgeon trained in its use, the intact canal wall procedure can produce a very satisfactory functional result.

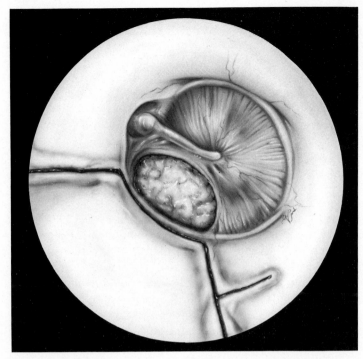

**Figure 16–9**  This illustration demonstrates the vascular strip incisions in the ear canal. Note the cholesteatoma debris in the middle ear as seen through the posterior-superior perforation. (Figs. 16–9 to 16–18 from Glasscock, M. E., III, and Miller, G. W.: Intact canal wall tympanoplasty in the management of cholesteatoma. Laryngoscope 86:1639–1657, 1976.)

The technique is as follows: The ear is prepared and draped in the usual manner and then the external canal is injected by the scrub nurse with Xylocaine with 1:100,000 epinephrine. A vascular strip incision is made as described in Chapter 15, and inferior and superior flaps are created (Fig. 16–9). Next, the postauricular incision is made about 5 mm. behind the fold (Fig. 16–10). By the time the incision is

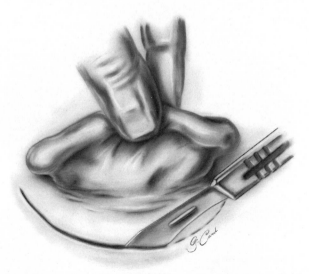

**Figure 16–10**  A routine postauricular incision is made about 5 mm. behind the postauricular fold.

made (10 minutes) the epinephrine has had time to become effective, and there is very little bleeding. A bovie is used to control any hemorrhage that might occur. A self-retaining retractor is inserted, and the areolar tissue overlying the temporalis fascia is taken for the grafting material (Fig. 16–11).

Tension is put on the auricle during the incision by pulling away from the head. This creates an avascular plane above the actual fascia as well as a layer of areolar tissue. By injecting this tissue with anesthetic solution it balloons up so a large piece can be readily removed. This is squeezed out on a Teflon block and placed under a gooseneck lamp on the back table.

Next a T-shaped incision is made in the subcutaneous tissue of the postauricular area, allowing the auricle and vascular strip to be lifted forward (Fig. 16–12) exposing the external auditory canal. The self-retaining retractor is reinserted to hold the vascular strip and auricle out of the surgeon's way, thus eliminating the need for a speculum holder and allowing the surgeon to see all areas of the middle ear. With the aid of the Zeiss operating microscope, irrigation suction and a dental-type drill, a simple mastoidectomy is performed (Fig. 16–13).

It is important to identify the middle fossa dura and the sigmoid sinus immediately after removing the cortex. Next the antrum is entered, and the cholesteatoma sac is usually encountered. It is opened and the contents evacuated (Fig. 16–13). The matrix is dissected free of the antrum, taking care to look for fistulas of the posterior horizontal and superior semicircular canals. The incus is identified (if present) and the facial recess opened (Fig. 16–14). As the incus and malleus head frequently are engulfed in cholesteatoma, it then becomes necessary to remove the ossicles in order to ensure complete removal of the disease. This is especially important when there is cholesteatoma anterior to the head of the malleus in the attic. First, the incudostapedial joint is disarticulated under direct vision and the incus extracted (Fig. 16–15). This allows the surgeon to further open the facial recess, remove the head of the malleus, and drill deeper into the root of the zygoma,

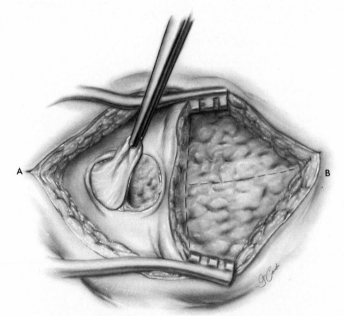

**Figure 16–11**  *A*, Superficial areolar tissue is removed from the temporalis fascia and put aside to be used later as a grafting material. *B*, A "T" shaped incision is made in the soft tissue over the mastoid.

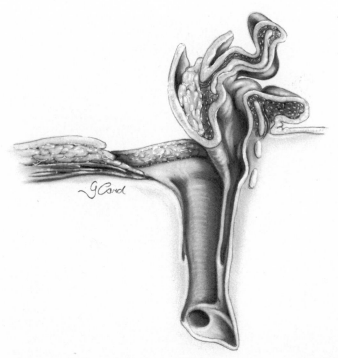

**Figure 16–12**  The vascular strip is elevated out of the ear canal and held in place with a Weitlaner retractor.

exposing the anterior attic area (Fig. 16–16). With this exposure and by working down the ear canal, in the majority of cases the surgeon can gain a very adequate view of the middle ear. Cholesteatoma is removed from the middle ear cleft along with diseased mucosa, and the undersurface of the annulus is denuded of mucosa. The ear canal flaps are created as previously described in Chapter 15 in the discussion of myringoplasty. If the perforation is limited to the posterior-superior

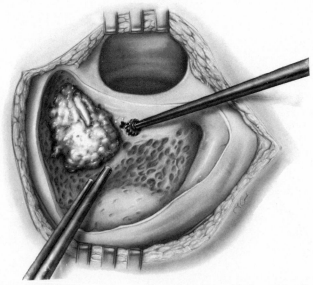

**Figure 16–13**  A simple mastoidectomy is performed, with the aid of a pneumatic drill and irrigation suction. Note the cholesteatoma lying in the antrum.

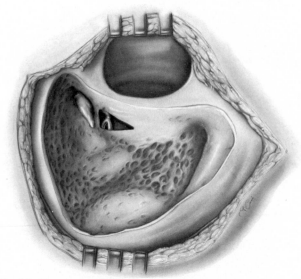

**Figure 16–14**   In this illustration the cholesteatoma debris and matrix have been removed from the antrum, and the facial recess has been opened.

quadrant, as in Figure 16–17, the normal drum remnant is preserved and the fascial graft placed under the remnant, supported by Gelfoam in the middle ear (Figs. 16–17 and 16–18). If the drum is absent or diseased, a total graft replacement is carried out, placing the fascia medial to the malleus handle and annulus. In some cholesteatomas it is not unusual to have large bony defects of the lateral attic wall and posterior canal. If these are not repaired, they create a condition for recurrence of the original problem. Tragal autogenous or septal homograft cartilage can be used successfully to bridge these areas and give support in the postoperative period.

The junior author stages all cases of cholesteatoma; therefore the ossicular chain

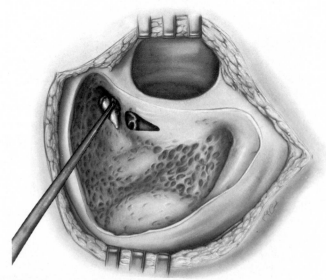

**Figure 16–15**   Once the incudostapedial joint has been disarticulated, a right angle hook is used to remove the incus.

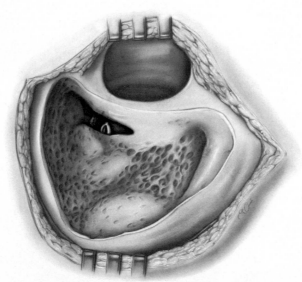

**Figure 16–16**  In this illustration the facial recess has been made continuous with the attic for better exposure of the oval window area.

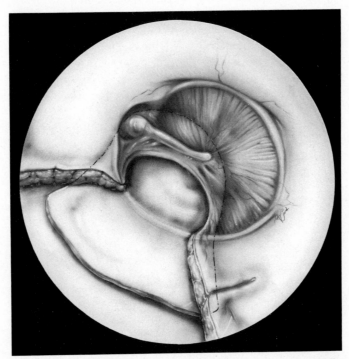

**Figure 16–17**  After all the cholesteatoma matrix has been removed, the middle ear is filled with Gelfoam, and the fascia graft is placed under the drum remnant and back over the posterior canal wall.

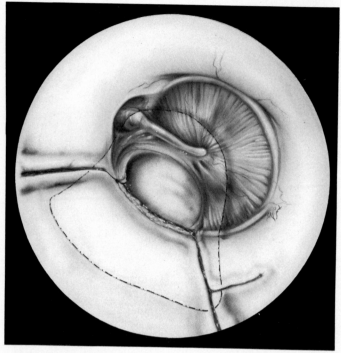

**Figure 16–18**   The vascular strip is put back into place and the ear canal filled with an antibiotic ointment. The postauricular incision is closed with subcuticular sutures.

is not reconstructed at the initial surgery. Many surgeons, however, perform primary ossicular reconstruction and usually do this before the graft is put into position. Depending upon the mucosal status, silastic sheeting is commonly used, from the eustachian tube orifice through the middle ear and facial recess into the attic and mastoid cavity.

The osteoplastic epitympanotomy developed by Sabina Wullstein[47] combines the advantage of wide surgical exposure of cholesteatoma in the attic and antrum with replacement of the superior bony canal wall to produce a normal external meatus. A similar technique had been advocated by Guilford[37] shortly before his untimely death.

Sabina Wullstein's method begins with wide exposure of the bone above and

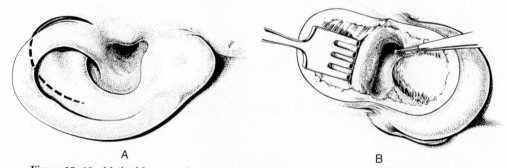

A                                                              B

**Figure 16–19**   Method for osteoplastic epitympanotomy developed by Sabina Wullstein. *A*, A curved incision is made above the auricle, which is turned downward. *B*, The bony superior and posterior meatal wall is thinned. (Figs. 16–19 to 16–22 courtesy of Dr. Sabina Wullstein.)

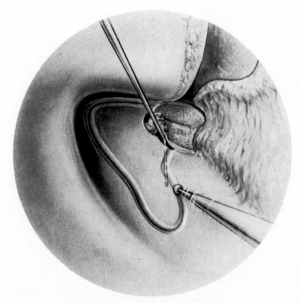

**Figure 16–20**   A lid of bone that will be removed is outlined with a fine diamond burr.

behind the external meatus. She uses a curved incision above the auricle, which is turned downward (Fig. 16–19). The usual endaural incision as described in Chapter 6 has been employed by the senior author for this operation. The meatal skin is separated from the superior and posterior bony wall as far as the notch of Rivinus. The bony superior and posterior meatal wall is thinned, thus enlarging the bony meatus, but not enough to enter air cells of the epitympanum and antrum (Fig. 16–19*B*). A lid of bone that will be removed is outlined with a fine diamond burr (Fig. 16–20) and deepened until the lid can be broken loose and lifted out (Fig. 16–21). The wide exposure of the attic and antrum and of the upper part of the

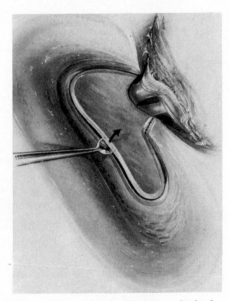

**Figure 16–21**   The outline is deepened until the lid can be broken loose and lifted out.

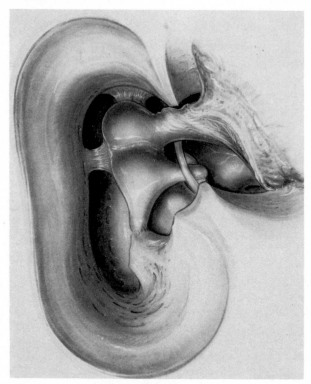

**Figure 16–22**   Wide exposure of the attic and antrum and upper part of the tympanic cavity seen through the operating microscope.

tympanic cavity thus achieved is seen through the operating microscope in Figure 16–22. Meticulous removal of all cholesteatoma matrix with whatever ossicular reconstruction is indicated is followed by replacement of the bony lid. A large fascial graft closes the tympanic membrane perforation and extends upward to cover the replaced superior bony meatal wall. The meatal skin is then replaced over the fascia and bony lid. In over 300 epitympanotomies by Sabina Wullstein and residents working under her direction, there was not one rejection of the replaced bony superior meatal wall. Advantages of this method include the wide surgical exposure of pathology in the attic, antrum and tympanum, with access to the facial recess, sinus tympani and eustachian tube. The senior author has had occasion to use this approach via an endaural incision in several cases with satisfactory results.

## COMPLICATIONS

The complications associated with tympanoplasty are usually the result of two factors: first, the extent of destruction caused by the disease, exposing vital structures to injury, and second, surgical accidents. These include either dead ears or vertigo caused by inadvertently uncapping a fistula of the horizontal canal or oval window. This complication is the result both of the disease itself (the fistula) and of a surgical accident in which the matrix was inadvertently removed before the presence of the fistula was known to the surgeon.

In like manner, facial nerve injuries usually occur when the nerve has been exposed by cholesteatoma or granulation tissue and no longer has its bony fallopian canal to protect it from the surgeon's knife or drill, and when disease or previous operation has distorted landmarks.

Some complications have to do with the type of technique employed. For instance, lateralization and anterior blunting of the graft occur most commonly with the overlay technique, as does stenosis of the external auditory canal.

Postoperative infections are considered a complication and can be due to poor aseptic technique or to the presence of bacteria in the ear at the time of surgery.

Graft failure is a complication that is often associated with postoperative infection. Faulty undersurface grafting technique will often result in graft failure.

Most complications can be prevented by paying careful attention to aseptic technique and anatomical landmarks and by exercising good clinical judgment throughout the operative procedure. However, even in the most capable hands, a certain percentage of complications will occur. It is important to recognize complications when present and to be prepared to deal with them in an expeditious and judicious manner.

## RESULTS

The two goals of tympanoplasty are to eliminate disease and to improve hearing. The results of tympanoplasty are measured in terms of success or failure of graft take and hearing improvement. In order to obtain a fair assessment of the success of chronic ear surgery it is best to separate the benign central perforation from cholesteatoma cases and atelectatic ears. Individuals with benign perforations and simple ossicular chain deficits (M+S+) have a very good to excellent chance of obtaining a dry ear with a hearing level within normal range. Such a patient should have a 96 to 97 per cent[43] chance for a good graft take and an 85 to 90 per cent[35] chance for a hearing gain to within 20 decibels of his bone level.

However, what of the individual with cholesteatoma, severe mucosal disease, poor eustachian tube function and total loss of the ossicular chain (M−S−)? As a group these patients will not fare as well. Some of the ears will do satisfactorily and others will not, depending upon the extent of disease present at the time of surgery and the manner in which the disease is managed. It must be remembered that a tympanoplasty may be considered partially successful if a dry, intact ear is obtained regardless of whether there is any hearing improvement.

In dealing with cholesteatoma cases, one must have a long follow-up period before results can be considered valid. Reports should not be made with anything less than five years' postoperative observation. In the junior author's experience, recurrent attic retraction cholesteatoma is a major problem and occurs in 14 per cent of his cases.[46] Residual disease can be controlled to some extent by staging or second-look surgery. In the junior author's hands the overall incidence of residual disease is 12 per cent, 7 per cent of which is unsuspected at the time of the second stage. The remaining 5 per cent was known to be present because it was left at the original operation. If one considers that most residual disease will be found at the second stage, then the real problem lies in the 14 per cent who have a recurrence. Some authors[43, 44] report less of an incidence of recurrent and residual cholesteatoma for canal up operations, while others report more.[40]

Ossicular reconstruction results are directly proportional to the amount of damage to the ossicles. In other words, Type A ears (M+S+) will have better results (85–90 per cent)[33] than Type D ears (M−S−) (60–70 per cent).[33] T.O.R.P. and

P.O.R.P. prostheses may influence these figures, but to date they have not been used long enough to prove their true value.

Those individuals with atelectatic ears and poor eustachian tube function will not do well unless something can be accomplished to aerate the middle ear. Tympanoplasty with a Wright eustachian tube prosthesis or tympanoplasty followed by a long-standing, indwelling ventilating tube is sometimes the answer.

The results of tympanoplasty have improved, so that, in the majority of cases, it is a reasonable procedure to recommend. The techniques practiced today have changed considerably from those advocated in the early 1950's. However, there remain many problems. Until the otologic surgeon can obtain a functional, dry ear in over 90 per cent of his cases of all types of disease, then tympanoplasty must still be improved. It is hoped that our best tympanoplasty results today will be considered inadequate 25 years from now.

## REFERENCES

1. Wullstein, H.: Die Tympanoplastik als gehörverbessernde Operation bei Otitis Media chronica und ihr Resultate. Proc. Fifth Internat. Congress Oto-Rhino-Laryng., 1953, p. 104.
2. Kessel, J.: Über das Mobilisieren des Steigbügels durch Ausschneiden des Trommelfelles, Hammers und Amboss bei undurchgängigkeit der Tuba. Arch. Ohrenh., 13:69, 1878.
3. Berthold, E.: Ueber Myringoplastik. Wein. med. Bl., 1:1627, 1878.
4. Kiesselbach, W.: Versuch zur Anlegung eines äusseren Gehörganges bei angeborener Missbildung beider Ohrmuscheln mit Fehlen der äusseren Gehörgänge. Arch. Ohrenh., 19:127, 1882.
5. Helmholtz, H. L. F.: Die Mechanik der Gehörknöchelchen und des Trommelfelles. Pflügers Arch. ges. Physiol., 1:1, 1868.
6. Boucheron, E.: La mobilisation de l'étrier et son procédé operatoire. Union méd., Paris, 46:412, 1888.
7. Miot, C.: De la mobilisation de l'étrier. Rev. laryng., 10:49, 83, 113, 145, 200, 1890.
8. Kerrison, P. D.: Diseases of the Ear. 4th ed. Philadelphia, J. B. Lippincott Co., 1930.
9. Ballance, C. A.: Surgery of the Temporal Bone. New York, The Macmillan Co., 1919.
10. Schwartze, H. H., and Eysell C. G.: Ueber die künstliche Eröffnung des Warzenfortsatzes. Arch. Ohrenh., 7:157, 1873.
11. Küster, E.: Ueber die Grundsätze der Behandlung von Eiterungen in starrwandigen Höhlen, mit besonderer Berücksichtigung des Empyems der Pleura. Deutsche med. Wchnschr., 15:254, 1889.
12. Zaufal, E.: Technik des Trepanation des Proc. mastoid nach Küsterschen Grundsätzen. Arch. Ohrenh., 30:291, 1890.
13. Stacke, L.: Stacke's Operationsmethode. Arch. Ohrenh., 35:145, 1893.
14. Holmgren, G.: Some experiences in surgery for otosclerosis. Acta oto-laryng., 5:460, 1923.
15. Nylén, C. O.: The microscope in aural surgery, its first use and later development. Acta oto-laryng., Suppl. 116, 1954.
16. Sourdille, M.: New technique in the surgical treatment of severe and progressive deafness from otosclerosis. Bull. New York Acad. Med., 13:673, 1937.
17. Lempert, J.: Improvement of hearing in cases of otosclerosis: new one-stage surgical technic. Arch. Otolaryng., 28:42, 1938.
18. Pattee, G. L.: An operation to improve hearing in cases of congenital atresia of the external auditory meatus. Arch. Otolaryng., 45:568, 1947.
19. Ombrédanne, M.: Surgery of deafness: fenestration in cases of congenital atresia of the external auditory canal. Oto-rhino-laryng. internat., 13:229, 1947.
20. Rosen, S.: Mobilization of the stapes to restore hearing in otosclerosis. New York J. Med., 53:2650, 1953.
21. Juers, A. L.: Observations on bone conduction in fenestrated cases. Ann. Otol. Rhin. & Laryng., 57:28, 1948.
22. Davis, H., and Walsh, T. E.: The limits of improvement of hearing following the fenestration operation. Laryngoscope, 60:273, 1950.
23. Moritz, W.: Hörverbessernde Operationen bei chronisch-entzündlichen Prozessen beider Mittelohren. Ztschr. Laryng. Rhin. Otol., 29:578, 1950.
24. Zöllner, F.: Die Radikal-Operation mit besonderem Bezug auf die Hörfunktion. Ztschr. Laryng. Rhin. Otol., 30:104, 1951.
25. Wullstein, H.: Funktionelle Operationen im Mittelohr mit Hilfe des freien Spaltlappen-Transplantates. Arch. Ohren- Nasen- u. Kehlkopfh., 161:422, 1952.

26. Kley, W., and Dra, F. W.: Histologic studies of autotransplanted ossicles and bone in the human middle ear. Acta oto-laryng., 59:593, 1965.
27. Hall, A., and Rytzner, C.: Stapedectomy and autotransplantation of ossicles. Acta oto-laryng., 47:318, 1957.
28. House, W. F., Patterson, M. E., and Linthicum, F. H.: Incus homografts in chronic ear surgery. Arch. Otol., 84:148, 1966.
29. Shea, J. J., and Homsy, C. A.: The use of proplast in otologic surgery. Laryngoscope, 84:1835, 1974.
30. Schmitt, H.: Über die Bedeutung der Schalldrucktransformation und der Schallprotektion für Hörschwelle. Acta oto-laryng., 49:71, 1957.
31. Committee on Conservation of Hearing, American Academy of Ophthalmology and Otolaryngology: Standard classification for surgery of chronic ear disease. Arch Otol., 81:204, 1965.
32. Wright, J. W., III, and Wright, J. W., Jr.: The eustachian tube prosthesis revisited. Otolaryngology, 86:834–837, 1978.
33. Austin, D. F.: Ossicular reconstruction. Arch. Otol., 94:525, 1971.
34. Guilford, F. R.: Repositioning of the incus. Laryngoscope, 75:236, 1965.
35. Pennington, C. L.: Incus interposition techniques. Ann. Otol. Rhinol., & Laryng., 82:518, 1973.
36. Derlacki, E. L., Harrison, W. H., and Clemis, J. D.: Congenital cholesteatoma of middle ear and mastoid: A second report presenting seven additional cases. Laryngoscope, 78:1050, 1968.
37. Guilford, F. R.: Personal communication.
38. Wullstein, S. R.: The surgical principles in cholesteatoma surgery. In Proceedings of the Shambaugh Fifth International Workshop on Middle Ear Microsurgery and Fluctuant Hearing Loss. Huntsville, Alabama, Strode Publishers, Inc., 1976, pp. 169–172.
39. Smythe, G. D. L.: Postoperative cholesteatoma in combined approach tympanoplasty. J. Laryng. Otol., 90:597, 1976.
40. Cody, D. T. R.: Personal communication.
41. Austin, D. F.: The retraction pocket in the treatment of cholesteatoma. Arch. Otol., 102:741, 1976.
42. Palva, T.: Mastoid obliteration. Arch. Otol., 101:271, 1975.
43. Jansen, C. L.: The combined approach for tympanoplasty. J. Laryng. Otol., 82:776, 1968.
44. Sheehy, J. L. and Patterson, M. E.: Intact canal wall tympanoplasty with mastoidectomy. Laryngoscope, 77:1502, 1967.
45. Wright, W. K.: Management of otitic cholesteatomas. Arch. Otol., 103:144, 1977.
46. Glasscock, M. E., and Miller, G. W.: Intact canal wall tympanoplasty in the management of cholesteatoma. Laryngoscope, 86:1639, 1976.
47. Wullstein, S. R.: Osteoplastic epitympanotomy. Ann. Otol. Rhinol. & Laryng., 83:663, 1974.

## SUGGESTED ADDITIONAL READING

Garcia-Ibánez, L.: Sonoinversion: A new audiosurgical system. Arch. Otol., 73:268, 1961.
Stevenson, E. W.: Conduction of sound by a round-window columella. Arch. Otol., 74:81, 1961.
Rambo, J. H. T.: The use of paraffin to create a middle ear space in musculoplasty. Laryngoscope, 71:612, 1961.
Ruggles, R. L., and Smith, K. P.: Tube graft tympanoplasty. Laryngoscope, 73:512, 1963.
Plester, D.: Problems of tympanoplasty. J. Laryng. & Otol., 75:879, 1961.
Wullstein, H.: Tympanoplasty today. Arch. Otol., 76:295, 1962.
Zöllner, F.: The prognosis of the operative improvement of hearing in chronic middle ear infections. Ann. Otol. Rhin. & Laryng., 66:907, 1957.
Joseph, R. B.: The effect of absorbable gelatin sponge preparations and other agents on scar formation in the dog's middle ear. Laryngoscope, 72:1528, 1962.
Doyle-Kelly, W.: Behavior of absorbable gelatin sponge in the animal middle ear. J. Laryng. & Otol., 75:152, 1962.
Guilford, F. R., and Wright, W. K.: Basic techniques in myringoplasty and tympanoplasty. Laryngoscope, 68:825, 1958.

## Joseph Toynbee

BORN 1815
DIED 1866

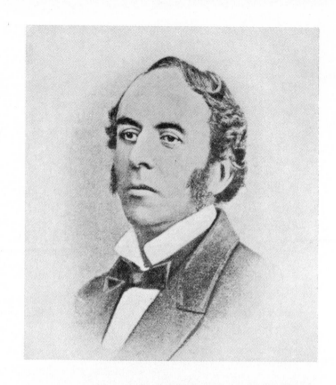

Demonstrated by anatomic dissections the common occurrence of stapes ankylosis as a cause of deafness.

## Lucius Rüedi

BORN 1900

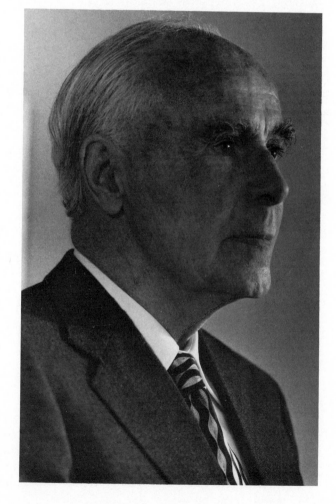

Leading histopathologist of the otosclerotic bone lesion and authority on the mechanism of sensorineural loss in cochlear otosclerosis.

# Chapter 17

# Diagnosis, Indications for Surgery and Medical Therapy of Otospongiosis (Otosclerosis)

HISTORICAL ASPECTS
GROSS PATHOLOGY OF OTOSPONGIOSIS
MICROSCOPIC PATHOLOGY OF OTOSPONGIOSIS
ETIOLOGY OF OTOSPONGIOSIS
NATURAL HISTORY OF THE OTOSPONGIOTIC LESION
DIAGNOSIS OF OTOSPONGIOSIS
SELECTION OF CASES FOR SURGERY
MEDICAL TREATMENT OF OTOSPONGIOSIS

Otospongiosis (otosclerosis) is the primary focal spongifying disease of the labyrinthine capsule. In the majority of cases, it remains symptomless and silent. In about 12 per cent of cases, it invades the oval window, causing fixation of the stapes. In some cases, it is associated with and presumably causes cochlear degeneration alone. In many cases of stapes fixation, cochlear degeneration disproportionate to the patient's age precedes, accompanies or follows some years after fixation of the stapes.

## HISTORICAL ASPECTS

Ankylosis of the stapes to the margins of the oval window was described by Valsalva[1] in 1735, on autopsy of a deaf patient. During the next century and a half, other reports appeared in the literature of stapes ankylosis discovered at autopsy in deaf patients, the most noteworthy report being that of Toynbee[2] in 1841, who

**455**

concluded, on the basis of 1659 ear dissections, that "osseous ankylosis of the stapes to the fenestra ovalis was one of the common causes of deafness."

The term "sclerosis" was first applied to stapes ankylosis by von Tröltsch[3] in 1881, in the belief that sclerosing changes in the tympanic mucosa were the cause of the stapes fixation.

How mistaken this view was became evident when Politzer[4] in 1893 described the histologic findings in sixteen cases of stapes fixation that he had examined during life. He concluded that "deafness that had previously been attributed to interstitial middle ear catarrh with secondary stapes ankylosis **is in reality a primary disease of the labyrinthine capsule.**"

Bezold, Siebenmann and others soon confirmed Politzer's revolutionary view, and Siebenmann[5] proposed that the correct name of otospongiosis should replace the misnomer "otosclerosis," since the diseased bone is more porous and less dense than the normal capsule that it replaces. Popular usage, however, except in France, has continued to employ the misnomer "otosclerosis" for this spongifying disease of the labyrinthine capsule. Now that medical therapy is available to promote recalcification and inactivation of an otospongiotic focus, there is added need to use the correct name, recognizing that the normal labyrinthine capsule is already of maximum density and cannot become more sclerotic.

## GROSS PATHOLOGY OF OTOSPONGIOSIS

The operating microscope enabled the fenestration surgeon to view the otospongiotic focus in the living patient for the first time, while its gross appearance in the oval window niche became familiar to the stapedectomy microsurgeon.

The **mature**, inactive otospongiotic focus as seen through the operating microscope contrasts with the slightly yellowish normal capsule by its whiter, chalk-like color, as well as by the distortion of the normal anatomy of the oval window niche. An **immature**, active otospongiotic focus will be covered by thickened vascular mucosa, giving a pinkish hue to the promontory (known as the Schwartze sign) when viewed through a normally translucent tympanic membrane.

The size of the otospongiotic focus observed during stapedectomy varies from a few millimeters, confined to the site of predilection just in front of the oval window, to an extensive focus involving most or all of the promontory and narrowing, but rarely obliterating, the round window niche. At first, a small focus fixes the footplate by impaction as it is pushed backward by the expanding lesion. Stapes mobilization has restored hearing lasting many years in some of such cases. In larger involvements, the spongiotic bone has invaded the upper and lower edges of the footplate from the site of predilection, producing a "lobster-claw" fixation. Less common is the surgically favorable situation of a primary focus beginning in and confined to the footplate, which then has a biscuit-like appearance without extension to the walls of the oval window. Stapedectomy can extract such a focus entirely, truly "curing" the disease provided other foci are not present elsewhere in the capsule. A less favorable situation is obliteration of the oval window niche by extensive otospongiosis requiring a drill-out to open the oval window. Least surgically favorable is a large focus narrowing or obliterating the oval window, and covered by thickened vascular mucosa, indicating a very active lesion likely to reclose the oval window after stapedectomy unless the patient has been pretreated with fluoride. The rare case of round window closure with stapes fixation requires special consideration under selection of cases for surgery.

## MICROSCOPIC PATHOLOGY OF OTOSPONGIOSIS

By light microscopy of hematoxylin-eosin–stained sections of the temporal bone, the active otospongiotic focus stains more deeply than the normal capsule around it. The otospongiotic focus lacks the islands of calcified cartilage that characterize the endochondral bone of the capsule in which it originates. The new pathologic bone varies from a loose spongy structure of irregularly arranged lamellae of bone separated by wide vascular spaces containing many histiocytes and osteoblasts, and some osteoclasts in the case of an immature active focus, to a denser structure of mature inactive bone with fewer cells, narrower vascular spaces and smaller blood vessels (Fig. 17–1). A single focus may show areas of varying activity, but as a general rule the degree of remodeling activity tends toward uniformity in an ear, and in both ears of an individual.

The slightly irregular, sharply defined margins of an otospongiotic focus may show finger-like projections along blood vessels into the surrounding normal capsule. A border or "mantle" of blue-staining bone may be seen around such vessels; these "blue mantles"[6] are believed to represent the earliest stage of the otospongiotic process. Small irregular areas of new bone formation near an active focus have been likened to "splashing" of bone-resorbing enzymes from the expanding focus.

In 80 to 90 per cent of ears with otospongiosis, a focus is found at the "site of predilection" just in front of the oval window. The next most frequent site for a focus is the border of the round window niche, found in 30 to 50 per cent of ears with the disease. The stapes footplate itself is next in frequency as the site of a primary focus, while an otospongiotic focus may be in the wall of the internal auditory canal, or less often, around a semicircular canal. About half the ears with the disease have a single

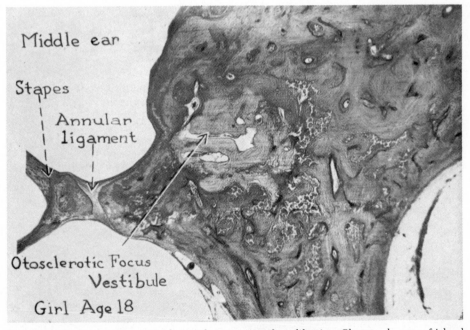

**Figure 17–1**  Small mature otosclerotic focus at site of predilection. Observe absence of islands of ossified cartilage in the focus. No evidence of activity. Such a focus of histologic otosclerosis without symptoms may be found at autopsy in about 10 per cent of white adults.

focus; half show two or more separate foci. In 70 to 85 per cent of cases, both ears of an individual are involved, with a tendency toward symmetry in size, location and histologic structure of the lesions.

A focus of otospongiosis always begins in the ivory-hard avascular endochondral bone of the labyrinthine capsule. As it expands, it can reach the oval window, fixing the stapes (Fig. 17–2) as well as the periosteum of the tympanic cavity, which becomes thickened and hyperemic in the active phase, imparting a positive Schwartze sign. An enlarging focus can reach the endosteum of the vestibule, semicircular canals or cochlea, causing thickening of the endosteal membrane and the formation of new abnormal vascular connections, "shunts," between the blood supply of the capsule and that of the cochlea (See Fig. 17–6A and B).

The large series of cases of otospongiosis studied by Guild,[7] and by Rüedi and Spoendlin[8] are instructive. In 1161 routine autopsies, Guild sectioned the temporal bones and found one or more foci of otospongiosis in 49. Under the age of five, only 0.6 per cent of autopsies revealed the disease. The incidence increased progressively with age until by late middle age 9.7 per cent (nearly 10 per cent) of white males and 18.5 per cent (close to 20 per cent) of white females had the disease. Guild classified the spongiotic lesions as active in 50 per cent of ears and inactive in 50 per cent, with active foci somewhat less often (in one third of ears) after the age of fifty.

Rüedi and Spoendlin divided eighty-eight ears with otospongiosis into five degrees of activity. Both active and inactive lesions occur at all ages, but high degrees of activity are more common under the age of fifty, while very low activity is much more common after the age of seventy. There is, thus, a mild tendency, neither strong nor consistent, for otospongiosis to become less active with advancing years. As we shall see, it is in the hope of promoting or encouraging this natural tendency that sodium fluoride treatment is recommended.

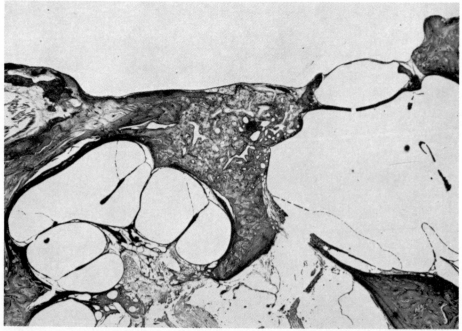

**Figure 17–2**     Stapedial moderately active otospongiosis with ankylosis of the anterior end of the stapes footplate in a patient in whom fenestration was successful but who died of multiple myeloma 2 years later.

A peculiarity of otospongiotic bone emphasized by Schuknecht[9] is that, unlike neoplasms, the lesion tends to conform to the original endochondral structure of the temporal bone. The senior author in his experience of thousands of fenestration operations observed an otospongiotic focus of the dome of the horizontal semicircular canal in 3 per cent of fenestrations. The enlarged lateral surface of the bony canal in such cases was covered with velvety thickened vascular mucosa. As the bony canal was enchondralized with the diamond burr under the operating microscope, the otospongiotic bone was clearly chalk-white, more friable and sometimes more vascular than the normal endochondral capsule from which it was sharply demarcated. The normally delicate endosteum was thickened and leathery where the focus reached the lumen. In no instance did the focus encroach upon the lumen of the horizontal semicircular canal.

Involvement of the wall of the fallopian aqueduct by otospongiosis is extremely common, yet, following Schuknecht's dictum, the lumen of the facial canal is not appreciably narrowed and facial weakness is not observed.

When otospongiosis reaches the endosteum of the cochlea, lamellae of new bone tend to be laid down along the spiral ligament, while the scala tympani in a few cases may be invaded and even obliterated by lamellar bone adjacent to the focus. Very rarely does otospongiotic bone project into the cochlea.

## ETIOLOGY OF OTOSPONGIOSIS

Many theories to explain the pathogenesis of this common and unique disease have been proposed. The key to the disease may well lie in the unique embryology and adult structure of the remarkably avascular, stony hard (petrous) endochondral bone of the capsule, which is almost devoid of the bone turnover and remodeling that occurs in all other parts of the skeleton.

Recalling the embryology of the labyrinth as described in Chapter 1, the inner ear, with its sensory end-organs in the semi-circular canals, vestibule and cochlea, attains full size and differentiation by midterm. This precocious maturation of the inner ear is required before ossification of the cartilaginous capsule occurs, for once the otic capsule is ossified, the rigidly encased inner ear can grow no further.

Ossification of the labyrinthine capsule occurs rapidly from fourteen centers between the sixteenth and twenty-third weeks of fetal life, until there remains only a narrow rim of cartilage around the annular ligament of the stapes footplate, a small area of cartilage yet to be ossified over the horizontal semicircular canal, and a rim of cartilage surrounding an irregularly shaped fissure filled with connective tissue, extending from the vestibule to the middle ear. This was named the "fissula ante fenestram" by Siebenmann, its discoverer (Fig. 17–3). As ossification of the primitive cartilaginous capsule is completed to form the endochondral capsule, a thin uniform layer of endosteal bone is laid down by the endosteum lining the labyrinth, while a much thicker layer of periosteal bone begins to be laid down outside of the endochondral capsule. Like periosteal bone elsewhere and quite unlike the endochondral capsule, active remodeling of the periosteal layer proceeds to form haversian bone with marrow spaces. Then, beginning just before birth and continuing into middle adult life, pneumatization of the periosteal layer proceeds by invasion of air cells from the typanic cavity.

The auditory ossicles and the endochondral labyrinthine capsule retain primitive endochondral bone throughout the life of the individual. Everywhere else in the skeleton, as in the ends of the long bones, endochondral bone initially formed in

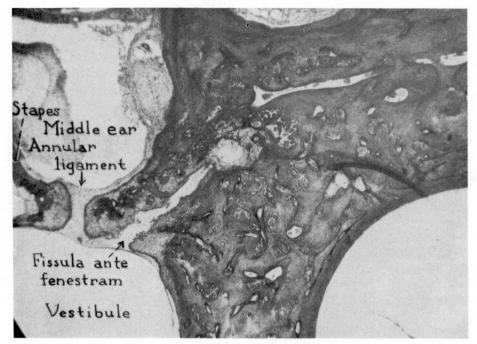

Stapes
  Middle ear
  Annular
    ligament

Fissula ante
fenestram

Vestibule

**Figure 17–3**   Fissula ante fenestram believed by Perozzi, Anson and Bast to be related to otosclerotic foci. In this section the vestibular orifice of fissula is seen but not the tympanic.

cartilage is soon removed and replaced by periosteal bone, where bone turnover and remodeling continue, though at a gradually diminishing pace, into old age.

Why does the primitive endochondral labyrinthine capsule persist unchanged from before birth until old age? Perhaps to maintain the configuration of the cochlea, vestibule and semi-circular canals with their contained sensory end-organs. A more compelling reason is that the unchanged capsule protects the inner ear fluids that bathe the hair cells from contamination by the toxic enzymes of bone resorption, such as collagenase and trypsin. The brilliant research of Chevance, Causse and Bergès[10] demonstrating such enzymes in the perilymph of patients with otospongiosis and with progressive sensory deterioriation lends credence to this idea.

The relative dearth of bone remodeling in the normal endochondral capsule accounts for the observation that fractures through it may remain unhealed for many years. Similarly, fractures of the stapes footplate and stapedial crura show little tendency to heal. The method of "enchondralization of the fenestra" described many years ago by the senior author of this text took advantage of the sluggish osteogenic response of endochondral bone, so that with this microsurgical technique, osseous closure of fenestrae rarely occurred.

It is in the avascular, ivory-hard endochondral bone nearly devoid of bone remodeling, that the pathologic bone of otospongiosis arises. Lindsay,[11] an astute observer of the labyrinthine capsule, notes that osteocytes tend to disappear from the endochondral capsule, leaving empty lacunae. Kakisaki[12] demonstrated an age-related disappearance of living bone cells in the endochondral capsule by age fifteen, corresponding to the frequent age of onset of otospongiosis. Rüedi, too, observed empty lacunae just ahead of the focus of otospongiosis. Thus, the new bone of otospongiosis may simply be nature's response to an area of devitalized bone, removing the dead bone and replacing it with new, vascular periosteal type bone subject to continued bone turnover, like periosteal bone elsewhere. The hydrolytic enzymes produced and liberated by osteoclasts and histiocytes in such a focus dissolve collagen and injure nearby osteocytes, causing such a focus to slowly expand. This attractive theory of pathogenesis was proposed by Rius and Mendoza[13] of Uruguay and Arslan and Ricci[14] of Italy at about the same time, in 1961. The demonstration by Chevance, Bretlau, Jørgensen and Causse[15] of hydrolytic enzymes in the numerous histiocytes of an active focus, with acid phosphatase activity in the periphery of an expanding focus, supports this concept.

The frequently mentioned absence of otospongiosis in domestic and laboratory animals may simply be due to the relative longevity of man. It would be interesting to examine the temporal bones of aging whales, elephants and tortoises where otospongiosis might be expected to occur if this theory of pathogenesis is correct.

Otospongiosis need not have a single etiology, but rather it may be a non-specific reaction to various etiologic factors that promote bone remodeling. Anson, Cauldwell and Bast[16] suggested that the fissula ante fenestram at the site of predilection is an area of instability with late formation in adult life of new cartilage and new bone that might be the start of otospongiosis (Fig. 17–4). Cartilage rests elsewhere in the capsule might account for foci beginning away from the site of predilection.

Puberty, pregnancy and menopause may influence bone turnover and increased activity of a focus of otospongiosis. The risk of increased hearing loss from any one pregnancy in a woman with stapedial otospongiosis, as observed by the senior author, was about one chance in four. A similar effect of birth control pills has been observed.

Osteogenesis imperfecta is so often associated with otospongiosis, the syndrome of van der Hoeve and de Kleijn,[17] that Simpson-Hall and Ogilvie[18] believe that the generalized inherited defect of osteoblasts causing frequent fractures also causes otospongiosis. They suggest that in cases of stapes fixation without fractures, the same defect of osteoblasts is localized to the labyrinthine capsule. Fowler's observation of abnormal blueness of the sclerae in many cases of stapes fixation without fractures supports this notion (Fig. 17–5).

Brief mention should be made of Wittmaack's[19] theory that localized venous congestion in the labyrinthine capsule incites new bone formation, refuted by Rüedi's[20] observation that the reverse seems to occur: the actively expanding focus attracts an increased blood supply (Fig. 17–6A and B).

Sercer[21] held that mechanical stress on the petrous bone by transition from four-legged gait to an upright posture and by growth of the brain and mandible causes spontaneous fractures of the capsule which then heal with the formation of new otospongiotic bone. Rüedi, Kelemen and Linthicum point out that spontaneous microfissures of the capsule do occur, but only rarely at the site of predilection for otospongiosis, while there is little tendency for fractures through the labyrinth ever to heal.

A resemblance between Paget's disease of bone (Fig. 17–7A) and otospongiosis has prompted a theory that the latter may be Paget's disease confined to the temporal bone. However, Valvassori emphasizes that otospongiosis begins in the endochondral capsule and expands outward, while Paget's disease of the temporal bone begins in the periosteal bone outside the capsule, and last of all, extends inward into the endochondral bone. Moreover, stapes fixation in Paget's disease is usually due to

*Text continued on page 465.*

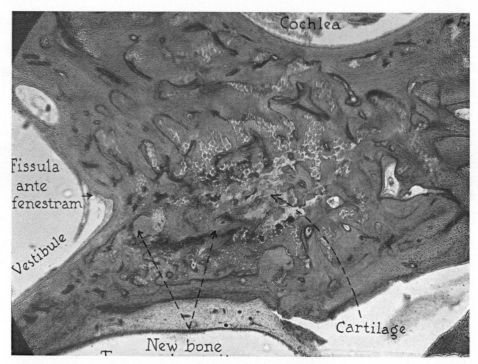

**Figure 17–4**  New bone in the fissular region, which may represent the earliest stage of otosclerosis.

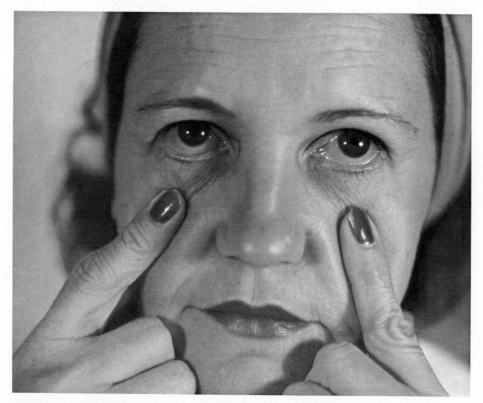

**Figure 17–5**  Patient with van der Hoeve's syndrome, with blue sclerae, recurring fractures and otosclerosis.

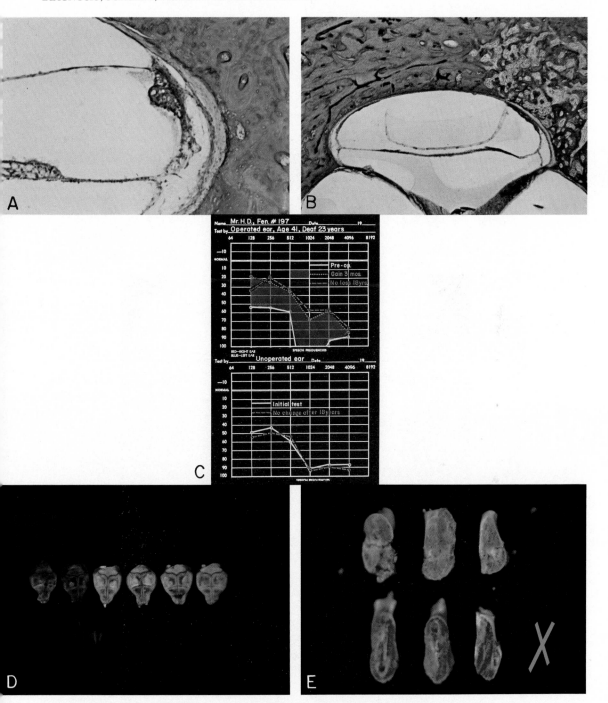

**Figure 17–6** *A*, Female, age 75, new lamellar bone in spiral ligament next to mature focus of otospongiosis with polypoid proliferation of stria vascularis. *B*, Female, age 65, active otospongiosis with enlarged vessels of stria vascularis. (17–6*A* and *B* from Rüedi, L.: Inner ear changes in otosclerosis. Acta. Otol., *57*: 236, 1964.) *C*, Upper audiogram: right ear showing improvement, shaded blue, 3 months and 18 years after fenestration of right ear. Lower audiogram: yellow unoperated ear, at age 41, red at age 59, showing stable high-tone sensorineural loss. Temporal bones showed extensive mature, mostly inactive, otospongiosis of both cochlear capsules. *D*, Calvaria of litter-mate rats, with tetracycline labeling of new bone, as seen under ultraviolet light. Two controls on left did not receive sodium fluoride; two in center received five daily injections of 0.002 mg. sodium fluoride; two on right received larger, less optimal dose of five daily injections of 0.05 mg. of sodium fluoride. *E*, Femurs of litter-mate rats after fracture. Upper row: treated with fluoride, showing calcification of callus after fluoride therapy. Lower row: controls.

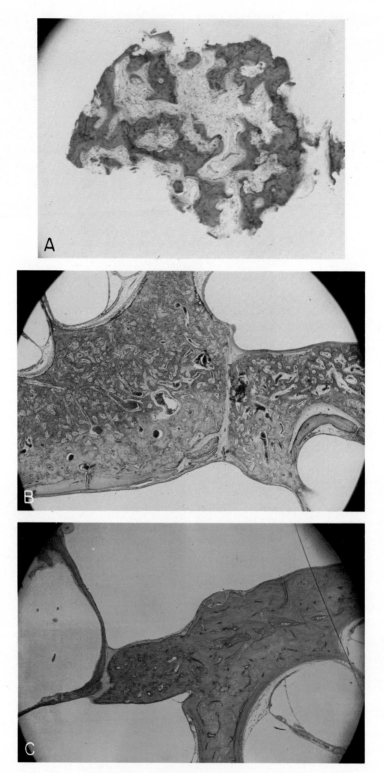

**Figure 17–7**  *A,* Bone from pyramidal process removed during stapes operation for fixation by Paget's disease of skull and long bones. *B,* Otosclerosis of active spongy type at site of predilection involving the stapes footplate resembling Paget's disease in its histologic structure. (Courtesy of L. Rüedi.) *C,* Mature otosclerosis at site of predilection. Sodium fluoride is used to promote recalcification and inactivation of *B* to *C.* (Courtesy of L. Rüedi.)

narrowing of the oval window niche pressing against the stapedial crura, rather than to involvement of the footplate itself. Nevertheless, the vigorous bone remodeling of active otospongiosis resembles the rapid bone turnover of Paget's disease, and both lesions tend to cause progressive sensorineural hearing loss, due presumably to hydrolytic enzymes entering the cochlear fluids.

The strong family incidence must be recognized: 50 per cent of cases of stapedial fixation otospongiosis have one\or more members of the family with the same condition. The impressive racial incidence must also be considered, the disease being common among Indo-Europeans (Caucasoids) but rare among Orientals in China and Japan (Mongoloids) and in American Indians, probably descended from Mongolians that migrated from Siberia to Alaska. Otospongiotic stapes fixation is quite rare among African Negroes and their descendants.

Genetic analysis of families with stapedial otospongiosis has suggested a "monohybrid autosomal dominant inheritance with a penetrance of the pathologic gene in 25 to 40 per cent." However, since stapedial fixation is like an iceberg, with the silent bone disease nearly ten times more frequent than stapedial fixation otospongiosis, final analysis of the true pattern of heredity must await sectioning of the temporal bones of all membranes of otospongiotic families.

The similar audiometric loss usually found in identical twins with stapes fixation is noteworthy, although in rare instances only one twin develops the condition. Finally, the incidence of stapedial otospongiosis by sex has been noted by histopathologists and by clinicians: it occurs nearly twice as often in women as in men. An exception is in India where more men than women seek surgical help, perhaps for cultural and economic reasons.

## NATURAL HISTORY OF THE OTOSPONGIOTIC LESION

Guild's study[7] indicating that the presence of silent histologic otospongiosis (Fig. 17–1) is eight times more frequent than clinical stapes fixation (Fig. 17–2), with the histologic lesion beginning in late childhood and increasing in frequency until middle adulthood, means that the disease begins at least several years before it is clinically manifest. Remember that in most cases the focus matures and becomes inactive before it ever reaches the oval window or the cochlea to produce hearing loss.

The experience of fenestration surgeons with operated patients that need to return annually or more often for cleaning of their fenestration cavities has afforded an unprecedented opportunity to observe the sensorineural component of loss in these cases. Stapedectomy surgeons have less of an opportunity to study the progress of the disease, as successfully operated patients are likely not to follow the advice to return for annual tests of their hearing.

The average age of onset of subjective hearing loss reported to the senior author by 2100 fenestrated patients was twenty years, with a few cases beginning under the age of twelve and a few cases beginning in middle adult life.

Noteworthy in a large series of cases of fenestration has been the eventual development in most, but not all, of progressive sensorineural loss disproportionate to their ages. As these patients are followed audiometrically year after year, the onset of progressive sensorineural loss may begin from several to twenty, thirty or forty years after successful fenestrations, with no increase in the small residual conductive loss always seen after successful fenestrations to suggest fenestral closure.

Polytome examination of the cochlear capsules in such cases usually (but not invariably) will discover a spongiotic lesion in the cochlear capsule. A positive Schwartze sign, increase in tinnitus and sometimes mild intermittent imbalance are additional evidence of an actively expanding focus.

All of these symptoms and findings of activity of the underlying otospongiosis tend not to progress steadily, but rather to progress step-like, with periods of stability alternating with periods of progression.

## DIAGNOSIS OF OTOSPONGIOSIS

It should be recalled that the clinical diagnosis of impaired hearing due to stapes fixation by otospongiosis was hardly ever made in America prior to Lempert's one-stage fenestration operation, so that in the senior author's residency at the Massachusetts Eye and Ear Infirmary from 1930 to 1932 not a single case of stapedial otosclerosis (otospongiosis) was diagnosed in the large outpatient clinic, all cases of conductive hearing loss with intact tympanic membranes and without fluid in the middle ear being diagnosed as "chronic catarrhal otitis media." Notable exceptions

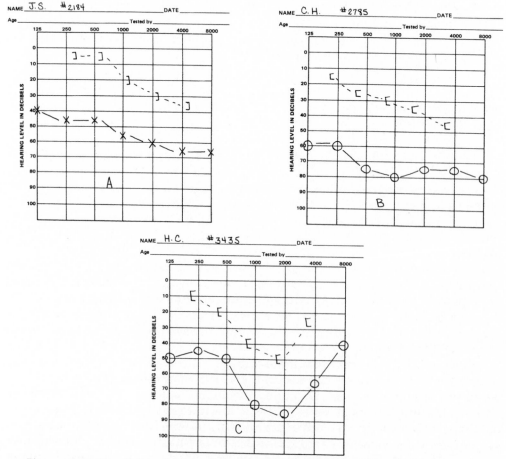

**Figure 17–8**  Stapedial combined with cochlear otosclerosis. *A*, Cochlear loss confined to high frequencies. *B*, Cochlear loss for all frequencies. *C*, "Bite-type" cochlear loss localized to the middle tone range.

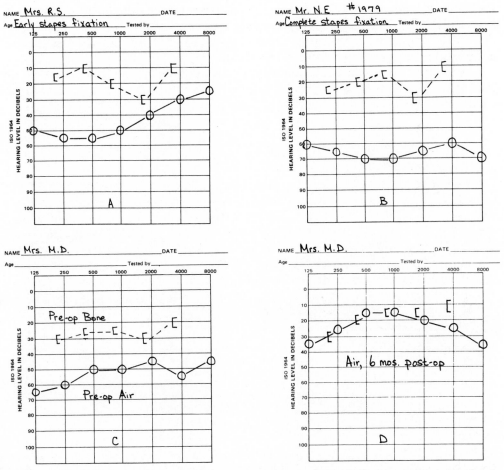

**Figure 17–9** *A,* Audiogram of early otosclerosis showing stiffness tilt. Note Carhart's otosclerotic notch in the bone curve. *B,* Audiogram of advanced stapes fixation showing mass flattening. *C,* Audiogram of clinical otosclerosis. Note Carhart's otosclerotic notch in the bone curve. *D,* Audiogram of the same patient as in *C,* 6 months after stapes mobilization. Note elimination of Carhart's notch in the bone curve.

to the reluctance of clinicians to diagnose primary stapes fixation were Arthur B. Duel and Edmund P. Fowler of New York and J. Gordon Wilson and George Shambaugh, Sr.[22] of Chicago. Only when Lempert's fenestration operation began to be employed, permitting inspection of the oval window during life, was it belatedly recognized that primary fixation of the stapes by osseous changes in the labyrinthine capsule is indeed the most common cause for progressive conductive hearing loss in adults.

The typical case of stapedial otospongiosis will develop a slowly increasing audiometric air–bone gap, confirmed by tuning fork tests with a negative Rinne test, first for the 256 fork, then for 512 and finally, as fixation becomes complete, for the 1024 tuning fork. Bilateral involvement is the rule, but with one side generally preceding the other in the onset and severity of the loss. Varying degrees of sensorineural impairment disproportionate to the patient's age are observed in a majority of patients (Fig. 17–8). The audiometric "otosclerotic Carhart notch" in the audiogram, with a small to moderate dip in the bone conduction audiogram (Fig. 17–10), induced by stapes fixation, must be discounted in assessing the sensorineural

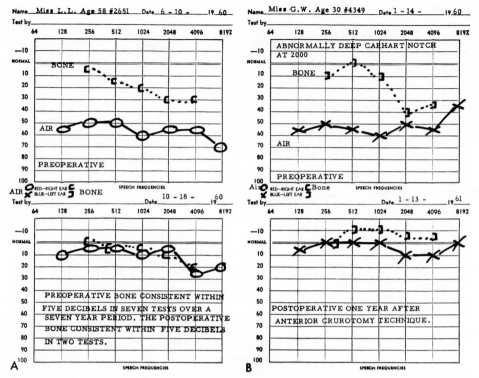

**Figure 17–10** *A*, Unusually large Carhart notch eliminated by stapedectomy. *B*, Abnormally deep Carhart notch at 2048 decibels eliminated by anterior crurotomy. (From Shambaugh, G. E., Jr.,' and Adamson, M.: Bone conduction changes following stapes surgery as related to indications for surgery. Laryngoscope, *74*:513, 1964.)

and conductive components of loss. In all cases, the tuning fork tests to confirm the audiometric air–bone gap should be employed with adequate narrow-band masking of the opposite ear.

Except when there is advanced sensorineural involvement or a superimposed endolymphatic hydrops, speech discrimination remains excellent in stapedial fixation otospongiosis. Tympanometry in the earliest stage of pre-clinical stapes fixation may show an "on-off effect," as described in Chapter 3. The maximum conductive loss of complete stapes fixation is generally around 50 decibels of air–bone gap after correcting the bone curve for Carhart's average notch. A greater air–bone gap suggests ossicular interruption rather than stapes fixation.

Malleus head fixation may cause the same conductive deficit as stapes fixation, while both malleus fixation and stapes fixation can occur at the same time. Perhaps a tendency toward malleus head fixation is induced by long-standing immobility of the ossicular chain when the stapes is ankylosed.

Congenital fixation of the stapes may occur with no other abnormality of the middle ear, and should be suspected when the loss of hearing was first noted in early childhood. An abnormally small tympanic membrane, partial meatal atresia or short manubrium suggests the possibility of congenital stapes fixation. Since the facial nerve in such cases often runs an abnormal course through the middle ear, the surgeon must proceed with extra caution.

Chronic secretory otitis media behind a thickened tympanic membrane might be mistaken for stapes fixation, but tympanometry should indicate the correct diagnosis.

Tympanosclerosis fixing one or all of the ossicles can produce the same conductive loss as primary otospongiotic stapes ankylosis. Marked thickening of the tympanic membrane, polytomography showing soft tissue masses in the attic and oval window and a stable, rather than slowly progressive, conductive hearing loss may lead to the correct preoperative diagnosis.

The rare case of round window closure, usually associated with stapes fixation, can be suspected in cases with profound hearing loss, combining conductive and sensorineural components. Polytomography is helpful in demonstrating closure of the round window. Narrowing of the round window niche will have no effect on hearing as long as a tiny opening "no larger than a red cell" remains. When both windows are found to be obliterated by otospongiosis, the oval window alone should be opened by stapedectomy, with the expectation of improvement in hearing to the level of the preoperative bone conduction.

The diagnosis of pure sensorineural hearing loss due to otospongiosis is today much like the diagnosis of stapedial otospongiosis forty years ago. Its existence is denied by a few otologists and ignored by many. It is generally acknowledged that varying degrees of sensorineural hearing loss disproportionate to the patient's age and without discernible cause are quite frequently combined with, or follow some years after, stapes fixation. The recent perfection by Valvassori of polytomographic detection of spongification of the cochlear capsule promises to do for the diagnosis of pure cochlear otospongiosis what fenestration did for stapedial fixation otospongiosis (Fig. 17–11).

In 1903 Shambaugh Sr.[22] reported the first case of pure sensorineural loss diagnosed during life as due to otosclerosis (otospongiosis) of the cochlear capsule. In 1926 Shambaugh Sr. and Holderman[23] predicted that cases of pure sensorineural hearing loss due to cochlear otospongiosis "are probably more common than is generally believed, as future histologic studies are likely to prove."

The still disputed etiology and diagnosis of sensorineural hearing loss in cases of otospongiosis of the cochlear capsule is due partly to considerable inconsistency between the degree of capsular replacement by pathologic bone and the degree of sensorineural impairment. Thus, sensorineural loss disproportionate to the patient's age may occur in lesions that do not reach the cochlear endosteum. At the other end of the spectrum, total replacement of the cochlear capsule by spongiotic bone may occur with essentially normal cochlear function. Nevertheless, there is a rough approximation of sensorineural loss to the size of foci and the degree of endosteal involvement.

A second reason that some doubt the otospongiotic origin of sensorineural loss is the lack of anatomical invasion of the cochlea in most cases, such as occurs in the oval window, fixing the stapes. The recent demonstration by Chevance, Causse and Bergès[10] of cytotoxic enzymes of bone resorption in the perilymph of stapedectomized patients with sensorineural progression (only rarely when there was no preoperative sensorineural loss) and Rüedi's[24] demonstration of abnormal vascular shunts between the focus and the cochlea (see Fig. 17–6A) provide a clear explanation for the mechanism of sensorineural loss. The reasons that this loss can occur from a small focus that does not reach the endosteum, and may not occur from a large focus replacing most of the cochlear capsule, may be related to the degree of bone remodeling activity of the focus more than to its size. The enzymes of bone remodeling conceivably could reach the perilymph via bone canaliculi when a focus has not reached the cochlear endosteum.

Now that sodium fluoride offers the possibility of retarding or arresting progressive sensorineural deterioration due to active otospongiosis, the clinical

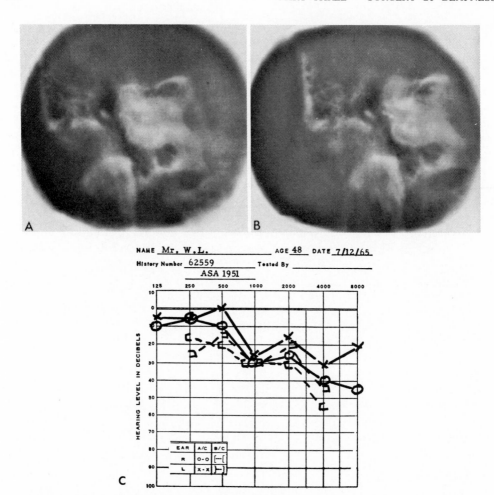

**Figure 17–11** Cochelar otosclerosis. Bilateral sensorineural loss. Mixed changes of delcalcification and sclerosis in basal turn of right cochlea. *A*, Tomogram through basal coil of cochlea showing partial loss of definition between lumen and capsule due to decalcified spongy otosclerosis. *B*, Tomogram after sodium fluoride treatment, showing normal appearing cochlear capsule. After 3 months of sodium fluoride, 60 mg. daily, cochlear capsule has returned to normal density. *C*, Audiogram. Solid lines: air conduction, right ear o—o, left ear x—x; dotted lines: bone conduction, right ear [, left ear].

diagnosis of pure cochlear otospongiosis becomes more urgent. The following six criteria were suggested by the senior author[25] in 1967 for suspecting the otospongiotic origin of a pure progressive sensorineural hearing loss:

1. A positive Schwartze sign in one or both ears, more commonly observed in younger individuals and tending to fade and disappear with increasing age. Do not be misled by a Schwartze sign in a crying infant or child!

2. A family history of surgically confirmed stapedial otospongiosis.

3. Symmetrical progressive sensorineural loss in both ears, with early or advanced stapes fixation in one ear.

4. A flat, "cookie-bite" rising or descending audiometric curve (see Fig. 17–8) with unusually good speech discrimination for a pure sensorineural loss.

5. Pure sensorineural loss beginning at the usual age for stapedial fixation and progressing without other discernible etiology.

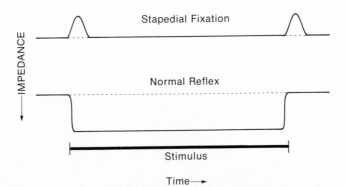

**Figure 17–12**   Time course of a normal reflex and one with a diphasic impedance change. Note that both show a negative deflection at the onset of the stimulus. In cases of stapedial fixation, a negative deflection is also seen at the termination of the stimulus.

6. Polytomography in a patient with one or more of the above criteria that shows clearly defined demineralization of the cochlear capsule. Negative polytomographic findings do not always exclude the possibility that a pure progressive sensorineural loss might be due to otospongiosis, for a mature focus that approaches the density of the normal capsule will no longer be detectable in the polytome.

7.  A seventh criterion is based on impedance audiometry for cases of suspected cochlear otospongiosis, as well as for stapedial fixation. In cases of very early, impending stapes fixation before an audiometric air–bone gap is present, acoustic reflexes are present and there may also be a unique diphasic impedance change, or on-off effect[26], characterized by a negative deflection or decrease in impedance at both the onset and termination of the stimulus (Fig. 17–12). Such a patient will later develop the classic audiometric pattern of stapes fixation. As stapes fixation increases, there may be a normal impedance profile, although more often there will be a Type A shallow tympanogram of low static compliance and absent reflexes. The combination of normal tympanogram and acoustic reflex results with a conductive hearing loss suggests stapes fixation as "there is virtually no other type of middle ear disorder that does not show some abnormality in the impedance battery."[27]

## SELECTION OF CASES FOR SURGERY

Fenestration of the horizontal semicircular canal always resulted in a small residue of conductive loss averaging 25 decibels for the speech frequencies, due to loss of the transformer ratio of normal middle ear sound conduction. When the air–bone gap, after correction for Carhart's notch in the bone conduction curve, was less than 35 decibels, fenestration was not indicated. Stapedectomy, on the contrary, should completely eliminate the conductive deficit, and can be considered whenever there is a handicapping loss due to partial or complete stapes fixation, with sufficient cochlear reserve to anticipate a useful improvement. Thus, stapedectomy has replaced horizontal canal fenestration except in very rare cases of congenital absence of the oval window, or in cases of repeated oval window closure after stapedectomy.

Of great importance in selecting cases for stapedectomy is the speech discrimination test, for if this is impaired out of proportion to the degree of loss, a superimposed endolymphatic hydrops must be suspected. Stapedectomy in such an ear is very likely to cause a permanent, severe further sensorineural loss.

The use of an old-fashioned speaking tube, while masking the opposite ear, is a useful adjunct to speech audiometry in deciding for or against surgery in severe loss of combined stapes fixation and cochlear otospongiosis. The possibility of improvement in such cases is limited by the bone conduction curve, after correcting for Carhart's notch.

As mentioned previously, in all cases the audiometric air–bone gap should be verified by the tuning fork tests while masking the ear opposite the one being tested.

## MEDICAL TREATMENT OF OTOSPONGIOSIS

In 1964 the senior author[28] proposed the use of moderate doses of sodium fluoride to promote recalcification and inactivation of an actively expanding focus of otospongiosis. Subsequent animal research by Petrovic[29] and organ cultures of otospongiotic bone removed during stapedectomy demonstrated the favorable action of sodium fluoride on the active phase of otospongiosis (see Fig. 17–6*D* and *E*). Clinical studies of sensorineural loss in surgically confirmed stapedial otospongiosis indicated stabilization of hearing in 4 out of 5 cases by this therapy[30] (Fig. 17–13). Polytomography of the cochlear capsule before and after treatment demon-

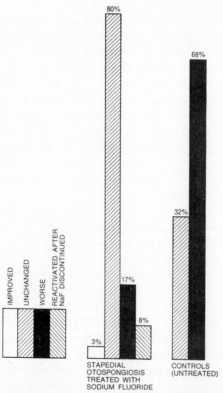

**Figure 17–13**  Results in 575 patients with surgically confirmed stapedial otospongiosis treated with sodium fluoride compared with 34 untreated controls. Sensorineural loss improved in 3 per cent, stabilized in 80 per cent after treatment. In 8 per cent the cochlear loss began again after stopping the fluoride. In all cases, progressing sensorineural loss with polytome evidence in most of spongiotic changes in the cochlear capsule preceded therapy.

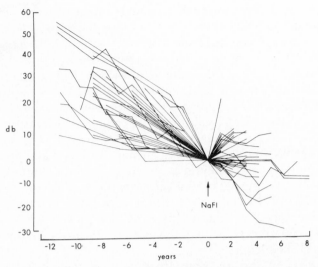

**Figure 17–14** Depicted here are the decibels of sensorineural loss occurring in 46 stapes-operated patients followed for 1 to 14 years. The course of the hearing after the fluoride began shows that there was an actual improvement in hearing in 23, stabilization in 10, and the sensorineural progression continued, despite fluoride therapy, in 13 (Courtesy of H. House).

strates stabilization of the spongifying process in most and actual recalcification of the spongy focus in some cases (see Fig. 17–11). Fading of a positive Schwartze sign, reduction in tinnitus, and improvement in mild imbalance are additional evidence of benefit by this medication. Figure 17–14 presents a visual summary of the effects of fluoride medication in 46 stapes-operated patients.

Well over 2000 patients with progressive sensorineural loss after successful fenestration or stapedectomy, as well as some cases of pure sensorineural loss believed due to cochlear otospongiosis, have been treated by the senior author with moderate doses of sodium fluoride, some for as long as ten years, generally, but not invariably, with the favorable results of stabilizing the hearing, and, in a few cases, of actually improving the hearing. Jean Causse of Beziers, France, has employed this therapy in more than 10,000 patients, most of them with surgically confirmed stapedial otospongiosis.

In no case treated with moderate doses of sodium fluoride observed by the senior author, by Causse,[31] by Linthicum and House,[32] or by Cody[33] has permanent harm to the patient resulted.

The following conditions require precautions in prescribing sodium fluoride: chronic nephritis with nitrogen retention, in which the urinary excretion of fluoride might be impaired, with toxic levels accumulating in the blood; allergy to the medication in the form of an itching skin rash each time it is taken, or asthma as occurred in one case; arthritic symptoms, which may be increased while on the medication, but return to their previous status within a month of discontinuance; gastric distress, which is unusual with the combination of sodium fluoride and calcium carbonate (sold as a dietary supplement by Mericon Industries, Peoria, Illinois, under the trade name Florical). Nevertheless, a few patients do not tolerate the medication because of gastric distress.

An x-ray of the spine should be taken at the onset and after two years of therapy, to detect the earliest evidence of skeletal fluorosis, with thickening of trabeculae. When the fluoride is stopped, this earliest fluorosis can return to normal. It is without symptoms, is harmless and is actually beneficial to women past the menopause who tend to develop vertebral collapse due to osteoporosis.

The optimum dosage and duration of therapy with sodium fluoride remains to be determined by long experience. A maximum dose of Florical is achieved by taking 3 capsules with each meal, or 9 a day, each capsule containing 8.3 mg. of sodium fluoride and 364 mg. of calcium carbonate, for a total of approximately 75 mg. of fluoride daily. Clinical experience suggests that a somewhat smaller dose of 50 mg. daily achieved by taking 2 capsules with each meal, may be as effective as the larger dose.

Since bone remodeling is more active during childhood and puberty, the effect of sodium fluoride medication should be greater then than in adults. Accordingly, under the age of 16 one capsule of Florical three times daily, for a daily dose of 25 mg. of fluoride, should be prescribed. During the last half of pregnancy, a still smaller dose of one capsule of Florical daily (8.3 mg. of sodium fluoride) might be prescribed, both to retard expansion of the mother's focus and to improve the caries resistance of the child's teeth.

After two years of therapy, the situation is re-evaluated by hearing tests, inspection for a Schwartze sign, status of tinnitus or imbalance and polytomography. If the condition has stabilized or improved, a maintenance dose of one capsule of Florical three times a day should be continued the rest of that patient's life. It was found that stopping the fluoride often results in reactivation of the otospongiotic focus two or three years later.

Mention should be made of a recent study of intestinal absorption of various fluoride preparations:[34] gelatin capsules or liquid sodium fluoride is absorbed the most readily, but causes severe gastric distress in most subjects. Enteric-coated sodium fluoride tablets are absorbed inconsistently and often very poorly. A combination of calcium carbonate and sodium fluoride is well tolerated and is absorbed fairly uniformly and well. This is marketed as a dietary supplement, Florical. To achieve 50 mg. of sodium fluoride daily, two of the capsules need to be taken three times a day, preferably with meals.

In conclusion, moderate dosage sodium fluoride is the only known treatment for the otospongiotic lesion. This treatment is both effective and **safe** for promotion of inactivation and recalcification of an actively expanding focus of otospongiosis.[35]

## REFERENCES

1. Valsalva, A. M.: Opera, hoc est, tractatus de aure humana. Venice, Pitteri, 1735.
2. Toynbee, J.: Pathological and surgical observations on the diseases of the ear. Medico-Chir. Tr., 24:190, 1841.
3. Tröltsch, A. F. von: Lehrbuch der Ohrenheilkunde, 7th ed. Leipzig, Vogel, 1881.
4. Politzer, A.: Ueber primäre Erkrankung der knöchernen Labyrinthkapsel. Ztschr. Ohrenh., 25:309, 1893.
5. Siebenmann, F.: Demonstration mikroscopischer und makroscopischer Präparate von Otospongiosis progressiva. Papers Internat. Otol. Cong., 9:207, 1912.
6. Manasse, P.: Neue Untersuchungen zur Otosklerosenfrage. Ztschr. Ohrenh., 82:76, 1922.
7. Guild, S. R.: Histologic otosclerosis. Ann. Otol. Rhin. & Laryng., 53:246, 1944.
8. Rüedi, L., and Spoendlin, H.: Histology of the otosclerotic ankylosis of the stapes. In Rüedi, L. (Ed.): Advances in Oto-Rhino-Laryngology. Vol. 4. New York, S. Karger, 1957.
9. Schuknecht, H. F.: Stapedectomy. Boston, Little, Brown & Co., 1971.
10. Chevance, L. G., Causse, J. R., and Bergès, J.: Alpha 1-antitrypsin activity of perilymph. Occurrence during progression of otospongiosis. Arch. Otol., 102:363, 1976.
11. Lindsay, J. R.: Otosclerosis. In Paparella, M. M., and Shumrick, D. A. (Eds.): Otolaryngology, Vol. II. Philadelphia, W.B. Saunders Co., 1973.
12. Kakizaki, I., Zechner, G., and Altmann, F.: The osteocytes of the human labyrinthine capsule. Arch. Otol., 94:139, 1971.

13. Rius, M., and Mendoza, D.: Nueva Teori Sobre La Etiopathogeniadela Otosclerosis. Montevideo, Garcia Morales-Mercant, 1961.
14. Arslan, M. and Ricci, V.: L'otosclerosi puo essere considerata come una malattia del collageno? Resultati direcerche istochimiche. Otorino-laryng. Ital., 30:81, 1961.
15. Chevance, L. G., Causse, J., Bretlau, P., Jørgensen, M. B., et al.: Otosclerosis: An electron microscopic and cytochemical study. Acta Oto-laryng. Suppl. 272, 1970.
16. Bast, T. H. and Anson, B. J.: The temporal bone and the ear. Springfield, Illinois, Charles C Thomas, 1949.
17. Der Hoeve, J. van and de Klein, A.: Blaue Skleren, Knochen bruckigkeit und Schwerhörigkeit. Arch. Ophthal., 95:81, 1918 (Berlin).
18. Simpson-Hall, I., and Ogilvie, R. I.: Otosclerosis in osteogenesis imperfecta. Acta Oto-laryng., 53:202, 1961.
19. Wittmaack, K.: Handbuch der speziellen pathologischen Anatomie und Histologie Vol. 12, Gehöror-gan 415, J. Springen, 1926.
20. Rüedi, L.: Pathogenesis of otosclerosis. Arch. Otol., 78:469, 1963.
21. Sercer, A.: Etiopathogenie de l'otosclerose. Progr. Otorhinol., 8:188, 1961.
22. Shambaugh, G. E., Sr.: Otosclerosis or spongifying of the capsule of the labyrinth. Ann. Otol. Rhin. & Laryng., 12:83, 1903.
23. Shambaugh, G. E., Sr., and Holderman, J. W.: Occurrence of otosclerosis in etiology of progressive deafness. Arch. Otol., 4:127, 1926.
24. Rüedi, L.: Discussion of Carhart: Labyrinthine otosclerosis. Arch. Otol., 78:499, 1963.
25. Shambaugh, G. E., Jr.: Surgery of the Ear. 2nd ed. Philadelphia, W.B. Saunders Co., 1967.
26. Bel, J., Causse, J., Michaux, P., et al.: Mechanical explanation of the on-off effect (diphasic impedance change) in otospongiosis. Audiology, 15:128, 1976.
27. Jerger, J.: Diagnostic use of impedance measures. In Jerger, J. (Ed.): Handbook of Clinical Impedance Audiometry. Dobbs Ferry, New York, American Electromedics Corp., 1975.
28. Shambaugh, G. E., Jr., and Scott, A.: Sodium fluoride for arrest of otosclerosis. Arch. Otol., 80:263, 1964.
29. Petrovic, A., and Shambaugh, G. E., Jr.: Promotion of bone calcification by sodium fluoride. Arch. Otol., 83:162, 1966.
30. Shambaugh, G. E., Jr., and Causse, J.: Ten years experience with fluoride in otosclerotic (otospongio-tic) patients. Ann. Otol. Rhin. & Laryng., 83:635, 1974.
31. Causse, J.: Personal Communication.
32. Linthicum, F. H., Jr., and House, H.: Personal Communication.
33. Cody, D. T. R., and Baker, H. L.: Otosclerosis: vestibular symptoms and sensorineural hearing loss. Ann. Otol. Rhin. & Laryng., 87:778, 1978.
34. Deka, R. C., Kacker, S. K., and Shambaugh, G. E., Jr.: Intestinal absorption of fluoride preparations. Laryngoscope, 88:1918, 1978.
35. Kacker, S. K. and Shambaugh, G. E., Jr.: Effect of fluoride on alpha-chymotrypsin. Arch. Otol. 106:260, 1980.

## Samuel Rosen
BORN 1897

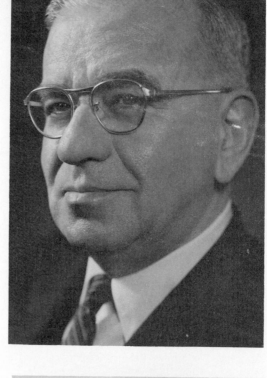

Had the vision to seize upon a chance mobilization and thus revived the direct operation upon the stapes. "The surgeon must . . . go along . . . step by step as the conditions unfold; trying . . . to preserve or reconstitute the transformer action of the middle ear, with preference always for using the patient's own tissues. . . ." (1960).

## John J. Shea
BORN 1924

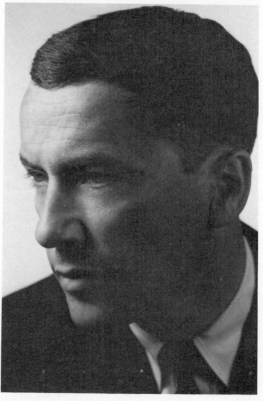

Revived stapedectomy more than half a century after Blake and Jack, adding prosthetic restoration of ossicular continuity from incus to tissue covering oval window.

# Chapter 18

# Stapes Operations for Otospongiosis (Otosclerosis)

HISTORICAL ASPECTS
PRINCIPLES UNDERLYING STAPES OPERATIONS
INDICATIONS FOR STAPEDECTOMY
TECHNIQUE OF STAPES OPERATION
    PREOPERATIVE PREPARATION
    LOCAL ANESTHESIA
    OBTAINING THE TISSUE GRAFT
    EXPOSURE OF THE OVAL WINDOW
    ANTERIOR CRUROTOMY MOBILIZATION
    STAPEDECTOMY
SPECIAL PROBLEMS DURING STAPEDECTOMY
    FLOATING FOOTPLATE PROBLEM
    OBLITERATIVE OTOSPONGIOSIS PROBLEM
    THE BISCUIT FOOTPLATE
    THE DEHISCENT, PROLAPSED FACIAL NERVE
    FIXED MALLEUS
    ROUND WINDOW CLOSURE
    FRACTURE OF LONG PROCESS OF THE INCUS
    PERILYMPH GUSHER
POSTOPERATIVE CARE
COMPLICATIONS OF STAPEDECTOMY
    POSTOPERATIVE PERILYMPH FISTULA
STAPEDECTOMY AFTER FENESTRATION
REVISION OF STAPES OPERATIONS
EARLY AND LATE SENSORINEURAL LOSS FOLLOWING
    STAPES SURGERY

## HISTORICAL ASPECTS

The earliest surgical attempts to improve hearing in stapes fixation were directed to the stapes itself. Over a century ago in 1878 Kessel[1] incised the posterior part of the tympanic membrane, separated the incus from the stapes, removed part of the bony meatal wall when necessary for proper exposure of the stapes and then tried to mobilize the stapes by applying pressure to its head in various directions.

In 1888 Boucheron[2] reported 60 mobilizations, with the best results in cases of early ankylosis without involvement of the sound-perceiving apparatus. Then in 1890 Miot[3] in a series of five articles reported 200 stapes mobilizations with techniques and results amazingly similar to Rosen's operation of 62 years later. Miot observed the improvement in bone conduction ("cranial perception") following successful mobilization due, we know now, to elimination of Carhart's notch. There were no deaths or labyrinthine complications in his series.

In 1892 Blake[4] of Boston removed a stapes to improve hearing, and in 1893 Jack[5] reported a series of cases of extraction of the stapes. Ten years later he described one of these as having maintained quite good hearing, noting that: "The drums have healed. The portion covering the seat of the operation is somewhat sunken forming a moveable membrane on the oval window. . . . Removal of the stapes does not destroy the hearing but sometimes improves it. The contrary statements in most textbooks . . . were incorrect."

In 1899 Faraci[6] published his results in 30 cases of stapes mobilization, and this was the last recorded stapes operation to improve hearing for more than half a century, for in 1900 at the International Congress Siebenmann[7] was joined by Politzer and other leaders in otology in condemning all surgical attempts to improve hearing in otospongiosis as both useless and dangerous. The reasons for the concerted and effective opposition is not clear, and one can but surmise that there were some unreported serious complications.

By 1952 several developments had set the stage for the revival of operations upon the fixed stapes: the success of Lempert's fenestration operation had overcome the prejudice against surgery for otospongiosis; antibacterial drugs afforded added protection against infection; electric illumination and magnification by loupe made endomeatal surgery more practical; audiometry to measure and report hearing results verified improvements; and last, but not least, Lempert's endomeatal approach to the tympanic cavity without perforation of the tympanic membrane proved ideal for operations upon the stapes.

In 1952 Rosen,[8] unaware of Miot's earlier work, began to use Lempert's endomeatal approach to the tympanic cavity to palpate the stapes and verify the degree of fixation prior to fenestration. In one such case the stapes suddenly mobilized, with a remarkable restoration of normal hearing, even better than fenestration would have yielded. Rosen followed this chance observation by purposeful attempts to mobilize the stapes, reporting hearing improved to the 30 decibel level (A.S.A.) or better for the speech frequencies in 22 per cent of 211 operations. Soon many fenestration surgeons were attempting preliminary stapes mobilization which, when successful, could surpass the hearing achieved by fenestration with a fraction of the time needed for convalescence and no need for lifetime fenestration cavity care.

In 1954 the senior author of this text, accustomed since 1940 to the operating microscope for fenestrations,[9] applied it to stapes mobilizations. The microscope made possible the development by Heermann[10] and Derlacki[11] of microchisels to loosen the footplate, of anterior crurotomy mobilization by Basek and Fowler,[12] and finally the revival of stapedectomy by Shea[13] in 1956. Unlike Blake and Jack, who failed to comprehend the need to reconstruct an ossicular chain and who left the oval window open, Shea closed the oval window after extraction of the stapes "with a thin slice of connective tissue" and inserted a prosthesis from incus to oval window to restore the normal mechanics of the middle ear.

Many modifications of Shea's stapedectomy have been designed and employed, all following the principles firmly established by Shea that the oval window needs to be sealed, and there must be ossicular continuity by using the posterior crus of the stapes or a prosthesis from incus to oval window. Among these modifications are a prosthesis of fat tied to a wire loop; a preformed wire loop against compressed Gelfoam, vein, fascia or perichondrium to seal the oval window; and a piston-type prosthesis of stainless steel, tantalum, platinum or teflon from incus to oval window. Most surgeons currently prefer a tissue graft, rather than Gelfoam, to seal the oval window, as being less likely to result in a perilymph fistula. The tendency for a preformed wire loop to become adherent to the edge of the oval window has prompted the use of a piston-type prosthesis of teflon or stainless steel. In contrast to results obtained when removing the entire stapes footplate or a major part of it, there appears to be less labyrinthine reaction when the prosthesis is inserted into a smaller opening in the footplate, using a very thin graft made from a pressed vein or from the dried loose areolar tissue superficial to the temporalis fascia. The latter technique will be described in this text, although other methods may be equally satisfactory.

## PRINCIPLES UNDERLYING STAPES OPERATIONS

A valuable pathologic study by Rüedi and Spoendlin[14] of 79 ears with otospongiosis involving the oval window showed bony fixation of the stapes footplate in only 28, whereas in 51, the enlarging anterior focus of otospongiosis had fixed the footplate by compression, impaction and often subluxation (Fig. 18–1). The otospongiotic foci were highly or very highly active as judged by their vascularity and cellularity in 27 per cent; 37 per cent of the otospongiotic lesions were of intermediate activity; and 35 per cent were recalcified mature foci of low or very low activity. These observations explain the initial success of simple transcrural mobilization of the stapes in 22 per cent of cases when it was fixed by pressure of the

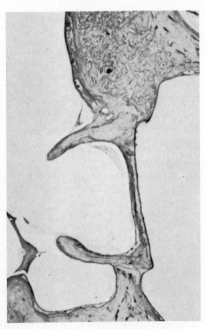

**Figure 18–1** Highly active vascular otosclerotic focus at site of predilection that has caused fixation of the stapes by impaction and subluxation against the posterior end of the oval window. Bony ankylosis has not yet occurred. (From Rüedi, L., et al.: Stapes Mobilization. Basel and New York, S. Karger, 1957.)

enlarging focus, but the probability that it will refix in two thirds of the cases as a moderately or highly active focus continues to expand.

It seems likely that surgical trauma to the focus by drill or scrapers will stimulate increased activity of otospongiosis, especially in a highly active focus. Preoperative therapy with sodium fluoride (as described in Chapter 17) for six months or a year to reduce the activity is advisable when there is a strongly positive Schwartze sign, or when exposure of the oval window reveals a highly vascular and thus very active focus.

The probability of regrowth of active otospongiosis eventually closing the oval window contrasts with horizontal semicircular canal fenestration, an area of the labyrinthine capsule only rarely invaded by otospongiotic bone. Thus, fenestration may be indicated when the oval window repeatedly closes after stapedectomy.

## INDICATIONS FOR STAPEDECTOMY

The clinical diagnosis of stapedial fixation otospongiosis was considered in Chapter 17. The degree of footplate fixation is estimated by the size of the air–bone gap, while the degree of cochlear hearing loss is measured by the bone conduction curve, taking into account the variable and unpredictable Carhart otosclerotic notch (see Fig. 17–10). In every case, to confirm the presence and size of a genuine air–bone gap, the clinician should use the 256, 512 and 1024 tuning fork Rinné tests, with narrow-band masking of the opposite ear, for the audiometer is not immune to mechanical error. While the preoperative hearing tests indicate the degree of fixation, they do not predict the pattern and extent of oval window involvement by otospongiosis. This can be determined only when the oval window and stapes are surgically exposed under the operating microscope.

Stapedectomy is indicated when the stapes is firmly fixed, as demonstrated by an air–bone gap of 35 to 40 decibels for the speech frequencies and a negative Rinné test for the 256 and 512, and sometimes the 1024 tuning forks. When there is very early partial fixation with Rinné tests negative for the 256 fork and positive for the 512 tuning fork, and a narrow air–bone gap of 20 or 25 decibels, stapedectomy is best delayed until fixation is more complete, for there is only a little hearing improvement to be gained, and much to be lost in case of a severe cochlear reaction. Should operation be considered for an early fixation, for example, to relieve or diminish annoying tinnitus, or when there is bilateral sensorineural involvement, an anterior crurotomy mobilization or a transcrural (Miot-Rosen) mobilization should be considered, rather than a stapedectomy.

Because of the residual conductive deficit after successful horizontal canal fenestration, this operation is rarely advised for stapes fixation with advanced cochlear nerve involvement. By contrast, fully successful stapes mobilization or successful stapedectomy not only corrects the entire conductive component of loss, but it also removes the variable Carhart notch with overclosure of the preoperative air–bone gap. Thus, stapedectomy can be useful for improving hearing aid usage in the presence of stapes fixation with a profound cochlear loss, provided there is good speech discrimination as determined by audiometry and a speaking tube. Poor speech discrimination or a history of vertigo in recent months are contraindications to stapedectomy, as they indicate the probability of hydrops of endolymph with the risk of further cochlear loss should the labyrinth be opened.

Operation on a patient's only useful hearing ear should be avoided, because of the small, but definite and unpredictable risk of a permanent cochlear loss.

# TECHNIQUE OF STAPES OPERATION

## Preoperative Preparation

Since the ideal patient for stapes surgery is also an ideal candidate for a hearing aid, he should be fully informed of this and of the uncertainties and risks of surgery. Since verbal explanations are notoriously misinterpreted by patients, a printed sheet should include this information.

If the ear has not been operated before and there is a large air–bone gap with good cochlear function, including excellent speech discrimination, the patient has at least 9 chances in 10 of a useful hearing improvement that will be maintained for several years. There is, however, one chance out of 100 that there may be a permanent loss instead of a gain, rendering that ear unsatisfactory for a hearing aid.

Dizziness of some degree follows nearly every stapes operation, lasting a few hours to several days and in rare cases, much longer. Taste is likely to be affected, whether or not the chorda tympani nerve was sectioned, gently pushed out of the way or not visibly traumatized. Permanent loss or distortion of taste can occur. An unhealed perforation of the tympanic membrane may require subsequent repair.

Paralysis of the facial nerve should be mentioned. It occurs in less than 1 per cent of operations, usually beginning several days to a week after operation, and is due to edema of the nerve in the fallopian canal. Much rarer, and more serious, is immediate facial paralysis when a dehiscent or aberrant nerve protrudes or crosses the footplate and may be injured during surgery (Fig. 18–2).

The patient in most cases can plan to return to work one week after his stapes operation.

Following successful stapes surgery, the patient should return each year for hearing tests to detect beginning cochlear involvement by the otospongiosis, which calls for sodium fluoride therapy. Should there occur at any time symptoms of hydrops of endolymph: imbalance, fullness in the ear, tinnitus, or hearing drop, the patient should return immediately, as this may indicate a perilymph fistula or a postoperative hydrops that will respond to medical therapy.

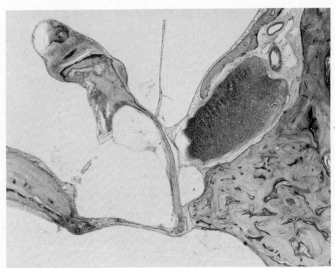

**Figure 18–2**  Dehiscent facial nerve canal, the protruding vulnerable nerve adherent to the stapes. (Courtesy of G. Kelemen)

The preoperative preparation of the patient includes inspection of the meatus for any evidence of outer or middle ear infection that requires postponement of the operation, and for selection of the ear for surgery. Application of tinted tincture of merthiolate to the outer meatus insures that the wrong ear will never be operated.

## Local Anesthesia

With rare exceptions, stapes operations are best performed under local infiltration anesthesia, with sufficient sedation to allay apprehension. Currently, the senior author prescribes Valium 5 mg. the night before if the patient has difficulty sleeping, and Valium 10 mg. by mouth two hours before the scheduled operation. One hour before operation, Talwin 30 mg. (or Demerol 50 mg.), Phenergan 25 mg. and atropine 0.4 mg. are given by intramuscular injection. Should the patient be wide awake on arriving in the operating room, an additional intramuscular injection of Talwin, 15 to 30 mg., or Demerol, 25 or 50 mg., is given.

Local infiltration of the skin just above the auricle and the skin of the external meatus with 2 per cent Zylocaine and 1 to 100,000 adrenalin, as described in Chapter 6, to a total of 2 or 3 cc. will produce quite satisfactory anesthesia after a few minutes.

## Obtaining the Tissue Graft

For the tissue graft that seals the oval window, the senior and junior authors both prefer the loose areolar tissue that lies lateral to the temporalis fascia. By making an incision close to the upper attachment of the auricle and forcibly pulling the auricle forward and downward, the tissue plane lateral to the temporalis fascia is established. Injection of 1 cc. of the Zylocaine and adrenalin solution into the loose connective tissue to "blow it up" helps in grasping and removing a portion of it that can then be teased out on a teflon block to a very thin uniform layer that, placed to dry under a lamp, becomes a marvelously thin intact tissue graft (see Fig. 16–11).

## Exposure of the Oval Window

After suturing the skin incision for the tissue graft, the operating microscope is moved into position, and from this point on the entire procedure is performed through an ear speculum and Lempert's endomeatal skin incision as described by Rosen.

Through the largest speculum that can be inserted into the meatus, the skin of the posterior osseous meatal wall is incised with the angled meatal knife applied with repeated pressure against skin and underlying bone to crush capillaries and lessen bleeding, thus producing a U-shaped flap beginning at 6 o'clock (were the patient upright) in the floor of the meatus just lateral to the annulus, sloping backward and upward to 6 or 8 mm. from the annulus at 10 o'clock for the right ear and 2 o'clock for the left ear, and then curving forward to above the pars flaccida at 12 o'clock (Figs. 18–3 and 18–4). This latter part of the incision through the vascular strip is conveniently made with the alligator-type Bellucci scissors.

The skin flap is elevated to the sulcus tympanicus with the same angled knife, and by placing a tiny cotton ball moistened in the Zylocaine and adrenalin solution and applying suction to it, a dry field is maintained.

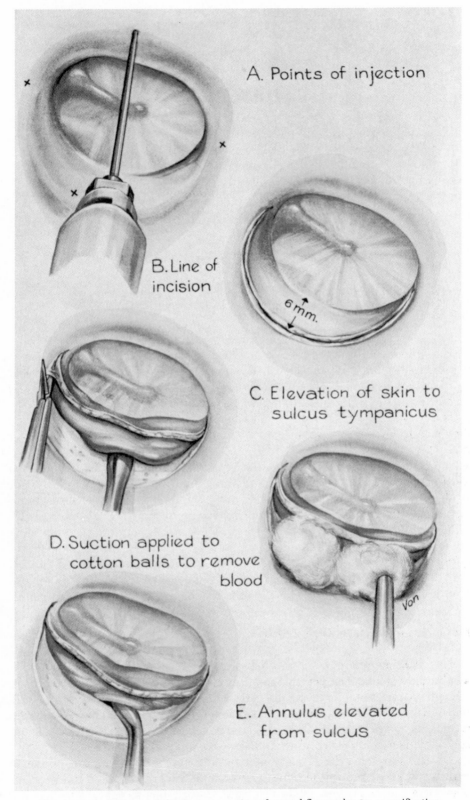

A. Points of injection

B. Line of incision

6 mm.

C. Elevation of skin to sulcus tympanicus

D. Suction applied to cotton balls to remove blood

Von

E. Annulus elevated from sulcus

**Figure 18–3**   Stapes mobilization — creation of meatal flap under 6× magnification.

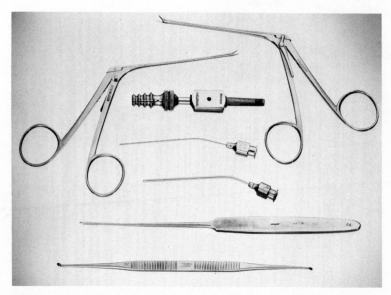

**Figure 18–4** Instruments for exposure of stapes (from top to bottom): Alligator scissors; alligator forceps; adapter for suction tips; suction tip made from No. 20 spinal tap needle; No. 17 suction tip; angled knife and elevator; angled curet.

The fibrous annulus tympanicus is elevated from the sulcus tympanicus with the same instrument, which is pushed down over the edge of the bony sulcus at repeated points. Especial care is needed in separating the attachment of the posterior fold of the pars tensa to the midpoint of the sulcus posteriorly.

The tympanic cavity is entered in a dry field obtained by suction against a moist cotton ball. In some cases light electrocoagulation may be needed to be applied to the metal #20 suction tip in contact with a bleeding point. As the delicate tympanic mucoperiosteum is entered, pain may be experienced, but it is quickly alleviated by instilling 0.25 to 0.5 cc. of Zylocaine and adrenalin solution into the middle ear and quickly aspirating it to minimize any round window membrane absorption, for anesthesia of the tympanic mucoperiosteum occurs instantaneously.

In most cases, to gain adequate exposure of the oval window and stapes, 2 to 4 mm. of posterosuperior bony meatal rim must be removed with the angled middle ear (Fowler) curet, with care not to section or injure the chorda tympani nerve (Fig. 18–5A). This nerve may need to be freed of filmy adhesions and gently displaced upward or downward to fully visualize the footplate.

### Anterior Crurotomy Mobilization

This conservative procedure of Basek and Fowler has the advantage over stapedectomy of less postoperative cochlear reaction and very rare permanent loss or fistula. It is indicated for cases of partial fixation with a narrow air–bone gap, where the fixation is by impaction from an anterior focus with little or no invasion of the footplate beyond the anterior crus attachment. This method, only occasionally used today, is accomplished in three steps (Fig. 18–5 and 18–6):

1. The anterior crus is sectioned by applying a curved sharp Derlacki or Heermann microchisel to the anterior surface of the crus close to the neck of the stapes. The chisel is then pushed inward toward the footplate to remove thin shavings of bone until the crus fractures. The distal fragment of crus is pushed forward to leave a gap between it and the proximal fragment to prevent healing from

reuniting the fractured crus. Sometimes the entire stapes and footplate become freely mobile before the anterior crus is sectioned, in which case nothing more need be done.

2.  The footplate is cut across its center by repeated light pressure of a fine pick or with a straight microchisel struck one or two very light blows with the handle of the angled knife by the assistant.

3.  The posterior half of the footplate, now separated from the anterior portion fixed by the anterior otospongiotic focus, is nearly always impacted against the posterior edge of the oval window and needs to be freed by gentle pressure on the

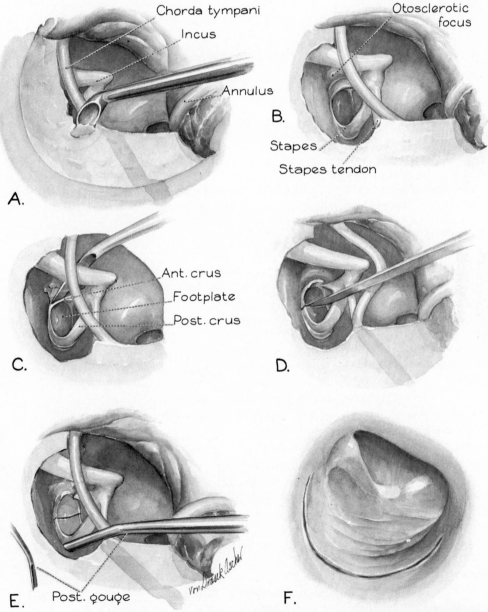

**Figure 18–5**   Anterior crurotomy mobilization. *A*, Removal of bony rim of meatus to expose stapes. *B*, Stapes fully exposed; otosclerosis confined to anterior crus attachment. *C*, Sectioning of anterior crus. *D*, Sectioning of footplate. *E*, Freeing impacted posterior end of footplate. *F*, Tympanic membrane replaced.

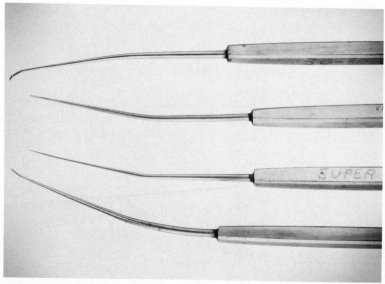

**Figure 18–6**  Instruments for anterior crurotomy mobilization (from top to bottom): angled Derlacki chisel; straight chisel; fine pick; posterior gouge.

head of the stapes, and by gentle application of Derlacki microchisels and gouge between the posterior crus and posterior wall of the oval window. A tiny connective tissue graft placed behind the posterior crus and another placed anteriorly at the site of footplate fracture will help to seal any perilymph leak.

## Stapedectomy

This method is preferred by most surgeons as it gives the highest levels of maintained hearing improvements, but it does carry a small risk, greater than anterior crurotomy or transcrural mobilization, of immediate or late cochlear loss due to cochlear reaction and perilymph fistula.

Stapedectomy after surgical exposure is accomplished in five steps (Figs. 18–7 and 18–8):

1.  A "safety-hole" is first made with a fine straight pick through a blue area of footplate to facilitate removal should the footplate mobilize and become "floating."

2.  The incudo-stapedial joint is separated with the capsule knife, and the stapedius tendon is severed with the alligator-type Bellucci scissors. The crura are fractured from the footplate by a sharp push upward or downward, and the stapes superstructure consisting of head and crura is extracted.

3.  The mucosa is removed from the footplate and margins of oval window with angled Harrison knives. Bleeding is controlled by applying pledgets of Gelfoam soaked in 1 to 1000 adrenalin. Very rarely a large persistent bleeding vessel needs to be stopped by light cautery to a suction tip applied to the bleeding point. Intramuscular Premarin 20 mg. appears helpful for capillary bleeding.

4.  In a dry field with the fine straight pick the posterior third or half of the footplate is cut across and a round hole made in it large enough to receive a 0.6 mm. teflon piston, 4.5 mm., rarely 4.75 mm., long, resting on the very thin connective tissue graft. With the Shambaugh fenestration microhook, fragments of the posterior half of the footplate are lifted out. Gentle irrigation with Tis-U-Sol clears the field of any blood and helps to bring footplate fragments to the surface. Any small fragment that remains depressed into the vestibule is not "fished for" but is left in place.

5.  The very thin dried areolar connective tissue graft, cut to size so as to

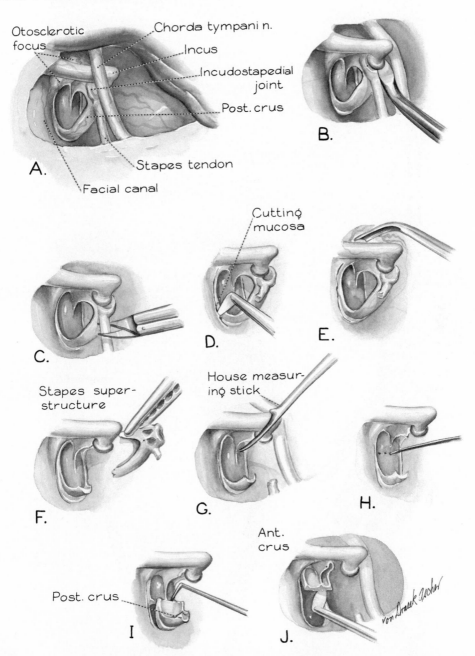

**Figure 18–7** Stapedectomy. *A*, Footplate exposed. *B*, Incudostapedial joint incised. *C*, Stapes tendon cut. *D*, Mucosa around footplate incised. *E*, Mucosa in front of anterior crus incised. *F*, Removal of stapes superstructure. *G*, Measuring from top of incus long process to footplate. *H*, Footplate perforated with fine pick. *I*, Extraction of posterior half of footplate. *J*, Extraction of anterior half of footplate. Note: In the text is described "small-hole" stapedectomy rather than complete footplate removal. Many surgeons prefer the smaller vestibular opening as causing less cochlear reaction.

generously overlap the footplate margins by at least one millimeter in all directions, is placed over the round opening, and the platinum-teflon piston of proper length, measured from top of incus to just below the footplate margin, is inserted and crimped onto the long process of the incus close to its tip. The tissue graft is smoothed out, the mobility of malleus and incus confirmed by gentle pressure on the undersurface of the manubrium, and the patency of the round window is verified by

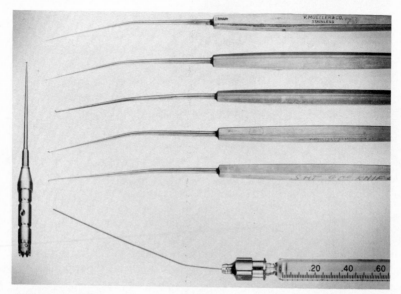

**Figure 18–8**  Instruments for stapedectomy (from top to bottom): fine pick; Shambaugh right-angled hook; right-angled spud; Harrison obtuse angle knife; Harrison right angle knife; suction tip to irrigate oval window; diamond burr.

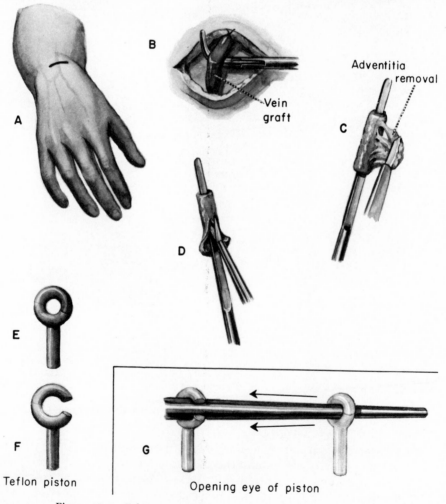

**Figure 18–9**  Taking vein graft for Shea technique of stapedectomy.

a positive round window reflex. The meatal skin flap is replaced, making certain that a cotton ball used earlier for hemostasis has been removed! A strip of surgical rayon placed against the tympanic membrane and posterior meatal wall and held in place by tiny dental cotton balls, moistened with Gantrisin otic solution and tied to a black thread so that they will not be lost, will provide light pressure for the next six days.

Shea's teflon piston placed against a vein graft is a method that has given very good results. The teflon appears to be less likely to adhere to the edge of the oval window than a wire prosthesis. The techniques of taking and preparing the vein graft and of opening the eye of the piston before insertion is shown in Figure 18–9. The vein graft, thinned by means of Shea's vein press, is depressed into the oval window with the Derlacki mobilizer, and the piston is then inserted and crimped onto the incus (Fig. 18–10).

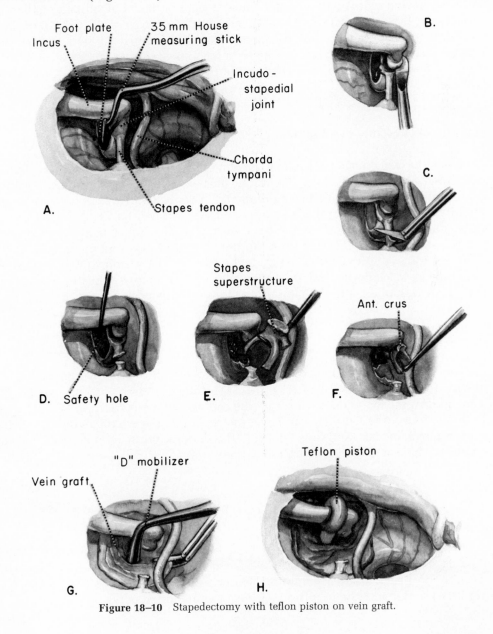

**Figure 18–10**   Stapedectomy with teflon piston on vein graft.

## SPECIAL PROBLEMS DURING STAPEDECTOMY

Malleus fixation, a floating footplate, obliterative otospongiosis, the "biscuit footplate," dehiscent facial nerve obscuring the footplate, round window closure, fracture of the long process of the incus and a perilymph "gusher" are special problems to be dealt with as described below.

### Floating Footplate Problem

The safety hole helps in the extraction of a footplate with minimal trauma to the vestibular contents should the footplate mobilize and become "floating." If necessary, a very tiny hole may be made with the diamond drill in the promontory margin to help in removing a floating footplate. Scheer has described a blood clot method of extracting a large footplate fragment depressed into the vestibule. A blood clot allowed to form and adhere to the footplate fragment is lifted out by a suction tip, with fragment attached.[16] In rare cases, the surgeon may elect to place his prosthesis against a floating footplate, first sealing the oval window with a very thin tissue graft.

### Obliterative Otospongiosis Problem

When the oval window is found to be obliterated by otospongiosis, a "drill-out" is required. The approximate location of the oval window is established by the crura and the fallopian canal. With a small diamond drill, the bone in the oval window is carefully thinned down until a blue area appears. Meanwhile Tis-U-Sol irrigation and suction removes all osteogenic bone dust. The final saucerized, thinned blue area is perforated and enlarged with the fine pick until a round opening is made about twice the width of the 0.6 mm. teflon piston. The piston in this case must extend about 0.5 mm. beyond the inner edge of the footplate opening. The thin tissue graft is applied, and the platinum-teflon piston is positioned as before.

### The "Biscuit Footplate"

This is the thickened footplate with well defined margins, produced by a primary focus in the footplate (Fig. 18–11). With the Harrison knife or a tiny diamond drill the footplate is cut across the center, and the margins of the footplate are thinned until the footplate can be extracted in two pieces, removing the entire focus of otospongiosis, and thus "curing" the disease, provided other foci are not present in this ear. The tissue graft and platinum-teflon piston are applied as before.

### The Dehiscent, Prolapsed Facial Nerve

At the first operation on an ear, there is little difficulty in identifying and avoiding injury to a dehiscent prolapsed facial nerve obscuring the footplate (Fig. 18–2). In most such cases, a small hole can be made in the footplate to receive the thin tissue graft and 0.6 mm. piston without trauma to the nerve.

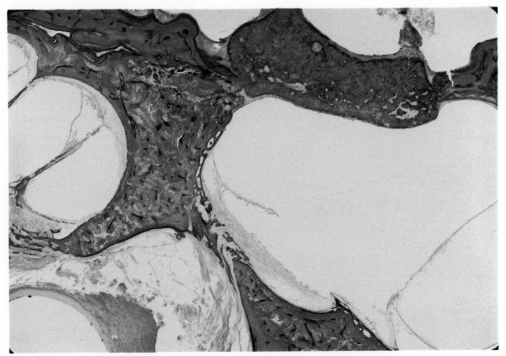

**Figure 18–11**   Primary otospongiotic focus in stapes footplate.

A more difficult and dangerous problem arises when a revision is performed on such an ear when the dehiscent facial nerve has become embedded and pulled down by fibrous tissue filling the oval window niche. Careful removal of the fibrous tissue resulted in injury to the facial nerve in four cases known to the senior author: one of his own resulted in a partial paralysis and three by other very experienced and skillful stapedectomy surgeons resulted in complete paralysis and pending malpractice lawsuits. Avoidance of facial nerve injury in such cases cannot always be avoided and must be ascribed to anatomical anomaly, not to surgical negligence.

### Fixed Malleus

Ankylosis of the malleus head to the attic wall can occur by itself or in combination with otospongiotic stapes ankylosis. It may be that prolonged immobility of the stapes predisposes to malleus ankylosis. In every stapedectomy, the mobility of the malleus and incus should be determined by palpation of the undersurface of the manubrium. Should the malleus be fixed, this should be corrected prior to inserting the prosthesis from incus to oval window, as vibrations from a drill or chisel used to free the malleus would be transmitted to the cochlea with permanent impairment.

Several methods are available for lysis of a fixed malleus. A sharp blow against a microchisel applied to the neck of the malleus may free it (method of J. Causse). If this fails or if the malleus after such a maneuver refixes, the head should be amputated with a microdrill or malleus clipper and removed using an endaural or endomeatal atticotomy. In some cases, a bony bridge between malleus head and anterior attic wall can be removed with a tiny drill without amputating the head.

The incus need not be removed in either of these methods. Only after lysis of a fixed malleus should the prosthesis from incus to oval window be inserted.

## Round Window Closure

Involvement of the margin of the round window niche by otospongiosis is very common, next in frequency to oval window involvement, but unlike the oval window, there is no effect on hearing until the niche is solidly closed. Physiologists of hearing tell us that a tiny opening, no larger than a red cell, suffices for to and fro vibrations of the cochlear fluid column between oval and round windows. The round window can be occluded by fibrous tissue without impairment of its function.

Complete bony closure of the round window, associated with stapes ankylosis, is quite rare and causes a severe combined sensorineural and conductive loss. Stapedectomy in such a case will result in some, but not a great amount of hearing improvement. Attempts to open the round window have been disappointing and should never be done at the same time as stapedectomy.

## Fracture of the Long Process of the Incus

Rarely, an unusually delicate and fragile long process of the incus will fracture as the prosthesis is crimped to it. Should the fracture be high up toward the body of the incus, it will be necessary to create a path between tympanic membrane and manubrium of the malleus to receive a malleus-to-oval window prosthesis. Fracture of the tip of the long process requires that the platinum band be crimped above the site of fracture, with insertion of a bit of folded tissue graft distal to it to promote adhesion to the tympanic membrane, thus avoiding future slippage of the platinum band.

## Perilymph Gusher

A rare, alarming and serious problem of stapes surgery is a profuse flow of perilymph the moment the vestibule is opened, due, as Schuknecht has shown, to abnormal patency of the cochlear duct. Elevation of the head of the table to reduce cerebrospinal fluid pressure lessens the flow of perilymph. Sealing the vestibular opening by a tissue graft held in place by a prosthesis, followed by bedrest while maintaining a 30 degree elevation of the head of the bed until the ear dressing remains dry, will result in cessation of the otorrhea after 2 to 6 days. A permanent cochlear loss is likely to result in such a case. Further surgery on this ear is contraindicated.

## POSTOPERATIVE CARE

A broad-spectrum antibiotic may be given the day of surgery and the next day. Immediately on return to bed after surgery and for the next 48 hours, the head of the bed should be elevated 30 degrees to reduce intracranial and perilymph pressure, thus reducing risk of a perilymph fistula. In most cases, the patient is ambulatory the evening of surgery and returns home the second day after operation.

The sutures and meatal packing are removed 6 or 7 days postoperative and the hearing tested by air and bone and speech discrimination. A loss by bone and discrimination compared to preoperative tests, often with diplacusis, indicates a cochlear reaction. See below under "Early and Late Sensorineural Loss Following Stapes Surgery" for further discussion of cochlear reaction following stapedectomy.

A hearing test made two weeks to a month after operation nearly always shows a good gain in hearing level and discrimination, but the best level of hearing is generally recorded three months postoperative. Before the second visit, a half dropperful of Johnson's Baby Oil in the ear for two nights will soften and facilitate removal of any dried crusts from the meatus.

## COMPLICATIONS OF STAPEDECTOMY

Severance of or trauma to the chorda tympani nerve often (not always) causes loss or distortion of taste on the side of the operation. Even when the nerve was not visibly traumatized, such a disturbance can follow stapedectomy. There is no treatment for this, but in most cases the symptom improves or disappears.

Perforation of the tympanic membrane becomes evident when there is a persistent conductive deficit and air escapes from the meatus on inflating the eustachian tube. If a perforation is seen at the time of surgery, the edges should be approximated and splinted with a patch of cigarette paper or with a connective tissue graft placed on the undersurface of the tympanomeatal flap.

Facial paralysis of the Bell's palsy type can occur several to ten days after an uneventful stapedectomy. In most cases, recovery begins in one to several weeks and will be complete, but in rare cases recovery is delayed and incomplete with synkinesis and spasm. Postoperative Bell's palsy should be treated with steroids like an idiopathic Bell's palsy. Decompression of the nerve might be indicated in rare cases (see Chapter 20).

Otitis media and suppurative labyrinthitis should not occur with careful sterile technique, and as Miot pointed out three quarters of a century ago, these complications indicate failure to maintain surgical asepsis.

### Postoperative Perilymph Fistula

A frequent, perhaps the most frequent, cause for immediate and late cochlear loss after stapedectomy is a slow leak of perilymph from the oval window. Tympanometry may help to indicate such a leak. The symptoms are identical to postoperative endolymphatic hydrops without a fistula. Exploration of the middle ear must be considered, with avoidance of entering the vestibule if a fistula is not found, for creating a fistula, no matter how tiny and how quickly sealed, will make hearing loss due to hydrops worse. If a certain or probable fistula is found, excess fibrous tissue in the oval window is carefully removed by Harrison knives, but the final membrane closing the oval window is left in place, and a generous tissue graft and prosthesis are applied to the oval window to seal the fistula. The prognosis for relief of persistent vertigo caused by a perilymph fistula is favorable after such a revision, but recovery of useful hearing is unusual and should not be promised the patient.

Perilymph fistula was most frequent in the senior author's experience when a polyethylene tube prosthesis was used. It also was common with compressed Gelfoam closure of the oval window, partial stapedectomy with Gelfoam closure, and fat and wire stapedectomy, and it could occur with sudden change in air pressure during a plane flight. Noteworthy have been the paucity of perilymph fistulas following Basek-Fowler anterior crurotomy and transcrural Miot-Rosen mobilizations, and the few fistulas after small hole stapedectomy with tissue graft as described in this text.

## STAPEDECTOMY AFTER FENESTRATION

Many patients who had a fenestration operation performed without the operating microscope subsequently developed recurrence of a large air–bone gap due to osseous closure of the fenestra. A satisfactory hearing improvement can be hoped for in such a case by stapedectomy with prosthesis from malleus handle to oval window. Osseous closure after fenestrations performed under the operating microscope has been quite rare. Stapedectomy in a horizontal canal fenestra that remains open with the average expected residual conductive deficit (see Chapter 19) will be of little value and should not be undertaken. Stapedectomy in an ear unsuccessfully fenestrated in the first place is doomed to failure, for the initial failure was due to serous labyrinthitis, and such an ear is very vulnerable to further hearing loss by surgery that opens the labyrinth. Of course, stapedectomy must not be done in an infected fenestration cavity no matter how localized and slight the infected area, and it must not be done while a perforation of the tympanic membrane is present.

The technique of stapedectomy after closure of a horizontal canal fenestration, as described by Sheehy, is to expose the oval window by a stapes type of meatal incision carried forward just above the prominence of the horizontal semicircular canal. The head and crura of the stapes and the mucosa covering the footplate and margins of the oval window are removed, but without disturbing the footplate as yet. The undersurface of the malleus handle is brought into view by further elevation forward of the tympanic membrane and by rotating the patient's head. A pocket between manubrium and tympanic membrane just below the short process is made using the right angle Harrison knife. A Sheehy incus replacement wire prosthesis (I.R.P.), a Shea malleus-to-oval window teflon prosthesis or a platinum-teflon prosthesis is inserted to grasp the manubrium without perforating the tympanic membrane, its other end measured so as to rest and depress slightly into the vestibule the tissue graft, which is inserted as soon as the posterior part of the footplate has been removed.

Sheer has employed an alternate and simpler method for attaching the prosthesis to the malleus handle.[17] After the footplate has been removed and the oval window closed with a tissue graft, the tympanic membrane is replaced and using a fine pick, holes are made on either side of the manubrium halfway between the umbo and the short process (Fig. 18–12). The teflon-wire prosthesis of proper length is inserted through the posterior hole from the meatal side of the tympanic membrane, and by working alternately underneath and outside the tympanic membrane, the prosthesis is positioned and then the wire loop is crimped onto the malleus handle from the outside of the tympanic membrane (Fig. 18–13). In all cases, the tympanic membrane holes had closed 12 days postoperative, and the wire appeared to be covered by a single epithelial layer.

The prognosis for maintained useful hearing after stapedectomy in a fenestrated ear is considerably poorer than stapedectomy in a virgin ear, for extrusion of the

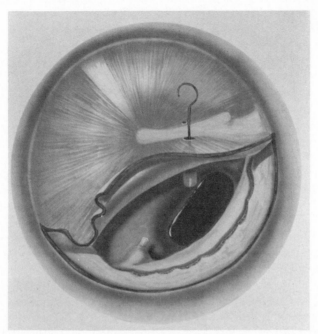

**Figure 18–12**  Holes through tympanic membrane for insertion of prosthesis. (Courtesy of Sheer, A. A. and Amjad, A. H.: A new method of incus bypass in stapedectomy. Arch. Otolaryngol. 100(4):322–323, 1974. Copyright 1974, American Medical Association.)

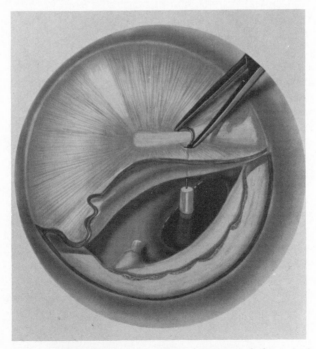

**Figure 18–13**  Crimping of prosthesis onto malleus. (Courtesy of Sheer, A. A. and Amjad, A. H.: A new method of incus bypass in stapedectomy. Arch. Otolaryngol. 100(4):322–323, 1974. Copyright 1974, American Medical Association.)

prosthesis through the tympanic membrane or displacement out of the oval window are frequent postoperative problems, while the procedure is technically difficult.

## REVISION OF STAPES OPERATIONS

Loss of initial gain in hearing after stapes mobilization or stapedectomy can be due to refixation of a mobilized footplate; gradual adherence of the prosthesis to the edge of the oval window (Fig. 18–14); displacement of the prosthesis onto the bony edge of the oval window; osseous closure of the oval window, fixing the prosthesis; aseptic necrosis of the tip of the long process of the incus; slippage of the prosthesis from the long process; loosening of the wire attachment to the incus or ankylosis of the malleus; and rarely ankylosis of the incus to the attic wall. Hearing tests, with special attention to the discrimination score, as well as air and bone testing, always confirmed by tuning forks, will establish whether there is recurrence of a large air–bone gap without sensorineural loss or whether the loss of hearing is largely or entirely sensorineural. Tympanometry will help to define the type of conductive deficit. Revision is indicated for all genuine conductive losses, occurring early or late after stapedectomy, with the probability of a useful hearing improvement. However, the prognosis for maintaining satisfactory hearing after a revision is less favorable than after operation on a virgin ear.

The technique of revision of a stapes operation is exactly the same as for the original operation (Fig. 18–14), except that the chorda tympani nerve is likely to be embedded in adhesions to the meatal skin flap, so that injury to it is probable in order to gain a satisfactory view of the oval window niche. Adhesions between tympanic membrane and incus and in the oval window niche are separated with the tiny right-angled Shambaugh hook or Bellucci scissors (Fig. 18–14B), keeping in mind the possibility of a dehiscent facial nerve that may have prolapsed into the oval window subsequent to the first operation.

Recurrence of a conductive deficit after successful stapedectomy with wire prosthesis is often due to adhesion of the wire to the edge of the oval window. Substituting a teflon piston in such a case usually reduces or eliminates the conductive deficit (Fig. 18–14I).

## EARLY AND LATE SENSORINEURAL LOSS FOLLOWING STAPES SURGERY

Immediate, sometimes irreversible, sensorineural loss after stapedectomy may occur following the most carefully performed, uneventful and atraumatic operation, due to serous nonsuppurative labyrinthitis, possibly with perilymph fistula formation or a middle ear granuloma. Therapy of immediate postoperative cochlear loss is as follows, as described and practiced by J. B. Causse,[15] today's busiest stapedectomy surgeon, and based upon his analysis of 1167 stapedectomies in one year.

1. When fullness in the ear and low frequency bone conduction loss is accompanied by a shift of the 256 Weber test to the unoperated ear 24 to 48 hours after operation, negative middle ear pressure due probably to blood in the eustachian tube was observed once in 50 cases. Purposeful yawning, Valsalva inflation or gentle Politzer bag inflation 24 to 48 hours postoperative immediately improved the symptoms and the Weber at once shifted back to the operated ear. Cortisone, as for a

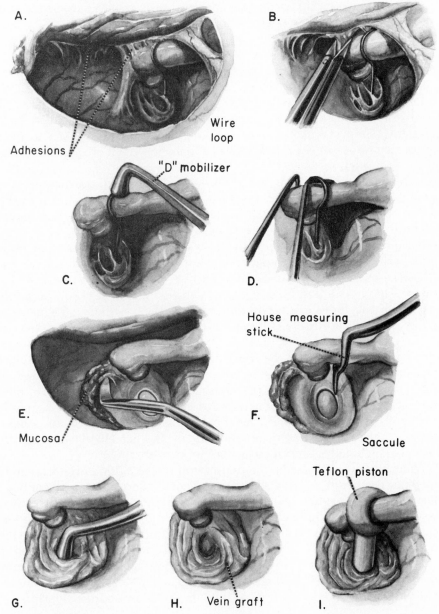

**Figure 18–14**　Stapedectomy revision for wire prosthesis adherent to the edge of the oval window.

Bell's palsy, to help edema of the eustachian tube is routinely prescribed by J. B. Causse after *all* stapedectomies. Preoperative tympanometry in all cases will alert the surgeon to a poorly functioning eustachian tube.

2. Another frequent cause for postoperative cochlear reaction, once in 100 stapedectomies according to J. B. Causse, was disequilibrium of labyrinthine fluids caused by too small a tissue graft with perilymph leak, or too long a prosthesis. The symptoms are those of endolymphatic hydrops and the therapy is expectant with probability of spontaneous recovery. Elevation of the head of the bed, low salt diet, avoidance of eustachian tube inflation, cessation of cigarette smoking, diuresis and dilute histamine (see Chapter 21) may be helpful. **Prevention** by use of a generous

sized areolar or pressed vein tissue graft and prosthesis carefully measured to barely extend beyond the rim of the oval window is the best therapy.

3. A less frequent cause of postoperative cochlear drop according to J. B. Causse, only once in 500 cases, was impaired blood supply to the cochlea by vertebral-basilar artery insufficiency. Preoperative test by electronystagmography (see Chapter 3) for this rare condition and avoidance of torsion of the neck during and following stapedectomy will prevent its occurrence. Carbogen inhalations for 30 minutes two to four times daily is indicated to dilate the cochlear blood supply.

4. Rare (one in a thousand) cases of allergic hydrops occur after stapedectomy. A brief course of steroids as for Bell's palsy and management of any food or inhalant allergy are indicated.

In a few cases (one in 500 in the series of J. B. Causse), all therapy fails, and the patient ends up with a permanent cochlear loss often referred to, erroneously, as a "dead ear." Since there are always remnants of cochlear function and always an active caloric response, the diagnosis of dead ear is incorrect.

Late sensorineural loss after initially successful stapedectomy may be of the sudden labyrinthine deafness type, often with symptoms of hydrops. When seen early these cases may recover with low salt diet, no smoking, diuresis and dilute histamine. The possibility of a perilymph fistula must be kept in mind and exploration of the middle ear without opening the vestibule considered when medical therapy of hydrops fails to control the vertigo and other symptoms of hydrops.

Much more common than the above after successful stapedectomy is a gradual sensorineural deterioration that is disproportionate to the patient's age. If the gradual sensorineural loss is simply consistent with the patient's age, one may assume that it is probably presbycusis. If the sensorineural loss is disproportionate to the patient's age, one should assume that it is the result of active otospongiosis of the cochlear capsule. These cases are more frequent when there was sensorineural involvement combined with stapes fixation prior to surgery.

The mechanism of the sensorineural loss of otospongiotic origin is the liberation into the perilymph of toxic enzymes of bone resorption, as so convincingly demonstrated by Chevance, Causse, et al. (see Chapter 17). A positive Schwartze sign, severe tinnitus and polytomographic visualization of a demineralized focus in the cochlear capsule favor this diagnosis. Moderate dosage sodium fluoride therapy as described in Chapter 17 should be prescribed for at least two years, and longer than this in most cases. As many of these patients are in the older age group with a tendency toward osteoporosis, their skeletal bone strength, as well as retardation or arrest of sensorineural deterioration, will be improved by sodium fluoride.

## REFERENCES

1. Kessel, J.: Über das Mobilisieren des Steigbügels durch Ausschneiden des Trommelfelles, Hammers und Amboss bei undurchgängigkeit der Tuba. Arch. Ohrenh., 13:69, 1878.
2. Boucheron, E.: La mobilisation de l'étrier et son procédé opératoire. Union méd., Paris, 46:412, 1888.
3. Miot, C.: De la mobilisation de l'étrier. Rev. Laryng., 10:49, 83, 145, 200, 1890.
4. Blake, C. J.: Middle ear operations. Tr. Am. Otol. Soc., 5:2, 306, 1892.
5. Jack, F. L.: Further observations on removal of the stapes. Tr. Am. Otol. Soc., 5:3, 474, 1893.
6. Faraci, G.: Importanza acustica e funzionale della mobilizzazione della staffa; Risultati di una nuova serie di operazioni. Arch. ital. otol., 9:209, 1899.
7. Siebenmann, F.: Sur le traitement chirurgical de la sclérose otique. Congr. internat. Méd., Sect. Otol., 13:170, 1900.

8. Rosen, S.: Palpation of stapes for fixation: preliminary procedure to determine fenestration suitability for otosclerosis. Arch. Otol., 56:610, 1952.

9. Shambaugh, G. E., Jr.: The surgical treatment of deafness. Illinois Med. J., 81:104, 1940.

10. Heermann, H.: Mobilisierung des Steigbügels durch Ausmeisseln und Eiwärtzverlagern der Fussplatte. Stschr. Laryng. u. Rhinol. 35:415, 1956.

11. Derlacki, E. L.: Chisel technics for stapes mobilization. Arch. Otol., 71:271, 1960.

12. Basek, M., and Fowler, E. P., Jr.: Anatomical factors in stapes mobilization operations. Arch. Otol., 63:589, 1956.

13. Shea, J. J., Jr.: Fenestration of the oval window. Ann. Otol. Rhin. & Laryng., 67:932, 1958.

14. Rüedi, L., and Spoendlin, H.: Histology of the otosclerotic ankylosis of the stapes. In Rüedi, L. (Ed.): Advances in Oto-Rhino-Laryngology. Vol. 4, New York, S. Karger, 1957.

15. Causse, J. B.: Personal Communication.

16. Sheer, A. A.: Retrieving the lost heavy footplate fragment. Arch. Otol., 91:412, 1970.

17. Sheer, A. A., and Amjad, A. H.: A new method of incus bypass stapedectomy. Arch. Otol., 100:322, 1974.

## Maurice Sourdille

BORN 1885
DIED 1961

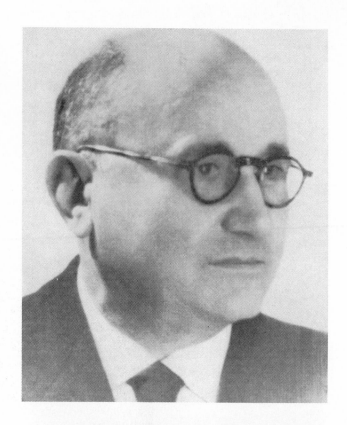

His ingenious tympano-labyrinthopexy permanently restored useful hearing for the first time in patients with otosclerosis and formed the basis for the one-stage fenestration operation of Lempert.

## Julius Lempert

BORN 1890
DIED 1968

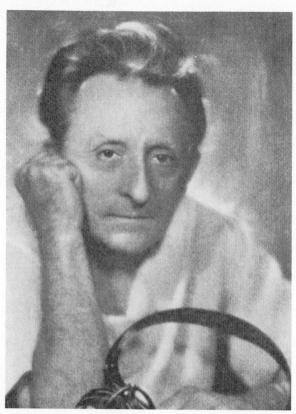

Foremost advocate of the endaural approach to the temporal bone. His one-stage fenestration operation led to the renaissance of reconstructive surgery for conductive hearing losses.

500

# Chapter 19

# Fenestration Operation for Otospongiosis (Otosclerosis)

INTRODUCTION
HISTORICAL ASPECTS
MECHANICS OF THE FENESTRATED EAR
INDICATIONS FOR THE FENESTRATION OPERATION
TECHNIQUE OF THE FENESTRATION OPERATION
SURGICAL ACCIDENTS DURING FENESTRATION
POSTOPERATIVE CARE
EARLY COMPLICATIONS AFTER FENESTRATION
LATE COMPLICATIONS AFTER FENESTRATION

## INTRODUCTION

The fenestration operation, hardly ever employed today for stapedial otospongiosis* and only occasionally for congenital malformations of the middle ear, will remain forever as a mighty landmark in the evolution of surgery to restore hearing. Clinical experience with thousands of fenestrated ears requiring annual or oftener cleaning of the fenestrated cavity continues to provide a unique opportunity to follow the course of otospongiotic disease by hearing tests over many years. Such an opportunity will never again occur, for successfully stapedectomized patients have no need for annual visits to their surgeon.

Studies of the cochlear reaction to opening of the labyrinth after fenestration, with occasional permanent impairment of cochlear function, help the otologist to understand the similar reaction that follows stapedectomy. The thousands of fenestrated patients who continue to require care of their modified radical mastoid cavities often develop infections of the cavity and, not infrequently, inner ear sensorineural losses that require therapy by the young otologists who have succeed-

---

*The last patient operated by the senior author by classical fenestration was in 1972. This young man with bilateral active and extensive oval window otospongiosis had undergone four stapedectomies, two on each ear, with loss of gain each time due to bony obliteration of the oval window. Fenestration of the horizontal semicircular canal, an area not involved by diseased bone, was successful in achieving a lasting improvement.

**501**

ed the surgeons who performed the operations. To deal effectively with these problems, an understanding of the surgical technique and complications of this once frequent operation is required, hence the space in this third edition of *Surgery of the Ear* devoted to classic fenestration of the horizontal semicircular canal.

## HISTORICAL ASPECTS

The one-stage fenestration operation introduced in 1938 by Lempert,[1] with the application to it of the operating microscope in 1940 by the senior author[2] of this text, marked the turning point from surgery for aural suppuration to the extraordinary blossoming of microsurgery in a clean field for the restoration of hearing.

As described in Chapter 17, prior to 1938 otospongiotic stapes fixation was rarely diagnosed in America and England, and when recognized was considered a dreadful, progressive disease for which there was no treatment, leading inexorably to profound deafness. The earliest and forgotten operations upon the fixed stapes by Kessel[3] in 1878, Miot[4] in 1890, and Blake[5] and Jack[6] in 1892 and 1893, mentioned in Chapter 18, might have begun a fruitful development of operations for stapedial otospongiosis had not Siebenmann's[7] pronouncement of 1900, joined by Politzer and other leaders in otology, that "attempts at mobilization of the stapes are not only useless but often harmful" effectively banned for more than half a century further surgery upon the fixed stapes.

Earlier, in 1897, Passow,[8] while discussing stapedectomy for otosclerosis, had mentioned that the same hearing improvement could be obtained by making a window in the promontory and then covering it by the tympanic membrane, and that such an operation had relieved tinnitus and slightly improved hearing.

The first report, after Siebenmann's pronouncement, of surgery for otospongiotic stapes fixation came from England in 1913 when Jenkins[9] made a fenestration in the horizontal semicircular canal and covered it by a Thiersch skin graft, with a slight improvement in hearing in two patients. Bárány[10] and then Holmgren[11] quietly dared to go against the prevalent opposition to surgery for stapedial otospongiosis in a long series of operations to "decompress the labyrinth" by making various fistulas, usually in a semicircular canal. Repeatedly, an immediate improvement in hearing was observed, but always it receded in the ensuing months.

The operations reported by Holmgren, who used careful sterile technique, gradually dispelled the dread of opening the labyrinth in a clean field. Using a binocular instrument, Holmgren had applied Nylén's operating microscope to otospongiosis surgery in 1922. He demonstrated that osseous closure of the labyrinthine window was the great stumbling block to permanent hearing improvements in these cases. He was the first to observe through the operating microscope the otospongiotic (otosclerotic) focus in front of the oval window fixing the stapes.

Holmgren's scientific integrity, backed by the experimental investigations of Engström[12] and the histologic observations of Nager,[13] helped to dispel the prejudice against surgery for otospongiosis. In 1924 Sourdille,[14] attracted by Holmgren's reports, visited his clinic, observed operations for constructing a horizontal canal fistula and returned to France where he devised the method of covering the fistula in the horizontal semicircular canal with a meatal skin flap attached to the tympanic membrane. For the first time, lasting improvements in hearing were achieved by fenestrating the labyrinth. In 1947 the senior author of this text examined two of Sourdille's early operations, one done in 1932, the other in 1935. In both patients, the healed cavity appeared exactly like one of Lempert's early fenestrations with the incus beneath the flap and the wide open fenestra clearly visible through the very thin skin covering it, and both patients had excellent hearing comparable audiometrically to successful Lempert fenestration operations.

In 1937 Sourdille[15] reported his technique and results before the New York Academy of Medicine. Lempert attended this lecture and was inspired to use this method in a series of cases of stapes fixation, but performed endaurally and in one stage, rather than in the two or three stages that Sourdille employed. Lempert followed Sourdille precisely in leaving the incus in place, amputating the head of the malleus and covering the horizontal semicircular canal fenestra with a tympanomeatal skin flap. Lempert called this the "fenestration operation," an easier name than Sourdille's "tympanolabyrinthopexy." Soon after Lempert's first publication in 1938,[1] the senior author of this text became his first pupil; then other otologic surgeons from America and abroad came to observe his skillful endaural technique and his favorable hearing results, and remained to learn the technique by cadaver dissections. Meanwhile, Lempert found that the incus was not needed as Sourdille had insisted "to carry sound across the mobile incus from the tympanic membrane to the horizontal canal window," and by removing the incus, a larger fenestra could be constructed over the ampulla of the horizontal canal. This Lempert[16] named the "fenestra nov-ovalis," as it resembled in size the oval window that it replaced.

Meanwhile, beginning in 1940 in a series of experimental fenestrations on monkeys by the senior author of this text[17] and his wife, a microsurgical technique began to be developed with enchondralization of the fenestra and continuous irrigation under an operating microscope to remove all bone dust particles. With use of the microscope, the tendency toward osteogenic closure of the fenestra was reduced to around 5 per cent of fenestrations. Wullstein and Zöllner were among the first to follow the senior author in using the microscope for fenestration operations, and then used it for their pioneer techniques of microsurgical tympanoplasty. Wullstein's lectures at the First Workshop in Chicago in 1959 convincingly established the techniques of tympanoplasty and the advantages of the operating microscope, until then opposed by Lempert who insisted that the microscope "made things larger, but not clearer." The Zeiss otomicroscope, demonstrated for the first time in 1953 at the International Congress in Amsterdam by Jongkees, soon became an essential tool in the new era of otologic microsurgery in a clean field to restore hearing.

## MECHANICS OF THE FENESTRATED EAR

The mechanical principle of the fenestration operation was simply stated by Passow[8] in 1897: it creates a sound pathway to the labyrinth to take the place of the oval window occluded by the otospongiotic stapes fixation. It is surprising that not until 1950 was the mechanics of the fenestrated ear more clearly understood, explaining its residue of unrestored conductive hearing loss as due to absence of the transformer mechanism of the middle ear. In 1948 on the basis of simple experiments on fenestrated patients Juers[18] had concluded that sound enters the labyrinth directly through the skin covering the fenestra, rather than being carried from the tympanic membrane to the fenestra, as maintained by Sourdille. Juers pointed out the necessity for an intact tympanic membrane "to protect the round window somewhat from direct exposure to sound," thus reviving the long forgotten

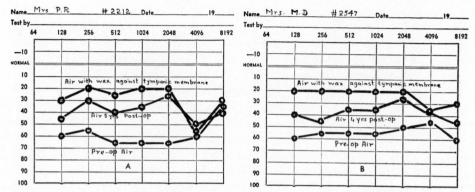

**Figure 19–1** Average result of fenestration in two patients whose hearing was improved by ointment blocking of the tympanic membrane.

concept of **round window protection** proposed by Kessel three quarters of a century earlier, and soon to be applied by Zöllner and Wullstein to their tympanoplasties. Juers also found that weighting or covering the tympanic membrane in the fenestrated ear with mercury or ointment affords an average gain of 5 decibels for the speech frequencies by reducing sound reaching the round window. The technique continues to be used by the senior author[19] to "sharpen the hearing" of many of his fenestrated patients who return every two or three months as the specially prepared ointment*migrates away from the tympanic membrane with a subjective decline in hearing (Fig. 19–1).

In 1950 Davis and Walsh[20] explained the residue of unrestored conductive loss after fenestration as due to absence of the transformer action of the large tympanic membrane connected by the ossicular chain to the small oval window. The senior author[21] found that this residual conductive loss averages 25 decibels for the speech frequencies.

## INDICATIONS FOR THE FENESTRATION OPERATION

Stapedectomy, because there is no residual conductive loss when completely successful, as well as because of the brief convalescence and absence of a postoperative radical mastoid cavity requiring life-long care, has replaced horizontal canal fenestration for stapedial fixation except for the following rare conditions: a prolapsed anomalous facial nerve covering the oval window; repeated closure of the oval window by active otospongiosis; and congenital absence of an oval window with good cochlear function.

In 1950 Carhart[22] discovered the average notching in the bone conduction audiogram that disappears after successful fenestration. The Carhart notch also disappears after stapedectomy, accounting for the frequent over-closure of the air–bone gap. In 1951 the senior author[21] proposed that the hearing result of fenestration could be predicted as 25 decibels poorer than the bone conduction curve corrected for Carhart's notch. Since this correction averages 10 decibels for the speech frequencies, one can predict the result of fenestration as simply 15 decibels

*The ointment is made of 2.5 per cent Neocortef ointment 45 gm., Polysorb 442.6 gm., beeswax 88.0 gm. and acetic acid 4.4 mm. It is warmed in a metal syringe and placed against the tympanic membrane through a 20 gauge blunt-end needle.

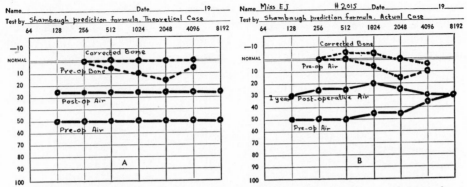

**Figure 19–2** Shambaugh formula for prediction of results of fenestration. *A*, Theoretical case. *B*, Actual case.

poorer than the preoperative bone audiogram. Patients were then classified according to the predicted postoperative hearing. An "A" case will be ideal for fenestration, having preoperative bone conduction within 25 decibels (I.S.O.) so that the predicted result will be within 40 decibels (I.S.O.) (Fig. 19–2). A case of "B" suitability with 26 to 35 decibels loss by bone should reach a level between 41 and 50 decibels after successful fenestration. A "C" case will have a bone curve poorer than 35 decibels and a predicted result poorer than 50 decibels.

The candidate for fenestration was informed that the properly selected hearing aid was an acceptable alternative to surgery and that surgery carried certain uncertainties and risks: 1 chance in 5 that the predicted hearing level would not be achieved, or if achieved, would not be maintained beyond two years; a 1 or 2 per cent chance of a further hearing loss in the operated ear such that a hearing aid might not be satisfactory in it; a hospital stay of 7 to 10 days with another 3 weeks away from work to recover equilibrium, at least 2 months of postoperative care of the fenestrated cavity, and thereafter visits once or twice a year for cleaning of the cavity and testing of the hearing. Mentioned also was the rare case of facial nerve paralysis coming on several to 8 days after operation, nearly always recovering spontaneously and completely; impairment of taste due to chorda tympani dysfunction; and occasional imbalance lasting beyond 3 or 4 postoperative weeks. When a patient was given all of the information and was unable to decide for or against surgery, he was encouraged to use a hearing aid for a year or two. Some of the most grateful fenestrated patients were those who had used a hearing aid and were freed from the need for this prosthesis.

The candidate for fenestration must, of course, have an ear with sufficient air–bone gap, confirmed by tuning fork Rinné tests with narow-band masking of the opposite ear, to predict a useful improvement. The ear must be free from outer or middle ear infection, the eustachian tube must be functioning and the tympanic membrane must be intact. Because of the 1 or 2 per cent chance of an irreversible cochlear loss, the poorer hearing ear should be selected for surgery.

## TECHNIQUE OF THE FENESTRATION OPERATION

The technique described below had been utilized by the senior author and his associates since 1946. It consists of Lempert's one-stage endaural nov-ovalis fenestration modified by use of an operating microscope, with use of continuous irrigation and a diamond drill to create an enchondralized bone-dust–free "micro-immaculate" fenestra covered by Sourdille's tympano-meatal skin flap, which is rotated so that the thinnest skin from the anterior meatal wall covers the fenestra and can be invaginated slightly into the fenestra.

The operation can be performed quite well under local anesthesia with adequate

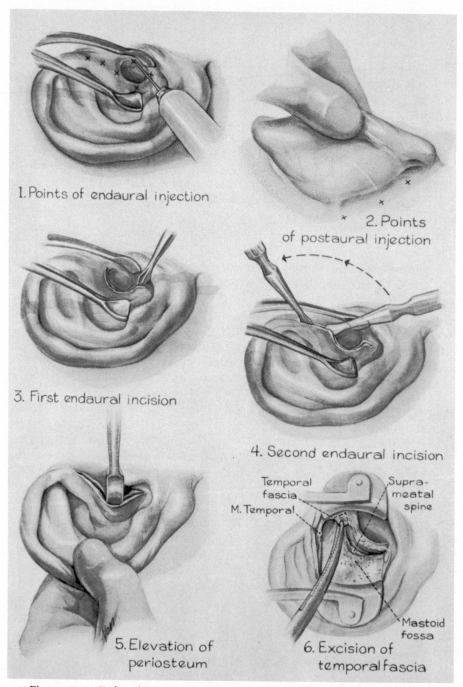

**Figure 19–3**    Endaural injection, incision and retraction for fenestration operation.

preoperative sedation. With this method, there is less bleeding and greater safety to the patient, over 5000 fenestrations having been performed under local anesthesia by the senior author and his associates, Juers and Derlacki, without an operative or postoperative fatality.

The steps in the fenestration operation are shown quite clearly in Figures 19–3, 19–4, 19–5, 19–6, 19–7 and 19–9. Complete removal of all mastoid cells is avoided,

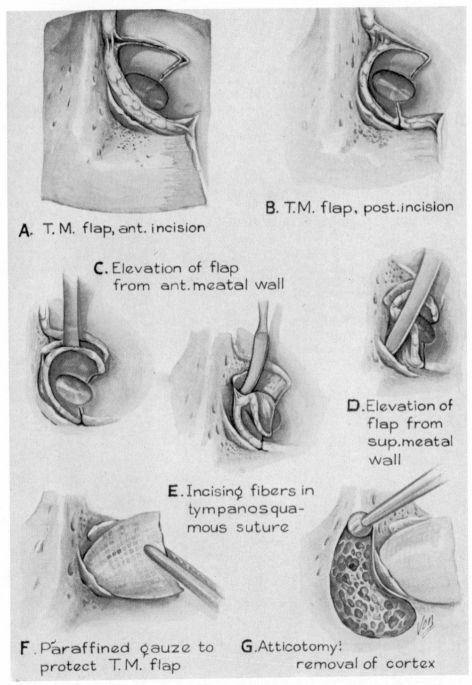

**A.** T.M. flap, ant. incision

**B.** T.M. flap, post. incision

**C.** Elevation of flap from ant. meatal wall

**D.** Elevation of flap from sup. meatal wall

**E.** Incising fibers in tympanosquamous suture

**F.** Paraffined gauze to protect T.M. flap

**G.** Atticotomy: removal of cortex

**Figure 19–4**   Construction of tympanomeatal (T.M.) plastic flap for fenestration operation.

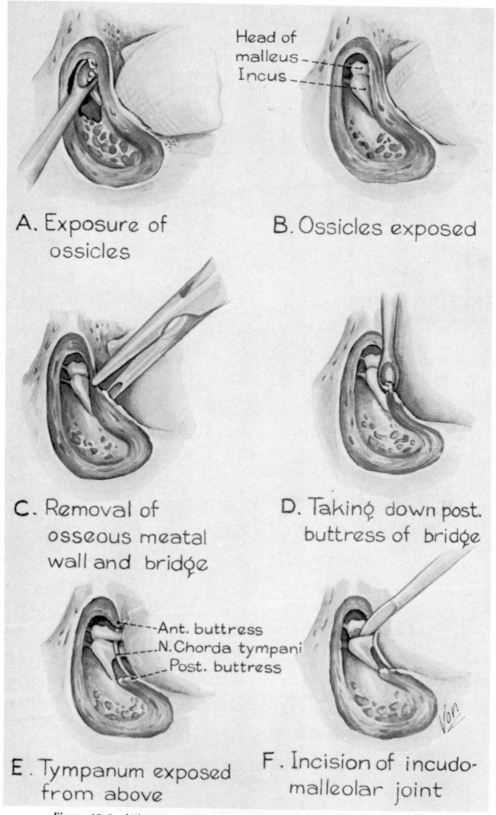

A. Exposure of ossicles

B. Ossicles exposed

Head of malleus
Incus

C. Removal of osseous meatal wall and bridge

D. Taking down post. buttress of bridge

E. Tympanum exposed from above

Ant. buttress
N. Chorda tympani
Post. buttress

F. Incision of incudo-malleolar joint

**Figure 19–5**   Atticotomy and removal of osseous meatal wall for fenestration.

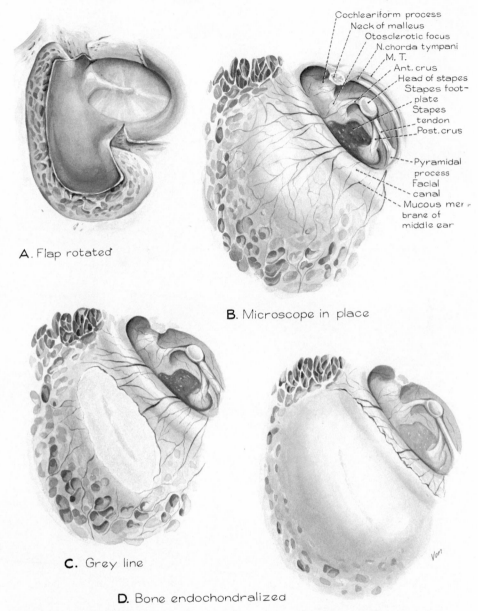

A. Flap rotated

B. Microscope in place

Cochleariform process
Neck of malleus
Otosclerotic focus
N. chorda tympani
M. T.
Ant. crus
Head of stapes
Stapes foot-
plate
Stapes
tendon
Post. crus
Pyramidal
process
Facial
canal
Mucous mer -
brane of
middle ear

C. Grey line

D. Bone endochondralized

**Figure 19–6**   Enchondralization of osseous horizontal semicircular canal (6× magnification).

as it creates an unnecessarily large cavity, which is more difficult to keep clean. Bone chips and bone dust packed into remaining open cells, with perfect sterile technique during the operation and in the postoperative care, will result in healthy granulations and then in skin lining the moderately sized radical mastoid cavity.

Since bone dust and chips are osteogenic (Fig. 19–8), it is necessary to remove under magnified vision every adherent particle of bone from the tympanomeatal flap (the "toilet of the flap") as well as from the fenestra. The senior author prefers the "eggshell technique" of removing fractured endosteal bone from the fenestra, rather than the "cupola technique," both of which are illustrated in Figure 19–9.

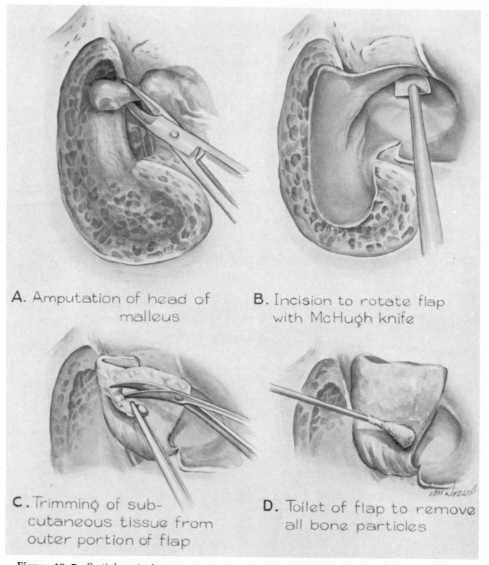

A. Amputation of head of
malleus

B. Incision to rotate flap
with McHugh knife

C. Trimming of sub-
cutaneous tissue from
outer portion of flap

D. Toilet of flap to remove
all bone particles

**Figure 19–7** Partial ossiculectomy and toilet of plastic flap for fenestration operation (2× magnification).

By widely removing the periosteal bone around the future fenestra with the diamond drill, the fenestra is "enchondralized," exposing the osteogenically inert endochondral layer of the labyrinthine capsule. The edges of the fenestra are left sharp (not curetted), the fenestra lies on top of a dome and the endosteal membrane within is not disturbed. The rotated tympanomeatal skin flap over the fenestra is covered with a wide strip of surgical rayon; then a small oval piece of photographer's grade synthetic sponge is placed on the fenestra to invaginate the skin flap slightly. A surgical rayon closed sleeve is placed in the cavity and packed snugly, but not tightly, with cotton balls or synthetic sponge. A single suture at the top of the endaural incision leaves the meatus two or three times wider than eventually desired.

## SURGICAL ACCIDENTS DURING FENESTRATION

The most frequent accident is tear of the tympanomeatal skin flap. The torn edges should be approximated and healing will be uneventful. Should the meatal flap be badly damaged or lost, the fenestra can be covered with a Thiersch skin graft taken from the undersurface, non-hair–bearing area of the upper arm.

Perforation of the tympanic membrane should be splinted by a patch of cigarette paper, taking care that the edges are not folded under. Should the perforation not heal, a future myringoplasty will be needed to give sound protection to the round window.

Tear of the endolymphatic labyrinth in the horizontal canal is more serious and is best avoided by using continuous irrigation and the operating microscope. A poor hearing result is likely, but not inevitable.

Exposure of the tympanic segment of the facial nerve, if done knowingly under adequate magnification, need cause no concern. Obvious trauma or section of the nerve requires decompression to normal nerve in both directions and rerouting approximation, or a nerve graft if there is a defect.

A laceration of the dura with escape of spinal fluid should be covered with a large piece of temporalis muscle after being certain there are no depressed bone fragments. The patient's head should be kept elevated for several days to reduce intracranial spinal fluid pressure, until the dressing remains dry.

Perforation of the sigmoid sinus causes alarming bleeding, which is quickly controlled by a large piece of compressed Gelfoam held in place with a one inch wide piece of iodoform gauze quickly applied until bleeding has stopped, usually 2 or 3 minutes by the clock. The iodoform gauze is removed cautiously, the Gelfoam is left in place, and the operation proceeds.

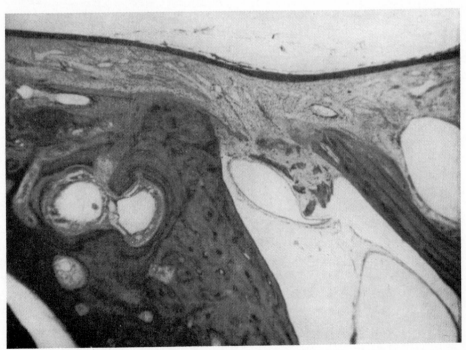

**Figure 19–8**   Bone dust particles surrounded by pale new bone, closing a fenestra of a monkey 6 weeks after operation.

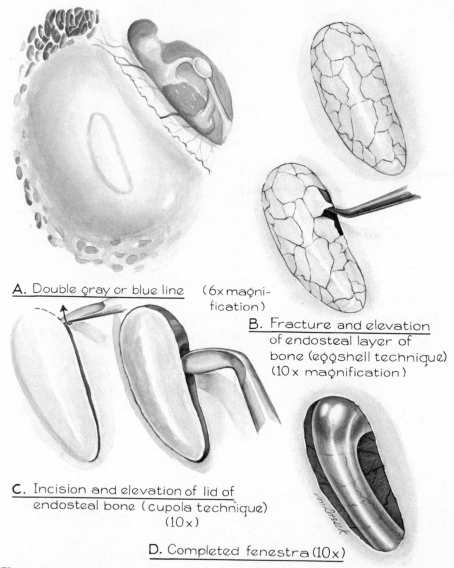

A. Double gray or blue line (6x magnification)

B. Fracture and elevation of endosteal layer of bone (eggshell technique) (10x magnification)

C. Incision and elevation of lid of endosteal bone (cupola technique) (10x)

D. Completed fenestra (10x)

**Figure 19–9** Creation of fenestra by fractured eggshell technique (Shambaugh) and by cupola technique (Lempert).

## POSTOPERATIVE CARE

Infection of the operated cavity leads to soft infected granulations, purulent discharge, delayed epidermization, infection of remaining mastoid and petrous air cells and the possibility of suppurative labyrinthitis and a totally dead ear. Therefore, not only the operation itself, but postoperative dressings for at least the first month must be accomplished with sterile technique, using freshly sterilized cotton and instruments, with thorough scrubbing of the hands of the surgeon and the use of sterile towels for drying. Serous drainage from the meatus can be removed with cotton applicators, and 2 per cent aqueous gentian violet applied to the lips of the endaural incision, which, to prevent postoperative atresia, should be spread open once a week to twice the size eventually desired. The cavity is not otherwise disturbed. After one month, the meatus will have healed at its desired size, and the patient is then instructed to place in his ear on retiring a dropperful of warmed 5 per cent boric acid in 70 per cent alcohol. When he returns two months after operation, the cavity will probably be nicely epidermized and dry. Should there be any unhealed area of granulations, the application of 2 per cent aqueous gentian violet encourages epidermization.

Some surgeons elect to apply split thickness skin grafts from the undersurface of the upper arm between 2 and 3 weeks postoperatively, these being placed on the bed of healthy granulations that have formed.

Primary skin grafting of the cavity at the time of fenestration, used in 100 consecutive cases by the senior author,[24] resulted in a very thin, unhealthy type of skin closely adherent to the underlying bone and lacking the usual layer of subepithelial connective tissue. These ears continue to cause trouble with excessive desquamation and tiny areas of granulations and moisture.

## EARLY COMPLICATIONS AFTER FENESTRATION

A Bell's palsy type of facial paralysis begins several to 8 to 10 days after operation in about 1 per cent of cases, a little less often if the facial nerve in its horizontal tympanic segment was not exposed. These cases should be treated conservatively with prednisone (see Chapter 20) and nearly always recover spontaneously and completely. The indications for surgical decompression (rarely required) are the same as for Bell's palsy.

Facial paralysis noted immediately after operation can be due to spread of the local anesthetic to the stylomastoid foramen. If it does not clear up in an hour or two, surgical injury to the nerve must be assumed, and the nerve should be uncovered, explored and decompressed the next day, and if a defect is found, it should be repaired by rerouting or a free nerve graft. Care must be taken not to disturb the portion of tympanomeatal skin covering the fenestra.

Postoperative labyrinthine reaction, termed serous labyrinthitis since it is reversible, occurs to some degree after every surgical opening of the labyrinth, whether fenestration of a semicircular canal or stapedectomy. Within 24 to 48 hours of fenestration, vertigo and spontaneous nystagmus reach their height; then four to six days after operation the vestibular sterile labyrinthitis is subsiding, but the reaction has spread to the cochlea with a decrease in bone-conducted hearing greatest for tones of high pitch, distortion and diplacusis. By 10 days to 2 weeks postoperative, the cochlear reaction is subsiding, with gradual improvement in bone and air hearing and disappearance of distortion and diplacusis. In cases of successful fenestration, the hearing continues to improve slowly to its best level, which is reached at around 3 months postoperative.

Various treatments were tried by the senior author[25] and Juers to combat postoperative serous labyrinthitis, none of statistical value. Since the labyrinthine reaction resembles and probably is an endolymphatic hydrops, the use of prednisone, carbogen inhalations 2 to 4 times a day (5 per cent carbon dioxide and 95 per cent oxygen), cessation of cigarette smoking, a low salt diet and a diuretic might be considered.

Postoperative femoral phlebitis with pulmonary emboli (none fatal, fortunately) occurred in two early fenestrated patients. Using Ochsner's routine of massage and elevation of the legs, with deep breathing every half hour for 6 hours, then every 3 hours until the patient was ambulatory, no further cases occurred.

## LATE COMPLICATIONS AFTER FENESTRATION

Suppurative labyrinthitis is, fortunately, exceedingly rare and was not seen immediately postoperative in the more than 5000 fenestrated patients operated by the senior author and his associates. Thus far, 4 cases have occurred 5 to 30 years after fenestration, due each time to neglected infection of the fenestration cavity, all 4 resulting in a completely dead ear and 1 ending in fatal meningitis. For this reason, every fenestrated patient must be impressed again and again with the necessity for regular cleaning of his cavity at least once a year, oftener if needed, and the immediate necessity for cavity cleaning should the ear begin to drain. Should suppurative labyrinthitis occur, an immediate labyrinthectomy is advisable to prevent intracranial spread.

To facilitate removal of adherent crusts from the fenestrated cavity, the patient is instructed to put a medicine dropperful of Johnson's Baby Oil into his ear for 3 or 4 nights before each visit. Should there be moisture under the crusts, 2 per cent aqueous gentian violet is applied to granulations and each night the patient instills a dropperful of warmed 5 per cent boric acid in 70 per cent alcohol. Such an ear should be cleaned and gentian violet applied frequently (once weekly) until perfectly dry and clean.

Occasionally these measures fail to obtain a dry ear, and mucopus can be seen repeatedly coming from a certain area of the cavity. This indicates an area of osteitis that requires curetting of the softened bone down to hard healthy bone. As years go by, there is a tendency in some cases for a deep retraction to develop toward the mastoid tip, which is difficult to keep clean. This may require a postaural approach to lower the facial ridge and to remove the deep tip cells filled with cholesteatoma debris, and then the use of a Palva type of fascial-muscle pedicle graft to obliterate the tip area, with care not to cover ány cholesteatoma matrix!

A rather frequent and poorly understood late complication of fenestration (and of stapedectomy) is an attack of endolymphatic hydrops in the operated ear. One may speculate that large protein molecules reaching the endolymphatic sac during the immediate postoperative serous labyrinthitis impair the future resorptive function of the sac. At any rate, years after a successful operation and maintained hearing improvement, the patient may experience a rather acute drop in hearing by air and by bone, with distortion, diplacusis, impairment of discrimination, tinnitus, pressure and even pain in the ear.[26] Imbalance and sometimes vertigo may be present. Most of these cases respond quickly to a low salt diet, a diuretic (Dyazide 1 or 2 tablets daily), cessation of cigarette smoking, and very dilute histamine given twice weekly by subcutaneous injection and by sublingual drops on days not injected. Quite often the very first injection of 0.1 cc. of 1:100,000,000 dilution of histamine is followed within hours by a miraculous improvement in symptoms. If so, this "optimum dose" is not increased. If the patient is no better, the dose is progressively increased until improvement occurs. The sublingual drops, 2 twice daily, are 10 times the strength of the injected histamine. The mode of action of dilute histamine for hydrops is not known. Perhaps it stimulates the production of the body's enzyme histaminase. At any rate, it works especially well in hydrops occurring months or years after successful fenestration or stapedectomy (Fig. 19–9). Endolymphatic sac drainage in a few cases was of no value.

Closure of the fenestra by osteogenesis is quite rare with the technique described. If it is going to occur, it does so generally within 2 years of the operation, but it can occur much later. There is a very gradual decline in hearing of the conductive type with recurrence of a large air–bone gap without impairment of discrimination, and there is a decrease or disappearance of the fistula test by gentle pressure over the site of fenestration. Stapedectomy may then be considered, using a prosthesis from malleus handle to oval window as described in Chapter 18. These operations are technically difficult, as the prosthesis must grasp the malleus handle close to the short process without perforating the tympanic membrane. The other end of the prosthesis should reach and depress a little into the vestibule the fascial or vein graft used to close the oval window. The senior author prefers to use a platinum and teflon prosthesis, which is more easily crimped onto the malleus than a stainless steel wire.

Stapedectomy on an ear with an open fenestra and the usual moderate conductive deficit is of little or no benefit.

Gradual sensorineural hearing deterioration occurs eventually in the majority of fenestrated ears followed for 20 to 40 years. In some, this is consistent with the patient's age and attributable to presbycusis; in others, often, in the experience of the senior author, it is accompanied by active expansion of the otospongiotic disease toward the cochlear endosteum. The diagnosis of active cochlear otospongiosis and its therapy with sodium fluoride is described fully in Chapter 17.

## REFERENCES

1. Lempert, J.: Improvement of hearing in cases of otosclerosis: new one-stage surgical technic. Arch. Otol., 28:42, 1938.
2. Shambaugh, G. E., Jr.: The surgical treatment of deafness. Illinois Med. J., 81:104, 1940.
3. Kessel, J.: Ueber das Mobilisieren des Steigbügels durch Ausschneiden des Trommelfelles, Hammers und Amboss bei undurchgängigkeit der Tuba. Arch. Ohrenh., 13:69, 1877.
4. Miot, C.: De la mobilisation de l'étrier. Rev. laryng., 10:49, 83, 113, 145, 200, 1890.
5. Blake, C. J.: Middle ear operations. Tr. Am. Otol. Soc., 5:306, 1892.
6. Jack, F. L.: Further observations on removal of the stapes. Tr. Am. Otol. Soc., 5:474, 1893.
7. Siebenmann, F.: Sur le traitement chirurgical de la sclérose otique. Congr. Internat. Med., Sect. Otol., 13:11, 1900.
8. Passow, H.: In Panse, R.: Discussion. Verhandl. deutsch. otol. Gesellsch., 6:141, 1897.
9. Jenkins, G. J.: Otosclerosis: certain clinical features and experimental operative procedures. Tr. XVIIth Internat. Congr. Med., London, 16:609, 1913.
10. Bárány, R.: Die Indikationen zur Labyrinthoperation. Acta oto-laryng., 6:260, 1924.
11. Holmgren, G.: Some experiences in surgery for otosclerosis. Acta oto-laryng., 5:460, 1923.
12. Engström, H.: Über das Vorkommen der Otosklerose nebst experimentellen Studien über chirurgische Behandlung der Krankheit. Acta oto-laryng., Suppl. 43, 1940.
13. Nager, F. R.: Demonstration der Schnitte einer Patienten mit Otosklerose. Acta oto-laryng., 26:342, 1938.
14. Sourdille, M.: Résultats primitifs et secondaires de quatorze cas de surdité par otospongiose opérés. Rev. laryng., 51:595, 1930.
15. Sourdille, M.: New technic in the surgical treatment of severe and progressive deafness from otosclerosis. Bull. New York Acad. Med., 13:673, 1937.
16. Lempert, J.: The permanently patent fenestra nov-ovalis. Laryngoscope, 61:215, 1951.
17. Shambaugh, G. E., Jr.: Fenestration operation for otosclerosis; experimental investigations and clinical observations. Acta oto-laryng., Suppl. 79, 1949.
18. Juers, A. L.: Observations on bone conduction in fenestration cases. Ann. Otol. Rhin. & Laryng., 57:28, 1948.
19. Shambaugh, G. E., Jr.: Technic for increasing sound pressure differential between fenestra and round window to enhance hearing improvement following successful fenestration. Tr. Am. Acad. Ophth., 58:454, 1954.
20. Davis, H., and Walsh, T.: The limits of improvement of hearing following the fenestration operation. Laryngoscope, 60:273, 1950.
21. Shambaugh, G. E., Jr.: Correlation of the predicted with the actual result of fenestration in 164 consecutive cases. Laryngoscope, 62:461, 1952.
22. Carhart, R.: The clinical application of bone conduction audiometry. Arch. Otol., 51:798, 1950.
23. Shambaugh, G. E., Jr., and Juers, A. L.: Surgical treatment of otosclerosis, preliminary report on an improved fenestration technic. Arch. Otol., 43:549, 1946.
24. Shambaugh, G. E., Jr.: Primary skin grafting of the fenestra and fenestration cavity. Arch. Otol., 64:46, 1956.
25. Shambaugh, G. E., Jr., and Takahara, S.: A clinical and experimental study of the effect of fenestration on the labyrinthine contents. Acta oto-laryng., Suppl. 123, 1955.
26. Shambaugh, G. E., Jr.: Histamine in treatment of certain types of headache and vertigo following the fenestration operation. Arch. Otol., 51:781, 1950.

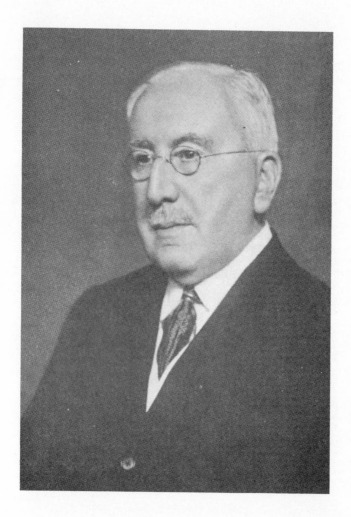

*Sir Charles Ballance*

BORN 1856
DIED 1936

Foremost pioneer aural surgeon of Britain; also founder
and first president of the Society of British Neurological
Surgeons. In experiments
with Arthur B. Duel of New
York he established the superiority of intratemporal facial
nerve grafts over anastomosis to other nerves.

# Part Four

*"Before describing the operation in the fallopian aqueduct, it is well to repeat that the operation is by no means easy to perform . . . the surgeon learned in anatomy, and with the knowledge and skill learned in the deadhouse, may safely traverse the perilous narrow ocean of the operation in the fallopian aqueduct."*

BALLANCE AND DUEL

# Surgery of the Facial Nerve, Endolymphatic Hydrops and Tumors of the Ear

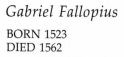

## Gabriel Fallopius

BORN 1523
DIED 1562

Described the fallopian aqueduct for the intratemporal portion of the facial nerve.

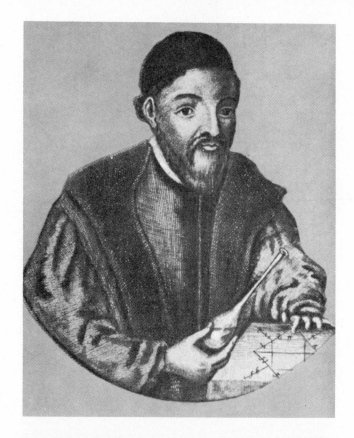

## Sterling Bunnell

BORN 1882
DIED 1957

Performed in 1927 the first successful intratemporal suture of the facial nerve, and, in 1930, the first successful facial nerve graft within the temporal bone.

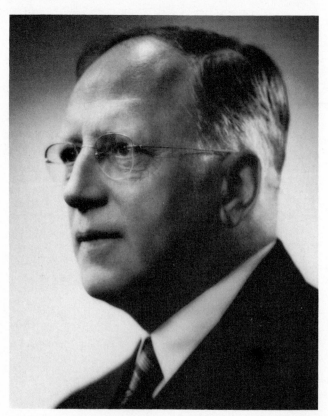

# Chapter 20

# Facial Nerve Decompression and Repair

INTRODUCTION
HISTORICAL ASPECTS
ANATOMY
PATHOLOGY OF PHYSIOLOGIC BLOCK AND AXONAL
   DEGENERATION
ETIOLOGY OF FLACCID FACIAL PARALYSIS
   TRAUMA
   TUMOR
   INFECTION
   IDIOPATHIC
DIAGNOSTIC STUDIES
   HISTORY AND PHYSICAL EXAMINATION
   AUDIOMETRY
   VESTIBULAR TESTS
   X-RAY EVALUATION
      PLAIN FILMS
      POLYTOMOGRAPHY
      ARTERIAL AND VENOUS STUDIES
      COMPUTERIZED AXIAL TOMOGRAPHY
   TOPOGRAPHIC STUDIES
      TEARING
      TASTE
      SALIVATION
      STAPEDIAL REFLEX
PROGNOSTIC STUDIES
   SALIVARY FLOW
   ELECTRODIAGNOSIS (NERVE EXCITABILITY
      STUDIES)
   ELECTROMYOGRAPHY
CARE OF THE EYE
SURGICAL INTERVENTION: DYNAMIC
   DECOMPRESSION OF THE FACIAL NERVE
      MIDDLE FOSSA APPROACH
      MIDDLE EAR AND MASTOID APPROACH
   NERVE GRAFTS
      GREATER AURICULAR NERVE
      LATERAL FEMORAL CUTANEOUS NERVE
      SURAL NERVE
   PRIMARY ANASTOMOSIS
   SECONDARY ANASTOMOSIS
   NEUROMUSCULAR TRANSFERS
SURGICAL INTERVENTION: STATIC
   SLINGS
   REGIONAL FACELIFTS
MISCELLANEOUS FACIAL NERVE PROBLEMS
COMPLICATIONS OF FACIAL NERVE SURGERY
RESULTS OF FACIAL NERVE SURGERY

## INTRODUCTION

The facial nerve is unique among motor nerves in that it has the **longest course** through a narrow bony canal of any nerve in the body, and because of this is **paralyzed more often** than any other nerve. The disability resulting from facial palsy is especially distressing because of the grotesque disfigurement accentuated by exactly those emotions that lend beauty to the normal countenance: smiling and laughter. Facial paralysis is above all an **otologic disease** because more than nine tenths of the cases are due to a lesion within the temporal bone. The family physician who often first sees the patient must be reminded of the dictum of the celebrated neurologist Sir William Gowers, that "a complete unilateral palsy of the face without other symptoms must mean disease of the nerve as it passes through the temporal bone."[1]

Facial paralysis may be the presenting symptom in conditions requiring urgent surgical intervention such as congenital cholesteatoma of the petrosa, tumor of the facial nerve or carcinoma of the ear, and it is an important warning symptom of bone invasion in chronic suppurative otitis media. The most frequent cause of facial paralysis, edema of the nerve, producing Bell's palsy, requires surgical decompression in certain cases to save the patient from a lifetime of anguished disfigurement. Too often the otologic surgeon is called in far too late to be able to avert this unhappy result.[2]

## HISTORICAL ASPECTS

In 1829 Charles Bell, anatomist and surgeon, read before the Royal Society of London an essay on the nerves of the face. That same year he was knighted for his neurophysiologic discoveries, including his distinction between the sensory innervation of the face by the fifth nerve and the motor innervation of the muscles of expression by the seventh nerve. As proof he cited three patients with facial palsy after division of the seventh nerve at or near the stylomastoid foramen, two accidental and the third during removal of a parotid tumor: "and the immediate effect has been the horrible distortion of the face by the prevalence of the muscles of the opposite side . . . and that distortion is unhappily increased when a pleasureable emotion should be reflected in the countenance." This picturesque description by Bell of seventh nerve paralysis cannot be improved upon. At first his name was applied to all cases of flaccid paralysis of the facial nerve, but as specific diseases affecting this nerve have been separated from cases of simple edema of the nerve in its bony canal, the name Bell's palsy has come to be applied only to the latter group.

Surgery to restore the function of the facial nerve began in 1879 when T. Drobnick is said to have anastomosed it at the stylomastoid foramen to the spinal accessory nerve in a patient with paralysis due to petrous suppuration.[3] However, the first published report of repair by anastomosis was in 1895 by Sir Charles Ballance, pioneer London otologic surgeon and neurosurgeon. At the age of 74, when most men are content to rest upon their laurels, he began a series of animal investigations with Arthur B. Duel of New York that demonstrated conclusively the superiority of nerve grafts over anastomosis to restore the function of the facial nerve.[4]

Repair of the severed facial nerve by approximation in its bony canal was first performed by Stacke in 1903.[5] Intratemporal suture and the successful insertion of a graft had both been performed by Sterling Bunnell[6, 7] a few years before the classic report of Ballance and Duel.

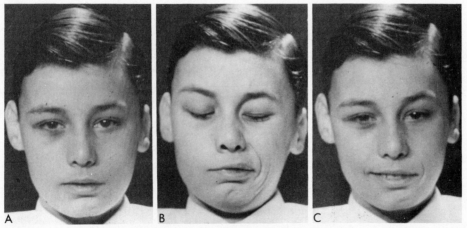

**Figure 20–1**   Result 15 months after extrapetrous graft following removal of a neurilemmoma of the left facial nerve. *A*, In repose. *B*, Voluntary contraction of left side of face. *C*, Smiling (emotional response). (From Drake, C. G.: Intracranial facial nerve reconstruction. Arch. Otol., *78*:456, 1963.)

The most recent advance in facial nerve repair is the insertion of a long graft from the stump of this nerve near the internal acoustic meatus, along the floor of the posterior fossa to the nerve after its exit from the stylomastoid foramen, thus by-passing the temporal bone. First performed in 1935 by Dott[8] when a facial nerve had to be sectioned during removal of an acoustic neurinoma, this procedure has been used successfully by others (Fig. 20–1).

Decompression of the facial nerve for certain cases of Bell's palsy was introduced in 1932 by Ballance and Duel.[4] Kettel[9] has furthered the cause of repair by a graft rather than anastomosis to another nerve (Fig. 20–2), and has demonstrated conclusively that the facial muscles after a successful facial nerve graft are

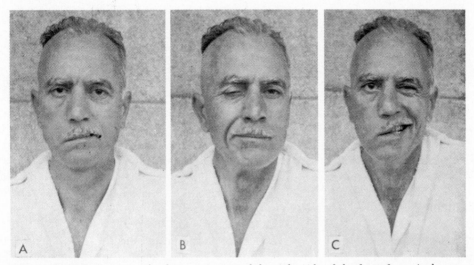

**Figure 20–2**   Restoration of voluntary motion of the right side of the face after spinal accessory-facial anastomosis but with complete absence of emotional response. *A*, Face at rest 6 years after operation. *B*, Voluntary closure of the eyes accompanied by the movement of the corner of the mouth. *C*, Patient laughs. Note the absence of emotional response on the right side. (Courtesy of Dr. Kartsen Kettle.)

innervated by this nerve and not by motor fibers from the trigeminal nerve, as suggested by Martin and Helsper.[10]

Surgery of the facial nerve made a long leap forward when Cawthorne in 1938 introduced the operating microscope for these operations, a method now used universally. The knighting in 1964 of Terence Cawthorne for his otologic contributions completes the recognition of three great London surgeons who have contributed so much to our knowledge about the facial nerve: Sir Charles Bell, Sir Charles Ballance and Sir Terence Cawthorne.

## ANATOMY

The unique journey of the facial nerve through its long, tortuous and narrow fallopian canal and its intracranial and extracranial relationship determine its vulnerability to disease, and the particular symptomatology of whatever segment of the nerve is involved.

The facial nerve originates in the pons in the facial motor nucleus with two portions: a superior portion that receives impulses from the precentral motor gyrus of **both** sides and sends fibers to the forehead and orbicularis oculi; and an inferior portion that receives impulses from the opposite precentral gyrus **only** and innervates the lower part of the face and the platysma of the neck. Therefore a lesion above the pons or of the motor cortex of one side causes paralysis only of the lower face of the opposite side, and the forehead and orbicularis oculi continue to function. Moreoever, this is a spastic rather than a flaccid type of paralysis.

The root of the facial nerve, after leaving its nucleus in the pons, hooks around the sixth nerve nucleus, and as a result a nuclear lesion with flaccid paralysis of the seventh nerve is nearly always accompanied by paralysis of the sixth nerve.

After leaving the pons, the facial nerve crosses the cerebellopontine angle in company with the eighth nerve and the intermedius nerve of Wrisberg, the latter carrying secretory fibers to the lacrimal gland and sublingual and submaxillary salivary glands, and carrying back to the pons taste and sensation from the anterior two thirds of the tongue, and pain, temperature and touch from the posterior wall of the external auditory meatus.

Upon entering the internal acoustic meatus, the facial and intermediate nerves join to form a common trunk that lies above the acoustic nerve (Fig. 20–3). A dural prolongation containing a narrow subarachnoid space with spinal fluid surrounds the seventh and eighth nerves to the bottom or lateral end of the internal acoustic meatus. At this point the facial nerve enters a separate bony canal, the **petrous segment of the fallopian canal**, that extends directly lateralward, just above the cochlea and just below the middle cranial fossa, to the middle ear. At the tympanic cavity the fallopian canal turns sharply posteriorly at the knee or genu (Fig. 20–4). Here a swelling of the nerve contains bipolar sensory ganglion cells for taste and sensation from the anterior two thirds of the tongue and a few sensory fibers from the external acoustic meatus. From this geniculate ganglion arises the first branch of the facial nerve, the greater superficial petrosal nerve that emerges through the hiatus of the fallopian canal onto the middle fossa surface of the temporal bone. The secretory fibers for the lacrimal gland leave the facial nerve at this point and proceed in the greater superficial petrosal nerve to the sphenopalatine ganglion. There is some uncertainty, according to Spalteholz,[11] as to whether taste from the anterior two thirds of the tongue may leave the facial nerve in the greater superficial petrosal nerve to join the maxillary division of the fifth before going to the pons, rather than going directly to the pons in the intermediate nerve as is generally believed.

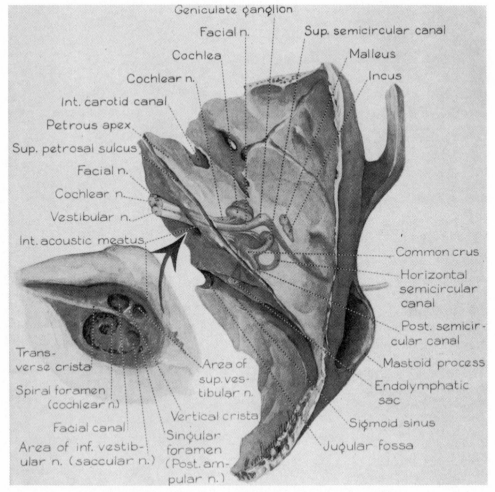

**Figure 20–3**  Internal acoustic meatus; anatomic relationships.

From the geniculate ganglion the facial nerve runs backward horizontally in a thin-walled bony canal just below the horizontal semicircular canal and just above the oval window, the **tympanic segment of the fallopian canal.** At the posterior wall of the tympanic cavity just above the pyramidal process the fallopian canal makes a second right-angle turn, more gentle than the genu, forming the **pyramidal segment,** and at this point arises the second branch of the facial nerve, the nerve to the stapedius muscle. From the pyramidal bend the fallopian canal proceeds vertically in the anterior wall of the mastoid process to the funnel-shaped stylomastoid foramen. About midway in its **vertical mastoid segment** the facial nerve gives off the chorda tympani nerve, bringing taste from the tongue and sensation for pain, temperature and touch from the posterior wall of the external auditory meatus and carrying secretory fibers to the submaxillary and sublingual glands.

The principal arterial supply of the facial nerve in its vertical mastoid segment is the stylomastoid artery, a branch of the external carotid artery that enters the stylomastoid foramen. It is joined by a second artery that enters the fallopian canal at the pyramidal bend. The stylomastoid artery continues in the tympanic segment where it anastomoses with the superficial petrosal branch of the middle

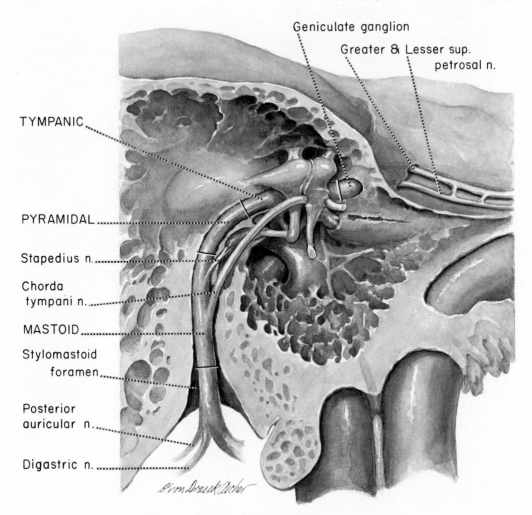

**Figure 20–4**   Facial nerve in the temporal bone.

meningeal artery that enters the fallopian canal through the facial hiatus. The arteries are accompanied by veins that run parallel with the nerve in the facial canal, both giving off twigs at right angles that perforate the sheath to supply the nerve trunk.

The sheath of the facial nerve begins in the internal acoustic meatus as a prolongation of the dura as the nerve enters the petrous segment of the fallopian canal and becomes especially strong and well developed as the nerve approaches the stylomastoid foramen. As in any peripheral nerve, each nerve fiber consists of a central protoplasmic process of the parent neuron, the axon, surrounded by an insulating layer of myelin, and then by the thin protoplasmic cytoplasm of the Schwann cells comprising the neurilemmal sheath of the nerve fiber. A single nerve fiber is enclosed by many Schwann cells, which deposit the myelin and convey oxygen to the axon. The axon, however, is dependent upon its parent neuron for replenishment of its axoplasm, which is normally used up by catabolism at a constant rate which would be sufficient to use up this material completely in 29 days were there not a constant flow of axoplasm from the parent neuron.[12] This flow proceeds at the rate of 1 mm. per day.

Around each nerve fiber is a thin connective tissue tubule; many tubules are held together in bundles, and the bundles are bound by connective tissue to form the nerve trunk. Normally the connective tissue that holds the bundles together is joined loosely with the connective tissue sheath of the nerve trunk, so that under the operating microscope the sheath of the normal nerve can be incised without cutting into the nerve trunk.

One of the most consistent anatomic relationships of the temporal bone is the course of the fallopian canal, yet minor variations and sometimes major anomalies do occur, especially in the tympanic, pyramidal and mastoid segments, that may lead to inadvertent and sometimes unavoidable surgical trauma by the most experienced and careful surgeon. The most frequent variation is a dehiscence of the bony canal, found in as many as half of all temporal bones.[13] The most frequent site of dehiscence is the tympanic segment, where an uncovered nerve may protrude downward, concealing the stapes footplate. Dehiscences between the petrous segment and the middle fossa dura and between the vertical mastoid segment and the retrofacial mastoid air cells are not uncommon. More serious for the surgeon are anomalies in the course of the fallopian canal, seen especially in congenital malformations of the middle and outer ear with microtia and atresia. But occasionally a markedly anomalous facial nerve is encountered with a normal outer ear and tympanic membrane. The senior author encountered and inadvertently sectioned a facial nerve that emerged from the surface of an aplastic mastoid process at the posterior end of its tympanic segment; the vertical mastoid segment of the fallopian canal was absent. In another case, fortunately not injured at surgery, an uncovered facial nerve crossed the tympanic cavity between the oval and round windows. A pronounced backward "hump" of the pyramidal segment may occur, making this area particularly vulnerable to surgical trauma during mastoidectomy, and variations in the depth of the pyramidal and vertical segments from the lateral surface of the mastoid may lead to damage when the bridge and facial ridge are being taken down. In rare cases the mastoid segment divides into two or three portions, each in its own bony canal. Accidental section of the facial nerve during an operation may be due to one of these variations or anomalies and not to negligence.[14]

## PATHOLOGY OF PHYSIOLOGIC BLOCK AND AXONAL DEGENERATION

Pressure on a peripheral nerve can block the transmission of nerve impulses without death and degeneration of the axon beyond the site of pressure, and may be associated with loss of myelin at the site of pressure. Release of pressure results in rapid and complete recovery of function without residuals. This type of paralysis is termed **neurapraxia.**

Section of an axon or sufficient pressure to block replenishment of axoplasm in the distal segment completely results in death of the distal segment, not at once but after several days. This is termed **axonotmesis.**

Section or disruption of the entire nerve trunk is termed **neurotmesis.** Surgical section of the entire facial nerve trunk produces "pure" neurotmesis. In many cases of trauma or of Bell's palsy there is a mixture of fibers with physiologic block or neurapraxia, fibers with degeneration of axons but intact neural tubules with axonotmesis and fibers disrupted by fibrosis or separation with neurotmesis.

As long as a little axoplasm can squeeze by a partial obstruction, the axon suffers only a physiologic block and neurapraxia. When the axon is severed or the obstruction to axoplasm flow is blocked completely, the distal segment survives for 2 or 3 days, with continued electrical excitability (see the next section), but without conduction of impulses across the block or section. Then, deprived of fresh axoplasm replenishment, the distal segment begins to die of starvation and to fragment and disintegrate, with a gradual decline in electrical excitability. The myelin simultaneously fragments, but the Schwann cells remain, proliferate and become phagocytic, removing axonal and myelin debris and filling the connective neural tubule with their cytoplasm. Meanwhile the parent neuron (in the pons in the case of the motor facial nerve) deprived of nutrients normally brought to it by the axon, sickens and undergoes changes known as chromatolysis, with loss of Nissl substance and swelling of cytoplasm. Sometimes such a neuron dies, but more often recovery begins as the end of the sectioned axon develops a growth cone and begins to bring back nutrients to its parent cell body. The furious protoplasmic activity of the growth cone of a young or regenerating axon is remarkable to observe in time-lapse cinematography as it throws out in all directions protoplasmic processes that imbibe nutrients that can be seen to travel back toward the cell body, resembling an ostrich swallowing an orange. As a protoplasmic process finds a favorable framework or pathway for growth, it proceeds outward, and other processes retract into the growth cone. Branching of a regenerating axon with protoplasmic threads entering several empty neural tubules is the rule rather than the exception, so that a single axon ends up innervating widely separated facial muscles. The result is synkinesis, or associated movements, whenever partial or complete degeneration is followed by regeneration of the facial nerve. When the patient closes his eyes the corner of his mouth on the affected side is drawn up, and when he smiles he winks (sometimes to his or her embarrassment!).

At first the regenerated axon is only a very thin protoplasmic thread, but as soon as it reaches the motor end-plate it proceeds to thicken as fresh axoplasm flows into it from the parent cell body. Only when it attains a certain thickness does it become myelinated. This creates the second residue of facial nerve regeneration: the large number of non-myelinated axons without insulation cause mass movements and spasm of the facial musculature. Many of the regenerated axons enter small tubules or tubules narrowed by fibrosis so that after regeneration there remains a permanent disproportion between myelinated and non-myelinated axons.

The authors and others have observed a return of tonus to the facial muscles preceding voluntary movement return. This may be because small axons not thick enough to transmit voluntary impulses can conduct tonic impulses.

## ETIOLOGY OF FLACCID FACIAL PARALYSIS

A flaccid paralysis of the muscles of facial expression occurs when there is some type of injury to the facial nerve. This may occur in the brainstem at the site of the nucleus, in the cerebellopontine angle (CPA), within the confines of the temporal bone or at a point after the nerve has exited the stylomastoid foramen. The paralysis may be the result of trauma, tumor involvement, infection, or idiopathic edema (Bell's palsy).

### Trauma

Traumatic injury to the facial nerve occurs when there is a fracture of the temporal bone involving the fallopian canal, at the hands of the surgeon (iatrogenic) during an operative procedure, or as the result of a penetrating wound.

Fractures of the temporal bone are classified as either longitudinal (along the axis of the petrous pyramid) or transverse (at right angles to the petrous pyramid) (Fig. 20–5). Ninety per cent of the fractures are longitudinal, and the remaining 10 per cent are transverse.[15]

As a general rule, hearing is spared in longitudinal fractures and lost in transverse; this is due to the fact that either the cochlea or the internal auditory canal (IAC) is involved in the fracture line when it lies at right angles to the petrous tip. Although the facial nerve may be injured in a longitudinal fracture, it is seldom severed (Fig. 20–6). Transverse fractures, however, almost always result in a severely damaged and often severed nerve.

In many instances of head trauma, it is difficult to establish whether there was an immediate onset of facial paralysis, because the patient may be brought into the hospital in an unconscious state. Only after the individual awakens does the paralysis become evident (perhaps three weeks after the injury). Occasionally, a bilateral paralysis will be missed for several days simply because there is no asymmetry of the face.

Immediate facial paralysis following head trauma indicates that the 7th nerve has been injured, but it does not necessarily imply a severence of the nerve. Most authors[16] feel the nerve should be explored if the onset of paralysis is immediate and if there is evidence of impending degeneration. Delayed onset assures that the nerve has obviously not been severed but does not preclude a severe injury that may well indicate surgical intervention. Again, impending nerve degeneration is the signal to explore the nerve.

When there has been an immediate onset of facial paralysis in a head trauma case, it is the junior author's belief that the nerve should be examined from the

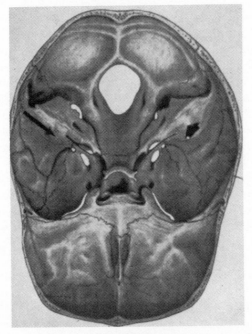

**Figure 20–5** Transverse fractures are perpendicular (short arrow on left side) and longitudinal fractures are parallel (long arrow on right side) to the long axis of the petrous bone. (From McHugh, H. E.: Facial paralysis in birth injury and skull fractures. Arch. Otol., 78:443, 1963.)

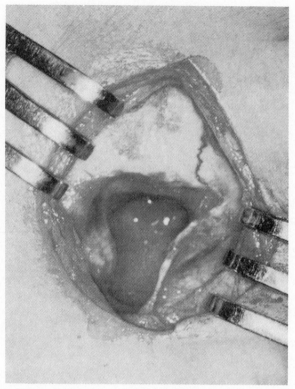

**Figure 20–6**  Facial paralysis following skull fracture with initial attico-antrotomy preparatory to exposure and decompression of the tympanic segment. Note the vertical fracture line, which involves the ossicles and tympanic facial canal. (Courtesy of Dr. Hollie E. McHugh.)

internal auditory canal to the stylomastoid foramen. The reason for this is that sophisticated x-ray examination (polytome) and topographic studies are simply not accurate enough to pinpoint the area of injury (or injuries) in all cases.

Less common than skull fractures are penetrating wounds of the skull and face that result in facial paralysis. These include wounds from gunshots and knives as well as from various other items, including knitting needles, automobile radio antennas, broken glass, and so on.

The third type of injury to the 7th nerve occurs during otologic surgery in the temporal bone or during tumor removal in the parotid. However, this text will be limited to intratemporal bone injuries.

During otologic surgery, the facial nerve is most commonly injured in the mastoid at the pyramidal or posterior bend or in its vertical course. In the middle ear, the most common site of injury is at the oval window. Approximately 50 per cent of the time there is a congenital dehiscence of the fallopian canal as it passes the oval window. This makes the nerve vulnerable to injury during any type of middle ear procedure but particularly during stapedectomy.

There are several reasons why the facial nerve is injured during otologic procedures. It may be the result of the surgeon's lack of technical skill or his inadequate knowledge of temporal bone anatomy. More commonly, however, the injury occurs as a result of congenital malformation of the anatomy with displacement of the nerve, or to destruction of the fallopian canal and other structures by cholesteatoma, granulation tissue, tumor or previous surgery.

The best method of preventing iatrogenic injury to the facial nerve is to identify the nerve in every case and use it as a landmark for finding other structures. When the surgeon can see the full course of the nerve in his operative field, he will not injure it. However, **unavoidable injuries to the facial nerve will occur from time to time even in the hands of the most qualified surgeon.** This possibility should accompany the preoperative discussion and prognosis of any ear operation, in writing.

Following otologic surgery, if a patient awakens in the recovery room with a facial paralysis, several steps must be taken. When a local anesthesia has been employed, wait two hours to allow its effects to subside. If the paralysis persists, the surgeon must decide in his own mind whether he feels there was a possible injury to the nerve. If during surgery he clearly identified the nerve and is certain that the nerve is intact, then the patient should be followed with prognostic tests to determine if degeneration is impending. The first signs of degeneration mean the patient should be returned to the operating room for exploration of the nerve. Should the surgeon have failed to properly identify the nerve during his operative procedure and therefore does not "know" whether the nerve is intact, then the fallopian canal *must* be immediately explored upon the recognition that there is a facial paralysis. "Immediately" means as soon as possible after the original surgery. This might mean the afternoon following morning surgery, or the next morning following an afternoon procedure.

A frequent cause of facial paralysis in newborn infants is forceps delivery. The palsy is immediately evident and easily seen as the child cries. The majority of these children have spontaneous recoveries, but they should be followed with prognostic studies, the same as in adults, to determine impending denervation. Should this occur, the nerve should be surgically explored, decompressed or repaired as necessary.

One point of differential diagnosis in the newborn is that there could be a congenital absence of the nerve itself. An examination by a neurologist using electromyography (EMG) is necessary to determine if the nerve is present or absent.

Regardless of the cause, traumatic injury to the facial nerve often requires decompression and repair of the nerve. Grafts are employed to bridge a gap in the continuity of the nerve. This subject will be discussed in more detail later in this chapter.


**Tumor**

Tumors can affect the facial nerve in the cerebellopontine angle (CPA), within the temporal bone, and in the parotid gland. This discussion will exclude those lesions involving the facial nerve beyond or distal to the stylomastoid foramen.

The classic symptom associated with tumors involving the facial nerve is a progressive paralysis of the face. In some benign lesions, this progression is extremely slow and may take as many as 6 to 12 months to become complete.

Benign tumors produce a facial paralysis by compressing the 7th nerve, whereas malignant lesions will actually invade the substance of the nerve itself. Therefore, in benign tumor removal, it is sometimes possible to gently dissect the mass away from the nerve and preserve its anatomical integrity. In dealing with malignant neoplasms, it is necessary to actually remove the nerve with the tumor.

*Differential Diagnosis:* There are numerous benign and malignant neoplasms that occur in and around the temporal bone. It is not possible to list all of them; however, the more common ones will be briefly discussed.

### Benign Tumors

1. *Neurolemmomas and Neurofibromas:* These benign lesions occur in the temporal bone or in the following cranial nerves in the cerebellopontine angle: 7th, 8th, 9th, 10th, 11th and 12th. If they become large enough, tumors on any of these nerves are capable of producing a facial paralysis; however, the most common are acoustic neuroma (8th) and facial nerve neuroma.

2. *Glomus Tumors:* Both glomus tympanicum and glomus jugulare tumors are capable of producing a facial nerve paralysis. Most commonly, the fallopian canal is invaded by the jugulare-type lesion.

3. *Hemangiomas:* These lesions occur both intra- and extradurally. They are slowly growing neoplasms and usually involve the facial nerve in the middle ear or cerebellopontine angle.

4. *Primary Cholesteatoma:* If the nerve is involved in the cerebellopontine angle, the primary cholesteatoma or pearly tumor classically produces a hemifacial spasm followed later by flaccid paralysis. When the lesion occurs in the petrous apex, the onset is usually an initial weakness progressing to flaccid paralysis associated with total cochlear and vestibular loss.

5. *Unusual Benign Lesions:* There are numerous other benign tumors that can produce facial paralysis depending upon where they arise within the temporal bone; these include giant-cell tumors, osteoblastomas, lipomas, adenomas and so on.

### Malignant Tumors

1. *Squamous Cell Carcinoma:* This lesion may be a primary tumor involving the temporal bone or a metastatic lesion from the lung, maxillary sinus, tonsil, oral cavity or skin of the face.

2. *Adenocarcinoma:* While extremely rare as a primary tumor of the temporal bone, it is not unusual to see a metastasis from the breast to the internal auditory canal producing a facial paralysis.

3. *Basal Cell Carcinoma:* Basal cell carcinoma is a locally invading lesion that is common on the auricle. The neoplasm would have to be badly neglected to produce a facial paralysis.

4. *Other Malignant Neoplasms:* Sarcomas are less common malignant tumors affecting the facial nerve within the temporal bone.

In summary, it is important to remember that a progressive facial weakness leading to a complete paralysis is a "Red Flag." Such a patient must be considered to have a tumor until proven otherwise. Should the diagnostic studies fail to locate a lesion, then the nerve should be explored from the cerebellopontine angle through the stylomastoid foramen into the parotid.

### Infection

Four major types of infection can cause facial paralysis — chronic middle ear infections with cholesteatoma and granulation tissue, malignant otitis externa, acute otitis media and mastoiditis, and herpes zoster oticus.

## Acute Otitis Media and Mastoiditis

Most commonly seen in children, facial paralysis associated with acute otitis media and mastoiditis seldom requires any surgery other than a myringotomy. Systemic antibiotics are required to bring the infection under control, and in most instances the facial recovery is complete. In some of these cases, the etiology of the paralysis is due to a congenital dehiscence of the fallopian canal in the area of the oval window. Such individuals should be followed closely for impending nerve degeneration while antibiotics are instituted. Should degeneration become evident, then surgical intervention in the form of mastoidectomy with decompression of the facial nerve is indicated.

## Chronic Middle Ear Infections

Facial paralysis associated with chronic ear disease is usually seen in cholesteatoma. Characteristically, the matrix destroys the fallopian canal and eventually exerts pressure on the facial nerve. Treatment consists of surgical removal of the cholesteatoma to relieve the pressure.

Occasionally, granulation tissue will destroy the bony canal and produce irritation of the nerve resulting in edema within the sheath. Again, surgical intervention with removal of the infected granulation tissue is necessary to eliminate the facial paralysis.

## Malignant Otitis Externa

This entity refers to a specific type of pseudomonas infection in debilitated diabetics beginning in the outer meatus and progressing to involve the temporal bone and skull base. It is almost always associated with facial paralysis. If not dealt with quickly and effectively, this is a fatal infection. In the strict sense, the term "malignant" should not be used except in describing invasive neoplasms; however, Chandler[17] felt this infection to be so fulminating and deadly that it warranted the use of the term malignant to convey its rapid course. At the time this infection was first identified, effective antibiotic therapy was not available and radical debridement of the temporal bone and skull base was necessary to save the patient's life. Recently, the antibiotic combination of gentamicin and carbenicillin have lessened the need for surgery.

## Herpes Zoster Oticus

Ramsay Hunt Syndrome (herpes zoster oticus) is a multicranial nerve involvement by the herpes zoster virus. Typically the individual manifests a sudden facial paralysis associated with severe pain in the ear and mastoid region. The auricle and ear canal become red and inflamed, and, in most instances, there are vesicles present (Fig. 20–7). The paralysis is thought to be due to edema of the facial nerve, particularly in the area of the geniculate ganglion. Quite often these patients present with a dry, irritated eye. In addition, the 8th cranial nerve is commonly involved, presenting as a sensorineural hearing loss and vertigo. Less often the other cranial nerves will produce signs and symptoms as well.

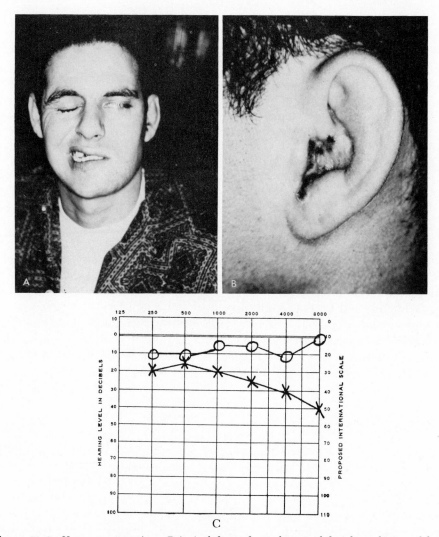

**Figure 20–7**  Herpes zoster oticus. Pain in left ear for 5 days, and facial paralysis and herpetic eruption of auricle for 3 days with mild sensorineural high-tone hearing loss and slight dizziness for 2 days. The facial palsy recovered completely in 3 weeks. (Courtesy of Dr. R. I. Barickman.)

## Idiopathic

When no cause for the paralysis can be determined, it is said to be idiopathic, and the term "Bell's palsy" is used to describe the patient's condition. Thus a diagnosis of Bell's palsy is made by exclusion.

A great deal of controversy surrounds this entity, and much has been written concerning its etiology and treatment. Most authors now believe that there is some type of viral involvement of the nerve itself, much as in the case of herpes zoster oticus. In fact, some feel the herpes simplex virus may be the offending organism. Blatt and May have suggested an inflammation of the chorda tympani nerve[18, 19] as the etiology of the paralysis. According to this theory, the chorda becomes edematous and as it enters the substance of the facial nerve produces pressure from within.

Fisch[20] places the site of involvement in the internal auditory canal and feels most of the edema occurs just as the nerve enters the fallopian canal medial to the geniculate ganglion. Anatomically there is a definite narrowing of the fallopian canal in this area.

At one time it was felt that Bell's palsy was due to spasm of the stylomastoid artery leading to ischemia and anoxic damage to capillaries with resulting edema.[21] This theory lead to the use of vasodilators in the treatment of early cases, but neither the theory nor the therapy are now thought to be valid.

In 80 to 85 per cent of Bell's cases a conductive block develops (neuropraxia) that is reversible. These individuals begin to have a return of function within a few days to a few weeks (average 8.5 days) following onset.[22] The majority of these patients recover without any residual symptoms of mass movement or synkinesis.

Whenever the etiology of a disease or syndrome is unknown, there are numerous opinions as how best to treat the problem; this is certainly true of Bell's palsy.

Over the years there has developed a continuing controversy as to whether patients with Bell's palsy should have no treatment, medical therapy or surgical intervention to decompress the nerve.

Although vasodilators have largely been abandoned in the treatment of Bell's palsy, the controversy concerning the use of steroids continues. The rationale for the use of steroids for Bell's palsy is based on their anti-inflammatory properties and their ability to reduce edema in affected tissue. However, in a double-blind study Taverner[22] concluded that cortisone had no effect on the speed or degree of recovery. On the other hand, Adour[23] subsequently presented evidence showing that when given early, steroids significantly reduced the tendency of the patient to develop degeneration of the nerve with subsequent sequelae.

May,[24] on the contrary, in a carefully controlled group of 51 patients, later was able to show that high doses of cortisone did not prevent degeneration.

While the medical therapy of Bell's palsy remains controversial, surgical decompression of the nerve provokes even more disagreement. To decompress the nerve, the fallopian canal must be opened and the nerve allowed sufficient room to swell. Some surgeons additionally slit open the sheath,[16] while others prefer not to do so.

Adour[23] has stated categorically that there is no indication for decompression in Bell's cases, but he is opposed by May[24] who feels, that to be effective, surgery must be performed before degeneration occurs. Fisch[20] advocates early decompression and feels that in most cases the nerve should be exposed in the middle fossa.

Most supporters of surgical intervention advocate early decompression prior to nerve degeneration. Jongkees[25] will operate up to three months following the onset, and Kettel[9] feels that operation seven months after onset is not unreasonable when recovery has been arrested or when there is marked contracture or residual paralysis.

Only when the etiology of Bell's palsy has been established will the proper therapy be agreed upon.


## DIAGNOSTIC STUDIES

To establish the etiology of a facial paralysis, the patient must undergo a series of diagnostic studies. The nerve itself, as well as adjacent structures, must be examined thoroughly in order to establish a diagnosis and to determine not only the cause of the paralysis but also the site of the lesion, the prognosis for spontaneous recovery and the type of therapy indicated.

### History and Physical Examination

There is no substitute for a thorough history and physical examination. Obviously a patient who has suffered a skull fracture from an automobile accident does not have a Bell's palsy when he presents with a flaccid paralysis of the face. Neither does the individual who states that his paralysis came on over a six to eight month period of time. In like manner, when one examines the ear and sees an attic cholesteatoma, the diagnosis of Bell's palsy is not valid. Most otolaryngologists have had the experience of being asked to see a patient in consultation with the diagnosis of Bell's palsy only to find that the patient has a cholesteatoma or middle ear tumor. The referring physician, in such an instance, has assumed the facial paralysis was the result of a Bell's palsy and failed to examine the patient's ear.

### Audiometry

Every otologic patient deserves the benefit of a pure-tone air and bone conduction audiogram with masking of the opposite ear and with speech discrimination scores. A unilateral sensorineural hearing loss on the same side of the facial paralysis makes one suspicious of a tumor in the petrous pyramid or cerebellopontine angle, while a conductive loss would indicate middle ear involvement.

Special audiometric studies will be covered in detail in Chapter 23 in the section on neurotologic evaluation. These studies are indicated when one is suspicious of retrocochlear pathology.

### Vestibular Tests

In the neurotologic evaluation of the patient with a facial paralysis, it is important to assess vestibular function as well as auditory acuity. The reason for this, of course, is that the vestibular nerve traverses the internal auditory canal with the cochlear and facial nerves. Not only is the vestibular nerve involved with tumors of the internal auditory canal and cerebellopontine angle, but not infrequently there are vestibular symptoms associated with the Ramsay Hunt Syndrome.

### X-Ray Evaluation

X-ray evaluation of the temporal bone and adjacent structures is essential in determining the presence of tumors, cholesteatoma and fractures.

### Plain Films

X-rays of the temporal bone must be taken on a special head unit such as the Franklin or Compere. If the petrous pyramid is not too pneumatized, these films will show the internal auditory canal quite clearly. However, they are seldom able to demonstrate fractures or lesions of the jugular bulb.

## Polytomography

The polytome apparatus is able to demonstrate quite clearly almost all of the structures within the temporal bone. This is accomplished by 1 mm. cuts in the anterior-posterior, lateral and oblique views. All structures above and below the focal point are blurred, resulting in a remarkably sharp representation of the structure under study. Not only can the internal auditory canal be seen easily in a pneumatized apex, but the fallopian canal can be delineated from the geniculate ganglion through the middle ear and mastoid to the stylomastoid foramen.

While the polytome is by far the best method of demonstrating fractures of the temporal bone, it is not infallible. Fractures in the floor of the middle fossa are particularly difficult to demonstrate.

The polytome can be of especial help in the diagnosis of facial nerve neuromas, since quite often localized enlargement of the fallopian canal can be demonstrated.

## Arterial and Venous Studies

In rare instances, carotid (internal and external) and vertebral arteriograms as well as retrograde venograms are indicated in the evaluation of the patient with a facial paralysis. The need for such studies is rare and depends upon the tentative diagnosis and the circumstances in each individual case.

## Computerized Axial Tomography

The Computerized Axial Tomography Scanner (CAT Scan) will be covered in detail in Chapter 23. This new type of brain scan is particularly useful in establishing the presence of lesions in the cerebellopontine angle. Sometimes a facial paralysis will be due to a metastatic tumor in the internal auditory canal or cerebellopontine angle.

## Topographic Studies

The site of a lesion may often be determined by topographic studies of facial nerve function. These include tearing, taste, salivation and the presence or absence of the stapedial reflex.

## Tearing

The greater superficial petrosal nerve leaves the geniculate ganglion in the floor of the middle fossa and supplies the lacrimal gland. Edema of the geniculate ganglion will result in involvement of the nerve of lacrimation. This results in a dry, irritated eye and pinpoints the site of the lesion in the facial nerve at or medial to the ganglion. When the eye is obviously dry, a Schirmer Test (tear test) may be performed. While helpful, this test is not always accurate and should be evaluated on an individual basis. The test is accomplished by placing litmus paper or a strip of filter paper, the end folded to fit, in the lower conjunctival fold of both eyes (Fig. 20–8A). The patient is then stimulated with a whiff of ammonia to initiate the

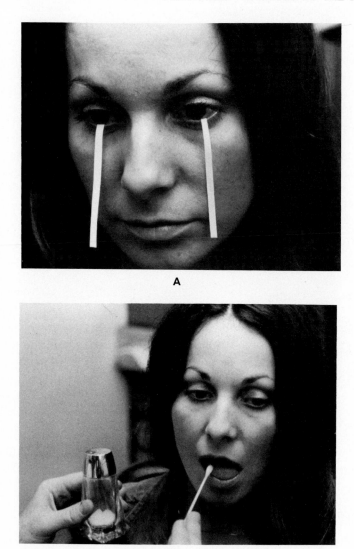

**Figure 20-8**  *A*, Tear test. *B*, Taste test.

tearing process. The normal side will tear profusely, causing the paper to become moist. By comparing the two sides, it is possible to demonstrate a lack of tearing on the paralyzed side. Fortunately, most patients with a truly dry eye complain bitterly about their discomfort, and there is little question in the surgeon's mind as to the involvement of the greater superficial petrosal nerve.

### Taste

The chorda tympani nerve supplies taste to the anterior two thirds of the tongue. By testing taste, the examiner can determine if the site of the lesion in the facial nerve is near the stylomastoid foramen. Salt, sugar, wintergreen and cloves may be selectively placed on that side of the tongue (Fig. 20–8B). The patient is asked to identify the substance without looking at it.

A more sophisticated method of testing taste is by the use of an electric gustometer. This device has an electrode that is placed on the tongue, and a reading is obtained when the patient develops a definite metallic taste. A meter reading on the involved side higher than the normal one demonstrates a lack of ability to taste. The results of any taste test are extremely variable and may be invalid if the patient is a heavy smoker or has had alcohol in the preceding 24 hours.

### Salivation

Salivary flow from the submaxillary gland is also a function of the chorda tympani nerve and provides another method of determining involvement near the stylomastoid foramen. This test is also extremely valuable in establishing impending denervation and will be discussed in more detail in the section on prognostic studies.

### Stapedial Reflex

Impedance audiometry can also be diagnostic of the severity of damage to the facial nerve. Since the efferent pathway of the auditory stapedial reflex is the 7th nerve, total or severe denervation will cause absence of the reflex in spite of other normal findings in the middle ear and 8th nerve. The reflex will be absent with the probe in the ear on the involved side, but it will be present when the sound is presented to the affected ear and the opposite efferent pathway is responding. If the lesion improves spontaneously, repeated impedance audiometry will indicate return of a measurable stapedial reflex.

### Summary

While site of lesion testing is not accurate in many cases, it does give the examiner some indication as to the location of the injury to the nerve. For example, if tearing and stapedial reflex are normal but taste and salivation are abnormal, the probable site of lesion is in the vertical segment of the facial nerve.

## PROGNOSTIC STUDIES

Prognostic testing of the facial nerve has as its primary goal the determination of impending degeneration. Salivary flow and various means of electrical stimulation of the nerve are used both to predict degeneration as well as to establish that the degeneration has already occurred.

### Salivary Flow

Salivary flow studies have proved to be accurate[19] and will precede a reduced electrical nerve excitability by several days. To perform this study, a length of #100 polyethylene tubing is threaded with the help of a punctum dilator into Wharton's Duct bilaterally (Fig. 20–9A). Test tubes are used to collect the saliva stimulated by a

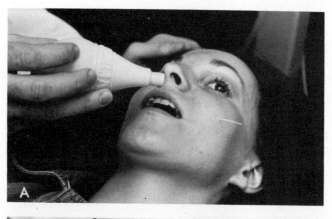

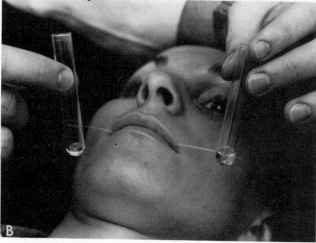

**Figure 20–9** *A*, Polyethylene tubes placed in Wharton's duct. Lemon juice dropped onto the tongue stimulates salivation. *B*, Test tubes are used to collect saliva.

lemon drop (Fig. 20–9*B*), and a comparison is made between the two sides. May has indicated that salivation on the side of paralysis reduced to less than 25 per cent of the normal side is a poor prognostic sign and implies the nerve is degenerating.

### Electrodiagnosis (Nerve Excitability Studies)

There are several battery operated nerve stimulators available commercially. Two of the most popular are the Hilger tester manufactured by W/R Medical Electronics Company and a much smaller apparatus made by Life-Tech Instruments. Others are sold by Xomed and Oto-Med.

To perform this study, it is important to cleanse the face in front of the ear with alcohol or acetone. An indifferent electrode is placed at the stylomastoid foramen, and an active one is used to selectively stimulate the individual branches of the facial nerve. A comparison is made between the two sides. If the nerves stimulate equally, then the involved nerve has a physiologic block, and the prognosis is excellent for a satisfactory recovery. A 3.5 mm. difference between the nerve responses of the two sides indicates degeneration is taking place. No response to electrical stimulation indicates that the nerve has already degenerated.

Even if the nerve is severed, it will continue to respond to stimulation for several days because there is about a four to seven day delay with this test. This is a limiting factor with nerve excitability studies and is the reason that a salivary flow study is more accurate as an early test.

As described by Hilger,[26] the stimulation is begun with the machine set at a *minimal* amount of milliamperage. The intensity is gradually increased until the muscles begin to move.

May[27] feels that it is best to stimulate the nerve with a *maximal* milliamperage, starting at the top of the scale. He further states that the maximal test improves reliability of electrodiagnosis and shortens the delay in detecting denervation.

Fisch[28] is of the opinion that a disadvantage of a minimal or maximal testing is that it is a *visualized* response observed by the tester who must compare the involved and normal sides of the face. Electroneuronography (ENOG) is an electrodiagnostic test that measures the compound action potential of facial muscles. A comparison between the two sides is made by measuring the amplitude of the summating potential and extrapolating a percentage of degenerated fibers on the abnormal side. This requires a special apparatus.

### Electromyography

Electromyography (EMG) is a method used to record electrical activity in any striated muscle via needle electrodes inserted into the muscle. Normally there is no electrical activity at rest, but with voluntary contraction, one can record **voluntary motor units.** In cases of facial paralysis, one looks for specific **fibrillation potentials** suggesting Wallerian degeneration.[29] These are usually present by the tenth day after onset of the paralysis. The absence of fibrillation indicates that degeneration is negligible. Conversely, the presence of active motor units (even with no facial movement) indicates that the nerve has not reached a point of severe degeneration.[30]

A favorable sign in facial paralysis that has been present for some time is the onset of polyphasic motor unit potentials that appear on EMG. These signal the onset of recovery from a conduction block several months before any visible muscle contraction.

### CARE OF THE EYE

Although a facial paralysis is disfiguring and cosmetically unpleasing, the only associated complication is with the eye. Because the eyelids do not blink, the conjunctiva is not lubricated normally, and there is a drying effect. These conditions, coupled with the absence of lacrimation or decreased corneal sensation or both, make corneal ulceration highly probable. When not properly managed, this can lead to blindness. For this reason, it is extremely important to instruct the patient in proper eye care, as described below. In most cases, the conscientious patient can prevent the need for a tarsorrhaphy.

If the nerve has been severed and a graft inserted, it will take eight to twelve months for the face to function. During this lengthy period of time, it is best to recommend a medial or lateral tarsorrhaphy, or both. An alternative is the insertion of a small spring into the upper eyelid to automatically close the eye.[31] The levator palpebra is innervated by the 3rd cranial nerve and is strong enough to raise the upper lid at will.

For those individuals who are expected to have a return of function in three to six weeks, care of the eye can be accomplished more easily. During the waking hours, the patient is instructed to close the eye frequently with the back portion of the bent index finger. In addition they are asked to instill one to two drops of artificial tears into the eye three times a day or more if the eye feels dry. When outdoors, the individual should wear sunglasses with a moisture chamber fixed to the temporal arm of the glasses. In the evening, upon retiring, a clear, plastic shield (commercially available) is placed over the eye to act as a moisture chamber. A less expensive method is to cut a square of clear plastic food wrap (Saran Wrap) and tape it into place with non-allergic adhesive tape.

## SURGICAL INTERVENTION: DYNAMIC

There are two basic surgical methods for rehabilitating the face following a facial paralysis. These are known as the dynamic and the static approaches, and the choice of procedure depends upon the circumstances present in each individual case.

Dynamic rehabilitation involves surgical exposure of the nerve, decompression, insertion of grafts, end-to-end anastomosis and nerve or neuromuscular transfers.

### Decompression of the Facial Nerve

The basic exposure of the facial nerve in the temporal bone is known as the decompression procedure. Regardless of what must be done to the nerve, it has to be exposed by opening the fallopian canal. Depending upon the site of the lesion, the nerve may be exposed in the middle fossa (internal auditory canal and geniculate ganglion), in the tympanic cavity, or in the mastoid.

### Middle Fossa Exposure of the Facial Nerve

The patient lies supine with the involved ear up. The surgeon sits at the head of the operating table and uses the Zeiss otomicroscope. A Frazier incision is made 1 cm. anterior to the tragus and carried through skin and subcutaneous tissue superiorly for approximately 6 cm. (Fig. 20–10). The temporalis muscle is incised and displaced with a self-retaining retractor. A craniectomy is performed in the squamous portion of the temporal bone using a cutting burr and irrigation suction (Fig. 20–11). Next, the dura of the temporal lobe of the brain is elevated and held in place by a House-Urban self-retaining retractor (Fig. 20–12). This allows the surgeon to have both hands free for operating and negates the need for a surgical assistant.

Once the bleeding from the dura has been controlled, the floor of the middle fossa is inspected for landmarks. The anterior limit of the exposure is the middle meningeal artery; posteriorly it is the arcuate eminence, which corresponds roughly to the superior semicircular canal. The greater superficial petrosal nerve is identified, and a diamond burr is used to follow the nerve posteriorly to the geniculate ganglion (Fig. 20–13). Once the ganglion has been found, the vital structures within the temporal bone, cochlea, semicircular canals, contents of the internal auditory canal, carotid artery and ossicles can be identified as follows.

*Text continued on page 544.*

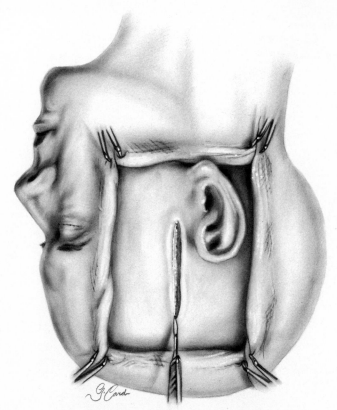

**Figure 20–10** A routine middle fossa incision is made from the level of the zygoma, extending superiorly about 6 cm.

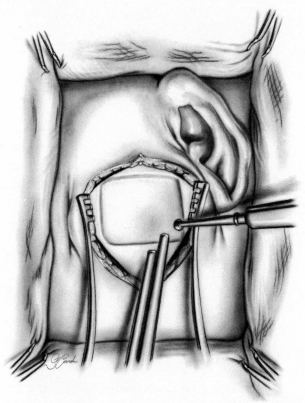

**Figure 20–11** Using a cutting burr, a craniotomy is performed in the squamous portion of the temporal bone.

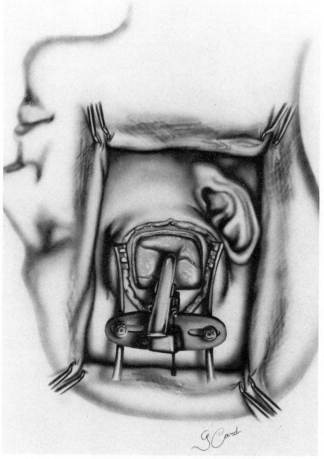

**Figure 20–12**   The House-Urban retractor is used to hold the temporal lobe off the floor of the middle fossa.

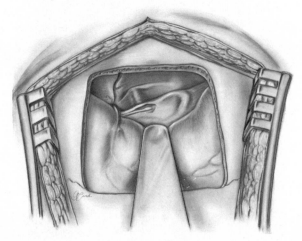

**Figure 20–13**   The greater superficial petrosal nerve is followed back to the geniculate ganglion to identify the facial nerve and the internal auditory canal.

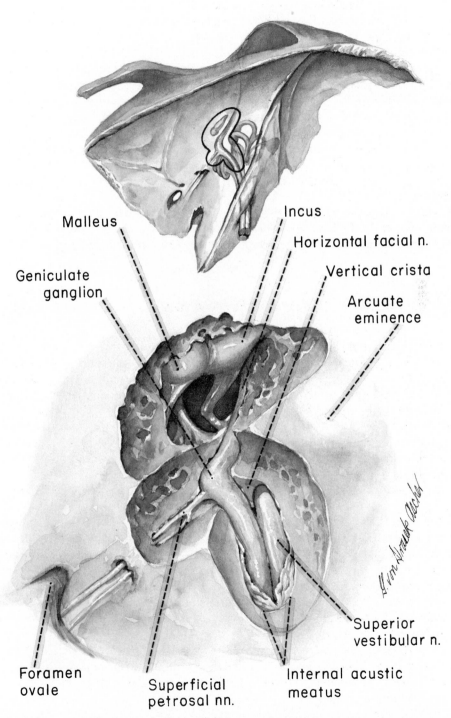

**Figure 20–14** Middle fossa exposure of facial nerve from the internal acoustic meatus to the pyramidal bend.

A blue line is obtained on the superior semicircular canal, and the facial nerve is followed into the internal auditory canal from the geniculate ganglion. Next, the thin bone of the middle ear tegmen is removed to expose the ossicles lying in the attic. The facial nerve is followed laterally from the geniculate into the middle ear as far as the cochleariformis process (Fig. 20–14).

This middle fossa exposure allows the surgeon to open the sheath of the nerve if he is decompressing it for a Bell's palsy or a Ramsay Hunt syndrome. It will also allow him to remove a tumor of the facial nerve in this area. Frequently fractures through the floor of the middle fossa will sever the facial nerve at the ganglion, thus requiring a graft or end-to-end anastomosis. Thus the middle fossa procedure is extremely important for obtaining the necessary exposure to accomplish this.

Once the facial nerve surgery itself has been done, the internal auditory canal is covered with temporalis muscle, and the retractor is removed. The temporal lobe expands, and the bone plug is either wired back into place or left out at the surgeon's discretion.

A bulky mastoid-type dressing is applied, and the patient is observed in the recovery room until late afternoon of the day of surgery. During this time, craniotomy checks are performed on a 15 minute to 1 hour basis.

### Middle Ear and Mastoid Exposure of the Facial Nerve

To expose the mastoid and middle ear segment of the facial nerve, one must perform a simple mastoidectomy and may then employ the facial recess approach.

A routine postauricular incision is made 3 to 5 mm. behind the postauricular fold. A self-retaining retractor holds the auricle forward, and a large cutting burr with irrigation-suction is used to remove the cortex of the mastoid process. A simple mastoidectomy is performed, exposing the middle and posterior fossa dural plates, the sinodural angle, sigmoid sinus and digastric ridge (Fig. 20–15). The landmarks for the vertical segment of the facial nerve are the horizontal semicircular canal and the fossa incudus superiorly, and the digastric ridge inferiorly.

A diamond burr is used to outline the course of the nerve by removing bone from its lateral, anterior and posterior surfaces. A thin layer of eggshell bone is left over the sheath. Next, the facial recess is exposed by removing the bone between the incudal fossa and facial and chorda tympani nerves (Fig. 20–16). This allows the surgeon access to the horizontal segment of the nerve. In some instances it might be necessary to remove the incus and head of the malleus to obtain adequate exposure. Should this be done, the facial recess is opened superiorly and the bone overlying the attic is removed. The hearing must be restored following this procedure and is best managed by using a fitted incus prosthesis from malleus handle to stapes head, as described in Chapter 16.

Once the nerve has been exposed in the described manner, the eggshell bone is removed and the sheath may be opened to decompress the nerve (Fig. 20–15). If surgery is being performed to insert a graft, this exposure is quite adequate for this purpose as well.

A small defect in the facial nerve can be corrected by section of the digastric and posterior auricular nerves, permitting the facial nerve to be mobilized at the stylomastoid foramen and brought upward in the fallopian canal, as shown in Figure 20–17.

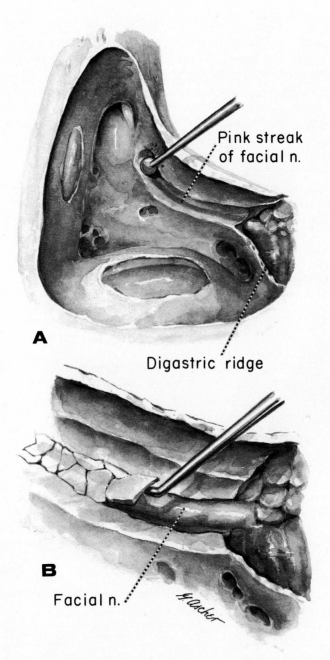

**Figure 20–15** Exposure of vertical (mastoid) segment of facial nerve.

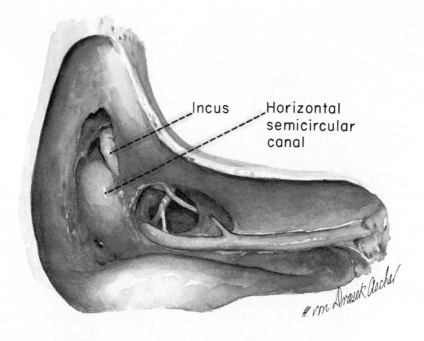

Incus

Horizontal
semicircular
canal

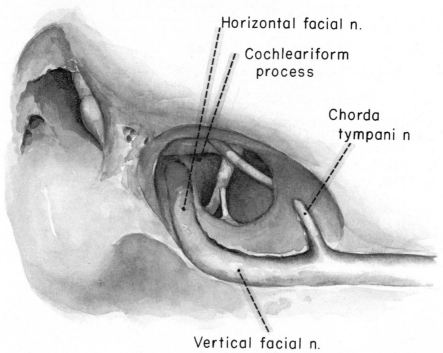

Horizontal facial n.

Cochleariform
process

Chorda
tympani n

Vertical facial n.

**Figure 20–16**   The facial recess is widened, and the vertical and tympanic segments of the facial
nerve are exposed.

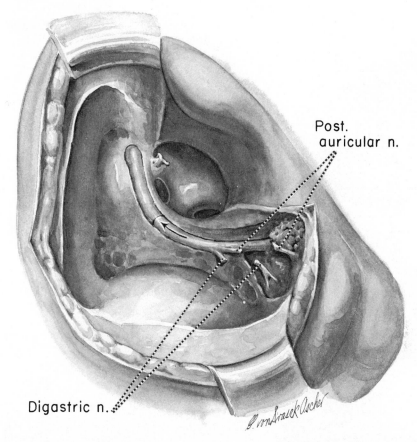

**Figure 20–17**   Facial nerve rerouted and approximated in the fallopian canal by section of digastric and posterior auricular nerves.

An alternative exposure by an atticotomy, employed by the senior author for a large facial nerve neuroma, is shown in Figures 20–18 and 20–19.

The middle fossa and mastoid approaches to the facial nerve may be used separately or in combination, depending upon the circumstances presented by each individual case. For example, if a facial nerve neuroma were limited to the vertical segment, a middle fossa exposure would not be necessary. However, should the tumor involve the course of the nerve from the geniculate ganglion to the stylomastoid foramen (as is often the case), a combined procedure would be mandatory.

### Nerve Grafts

When a segment of facial nerve is missing, owing to tumor involvement or injury from a fracture, the best functional result can be obtained by inserting a nerve graft. The graft is placed in the fallopian canal and aligned with the severed ends of the facial nerve. It is best to make a fresh cut of both the nerve and graft with a sharp knife. In most instances, if the graft can lie within the fallopian canal, it is not necessary to suture it in place. However, if the graft extends from the vertical segment out into the face, it is best to use sutures to prevent possible tension from separating the anastomosis.

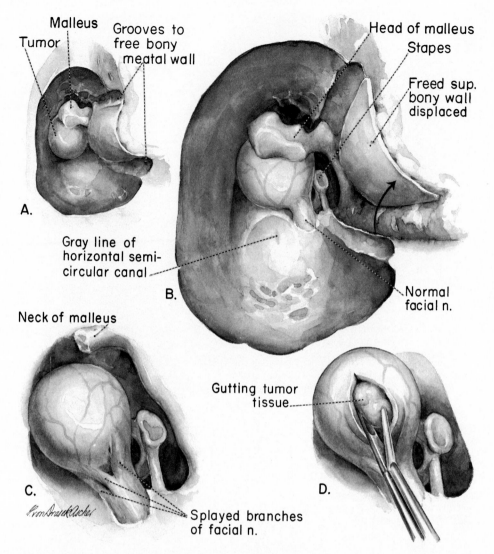

**Figure 20–18** Neuroma of facial nerve involving tympanic and petrous segments, requiring a long graft.

While most grafts are placed between the proximal and distal segments of the facial nerve, there has been some recent work done in which cable grafts (sural nerve) have been routed across the face[32] from severed branches of the normal nerve. The concept is to sacrifice some of the interlacing fibers of the normal nerve and anastomose these by means of the graft to the major branches of the non-functioning nerve.

Fisch feels that these interlacing fibers should be severed on the normal side in all cases of nerve grafts in order to further equalize the appearance of the face. In most instances, the normal side remains much stronger than the involved one and always makes for asymmetry. By slightly weakening the normal side, the cosmetic result is supposedly improved.

There are three major sensory nerves that are used in facial nerve grafting: the greater auricular, lateral femoral cutaneous and sural nerves.

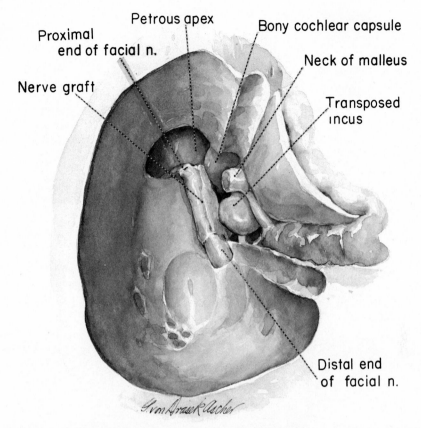

Proximal
end of facial n.

Petrous apex

Bony cochlear capsule

Neck of malleus

Nerve graft

Transposed
incus

Distal end
of facial n.

**Figure 20–19** Nerve graft from pyramidal segment to internal auditory meatus inserted by endaural atticotomy approach after removing neuroma. Recovery of facial function began in six months.

### Greater Auricular Nerve

This sensory nerve is the one of choice for most facial nerve repairs. Its advantages are that it approximates the size of the facial nerve and is in the otologic field. This nerve is readily obtained by drawing two imaginary lines, one approximately 4 cm. down from the external auditory canal and the other from the tip of the mastoid to the angle of the mandible (Fig. 20–20). Where these two lines cross, the nerve will be found lying on the sternomastoid muscle. The incision should be made in a neck crease for cosmetic reasons, and the nerve will be identified just under the platysma muscle. It will be seen coursing from posterior to anterior. Care should be used in handling the graft, and once it has been taken, it should be placed in a solution of Tis-U-Sol.

A facial nerve neuroma that involved the horizontal and petrous segments of the nerve, with a long graft from the greater auricular nerve, is shown in Figures 20–18 and 20–19. There was average recovery of facial nerve function after six months.

### Lateral Femoral Cutaneous Nerve

The advantage of this nerve is that a long segment can be taken for cross-face anastomosis. It is best to do this before the otologic procedure is started.

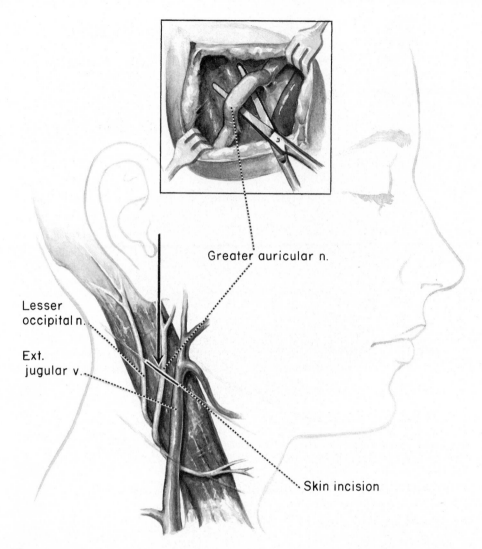

**Figure 20–20**  Skin incision and anatomical relationships in obtaining a graft of the great auricular nerve.

An incision is made in the upper thigh (Fig. 20–21) just below and medial to the ischial crest. Just beneath the fascia, the nerve will be found coursing inferiorly across the sartorius muscle.

### Sural Nerve

Another long sensory nerve that can be employed in cross-face anastomosis is the sural nerve. To identify this nerve, the surgeon palpates the lateral malleolus, as this nerve supplies the posterior-lateral aspect of the leg. It lies adjacent to the lesser saphenous vein (Fig. 20–22).

### Primary Anastomosis of the Facial Nerve

At one time it was customary to reroute the facial nerve across the middle ear in order to obtain an end-to-end anastomosis so as to avoid a nerve graft. The current

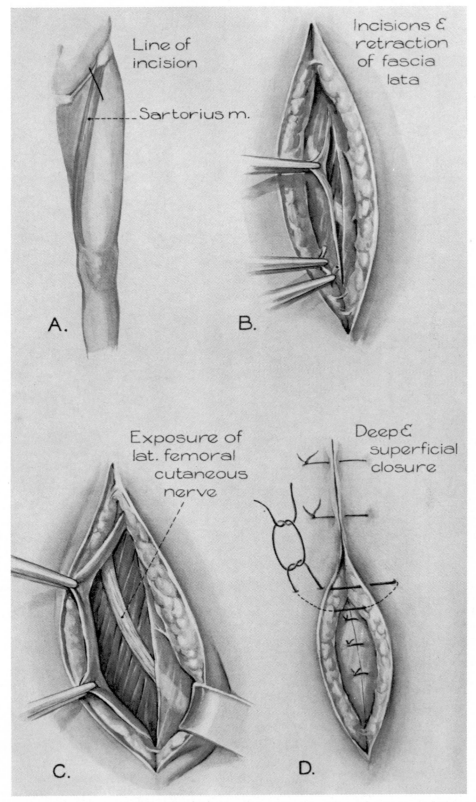

**Figure 20–21** Technique of obtaining a graft from the lateral femoral cutaneous nerve.

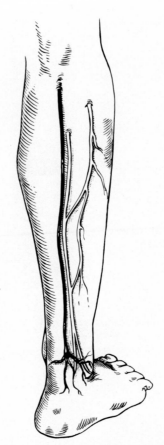

**Figure 20–22**   The sural nerve can be found lying adjacent to the saphenous vein in the lower leg.

feeling, however, discourages this method of nerve repair. On occasion, the junior author has rerouted the facial nerve from the internal auditory canal to the vertical segment by means of a primary anastomosis. There was no tension on the suture line, and the cosmetic result was similar to what would have been expected from a graft.

### Secondary Anastomosis

When a graft of the facial nerve is not practical (injury at the brainstem), an alternate method of repair is to anastomose the distal segment of the facial nerve to the proximal portion of the hypoglossal (12th) or spinal accessory (11th) nerve.

The junior author much prefers the 7 to 12 anastomosis to the 7 to 11 procedure, as the disability from loss of the spinal accessory nerve is formidable. Most patients tolerate a unilateral weakness of the tongue without difficulty.

The operative procedure is performed through a linear incision that should be placed in a neck crease just along the anterior border of the stylomastoid muscle (Fig. 20–23A). The facial nerve is located at the stylomastoid foramen in the routine manner and is tagged with a suture. Next, the hypoglossal nerve is identified as it crosses the external carotid artery and is followed as far distally as possible (Fig. 20–23B). At this point, the nerve is severed and brought back to be anastomosed with the cut end of the facial nerve. Employing the operating microscope, the surgeon places several small sutures in the sheaths of the two nerves to approximate their ends (Fig. 20–23C). The skin incision is closed with a drain and a bulky dressing applied. Motion in the face will occur within five to eight months following the operative procedure.

### Neuromuscular Transfers

Recently Tucker[33] has been implanting the ansa-hypoglossal nerve with attached muscle into the muscles at the corner of the mouth and nose. Within three to four weeks, there is motion in these muscles. The eye is managed by inserting a temporalis muscle flap into the orbicularis muscle.

This type of neuromuscular transfer has performed well in the larynx and has exciting possibilities as a means of rehabilitating the paralyzed face.

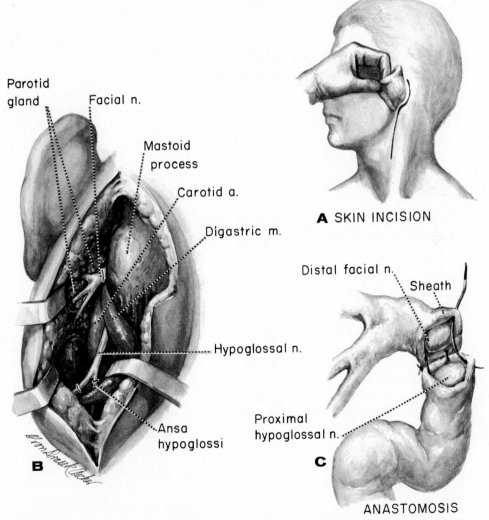

**Figure 20–23** A, Incision. B, Exposure of facial hypoglossal nerves. C, Anastomosis under the operating microscope.

## SURGICAL INTERVENTION: STATIC

Static rehabilitation of the paralyzed face includes the use of fascia lata and tendon slings as well as regional facelifts to improve the static (at rest) function of the face.

### Slings of Fascia Lata or Tendon

The patient who is not a candidate for either a nerve graft or 7 to 12 anastomosis can be helped with static support of the sagging muscles of the face. An example of such a patient would be an individual who has a bilateral brainstem injury or who was born without a facial nerve. In either case, a sling of fascia lata can be attached to the zygoma and run subcutaneously to the corner of the mouth where it is attached to the orbicularis oris muscle. With the face in repose, the mouth does not sag and is cosmetically acceptable. When the individual smiles, however, the extent of his handicap becomes quite evident.

### Regional Facelifts

Just as the fascia lata sling will improve the face at rest, a regional facelift procedure can correct the sagging face. Blepharoplasty combined with tarsorrhaphy will improve the appearance of the eye and help to protect it, while regional flaps are employed to raise the corner of the mouth. However, these methods are inferior to nerve repair and anastomosis and thus have limited value.

## MISCELLANEOUS FACIAL NERVE PROBLEMS

There are two types of facial nerve problems that do not fit well into the general scheme presented and for that reason are mentioned separately.

### Melkersson's Syndrome

A rather rare and interesting association of recurring facial palsy and chronic or recurring edema of the face was described by Melkersson in 1928.[34] Three years later, Rosenthal[35] reported a series of these cases, noting that in one third a fissured tongue was present. Most cases of Melkersson's Syndrome begin before the age of 16 years (sometimes as early as 18 months); bilateral involvement is not uncommon and recurrences are frequent. The facial edema usually involves the distribution of the motor facial nerve and affects especially the upper lip. The treatment of this syndrome is the same as that for Bell's palsy.

### Clonic Hemifacial Spasm

This debilitating condition is very disturbing for the patient and makes him very uncomfortable. In some cases only the eye muscles are involved, and in others the whole face displays rhythmic spasm. The condition makes it difficult for the individual to eat and talk, and is embarrassing as well.

Gardner[36] has stated that in 50 per cent of the cases, some cause for this condition could be found in the cerebellopontine angle, such as primary cholesteatoma or other tumor. Jannetta[37] has recently linked this problem to a loop of the anterior-inferior cerebellar artery pressing on the facial nerve. He places muscle or synthetic sponge between the vessel and nerve and has reported excellent relief of symptoms.

McCabe[38] has taken a different approach to the surgical management of this problem in that he selectively lyses the fibers to the eye, nose and mouth. This prevents the spasm but does not produce a complete facial paralysis.

Because of the high association of this condition with lesions in the cerebellopontine angle, all patients with hemifacial spasm should undergo a thorough neurotologic evaluation.

## COMPLICATIONS OF FACIAL NERVE SURGERY

The major complications in facial nerve surgery are injury to either the nerve itself (during decompression), to the semicircular canals (resulting in postoperative sensorineural hearing loss or vertigo), to the ossicles (conductive hearing loss) or to the cochlea (sensorinerual hearing loss or "dead ear").

There are some potential dangers to the middle fossa procedure,[39] such as extra- and subdural hematoma, hemiparesis and other neurologic deficits. However, from

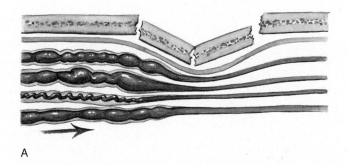

A

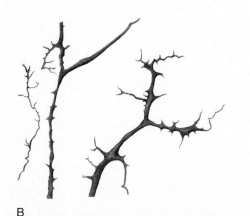

B

**Figure 20–24** *A*, How a depressed fracture of the fallopian canal causes damming of axoplasm with neuropraxia paralysis. *B*, Branching of growing axons in tissue culture, accounting for synkinesis and mass movement after regeneration of a cut or degenerated (axonotmesis) facial nerve.

the practical standpoint, these are extremely rare and are of such low incidence in the hands of the trained neuro-otologic surgeon as to make them negligible.

## RESULTS OF FACIAL NERVE SURGERY

When discussing a postoperative result with a patient prior to surgery, it is extremely important that he have a realistic concept regarding the surgical result. The surgeon must be very careful not to promise the patient too much in the way of returned function.

The best results of facial nerve surgery will be in those cases of early decompression for Bell's palsy when impending degeneration is evident. Once the axons have degenerated, whether due to a severe block or an actual severance of the nerve trunk, the result may be cosmetically acceptable, but it cannot be considered normal.

Any nerve graft or 7 to 12 anastomosis will result in a certain amount of mass motion and synkinesis. At repose, the face may show little asymmetry but on motion this is accentuated. Fisch's idea of severing some fibers in the good (opposite) nerve would seem to have merit. Until the orientation of the individual axons can be directed at will by the surgeon, patients with severe facial nerve injuries will have to accept mass movement and synkinesis (Fig. 20–24) as a necessary evil in order to regain movement of their paralyzed face.

Reinnervation experiments involving the facial nerve remain a fertile field for otologic research.

## REFERENCES

1. Cawthorne, T.: Indications for intratemporal facial nerve surgery. Arch. Otol., 78:429, 1963.
2. Walsh, T. E.: Bell's palsy: a much misused diagnosis. Laryngoscope, 71:761, 1961.
3. Cited by Sawicki, B., In Chepault: The Status of Neurosurgery. Paris, J. Rueff, 1902.
4. Ballance, C., and Duel, A. B.: The operative treatment of facial palsy. Arch. Otol., 15:1, 1932.
5. Stacke, L., quoted by Alt, F.: The operative treatment of otogenic facial palsy. Verhandl. deutsch. Otol. Gesellsch., 17:190, 1908.
6. Bunnell, S.: Suture of facial nerve within temporal bone with report of first successful case. Surg. Gynec. & Obst., 45:7, 1927.
7. Bunnell, S.: Surgical repair of facial nerve. Arch. Otol., 25:235, 1937.
8. Dott, N. M.: Facial nerve reconstruction by graft by-passing the petrous bone. Arch. Otol., 78:426, 1963.
9. Kettel, K.: Peripheral Facial Palsy. Copenhagen, Munksgaard, 1959.
10. Martin, H., and Helsper, J. T.: Spontaneous return of function following surgical section or excision of the seventh cranial nerve in the surgery of parotid tumors. Ann. Surg., 146:715, 1957.
11. Spalteholz, W.: Hand-atlas of Human Anatomy. 13th ed. Philadelphia, J. B. Lippincott Co., 1944.
12. Weiss, P.: Experiments on the mechanism of nerve growth. J. Exper. Zool., 107:315, 1948.
13. Dietzel, K.: Concerning dehiscences of the facial canal. Ztschr. Laryng. Rhin. Otol., 40:366, 1961.
14. Fowler, E. P., Jr.: Variations in the temporal bone course of the facial nerve. Laryngoscope, 71:937, 1961.
15. McCabe, B. F.: Symposium on trauma in otolaryngology: Injuries to the facial nerve. Laryngoscope, 84:1891, 1974.
16. Glasscock, M. E., III, et al.: Rehabilitation to the face following traumatic injury to the facial nerve. Laryngoscope, 1979 (In press).
17. Chandler, J. R.: Malignant external otitis. Laryngoscope, 78:1259, 1968.
18. Blatt, I. M.: Bell's palsy: Diagnosis and prognosis of idiopathic peripheral facial paralysis by submaxillary flow — Chorda tympani nerve testing: A study of 102 patients. Laryngoscope, 75:1081, 1965.
19. May, M., Hardin, W. B. Jr., Sullivan, J., and Wette, R.: Natural history of Bell's palsy: The salivary flow test and other prognostic indications. Laryngoscope, 86:704, 1976.
20. Fisch, U.: Transtemporal surgery of the internal auditory canal. Adv. Otorhinolaryngol., 17:203, 1970.

21. Hilger, J. A.: The nature of Bell's palsy. Laryngoscope, 59:228, 1949.
22. Taverner, D.: The treatment of facial palsy. Arch. Otol., 81:489, 1965.
23. Adour, K. K., et al.: Prednisone treatment for idiopathic facial paralysis (Bell's palsy). New Engl. J. Med., 287:1268, 1972.
24. May, M., Wette, R., Hardin, W. B., and Sullivan, J.: The use of steroids in Bell's palsy: A prospective controlled study. Laryngoscope, 86:1111, 1976.
25. Jongkees, L. B. W.: Bell's palsy a surgical emergency? Arch. Otol., 81:497, 1965.
26. Hilger, J. A.: Facial nerve stimulator. Trans. Am. Acad. Ophthalmol. and Otolaryngol., 68:74, Jan-Feb. 1964.
27. May, M., Harvey, T., Marovitz, W. F., and Stroud, M.: The prognostic accuracy of the maximal stimulation test compared with that of the nerve excitability test in Bell's palsy. Laryngoscope, 81:931, 1971.
28. Fisch, U.: In Proceedings of the Shambaugh Fifth International Workshop on Middle Ear Microsurgery and Fluctuant Hearing Loss. (George E. Shambaugh, Jr. and John J. Shea, Eds.) Huntsville, Alabama, Strode Publishers, 1977, p. 219.
29. Ballantyne, J., and Grover, J. (Eds.): Scott-Brown's Diseases of the Ear, Nose and Throat. 3rd ed. Philadelphia, J. B. Lippincott Co., 1971, p. 295.
30. Fisch, U.: Editorial comment on "Maximal nerve excitability testing (NET) versus neuromyography (NMG): Comparative prognostic value of tests in patients with facial paralysis." Arch. Otol. (In press).
31. Levine, R.: Managment of the eye in facial paralysis. Otolaryngol. Clin. North Amer., 8:531, 1974.
32. Scaramella, L. F.: Preliminary reports on facial nerve anastomosis. Third International Symposium on Facial Nerve Surgery, Osaka, Japan, September 27–30, 1970.
33. Tucker, H.: New concepts in rehabilitation of long-standing facial paralysis: Selective reinnervation through neuromuscular transfers. In Fisch, U. (Ed.): Facial Nerve Surgery. Birmingham, Alabama, Aesculapius Publ. Co., 1977, pp. 276–283.
34. Melkersson, E.: A case of relapsing facial palsy accompanied by angioneurotic edema. Hygiea, 90:737, 1928.
35. Rosenthal, C.: Simultaneous occurrence of facial paralysis, angioneurotic edema and furrowed tongue in a family. Ztschr. ges. Neurol. u. Psychiat., 131:475, 1931.
36. Gardner, W. J., Sava, G. A.: Hemifacial spasm — A reversible pathophysiologic state. J. Neurosurg. 19:240, 1962.
37. Jannetta, P. J.: The cause of hemifacial spasm: Definitive microsurgical treatment at the brainstem in 31 patients. Trans. Am. Acad. Ophthalmol. Otolaryngol., 80:319, 1975.
38. McCabe, B. F.: Management of hyperfunction of the facial nerve. Ann. Otol. Rhinol. Laryngol., 79:252, 1970.
39. Glasscock, M. E. III: The middle fossa approach to the temporal bone: An otologic frontier. Arch. Otol., 90:41, 1969.

## SUGGESTED ADDITIONAL READING

Jepson, O.: Topognosis (topographic diagnosis) of facial nerve lesions. Arch. Otol., 81:446, 1965.
Maxwell, J. H.: Repair of the facial nerve after facial lacerations. Tr. Am. Acad. Ophth., 58:733, 1954.
Conley, J. J.: Facial nerve grafting in treatment of parotid gland tumors. Arch. Surg., 70:359, 1955.
Cawthorne, T. E.: The surgery of the temporal bone. J. Laryng. & Otol., 67:437, 1953.
Shambaugh, G. E., Jr., and Orr, M. F.: The problem of regenerating nerves as studied in tissue culture. Ann. Otol. Rhin. & Laryng., 72:1124, 1963.
Campbell, E. C. R., Hickey, R. P., Nixon, K. H., and Richardson, A. T.: Value of nerve-excitability measurements in prognosis of facial palsy. Brit. M. J., 2:7, 1962.
Danforth, H. B.: Familial Bell's palsy. Ann. Otol. Rhin. & Laryng., 73:179, 1964.
Laumans, E. P., Jr.: Nerve excitability tests in facial paralysis. Arch. Otol., 81:478, 1965.
Hunt, J. R.: The symptom-complex of acute posterior poliomyelitis of the geniculate, auditory and pneumogastric ganglion. Arch. Int. Med., 5:631, 1910.
Cawthorne, T.: Geniculate ganglion facial palsy. Arch. Otol., 81:502, 1965.

## Prosper Meniere

BORN 1799
DIED 1862

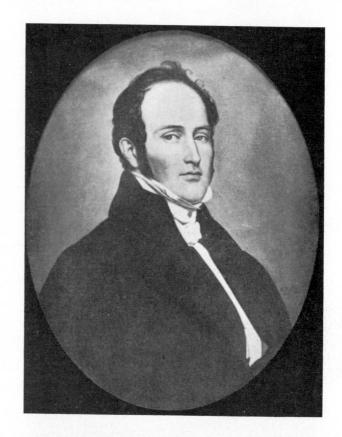

Described the symptomatology and proved the labyrinthine origin of episodic vertigo with deafness.

## Georges Portmann

BORN 1890

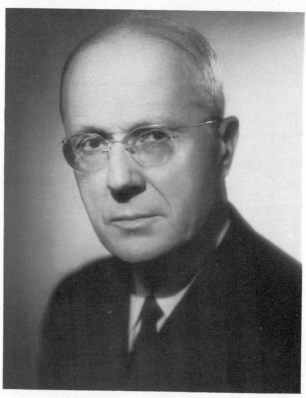

Proposed the endolymphatic hypertension hypothesis of Meniere's disease with surgical drainage of the endolymphatic sac.

# Chapter 21

# Surgical Treatment of Endolymphatic Hydrops

HISTORICAL ASPECTS
PATHOLOGY OF MENIERE'S DISEASE
ETIOLOGY OF ENDOLYMPHATIC HYDROPS
HYDRODYNAMICS OF THE LABYRINTHINE FLUIDS
DIAGNOSTIC SIGNS AND SYMPTOMS
NEUROTOLOGIC EVALUATION
DIFFERENTIAL DIAGNOSIS OF ENDOLYMPHATIC
    HYDROPS
MEDICAL TREATMENT OF ENDOLYMPHATIC HYDROPS
    SALT RESTRICTION
    DIURETICS
    LABYRINTHINE SEDATIVES
    HISTAMINE
    ALLERGIC MANAGEMENT
    SMOKING AND STRESS
    STREPTOMYCIN THERAPY
    RESULTS OF MEDICAL TREATMENT
SURGICAL TREATMENT OF ENDOLYMPHATIC HYDROPS
    INDICATIONS FOR SURGERY
    SURGICAL PROCEDURES
    POSTOPERATIVE COURSE
    RISKS AND COMPLICATIONS
    RESULTS OF SURGERY FOR ENDOLYMPHATIC
        HYDROPS

## HISTORICAL ASPECTS

In 1861 Prosper Meniere[1] in a series of five articles described, as a clinical entity related to the inner ear, the disease that goes by his name. The symptoms, according to Meniere, include **repeated attacks of vertigo** with nausea and vomiting, **occurring frequently** during weeks, months or years, but leaving the patient in perfect health between attacks except for **hearing impairment.** Meniere noted that the **loss of hearing** might be bilateral but more often is unilateral; it is of the **nerve type** but involves the **low frequencies more than the high;** and it is accompanied by **tinnitus** in the affected ear. He noted that the violent symptoms of an attack had often been mistaken for those of a brain lesion, but that there is no paralysis and following the attack the patient is perfectly well.

As evidence that the symptoms are of labyrinthine rather than, as previously thought, of cerebral origin, he cited the case of a young girl who after traveling on a cold night on top of a stage coach developed complete and sudden deafness with continual vertigo and vomiting. Death occurred 5 days later, and autopsy showed no lesion of the brain, but a blood-tinged exudate in the semicircular canals. Contrary to an oft-repeated statement, Meniere did **not** imply by this case that the syndrome of **repeated** attacks of vertigo is due to labyrinthine hemorrhage.[2] The case he cited, possibly of leukemia, was to prove to his confreres that the labyrinth, not the brain, is the source of vertigo.

To Meniere's original and thorough description of the symptomatology of the disease little further was added until 1923 when Shambaugh, Sr. and Knudson[3] called attention to the frequent occurrence of **diplacusis;** the marked **fluctuations** in the hearing impairment were noted in 1938 by Crowe[4] and by Mygind and Dederding;[5] **recruitment of loudness** in the affected ear, first described by Fowler[6] in 1937, was found by Dix, Hallpike, and Hood[7] to be especially characteristic of Meniere's disease as compared to other forms of sensorineural loss, while a sense of **fullness and pressure** or of actual pain in the affected ear was emphasized by Cawthorne[8] and Lindsay.[9]

In 1962 Jerger[10] proposed a battery of special hearing tests for differentiating cochlear hearing losses such as Meniere's disease from eighth nerve lesions such as acoustic neurinoma.

The actual pathology of Meniere's disease was suspected nearly 90 years ago by Knapp[11] who suggested that the symptoms might be due to an increase of pressure in the labyrinth comparable to glaucoma in the eye. Again in 1926 Portmann[12] referred to Meniere's disease as an "aural glaucoma" for which he advocated decompression by incision of the endolymphatic sac. In early 1938, Crowe[4] postulated, "Meniere's disease is the result of pressure or chemical changes in the endolymph." However, the non-fatal course of the condition prevented the accumulation of pathologic confirmation until intracranial section of the eighth nerve became popular for the relief of vertigo. In 1938 Hallpike and Cairns[13] examined the temporal bones of two patients who died following this operation. They found a marked dilatation of the endolymphatic labyrinth in the cochlea and vestibule (Fig. 21–1). Subsequent cases examined pathologically confirmed this finding, with the result that the term "endolymphatic hydrops" (or labyrinthine hydrops) has come to be used synonymously with Meniere's disease.

The history of the **treatment** of Meniere's disease has been noteworthy for the multiplicity of methods advocated. These have ranged from depressant drugs for the symptomatic relief of vertigo, through destructive procedures to abolish the function of the semicircular canals, to medical and surgical measures to cure the excess endolymph causing the symptoms.

The first surgical procedures to relieve the vertigo were destructive. In 1904 Parry[14] divided the eighth nerve intracranially and Milligan[15] and Lake[16] that same year opened the horizontal semicircular canal and vestibule.

Operations to relieve the excess endolymph began with Portmann's[12] drainage of the endolymphatic sac in 1926, when with rare prescience he conceived of Meniere's disease as being due to hypertension of the endolymph, 12 years before Hallpike and Cairns established the actual pathology by their classic report.

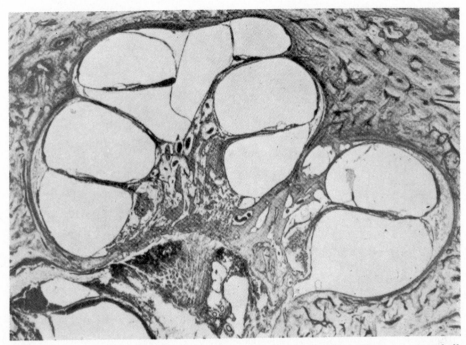

**Figure 21–1** First pathologic proof of endolymphatic hydrops in Meniere's disease. Note ballooning of Reissner's membrane. (From Hallpike, C. S., and Cairns, H.: Observations on the pathology of Meniere's syndrome. J. Laryng. & Otol., 53:625, 1938.)

## PATHOLOGY OF MENIERE'S DISEASE

By 1965 pathologic studies of 27 patients with Meniere's disease, bilateral in 5, had been reported. In every one of the 32 ears there was dilatation of the endolymphatic system in the cochlea, with bulging of Reissner's membrane into the scala vestibuli, greatest in the apical turn where the cecum cupulare forming the closed blind upper end of the cochlear duct was greatly elongated and prolapsed through the helicotrema. Dilatation, usually marked, of the saccule was present in all but 4 of the ears (Fig. 21–2); the utricle was described as dilated in slightly more than half, but in some of these a normal-sized utricle may simply have been displaced by the markedly dilated saccule.[17] Circumscribed outpouchings of the walls of the saccule and sometimes of the utricle were sometimes accompanied by ruptures. Herniations of the saccule or utricle into the lean or ampullated end of a semicircular canal were common. The semicircular canals themselves were unchanged, presumably because of the stouter walls of their endolymphatic ducts.

In striking contrast to the dilatation, usually marked, of portions of the endolymphatic system, has been the absence of degeneration of the nerve elements of the labyrinth whenever these have been sufficiently free from postmortem degeneration to be evaluated. Despite a hearing impairment of many years the spiral ganglion cell population (Figs. 21–3 and 21–4) and the hair cells of Corti's organ, the maculas of the utricle and saccule and the ampullas of the semicircular canals all fail to show alterations attributable to the disease.[9]

The mechanism of a severe attack of vertigo in Meniere's disease could be rupture of the saccule, but repeated attacks of milder degree are more likely due to pressure on the cupula by herniation of the saccule and utricle into the ampulla (Fig.

*Text continued on page 565.*

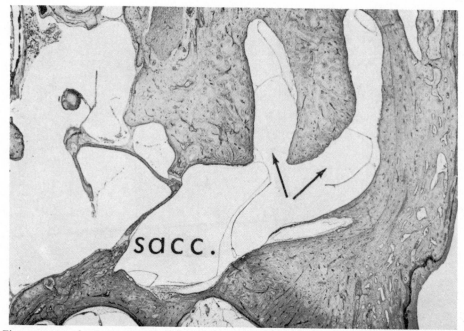

**Figure 21–2** Photomicrograph of the vestibule almost completely filled by dilated saccule and utricle in a patient with endolymphatic hydrops. Arrows show herniation of the utricle into the horizontal semicircular canal and into the common crus of the posterior and superior canals. (Figures 21–2 to 21–7 from Lindsay, J. R.: Labyrinthine dropsy. Laryngoscope, 56:325, 1946.)

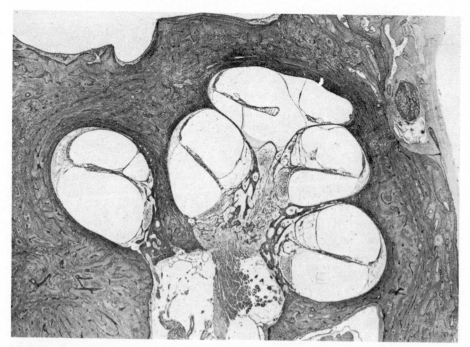

**Figure 21–3** Typical cochlear changes in endolymphatic hydrops. Marked dilatation of the cochlear duct with displacement of Reissner's membrane in all turns.

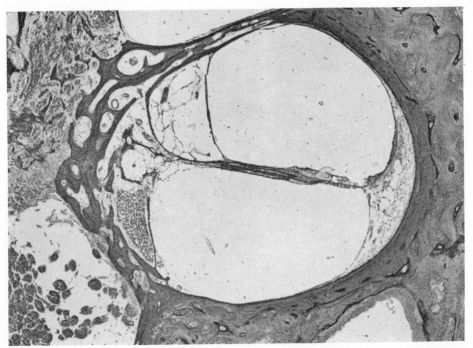

**Figure 21–4**   Enlargement showing intact spiral ganglion cells (same patient as in Figure 21–3).

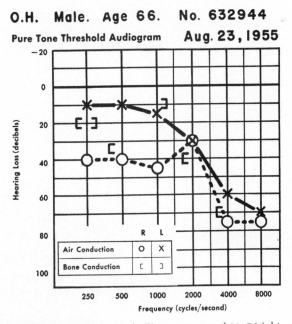

**Figure 21–5**   Audiogram of same patient as in Figures 21–6 and 21–7 (right ear: circles). Presbycusis in both ears with secondary endolymphatic hydrops in the right ear. (Courtesy Dr. J. R. Lindsay.)

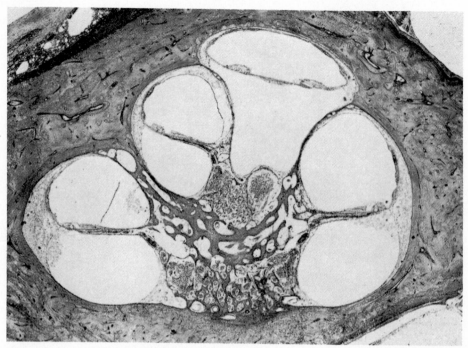

**Figure 21–6**   Cochlea of same patient as in Figures 21–5 and 21–7. Note the loss of ganglion cells in the basal turn due to presbycusis.

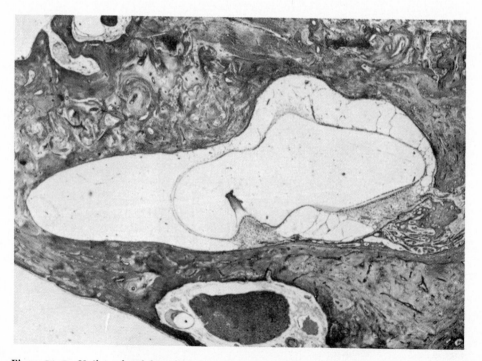

**Figure 21–7**   Unilateral endolymphatic hydrops without vertigo and without distortion of the ampulla of the horizontal semicircular canal in a 65 year old patient with presbycusis.

21–2). The mechanism of the fluctuating hearing impairment is less clear but may be related to deformation of the wall of the ductus cochlearis, greatest in the apical turn and thus causing the greater loss for low-frequency tones. The hydrops may be confined to the cochlea with fluctuating low frequency hearing loss (Figs. 21–5, 21–6, 21–7) or may be vestibular only, at first.

In the first patient described by Hallpike and Cairns, diminution in the amount of loose connective tissue around the endolymphatic sac was noted. Subsequent studies did not mention any changes in the endolymphatic duct or sac, nor in the stria vascularis in the cochlea. The senior author[18] observed the rich blood supply of the normal sac wall, exposed while acoustic neurinomas were being removed by the translabyrinthine method. In contrast he found the sac wall in some patients with Meniere's disease to be markedly ischemic; in other patients the lumen of the sac was greatly reduced or obliterated by adhesions of the walls, in a minority of patients the sac appeared normal and in a few cases it could not be found, indicating marked aplasia or absence of this structure. These clinical observations of frequent abnormalities of the endolymphatic sac in Meniere's disease are beginning to be confirmed by postmortem studies.

## ETIOLOGY OF ENDOLYMPHATIC HYDROPS

The distinguishing pathologic characteristic of Meniere's disease is certainly the increased volume of endolymph, yet why and how it is increased is not known. Wright[19] thought that focal infection, especially in the teeth and tonsils, was an important etiologic factor in Meniere's disease, but others have failed to find such a factor in the majority of cases.[8] Duke[20] described cases of typical Meniere's disease due to allergy, and Derlacki[21] found that 6 of 55 cases of unquestionable Meniere's disease were due to a specific food or inhalant allergy. But in the majority of cases a specific extrinsic allergic factor cannot be demonstrated. The senior author[22] obtained improvement by correcting a thyroid deficiency in some cases that had resisted medical treatment. To explain the majority of cases in which neither focal infection nor allergy nor thyroid deficiency can be implicated, Lermoyez[23] postulated an underlying vasomotor dysfunction with arteriolar spasm and atonic capillary dilatation, accompanied by increased permeability, presumably in the stria vascularis. Recently deficient resorptive function of the endolymphatic sac has been implicated.[24]

## HYDRODYNAMICS OF THE LABYRINTHINE FLUIDS

Pertinent to the etiology and therapy of endolymphatic hydrops is a consideration of the hydrodynamics of the labyrinthine fluids. More than a century ago Reissner demonstrated that the endolymphatic membranous labyrinth is a closed system, **nowhere in communication with perilymph** or spinal fluid. It "floats" in perilymph in much the same way that the brain and spinal cord float in cerebrospinal fluid, save for the areas of attachment of the sensory epithelium, where the sensory nerve fibers of the vestibular nerve penetrate the bony capsule, in the cochlea where the endolymphatic cochlear duct has perilymph on only two of its four sides, and in the endolymphatic duct and sac. A delicate arachnoid connective tissue mesh, a remnant of periotic tissue, fills the perilymphatic space in the vestibule and

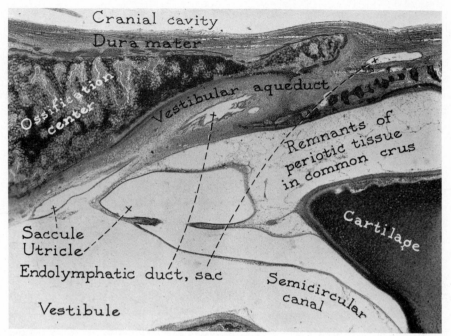

**Figure 21–8**  Intermediate stage in the ossification of the otic capsule in the region of the vestibular aqueduct. The aqueduct is formed around the already-present endolymphatic duct. Fetus of 5 months. (Courtesy of Dr. Barry J. Anson.)

semicircular canals (Fig. 21–8) analogous to the arachnoid of the cerebrospinal space. In the cochlea, where such tissue would impede the transmission of sound waves, it is lacking.

### Formation and Resorption of Perilymph

The perilymphatic space of the labyrinth communicates with the posterior fossa subarachnoid space via the cochlear aqueduct (cochlear canaliculus or perilymphatic duct), normally quite narrow in its midportion and filled with loose arachnoid-like connective tissue (Figs. 21–9 and 21–10) so that it can transmit spinal fluid only by seepage slowly into the scala tympani of the cochlea to augment the perilymph. Rarely, the cochlear aqueduct is abnormally wide (see Fig. 1–7) and patent, permitting free flow of spinal fluid when the labyrinth is opened, as in stapedectomy with a "gusher."

There are other channels besides the cochlear aqueduct through which spinal fluid can reach the perilymphatic spaces of the labyrinth. One is the loose connective tissue around the cochlear nerve bundles as they traverse the tractus spiralis foraminosa at the fundus of the internal acoustic meatus. Even red cells from an intracranial hemorrhage may reach the cochlea via these channels.[25] The loose connective tissue around the endolymphatic duct and sac has a texture similar to that of the cochlear aqueduct and probably contains perilymph, but whether these fluid spaces actually extend through the dense dura that envelops the distal portion of the endolymphatic sac to allow the exchange of perilymph and spinal fluid has not been determined.[26]

Additional perilymph may be produced by the upper portion of the stria vascularis adjacent to the scala vestibuli.[27] Resorption of perilymph is believed to

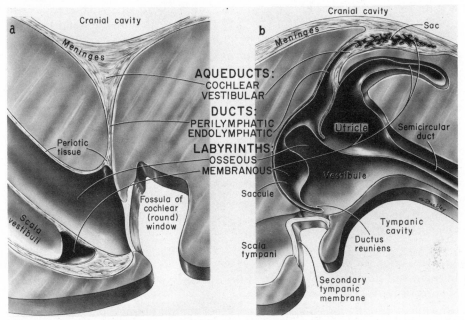

**Figure 21–9** The cochlear (perilymphatic) and vestibular (containing endolymphatic duct) aqueducts. Semischematic. (From Anson, B. J., Donaldson, J. A., Warpeha, R. L., and Winch, T. R.: A critical appraisal of the anatomy of the perilymphatic system in man. Laryngoscope, 74:945, 1964.)

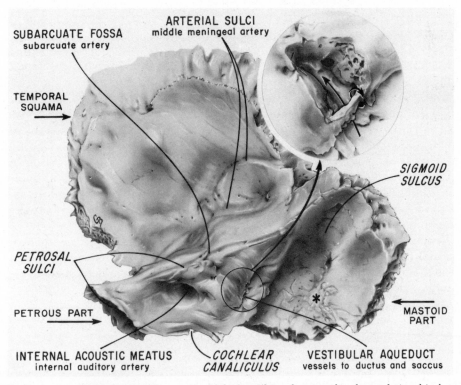

**Figure 21–10** Right temporal bone viewed from within, showing the close relationship between the intracranial orifices of the cochlear canaliculus (aqueduct) and the vestibular aqueduct. In the enlarged drawing the "roof" of the vestibular aqueduct has been partially removed; the long arrow follows the course of the endolymphatic sac and duct. (Courtesy of Dr. Barry J. Anson.)

occur partly via the perivascular spaces around the spiral veins that communicate in turn with similar spaces around the vein of the cochlear aqueduct and the veins of the internal acoustic meatus into both of which the spiral veins empty. Perilymph is probably resorbed also, and perhaps in largest part, from the loose vascular connective tissue that surrounds the endolymphatic sac.[28] In general the production and resorption of perilymph is believed to be much slower than of endolymph.

### Production and Resorption of Endolymph

The sensory cells of the cristae of the semicircular canals, the maculae of the utricle and saccule and the organ of Corti depend upon endolymph for oxygenation and nutrition. (Recently a third type of fluid, "cortilymph,"[28] has been postulated for nutrition of the hair cells of the cochlea.) More than a century ago Corti described the stria vascularis in the cochlea and suggested that it might secrete endolymph. In 1908 Shambaugh, Sr.,[29] described a gland-like tubule, "Shambaugh's gland," in the lower portion of the stria as further evidence of its secretory function. In 1927 Guild[30] showed that material injected into the scala media of guinea pigs could be found after an interval of time in the walls of the endolymphatic sac. Although there have been conflicting opinions, recent experiments strengthen the concept that endolymph produced by the stria vascularis flows through the canalis reuniens into the saccule and thence via the short saccular duct into the endolymphatic duct and sac, where it is resorbed.[31]

A knowledge of the embryology and adult anatomy of the endolymphatic duct and sac is important in considering their function. The entire labyrinth reaches adult size and differentiation in the fifth month of fetal life when its capsule ossifies, with the single exception of the endolymphatic sac. This portion of the membranous labyrinth protrudes posteriorly outside the otic capsule, and continues to grow and expand not only through the remainder of fetal life but throughout infancy and childhood, until in the adult the endolymphatic sac is threefold larger than at birth, and with its duct it may equal in length the entire labyrinth.

The endolymphatic duct begins with a fold described by Bast[32] that appears to have a valve-like action permitting endolymph to flow into the duct from the utricle but not in the other direction. Bast and Shambaugh, Jr.[24] observed a pinkish precipitate by hematoxylin and eosin stain within the sac and duct as far as the utriculo-endolymphatic valve, indicating fluid resorption by the sac and duct with larger protein molecules left behind. The saccular duct enters the endolymphatic duct quite close to the valve of Bast, and there is no valve-like fold between the saccule and the endolymphatic duct.

The endolymphatic duct and proximal portion of the sac lie in a bony channel, the vestibular aqueduct, somewhat wider than that of the cochlear aqueduct, so that there is room for a moderate amount of loose vascular connective tissue between the bony walls and the endolymphatic duct and sac (Figs. 21–8 and 21–11). The bony walls themselves are quite vascular, their blood vessels connecting with those of the connective tissue in the vestibular aqueduct.[25] The fairly large veins of this connective tissue drain into the adjacent sigmoid sinus.

The walls of the endolymphatic duct and proximal portion of the sac are rugose, villous and lined by columnar epithelial cells whose nuclei lie near their free end, as in resorptive epithelium elsewhere. The distal portion of the endolymphatic sac has smooth walls, is lined by cuboidal epithelium and lies between layers of the dura, which appears white and thick when exposed at operation, contrasting with the thin

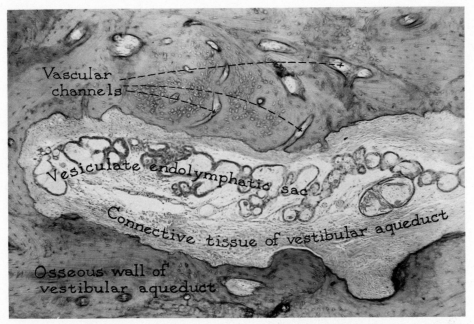

**Figure 21-11** Resorptive portion of endolymphatic duct and sac.

bluish-appearing posterior fossa dura elsewhere. The outer (mastoid) wall of the endolymphatic sac is considerably thicker than the inner (posterior fossa) wall.

In the fetus and at birth the dural portion of the endolymphatic sac overlies the sigmoid sinus with its veins draining directly into the sinus, a design that would appear especially favorable for rapid fluid resorption in view of the negative venous pressure in this sinus in the upright position. In the adult the growth of the posterior fossa and mastoid process has pulled the sinus away from the sac in some cases, although in others it remains in contact, but in either event the rich venous drainage from the sac continues to flow into the sinus.

### Pressure Equilibration in the Labyrinth

The need to maintain equal pressure between endolymph and perilymph is obvious, considering the extremely thin unsupported walls of the utricle and saccule, and the nearly as thin Reissner's membrane. The continuous column of perilymph between the cerebrospinal fluid of the posterior fossa and the labyrinth provided by the cochlear aqueduct is balanced by the column of endolymph between layers of posterior fossa dura and vestibule. The constant fluctuations of posterior fossa pressure induced by arterial pulse, the larger fluctuations with respiration and the enormous fluctuations produced by coughing, straining and change of position from recumbent to upright are transmitted instantly and equally to endolymph and perilymph without need for any appreciable flow of fluid in either direction, since water is virtually non-compressible. It is only necessary that there be bony channels filled with columns of fluid. It is significant that the intracranial apertures of the cochlear and vestibular aqueducts lie in the same horizontal plane and only a few millimeters apart (Fig. 21-10), so that the effects of gravity on posterior fossa pressure will be exerted equally on endolymph and perilymph.

The possibility that deficient resorption of endolymph by the sac is responsible for endolymphatic hydrops is suggested by the anatomic peculiarities of this structure, its normal resorbing function and the abnormalities noted by Shambaugh, Jr.[24] when the sac was exposed and incised for cases of Meniere's disease. Kimura and Schuknecht[33] produced endolymphatic hydrops experimentally in guinea pigs by obliterating the duct (Figs. 21–12 and 21–13). This provided confirmatory evidence that deficient resorption of endolymph may be the fault in Meniere's disease rather than, as formerly thought, increased production by the stria vascularis. Valvassori[34] observed by tomography absence of the groove for the endolymphatic duct in some patients with Meniere's disease, and the senior author failed to find an endolymphatic sac at operation in such a patient.

The volume of endolymph in the normal ear of man is about 3 microliters (0.3 cc.) and is believed to have a fairly rapid half-time fluid turnover of about one hour,

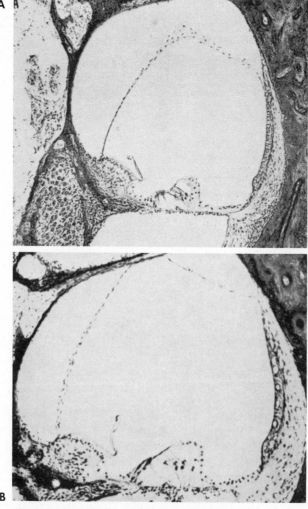

**Figure 21–12** Dilatation of the ductus cochlearis with displacement of Reissner's membrane after obliteration of the endolymphatic duct in a guinea pig. *A*, Three weeks, *B*, Two weeks. The sensory and spiral ganglia cells and stria vascularis are normal. Compare with Figures 21–3, 21–4, and 21–6. (From Kimura, R. S., and Schuknecht, H. F.: Membranous hydrops in the inner ear of the guinea pig after obliteration of the endolymphatic sac. Pract. oto-rhino-laryng., *27*:343, 1965.)

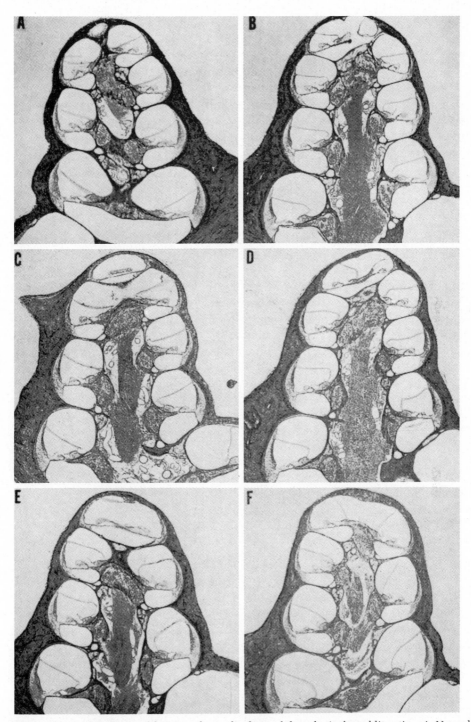

**Figure 21–13** Progressive dilatation of saccule after endolymphatic duct obliteration. *A*, Normal. *B*, One day. *C*, Three days. *D*, Two weeks. *E* and *F*, Three weeks. (From Kimura. R. S., and Schuknecht, H. F.: Membranous hydrops in the inner ear of the guinea pig after obliteration of the endolymphatic sac. Pract. oto-rhino-laryng., *27*:343, 1965.)

if assumed to be formed from perilymph.[35, 36] If formed from blood, the turnover time is much longer.

## DIAGNOSTIC SYMPTOMS AND SIGNS

The positive diagnosis of endolymphatic hydrops or Meniere's disease is made from the characteristic **symptoms** and the distinctive **hearing alterations.** The four cardinal symptoms of this disease are: vertigo, hearing impairment, tinnitus and fullness or pressure.

### Vertigo

The most dramatic, and in many cases the most disabling, symptom is the vertigo, which occurs in **repeated attacks,** and is usually **severe,** with intervals of complete freedom from dizziness between attacks. The attacks tend to occur in groups of several within a matter of weeks or months, followed by freedom from vertigo for months or years. Very typical of the vertigo is that it may occur **at any time,** unrelated to posture or activity. There may be a brief warning, but in at least half the cases the vertigo strikes suddenly without warning of any kind, a particularly disconcerting feature.[8] A few patients may have a more or less constant imbalance instead of, or in addition to, the severe attacks of vertigo.

As the term implies (Latin for whirling) the vertigo is accompanied by a sense of rotation, either of the patient himself or of his environment. Particularly important for differential diagnosis is that the vertigo of Meniere's disease, except in the very mildest attacks, is **always accompanied by nausea and vomiting, nystagmus and ataxia.** The spread of nerve impulses in the brain stem from the vestibular to the vagus nucleus may also cause abdominal pain, increased peristalsis and slowed pulse. Pallor and cold sweating add to the picture of shock. These various symptoms not only invariably accompany vertigo of labyrinthine origin but are **always proportionate to the severity of the vertigo.**

### Caloric Tests

Although the history of attacks of recurring vertigo is so characteristic of endolymphatic hydrops as to be of great diagnostic value, tests of the function of the semicircular canals do not show consistent changes. In the great majority of cases the caloric response on the affected side is diminished; in a few it is within normal limits; and rarely it is hyperactive.[2] Complete absence of caloric response on the side of the hearing impairment can occur in endolymphatic hydrops, but it is much more likely to occur in acoustic neurinoma (see Chapter 23).

Of some diagnostic help is the fact that the subjective sensations induced by the caloric test are identical in character though usually less severe than those experienced during an attack of vertigo due to Meniere's disease. The caloric test is also helpful in indicating the ear causing the vertigo in cases of hydrops with bilateral hearing impairment, the side with the reduced caloric response being the probable source of the vertigo.[8]

## Hearing Changes

The hearing impairment of Meniere's disease is so characteristic and distinctive that it is possible to make the positive diagnosis of endolymphatic hydrops from the hearing alterations alone without attacks of vertigo. Some of these patients will eventually develop the typical attacks of vertigo, completing Meniere's classic syndrome. The most constant pathologic alteration is in the cochlea, with ballooning of Reissner's membrane (see Figs. 21–1 and 21–2), and the alterations in hearing usually precede the attacks of vertigo and generally persist during remissions in the vertigo; therefore in most cases **the disease of endolymphatic hydrops is first a cochlear disturbance and secondarily vestibular.**

The hearing impairment of endolymphatic hydrops consists of a **sensorineural loss** with positive Rinne tests to all tuning forks when adequate masking is used, but with the loss **greater for low frequencies** than for high in the early stages. Later a flat audiometric curve is more characteristic, with a nearly equal loss for all frequencies. **Distortion and diplacusis** are very characteristic, **with impaired discrimination** (but not as severe as in acoustic neurinoma), and **recruitment of loudness** is usually but not invariably present. Békésy audiometry shows a type II curve; the SISI test reveals a markedly greater ability to detect small increases in intensity (see Chapter 3). Although endolymphatic hydrops nearly always begins in one ear, eventual involvement of both ears occurs in many cases.

The **tinnitus** of endolymphatic hydrops accompanies the hearing impairment and, like the hearing loss, is especially severe for the low frequencies, producing a **roaring** type of tinnitus. **All of the hearing alterations** and the tinnitus characteristically **fluctuate.** Perhaps the greatest fluctuations occur in the speech discrimination ability, and a definite improvement in the discrimination score may be the first evidence of clinical improvement. The patient with endolymphatic hydrops who wears a hearing aid will report that on some days he can understand fairly well with the aid, but that on other days everything is so distorted that he can understand nothing with it, despite an audiometrically stable pure tone loss.

It should be noted that binaural dysharmonic diplacusis, usually with an elevation of pitch in the diseased as compared to the normal ear,[38] can be demonstrated in patients with hydrops who possess good pitch perception, especially in musicians and people who enjoy music. Diplacusis is probably present in others with endolymphatic hydrops, but is described by the non-musical patient as a distorted or buzzing sound in the diseased ear as compared to a pure tone in the normal ear.

**Fullness or pressure** in the affected ear is present in the majority of cases of endolymphatic hydrops, and like the other symptoms it fluctuates in severity. Relief from the sense of fullness often heralds improvement, and an increase in the fullness and pressure accompanies or is followed by worsening of the other symptoms. In some cases an actual pain or headache on the affected side accompanies the fullness and pressure.[8, 39]

## DIFFERENTIAL DIAGNOSIS OF ENDOLYMPHATIC HYDROPS

The term Meniere's disease has often been used loosely and inaccurately to apply to any case of labyrinthine vertigo, with further confusion added by the terms "pseudo-Meniere" and "Meniere syndrome." Since the pathologic lesion of the disease described by Meniere is now known to be a dilatation of the cochlear, saccular and sometimes utricular endolymphatic spaces, the name "endolymphatic hydrops" is less likely to cause confusion.

The typical case of endolymphatic hydrops with recurring vertigo, nausea, vomiting and ataxia, a unilateral **fluctuating** sensorineural low-tone hearing loss accompanied by diplacusis, recruitment and impaired speech discrimination, roaring tinnitus and a sense of fullness, offers no particular problem in diagnosis, for there is no other form of sensorineural hearing loss with these peculiarities. The early or less typical case with some but not all of these symptoms may be confused with the following conditions: eustachian tube occlusion, cerebral ischemia, lesion of the central vestibular nuclei or tracts in the brain stem or cerebellum, serous or suppurative labyrinthitis, postural vertigo, cerebellopontine angle tumor, most often acoustic neurinoma, and sudden labyrinthine deafness. Differentiation is as follows:

**Eustachian Tube Occlusion.** Eustachian tube occlusion produces a conductive rather than a sensorineural type of loss. There is no diplacusis, recruitment or impairment of speech discrimination, and only very rarely, perhaps when there is an abnormally mobile stapes footplate, will alterations in intratympanic pressure result in momentary vertigo. Many patients with endolymphatic hydrops, simply because of fullness in the ear, have been subjected to a series of useless tubal inflations. To quote Hilger: "The eager and repetitious catheter has been a poor substitute for diagnosis much over-long."[40]

**Cerebral Ischemia.** Cerebral ischemia produces dizziness which is described as a sensation of faintness or "blackout" induced by an upright posture or by bending over and straightening up. It may be the result of an overactive carotid sinus reflex or of arteriosclerotic narrowing of the vertebral or internal carotid arteries. Cerebral ischemia dizziness lacks the sense of rotation and should not be confused with a true labyrinthine vertigo.

**Central Vestibular Lesion.** A central vestibular lesion of the brainstem or cerebellum, such as multiple sclerosis or a tumor, may produce attacks of vertigo, but between attacks the equilibrium continues to be disturbed. Nystagmus, nausea and vomiting and ataxia are lacking or are disproportionate to the severity of the vertigo; the hearing if impaired does not exhibit the characteristic alterations of endolymphatic hydrops.

**Serous or Suppurative Labyrinthitis.** Serous or suppurative labyrinthitis is nearly always secondary to acute or chronic otitis media, usually with a fistula of a semicircular canal, and should occasion no diagnostic problem.

**Postural Vertigo.** Postural vertigo is a puzzling and not infrequent condition of brief but definite and often violent vertigo and nystagmus with ataxia, nausea and sometimes vomiting, induced by turning or placing the head in certain positions. Cawthorne[41] points out that in the majority of cases the first time the head is placed in the particular position very marked nystagmus and sense of rotation are induced, but that when the head is placed in the same position a few moments later the symptoms are diminished or do not recur. He suggests that postural vertigo of this fatigable type may be of utriculosaccular origin, perhaps in some cases the result of viral vestibulitis. Non-fatigable postural vertigo may be due to a midline cerebellar lesion. Since the vertigo of endolymphatic hydrops is unrelated to posture, and postural vertigo usually lacks a hearing impairment, there should be no difficulty in differentiating the two conditions.

**Cerebellopontine Angle Tumor.** Cerebellopontine angle tumor, generally an acoustic neurinoma, may be confused with endolymphatic hydrops because there is a unilateral sensorineural loss with marked loss of speech discrimination, dizziness and headache. Absence of recruitment, of attacks of severe vertigo and of marked fluctuations in the hearing in cerebellopontine angle tumor, accompanied by radiologic osseous changes at the internal auditory meatus, involvement of the facial, trigeminal or other adjacent cranial nerves, cerebellar ataxia and complete loss of caloric response of the affected side, all help to differentiate cerebellopontine angle tumor from endolymphatic hydrops. The greatest diagnostic difficulty arises when endolymphatic hydrops is secondary to an acoustic neurinoma due to pressure on the internal auditory artery and vein (see Chapter 23). In doubtful cases a posterior fossa myelogram may be required to differentiate between the two conditions. Any patient with unilateral sensorineural hearing loss and tinnitus must undergo a thorough neurotologic examination, as described in Chapter 23.

**Sudden Labyrinthine Deafness.** Sudden labyrinthine deafness[42] is the condition most easily confused with endolymphatic hydrops since the initial symptoms of the attack closely resemble those of Meniere's disease. Sudden labyrinthine deafness occurs in young, or more often middle-aged and sometimes elderly adults, with the abrupt onset in one ear of **tinnitus** and **severe deafness,** followed in many cases in a few minutes or hours by **vertigo.** Diplacusis, distortion, recruitment and impaired speech discrimination usually accompany the severe loss of hearing. After the acute episode the vertigo gradually subsides and the hearing may slowly improve and occasionally returns to normal. It is known that sudden labyrinthine deafness may be the result of rupture of the oval or round window or a hemorrhage into the labyrinth, as in the case described by Meniere. It is assumed that occlusion of the internal auditory artery or of one of its branches by a thrombus, embolus or spasm can also be the cause. The use of nylidrin hydrochloride (Arlidin) as a vasodilator has been recommended.[43] A viral etiology is probably responsible for many of these cases, mumps being the prime example. Rupture of a dilated saccule due to hydrops may produce the picture of sudden labyrinthine deafness. **The absence of any further attacks of vertigo or further loss of hearing** differentiates sudden labyrinthine deafness from endolymphatic hydrops.

## Atypical Endolymphatic Hydrops

The complete syndrome of repeated vertigo, tinnitus, pressure and sensorineural hearing impairment is helpful but not necessary to make the positive diagnosis of endolymphatic hydrops. Since the condition often begins mildly and intermittently there will be patients in whom for a time the only symptom is a **sense of fullness** or tinnitus or an early but mild hearing impairment. Rarely vertigo is the first symptom. These patients, and patients with bilateral hydrops without vertigo, patients with a less typical high-tone rather than a low-tone sensorineural loss, and patients with mild imbalance without nausea and vomiting rather than the more typical severe vertigo, may require a period of observation with repeated hearing tests before the marked fluctuations in hearing with diplacusis, distortion and recruitment so diagnostic of endolymphatic hydrops can be demonstrated.

## Secondary Endolymphatic Hydrops

Although Meniere's disease typically occurs in an otherwise healthy person without previous ear disease, exactly the same symptoms may arise in a patient with congenital nerve deafness, noise-induced hearing loss, labyrinthine concussion, congenital luetic nerve deafness, otosclerosis (otospongiosis) and presbycusis. Lindsay[9] has shown that such a patient with secondary hydrops has the same dilatation of the endolymphatic system as in the more usual primary hydrops (see Figs. 21–5, 21–6 and 21–7). Endolymphatic hydrops has become one of the frequent late postoperative complications of fenestration and stapedectomy surgery. These cases often respond to medical treatment with dilute histamine.[37]

## MEDICAL TREATMENT OF ENDOLYMPHATIC HYDROPS

While it is interesting to review the historical management of Meniere's disease, it is not within the scope of this chapter to mention all methods of medical management. An attempt will be made, however, to describe the more common approaches.

### Salt Restriction

There is ample evidence that the histopathology of Meniere's disease is a hydrops of the endolymphatic system. It would be rational to assume, therefore, that reduction of general body fluids would decrease the amount of endolymph in the scala media and saccule. Salt restriction has been employed as a major method of controlling body fluid for years and has been a standard therapeutic approach for Meniere's disease.

The most famous salt-free diet is that of Furstenberg.[44] In addition to marked reduction of salt intake, the patient is administered ammonium chloride 3 gm. t.i.d. for three days; then it is omitted for two days. Similar salt reduction diets have been advocated by Mygind and Dederding[5] as well as Cawthorne.[8]

The junior author has found that the less complicated the diet instructions, the more apt the patient is to follow the regime. For this reason, the individual is simply instructed to refrain from eating ham, bacon and sausage as well as potato chips, peanuts, pretzels and other similar foods. For cooking, Morton's Litesalt is recommended in small amounts, and the patient is instructed not to salt the food at the table. A salt substitute such as KCl may be used at anytime.

### Diuretics

The rationale for salt restriction is the same basis upon which diuretics are administered. The ammonium chloride recommended in the Furstenberg diet has been replaced by mild diuretics such as Diuril and Dyazide, which may be sufficient to control Meniere's disease. Occasionally a more potent drug such as Lasix is indicated.

The authors have found Dyazide to be a useful preparation, as it is a potassium-sparing drug. Potassium loss is a problem with other diuretics, and for that reason, patients may occasionally need daily supplements, such as Slow-K or K-lyte. The latter drug comes in the form of an effervescent tablet, and when placed in a glass of water supplies 20 meq. of potassium. All patients placed on diuretics are asked to take their medication with a glass of orange or tomato juice or to eat at least one banana per day, as these foods contain natural potassium.

When placing a patient on a diuretic for the first time, it is important to explain that the extracellular fluid volume as well as the blood pressure will be lowered, often resulting in leg cramps and a general feeling of extreme weakness. Should these problems arise, it may be necessary to cut back on the medication and take it every three to four days rather than daily.

Many patients with Meniere's disease can control the pressure or fullness in their ears simply by taking a diuretic for a few days when the symptom first occurs. Many of these individuals titrate themselves, by only using drugs when they need them.

## Labyrinthine Sedatives

While salt restriction and diuretics are used to treat the underlying pathologic condition of Meniere's disease, the symptoms of vertigo, nausea and vomiting must be managed by the use of labyrinthine sedatives. These are usually given when the attack occurs or seems imminent. Occasionallly, if the symptoms have been occurring on a regular basis, a patient will be given these medications on a daily basis for several months. There are numerous drugs that fall into this category, but only the more common ones will be discussed here.

Of all the labyrinthine sedatives available, Valium is by far the most potent. McCabe[45] has shown that this drug is extremely valuable in treating all types of end-organ vertigo. It is such a powerful suppressant that it is almost impossible to obtain a caloric response in a patient who has had the medication within a 24 to 48 hour time period preceding an electronystagmography (ENG) test.

The usual dose is 5 mg. three times a day. Some individuals are very sensitive to drugs, and to Valium in particular. For that reason, it is important to adjust the dosage to each particular patient. They should be given written instructions with their prescriptions explaining the side effects of the drug. If they become drowsy or weak, they are asked to divide the tablet and take one half of a tablet (2.5 mg.) t.i.d. instead of the full 5 mg. Occasionally, a patient will become depressed and cry, owing to an idiosyncratic reaction to the drug. In this instance they must discontinue the medication, and a substitution will be made.

When Valium must be discontinued, the junior author prefers to use Bucladin as a second choice. There are numerous other antimotion and antinausea drugs available, such as Dramamine, Bonamine, Torecan, Compazine, Antivert and Meclazine.

Anticholinergic drugs such as Atropine, Probanthine, and Robinul are excellent for use in conjunction with Valium, Bucladin and so on. These drugs not only have a labyrinthine sedative effect but also help to control the vegetative symptoms of nausea, vomiting and perspiration that occur with an acute attack. In fact, Atropine 1/150 gr. subcutaneously will occasionally abort an attack if given early enough. The junior author prefers Probanthine and Robinul because of their sustained action dosage that only requires a b.i.d. administration.

## Histamine

Histamine acid phosphate has been a standard method of therapy in Meniere's disease for many years. It is given intravenously in the management of acute attacks and by subcutaneous injection and sublingual drops on a routine basis.

When used intravenously, 2.75 mg. of histamine acid phosphate (Eli Lilly) is diluted in 250 cc. of Ringer's solution and given at a rate of between 16 and 60 drops per minute. The rate of administration should be titrated to produce a flush of the face, but not a headache. The blood pressure should be taken frequently during administration of the drug. Two injections are given daily for three days.

The use of dilute histamine* on a daily increasing basis is advocated by the senior author as follows. The patient is given an initial subcutaneous injection of 0.1 cc. of histamine 1 to 100,000,000 dilution with a bottle of 1 to 10,000,000 dilution, two drops to be placed under the tongue twice daily except on the day of injection. If there has been no improvement by the time the weekly or biweekly dose has reached 0.1 cc. of 1 to 100,000 dilution by injection and 1 to 10,000 dilution by sublingual drops, this method of treatment is discontinued. If the symptoms are increased following any dose, the next dosage is reduced. When the effective "optimum" dosage is reached, it is continued once a week for 2 months, or longer as required.

## Allergic Management

In a small number of patients with Meniere's disease, the etiologic factor appears to be related to allergy. In such a case, the shock organ seems to be the inner ear. Often clear-cut seasonal exacerbations due to inhalant and pollen allergies manifest themselves. These individuals are managed by skin testing followed by desensitization injections of the specific allergen, according to Rinkel's skin titration for the optimum dosage.

A less easily managed problem occurs with food allergies. Some individuals can precipitate an attack of Meniere's disease by ingesting certain foods. Elimination diets are helpful in treating this type of Meniere's patient, as determined by provocative testing and cytotoxic studies[46] to determine the offending foods.

## Smoking and Stress

There is little doubt that stress, whether it be physical (infections, fatigue, and so on) or emotional, can precipitate an attack of Meniere's disease. Trying to eliminate stress from a patient's life may not be possible, but an attempt should be made to explain to the patient the role that stress plays in his disease. An obviously anxious or psychoneurotic individual might improve with psychiatric care.

As a rule, smokers are individuals who do not deal well with stress and use their addiction as a method of calming their "nerves." Unfortunately, the vasoconstrictive nature of nicotine probably affects the microvasculature of the endolymphatic sac

---

*Dilute histamine for subcutaneous injection is prepared from Eli Lilly's histamine acid phosphate 2.75 mg. in 5 cc., a 1 to 5,000 dilution. By taking 2 cc. of this solution and adding 2 cc. of Coca's solution (buffered saline with 0.4 per cent phenol as preservative), one obtains a 1 to 10,000 dilution. To make successively weaker dilutions, each ten times more dilute, take 0.5 cc. of 1 to 10,000 histamine and add 4.5 cc. of Coca's to make 1 to 100,000 dilution and so on to make the 1 to 100,000,000 dilution for the initial dose of 0.1 cc.

The oral sublingual drops are made by dissolving a 3 mg. histamine tabloid (1 mg. of histamine base) of Burroughs Wellcome Company in 1 cc. of Coca's to produce a 1 to 1,000 solution. This is diluted as above to the 1 to 10,000,000 dilution for the initial dose of sublingual drops.

The response to dilute histamine by subcutaneous injection and sublingual drops is often dramatic in early cases of endolymphatic hydrops. If symptoms are no better, increase the dose; if made worse, decrease the dose; if improved, remain at that "optimum" dose for 2 months.

and decreases the absorption of endolymph. All patients with Meniere's disease should be required to refrain from smoking.

Diamox and Neptazane have been used for glaucoma and hydrocephalus. They are carbonic anhydrase inhibitors and decrease production of aqueous humor in the anterior chamber of the eye and of cerebral spinal fluid. The enzyme carbonic anhydrase is found in especially high concentration in the stria vascularis. Neptazane 50 to 100 mg. t.i.d. may control the hydrops of endolymph in some cases. Not all patients will tolerate this dosage.

## Streptomycin Therapy

The individual with bilateral endolymphatic hydrops presents a unique problem. Often these patients do not respond well to medical management and because of the bilateral nature of their disease are not good candidates for destructive vestibular surgery.

Intramuscular injections of streptomycin may offer the patient with bilateral disease a chance for a satisfactory relief of vertigo. First advocated by Fowler[47] and later by Schuknecht,[48] streptomycin therapy will ablate the vestibular labyrinth while sparing the cochlea.

One gram of streptomycin is given twice a day for 10 to 20 days by intramuscular injection. After the 10th day, caloric examinations are administered every other day and audiograms daily. The patient is instructed to mention an increase in tinnitus or a further decrease in hearing level. When the caloric response has been completely depressed, the injections are discontinued. These individuals no longer have episodic vertigo but are left with a residue of ataxia, which usually diminishes with time, but may not disappear completely.

## Results of Medical Treatment

The spontaneous exacerbations and remissions characteristic of endolymphatic hydrops make interpretation of response to therapy, whether it be medical or surgical, uncertain and difficult. Certainly, in evaluating the results of either method, it is important to use the same criteria: the hearing should be stabilized, the pressure or fullness reduced, the tinnitus improved and the vertigo eliminated. Any result less than this is not acceptable.

Many authors have stated that medical management will control from 70 to 85 per cent of their patients with endolymphatic hydrops. Unfortunately, in most of these reports, hearing results are not considered.

## SURGICAL TREATMENT OF ENDOLYMPHATIC HYDROPS

### Indications for Surgery

The surgical treatment of endolymphatic hydrops should be reserved for those patients who are considered medical failures, such as individuals whose hearing is fluctuating widely and who are having frequent attacks of vertigo in spite of salt restriction, diuretics and labyrinthine sedatives. These patients are usually incapacitated by their symptoms and are desperate to obtain relief. Surgical treatment is preferable for those with unilateral disease.

There are two major classifications of operations that are available — destructive and conservative procedures. Destructive procedures are those in which the vestibular labyrinth is destroyed and the residual hearing is sacrificed. Conservative operations are those in which an attempt is made to preserve whatever hearing the patient has at the time of surgery.

To select the proper type of procedure for a given patient, there are certain criteria that must be weighed in arriving at a decision. First, it is important to establish what is to be considered serviceable hearing in the involved ear. The junior author feels that this hearing level should be sufficient for use with a hearing aid. Because of recruitment, it is often difficult to fit an aid on a patient with Meniere's disease, but the ear should have at least 60 dB SRT and a discrimination score of not less than 80 per cent.

Once this has been determined, then the decision to destroy or preserve the residual hearing can be made. What if the involved side represents a better hearing or only hearing ear? This will make the decision to perform any type of surgical procedure a most difficult one. Certainly, the surgeon then should only advise a conservative operation, if he is considering surgery at all. Probably most physicians would procrastinate as long as possible in hopes that a natural remission might occur. The junior author has performed conservative surgery in 12 patients' only hearing ears when it was judged highly probable that the disease would destroy the hearing if nothing was done. However, this surgery is extremely risky because the incidence of dead ears is at least 5 per cent in conservative operations for Meniere's disease.

An alternative to vestibular surgery is the injection of streptomycin as mentioned previously.[48] Not only is the vertigo controlled in a high percentage of the patients, but, in a fair number, hearing stabilizes.

## Surgical Procedures

Over the years numerous operative procedures have been recommended for the surgical control of endolymphatic hydrops; all can be classified as either destructive or conservative. The techniques of these procedures have been described in the literature. In what follows the highlights of each operation will be covered, with a summary concerning the results of each.

### Destructive Procedures

Known as labyrinthectomies or labyrinthotomies if incomplete, these operations sacrifice the residual hearing. The operations can be performed under local anesthesia as preferred by the senior author or under a general anesthetic as preferred by the junior author.

*Oval Window Labyrinthotomy.* This operation is performed through the ear canal reflecting the tympanic membrane in the same manner as a stapedectomy. The incus and stapes are disarticulated, and both are extracted. The incus is placed in the bone bank. The contents of the vestibule are then removed with a suction tip. Schuknecht[48] advocates placing Gelfoam soaked in streptomycin into the vestibule to further ablate the neuroepithelium in the ampullae of the three semicircular canals (Fig. 21–14).

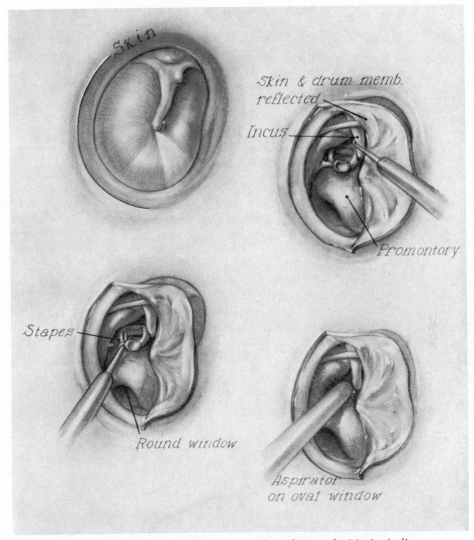

**Figure 21–14**  Schuknecht transtympanic labyrinthotomy for Meniere's disease.

*Horizontal Canal Labyrinthotomy.*   Described by Cawthorne,[49] this procedure requires either a mastoidectomy or atticotomy to expose the horizontal semicircular canal. Once this is accomplished, a fistula is created near its ampullated end, and a small right-angle hook is inserted into the horizontal and superior ampullae as well as the vestibule to remove the cristae and utricle. Bone chips are then placed into the fistula (Fig. 21–15).

*Translabyrinthine Labyrinthectomy.*   The junior author prefers the translabyrinthine labyrinthectomy to any of the previously mentioned operations because with this procedure all of the neuroepithelium of the vestibular labyrinth is systematically removed under direct vision. In any other type of procedure, the posterior ampulla is not opened and its neural elements destroyed. Streptomycin placed into the vestibule may or may not accomplish this. Therefore, anything less than a total labyrinthectomy will probably leave the patient with a functioning posterior semicircular canal ampulla. While this may not bother some individuals, it leaves others unsteady and with positional symptoms.

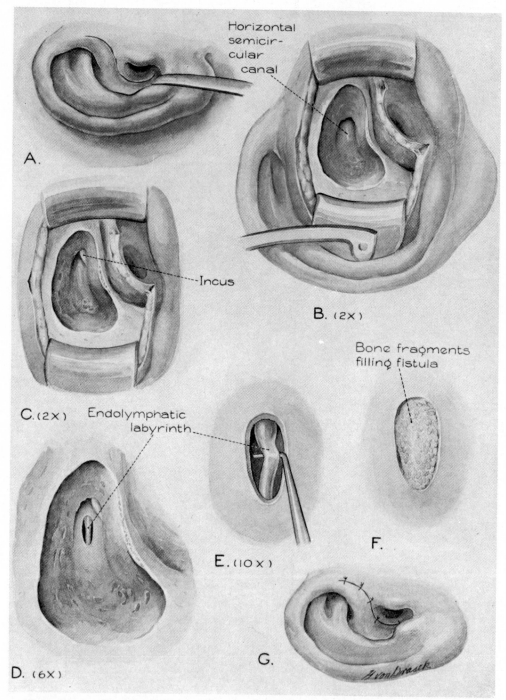

**Figure 21–15** Cawthorne's labyrinthotomy for Meniere's disease. *A,* Endaural incision. *B,* Attico-antrotomy. *C,* Exposure of the bony horizontal semicircular canal and edge of the incus. *D,* Fistulization of the canal under the operating microscope. *E,* Extraction of the endolymphatic horizontal semicircular canal. Insertion of the hook inferiorly extracts the utricle and saccule. *F,* Obliteration of the fistula with bone chips. *G,* Closure of the incision.

The technique of translabyrinthine labyrinthectomy requires that a simple mastoidectomy be performed. The incus is then removed and placed into the bone bank. The three semicircular canals are then drilled away exposing all three ampullae and the vestibule, as in the first step in translabyrinthine exposure of the internal auditory meatus (see Chapter 23). All neuroepithelium is removed and the incision closed.

*Translabyrinthine Cochlear and Vestibular Nerve Section.*    When severe tinnitus is a major complaint of the patient with endolymphatic hydrops and a labyrinthectomy is considered, section of the cochlear nerve may offer relief in some cases. Some individuals seem to have less unsteadiness following surgery if the vestibular nerve is sectioned medial to Scarpa's ganglion. This procedure also prevents the formation of small traumatic neuromas at the ends of the vestibular nerve following vestibular labyrinthectomy.

Translabyrinthine cochlear and vestibular nerve section is performed in the following manner. Once the mastoidectomy and labyrinthectomy have been performed as previously described, the bone is removed from the superior, posterior and inferior aspects of the internal auditory canal. Next, the lateral end of the superior vestibular nerve posteriorly is found (see Chapter 23). Once the facial nerve has been located, the superior and inferior vestibular nerves are lifted out and sectioned medial to Scarpa's ganglion. At this point, a right-angle hook is placed into the inferior anterior quadrant of the internal auditory canal and the cochlear nerve is pulled out and severed with a pair of scissors as it enters the internal auditory canal. The open canal is covered with temporalis fascia, and the mastoid cavity is filled with abdominal fat to prevent a cerebrospinal fluid leak.

### Conservative Procedures

Conservative procedures that attempt to preserve residual hearing include:

*Sacculotomy.*    According to histopathology slides of patients who had endolymphatic hydrops, the saccule is greatly distended and lies directly beneath the footplate of the stapes. This fact led Fick[50] to recommend puncturing the footplate with a sharp pointed needle in order to rupture the underlying saccule thus equalizing the pressure between the endolymphatic and perilymphatic systems.

Cody[51] carried Fick's idea further by designing a stainless steel tack that could be placed through the footplate of the stapes and left in place. Theoretically, each time the saccule enlarged as a result of the endolymphatic hydrops, it would automatically rupture itself on the sharp point of the tack, thereby equalizing the pressure between the two fluid systems.

Both of these procedures are performed through the ear canal and employ the stapes type flap.

*Ultrasound.*    The effect of ultrasound on the inner ear is not well understood. The first generators were large and bulky, and the amount of ultrasound radiation was not well calibrated. For this reason, there was an unacceptable incidence of facial nerve paralysis associated with the procedure.[52] The newer generators are much smaller and more readily calibrated and have markedly reduced the number of facial nerve injuries.

There are two methods by which the ultrasound probe can be applied to the inner ear. One way is to obtain a blue line on the horizontal canal[52] and place the probe on the canal until the nystagmus reverses. Obviously, the patient must be under local anesthesia to make this observation. Another method is to place the probe on the round window membrane through a stapes approach through the ear canal. Pennington[53] and Tabb[54] have used this procedure extensively in the United States, although the original work was performed by Arslan[52] in Europe.

*Cryosurgery.*    Similar to ultrasound, the effect of cryosurgery on the inner ear is not known. It can be applied to the horizontal canal as described by Wolfson[55] or at the round window niche in the manner of House.[56] This procedure has not gained general acceptance and is not widely used.

*Endolymphatic Sac Surgery.*    Of all the conservative operative procedures for the relief of Meniere's disease, those on the endolymphatic sac appear to be the most physiologic. The goal of sac surgery is to relieve the hydrops by decompressing the sac and draining it into the subarachnoid space[57] or mastoid cavity.[58, 59, 60]

The basic operative procedure consists of performing a simple mastoidectomy, identifying the middle and posterior fossa dural plates, the sinodural angle, the sigmoid sinus and the antrum (Fig. 21–16*A* and *B*). Next, the horizontal semicircular canal, digastric ridge and course of the facial nerve are found. It is best at this point to use a diamond burr and positively identify the facial nerve through thinned bone as it passes the horizontal canal; the nerve is followed but not exposed to the digastric ridge. It is important to make this identification because the endolymphatic sac lies below the facial nerve just medial to the retrofacial cell tract. In order to safely remove these cells, the facial nerve must be thoroughly visualized in its entire vertical portion.

The next step requires identifying the posterior semicircular canal. In a well pneumatized petrous apex, this is best accomplished by removing the cell tract superior to the canal with a cutting burr and tracing the canal around the facial nerve. In a sclerotic bone, it is much safer to find a blue line on the posterior canal, but with care not to fracture its wall.

When this has been accomplished, the bone overlying the posterior fossa dura between the sigmoid sinus and posterior semicircular canal is removed. The surgeon then traces an imaginary line through the center of the horizontal canal. The point where this line bisects the posterior canal corresponds to the upper edge of the sac. Once the sac has been identified in this matter, it is then decompressed as described by the senior author[18] (Fig. 21–16). Incision, freeing of intraluminal adhesions and insertion of a Silastic film extending into the mastoid complete the procedure.

(Both authors have had the experience of comparing the normal sacs of patients during translabyrinthine acoustic tumor removal to the atrophic and avascular ones of individuals undergoing surgery for Meniere's disease. The appearance of the endolymphatic sac in Meniere's patients suggests deficient resorptive function.)

Portmann's[12] initial procedure in 1926 was performed with a mallet and gouge, and the sac was simply incised for 2 to 3 mm. with a small knife. Modern day endolymphatic sac surgery had its beginning when William House[56] became interested in Portmann's early work. House began a series of dissections in the early 1960's, and subsequently he devised the surgical procedure previously described for identifying the sac. He felt it necessary to drain the endolymphatic system into the subarachnoid space in an attempt to equalize the system. House does this with a specially designed Silastic shunt tube that over the years has undergone numerous modifications (Fig. 21–17). Because the subarachnoid space is entered, there is the potential for a postoperative cerebrospinal fluid leak or other complication. To prevent this occurrence, temporalis muscle is sutured over the sac or abdominal fat is used to obliterate the mastoid.

House's first attempts at sac surgery drained the endolymph into the mastoid cavity. He later abandoned this procedure in favor of the subarachnoid shunt. Shea[58]

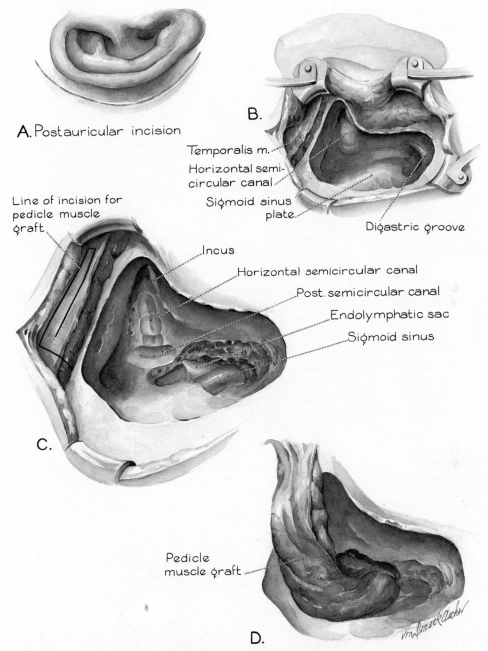

A. Postauricular incision

B.

Temporalis m.
Horizontal semi-
circular canal
Sigmoid sinus
plate

Digastric groove

Line of incision for
pedicle muscle
graft

Incus

Horizontal semicircular canal

Post. semicircular canal

Endolymphatic sac

Sigmoid sinus

C.

Pedicle
muscle graft

D.

**Figure 21–16**  Endolymphatic sac decompression. *A*, Postauricular incision. *B*, Mastoidectomy. *C*, Gray line of horizontal and posterior semicircular canals, exposed endolymphatic sac, sigmoid sinus and line of incision for pedicle temporal muscle graft. *D*, Muscle graft covering exposed sac and sigmoid sinus.

and later Paparella[59] favored the mastoid shunt. Recently Arenberg et al.[60] have developed a one-way valve that is placed into the endolymphatic sac with a limb of Silastic sheeting extending into the mastoid. Morrison's method is shown in Figure 21–18.[66] All forms of mastoid shunts require either Silastic, Teflon, or Gelfoam sheeting to create a fistula in the wall of the sac. Most surgeons cover the exposed sac with temporalis muscle or fascia.

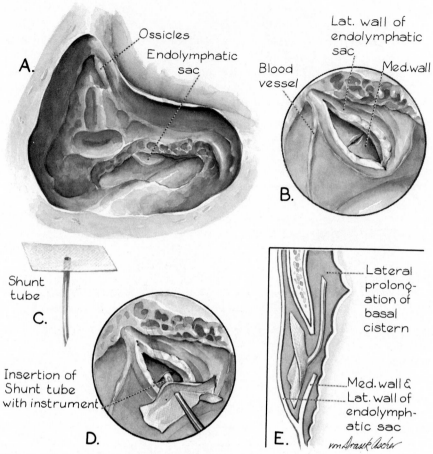

**Figure 21–17**   Endolymphatic-subarachnoid shunt. *A*, Gray line of horizontal and posterior semi-circular canals endolymphatic sac and sigmoid sinus exposed. *B*, Under microscope: Incision of sac outer and inner walls. *C*, Under microscope: shunt tube (W. House). *D*, Under microscope: shunt tube inserted. *E*, Diagram showing location of shunt tube.

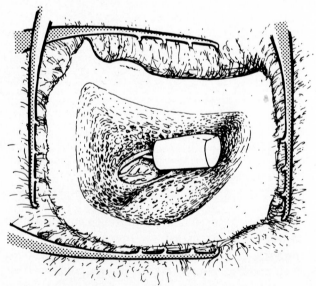

**Figure 21–18**   Capillary tube inserted into the lateral end of the endolymphatic duct with its distal tip inserted into Silastic sponge, technique of Andrew Morrison. (Right ear)

*Vestibular Nerve Section.* Section of the superior and inferior vestibular nerves is a conservative procedure because, in most cases, it preserves hearing; in one sense it could be considered a destructive operation in that it completely denervates the vestibular inner ear. Historically, there are two basic approaches that have been employed. Dandy[61] was the first surgeon to section the vestibular nerve for Meniere's disease, and this was done through a suboccipital exposure similar to the one used for the removal of acoustic tumors.

The primary disadvantage of this approach is the fact that it is extremely difficult to distinguish between the cochlear and vestibular divisions of the statoacoustic nerve in the posterior fossa. Another disadvantage is that there are definite, innate dangers in operating in the posterior fossa, due to the blood supply of the brainstem.

The most popular and most widely used approach to the vestibular nerve is through the middle fossa; it was first used by Clerc and Batisse.[62] The ingenuity of William House[63] has popularized this approach. He perfected this operative procedure in the early 1960's, but it is only in more recent years that it has gained wide acceptance. Fisch[64] and Glasscock[65] have each reported a series of Meniere's patients who have undergone this operation.

The approach is the same as that used for decompression of the facial nerve through the middle fossa, as described in Chapter 20. However, there are obviously some major differences once the internal auditory canal has been identified.

It should be assumed that the House-Urban self-retaining retractor is in place and the temporal lobe is elevated. The geniculate ganglion has been identified and a blue line obtained on the superior semicircular canal. A diamond burr with irrigation suction is used to follow the facial nerve into the internal auditory canal. The bone is carefully drilled away from the canal so that only the dura remains. It is important to carry the dissection to the most lateral extent of the internal auditory canal, separating the facial nerve anteriorly and the superior vestibular nerve posteriorly in order to identify "Bill's Bar." Next, a right-angle hook is placed into the posterior portion of the canal, and the dura is incised. The reason for this is to keep the hook away from the facial nerve. The dura is removed from the exposed canal so the surgeon can see the nerves lying side-by-side. At this point, the hook is placed into the superior vestibular nerve canal (using "Bill's Bar" as a landmark), and the nerve is lifted out (Fig. 21–19). It is held back with an 18-gauge suction, and the fibers of Rasmussen (olivocochlear bundle) that connect the superior vestibular and facial nerves are clipped. Continuing to hold the superior nerve out of the way, the surgeon reaches into the posterior inferior aspect of the internal auditory canal and lifts out the inferior vestibular nerve, taking care to avoid the internal auditory artery and cochlear nerve. Once both nerves have been lifted out, sharp scissors are used to sever them proximal to Scarpa's ganglion. The internal auditory canal is covered with a pledget of Gelfoam, followed by a plug of temporalis muscle. Craniotomy checks are performed in the routine manner, and the patient is kept in the recovery room until early evening.

## Postoperative Course

The postoperative course for endolymphatic sac procedures is usually benign. The hospital stay is from one to three days after surgery, depending upon whether the subarachnoid space was entered.

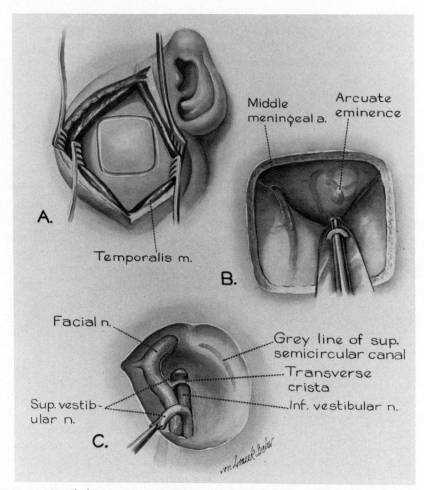

**Figure 21–19**  Vestibular nerve is avulsed with a right angle hook via the middle fossa approach.

Sacculotomy, ultrasound and cryosurgery patients are prone to have some degree of postoperative vertigo and may be bedridden for three or more days. Labyrinthectomy and vestibular nerve section patients usually have a stormy postoperative course and in most cases are confined to the hospital for at least one week. The first two to three days the individual is vertiginous and nauseated by head movement. Once these pass, the patient usually makes steady improvement on a daily basis. By the end of one week, the individual can walk well unassisted but requires at least three to four weeks to become completely steady. Older patients have greater difficulty adjusting to the loss of a labyrinth and may have some degree of unsteadiness for several months. It is important to explain all of these postoperative events to the patient prior to surgery. In fact, the junior author stresses to the patient that he may always experience some degree of unsteadiness when extremely tired or when he moves quickly. However, all of this depends upon the amount of residual function present in the vestibular system when it is ablated. Those individuals with nearly normal caloric responses are obviously going to have more trouble adjusting to the loss of their labyrinth than is a patient who already has a markedly reduced caloric response.

Cawthorne[8] described a series of head exercises designed to help the patient who has recently lost labyrinthine function as a result of some type of surgical procedure. The basic goal of the exercise is to fatigue the good (functioning) side so that the patient is more comfortable and can regain balance more readily.

### Cawthorne's Head Exercises

Exercises to be carried out for 15 minutes twice a day, increasing to 30 minutes.

| | |
|---|---|
| Eye Exercises: | Looking up, then down — at first slowly then quickly. 20 times. |
| | Looking from one side to other — at first slowly, then quickly. 20 times |
| | Focus on finger at arm's length, moving finger one foot closer and back again. 20 times. |

| | |
|---|---|
| Head Exercises: | Bend head forward then backward with eyes open — slowly, later quickly. 20 times. |
| | Turn head from one side to other side — slowly, then quickly. 20 times. |
| | As dizziness decreases, these exercises should be done with eyes closed. |

| | |
|---|---|
| Sitting: | While sitting, shrug shoulders. 20 times. |
| | Turn shoulders to right, then to left. 20 times. |
| | Bend forward and pick up objects from ground and sit up. 20 times. |

| | |
|---|---|
| Standing: | Change from sitting to standing and back again. 20 times with eyes open. Repeat with eyes closed. |
| | Throw a small rubber ball from hand to hand above eye level. |
| | Throw ball from hand to hand under one knee. |

| | |
|---|---|
| Moving About: | Walk across room with eyes open, then closed. 10 times. |
| | Walk up and down a slope with eyes open, then closed. 10 times. |
| | Walk up and down steps with eyes open, then closed. 10 times. |
| | Any game involving stooping or turning is good. |

The patient who has lost both labyrinths such as by streptomycin injection experiences some unique difficulties. These individuals will have frank ataxia for several months before a gradual improvement enables them to ambulate without difficulty. Their period of compensation is simply longer than with loss of one labyrinth, and they may never compensate completely.

One unusual symptom these patients often complain of is Dandy's syndrome. As the individual walks down a street, objects at a distance appear to "jiggle" up and down. While this is an annoying problem, most patients accommodate to it, as they do to their other problems.

### Risks and Complications of Surgery for Endolymphatic Hydrops

The risks and complications of vestibular surgery depend upon the procedure employed. All of the conservative operations are classified as such because an attempt is made to save the residual hearing; however, there is at least a 5 per cent chance for a "dead ear" with any of them. Facial nerve weakness has been reported following sac surgery, vestibular nerve section, ultrasound and cryosurgery. When the subarachnoid space is entered, as in the House shunt,[57] there is the potential for a cerebrospinal fluid leak. The same is true for middle and posterior fossa vestibular nerve section.

Any operative procedure may be complicated by a wound infection, and the potential for meningitis is always present when the cerebrospinal fluid space has been exposed.

The middle and posterior vestibular nerve sections have the added risk of neurosurgical complications such as extra- and intradural hemorrhage, hemiparesis and coma. However, these theoretical complications have not occurred in any of the reported series of middle fossa vestibular nerve sections.

## Results of Surgery for Endolymphatic Hydrops

The best and most consistent results, particularly regarding vertigo, have been with labyrinthectomies and vestibular nerve sections. The middle fossa nerve section has the advantage of producing complete denervation of the vestibular labyrinth without destroying the hearing in the majority of cases. Glasscock[65] and Fisch[64] have reported 94 per cent relief of vertigo, 70 per cent improvement in tinnitus and pressure and a preservation of the preoperative hearing level in 80 per cent. There is an incidence of from 4 to 5 per cent of dead ears.

It is the junior author's belief that middle fossa vestibular nerve section is the procedure of choice in the majority of patients with severe endolymphatic hydrops. The results are predictable and consistently good. There are drawbacks to the operation, as the potential risks are greater and a half-head neurological prep must be performed. Deciding whether to perform an endolymphatic shunt or vestibular nerve section depends upon whether the hearing is fluctuating widely, the stage of the disease and the preference of the patient. Some individuals are extremely frightened at the thought of a craniectomy with elevation of the temporal lobe.

Endolymphatic sac procedures have been reported to have success rates from 65 to 90 per cent[57, 59] for the relief of vertigo. The junior author has found that in the endolymphatic subarachnoid shunt the vertigo was relieved in 65 per cent, tinnitus and pressure 48 to 50 per cent, and hearing was stabilized in 65 per cent. These figures are comparable with the reports of others and with endolymphatic mastoid shunts.

Pennington[53] has reported 80 per cent relief of vertigo with ultrasound. Tinnitus and pressure were unchanged, and hearing stabilized in most cases.

Wolfson[55] and House[56] had similar results with cryosurgery in that vertigo was relieved in 70 per cent, tinnitus and pressure improved in 50 per cent and hearing stabilized in 70 per cent.

Fick[50] and Cody[51] have reported very similar results with sacculotomy, but others have failed to obtain such improvements.

The important fact to remember about surgery for Meniere's disease is that these procedures are reserved for patients who are refractory to medical therapy.

Vestibular surgery has come of age. It must no longer be ignored but rather should be made more available to the patient suffering from uncontrolled Meniere's disease. Certainly no patient should be denied the benefit of vestibular surgery unless his general health is poor. The junior author has seen a number of incapacitated individuals with nearly dead ears who simply were in need of a labyrinthectomy, yet their doctors continued to treat them medically even in the face of recurring and frequent attacks of violent vertigo. These patients are eternally grateful when someone finally takes an interest in them and performs a destructive labyrinthine procedure.

# REFERENCES

1. Meniere, M. P.: Maladies de l'oreille interne offrant les symptomes de la congestion cérébrale apoplectiforme. Gaz. Méd. Paris, 16:55, 88, 239, 279, 597, 1861.
2. Williams, H. L.: Meniere's Disease. Springfield, Ill., Charles C Thomas, 1952.
3. Shambaugh, G. E., and Knudson, V. O.: Report of an investigation of ten cases of diplacusis. Tr. Am. Otol. Soc., 16:397, 1923.
4. Crowe, S. J.: Ménière's disease. Medicine, 17:1, 1938.
5. Mygind, S. H., and Dederding, D.: The diagnosis and treatment of Meniere's disease. Ann. Otol. Rhin. & Laryng., 47:763, 1938.
6. Fowler, E. P.: Measuring sensation of loudness: a new approach to the physiology of hearing and functional and differential diagnostic tests. Arch. Otol., 26:514, 1937.
7. Dix, M. R., Hallpike, C. S., and Hood, J. D.: Observations upon loudness recruitment phenomenon. J. Laryng. & Otol., 62:671, 1948.
8. Cawthorne, T. E.: Meniere's disease. Ann. Otol. Rhin. & Laryng., 56:18, 1947.
9. Lindsay, J. R.: Labyrinthine dropsy. Laryngoscope, 56:325, 1946.
10. Jerger, J.: Hearing tests in audiologic diagnosis. A.S.H.A., 4:139, 1962.
11. Knapp, H.: A clinical analysis of the inflammatory affections of the inner ear. Arch. Ophthal., 2:204, 1871.
12. Portmann, G.: The saccus endolymphaticus and an operation for draining the same for the relief of vertigo. J. Laryng. & Otol., 42:809, 1927.
13. Hallpike, C. S., and Cairns, H.: Observations on the pathology of Meniere's syndrome. J. Laryng. & Otol., 53:625, 1938.
14. Parry, R. H.: A case of tinnitus and vertigo treated by division of the auditory nerve. J. Laryng. & Otol., 19:402, 1904.
15. Milligan, W.: Meniere's disease, a clinical and experimental inquiry. J. Laryng. & Otol., 19:440, 1904.
16. Lake, R.: Removal of the semicircular canals in a case of unilateral aural vertigo. Lancet, 1:567, 1904.
17. Altmann, F., and Kornfeld, M.: Histological studies of Meniere's disease. Ann. Otol. Rhin. & Laryng., 74:915, 1965.
18. Shambaugh, G. E., Jr.: Surgery of the endolymphatic sac. Arch. Otol., 83:302, 1966.
19. Wright, A. J.: Meniere's disease. Proc. Roy. Soc. Med., 41:801, 1948.
20. Duke, W. W.: Meniere's syndrome caused by an allergy. J.A.M.A., 81:2179, 1923.
21. Derlacki, E. L.: Non-surgical management of Meniere's disease. Laryngoscope, 64:271, 1954.
22. Shambaugh, G. E., Jr.: Endocrine aspects of Meniere's disease. Laryngoscope, 69:1027, 1959.
23. Lermoyez, M.: Le vertige qui fait entendre. (Angiospasme labyrinthique). Ann. mal. oreille, larynx, 48:575, 1929.
24. Shambaugh, G. E., Jr.: Surgery on the endolymphatic sac. Arch. Otol., 83:305, 1966.
25. Nager, F. R.: Personal communication, 1965.
26. Anson, B., Donaldson, J. A., Warpeha, R. L., and Winch, T. R.: Surgical anatomy of the endolymphatic sac and perilymphatic duct. Laryngoscope, 74:480, 1964.
27. Kirikae, I., et al.: A consideration of the circulation of the perilymph. Ann. Otol. Rhin & Laryng., 70:337, 1961.
28. Engström, H.: The cortilymph, the third lymph of the inner ear. Acta Morphol. Neerl. Scandinav., 3:195, 1960.
29. Shambaugh, G. E.: On the structure and function of the epithelium in the sulcus spiralis externus. Arch. of Otology, 37:538, 1908.
30. Guild, S. R.: The circulation of the endolymph. Am. J. Anat., 39:57, 1927.
31. Lundquist, P.: The endolymphatic duct and sac in the guinea pig. Acta oto-laryng., Suppl. 201, 1965.
32. Bast, T. H., and Anson, B. T.: The Temporal Bone and the Ear. Springfield, Ill., Charles C Thomas, 1949.
33. Kimura, R. S., and Schuknecht, H. F.: Membranous hydrops in the inner ear of the guinea pig after obliteration of the endolymphatic sac. Pract. oto-rhino-laryng., 27:343, 1965.

34. Valvassori, G.: Personal communication, 1967.
35. Konishi, T., Hamrick, P. E., and Walsh, P. J.: Ion transport in guinea pig cochlea. I. Potassium and sodium transport. Acta Otolaryng., 86:22, 1978.
36. Konishi, T., and Hamrick, P. E.: Ion transport in the cochlea of guinea pig. II. Chloride transport. Acta Otolaryng., 86:176, 1978.
37. Maren, T. H.: Personal communication, 1979.
38. Shambaugh, G. E., Jr.: Diplacusis: a localizing symptom of disease of the organ of Corti. Arch. Otol., 31:160, 1940.
39. Shambaugh, G. E., Jr.: Histamine in treatment of certain types of headache and vertigo following the fenestration operation. Arch. Otol., 51:781, 1950.
40. Hilger, J. A.: Otolaryngologic aspects of hypometabolism. Ann. Otol. Rhin. & Laryng., 65:395, 1956.
41. Cawthorne, T. E.: Positional nystagmus. Ann. Otol. Rhin. & Laryng., 63:481, 1954.
42. Hallberg, G. E.: Sudden deafness of obscure origin. Laryngoscope, 66:1237, 1956.
43. Rubin, W., and Anderson, J. R.: The management of circulatory disturbances of the inner ear. Angiology, 9:256, 1958.
44. Furstenberg, A. C., Lashmet, F. H., and Talbot, F.: Meniere's symptom complex: medical treatment. Ann. Otol. Rhin. & Laryng., 43:1035, 1954.
45. McCabe, B. F., and Bernstein, P.: The effect of Diazepam on vestibular compensation. Laryngoscope 84:267, 1974.
46. Bryan, W. T. K., and Bryan, M. P.: The application of in vitro cytotoxic reactions to clinical diagnosis of food allergy. Laryngoscope, 70:810, 1960.
47. Fowler, E. P., Jr.: Streptomycin treatment of vertigo. Tr. Am. Acad. Ophth., 52:239, 1948.
48. Schuknecht, H. F.: Ablation therapy in Meniere's disease. Acta oto-laryng., Suppl. 132, 1957.
49. Cawthorne, T. E.: Personal communication.
50. Fick, I. A.: Decompression of the labyrinth. Arch. Otol., 79:447, 1964.
51. Cody, D. T. R.: The tack operation for endolymphatic hydrops. Laryngoscope, 79:1737, 1969.
52. Arslan, M.: Direkt Applikation des Ultrashalls auf das knöcherne Labyrinth zur Therapieder Labyrinthose (Morbus Meniere). H. N. Ohrenh., 4:166, 1954.
53. Pennington, C. L., and Stevens, E. L.: Ultrasonic ablation of the labyrinth in the treatment of endolymphatic hypertension (Meniere's disease). South. Med. J., 60:34, 1969.
54. Tabb, H. G., Norris, C. H., and Hagan, W. E.: Round window ultrasonic irradiation for Meniere's disease with ENG monitoring. Laryngoscope, 88:1460, 1978.
55. Wolfson, R. J., Cutt, R. A., Ishiyama, E., and Myers, D.: Cryosurgery for Meniere's disease. Laryngoscope, 78:632, 1968.
56. House, W. F.: Cryosurgical treatment of Meniere's disease. Arch. Otol., 84:616, 1966.
57. House, W. F.: Subarachnoid shunt for drainage of endolymphatic hydrops. Laryngoscope, 72:713, 1962.
58. Shea, J. J.: Teflon film drainage of the endolymphatic sac. Arch. Otol., 83:316, 1966.
59. Paparella, M. M., and Hanson, D. G.: Endolymphatic shunt for drainage for intractable vertigo (method and experiences). Laryngology, 85:697, 1978.
60. Arenberg, I. K., Rask-Andersen, H., Wilbrand, H., and Stahle, J.: The surgical anatomy of the endolymphatic sac. Arch. Otol., 103:1, 1977.
61. Dandy, W. E.: The surgical treatment of Meniere's disease. Surg. Gynec. & Obst., 72:421, 1941.
62. Clerc, P., and Batisse, R.: Access to the intrapetrous structures from the intracranial aspect. Ann. oto-laryng., 7:20, 1954.
63. House, W. F.: Surgical exposure of the internal auditory canal and its contents through the middle cranial fossa. Laryngoscope, 71:1363, 1961.
64. Fisch, U.: Vestibular and cochlear neurectomy. Trans. Am. Acad. Ophthalmol. and Otolaryngol., 78:252, 1974.
65. Glasscock, M. E., and Miller, G. W.: Middle fossa vestibular nerve section in the management of Ménière's disease. Laryngoscope, 87:529, 1977.
66. Morrison, A. W.: Surgical drainage for hydrops. Sixth Shambaugh-Shea Workshop. In Press.

## SUGGESTED ADDITIONAL READING

Talbott, J. H., and Brown, M. R.: Meniere's syndrome: acid-base constituents of the blood: treatment with potassium chloride. J.A.M.A., 114:1035, 1954.
Williams, H. L., Horton, B. T., and Day, L. A.: Endolymphatic hydrops without vertigo: its differential diagnosis and treatment. Tr. Am. Otol. Soc., 35:116, 1947.
Jongkees, L. B. W.: Medical treatment of Meniere's disease. Acta oto-laryng., Suppl. 192, 1964.
Peacock, R.: Alcoholic labyrinthine injection through the oval window in the treatment of aural vertigo. Lancet, 1:421, 1938.

Wright, A. J.: Labyrinthine destruction in the treatment of vertigo by the injection of alcohol through the oval window. J. Laryng. & Otol., 53:594, 1938.

Day, K. M.: Labyrinth surgery for Meniere's disease. Laryngoscope, 53:617, 1953.

Mogan, R. F., and Baumgartner, C. J.: Meniere's disease complicated by recurrent interstitial keratitis; excellent result following cervical ganglionectomy; report of a case. West. J. Surg., 42:628, 1934.

Passe, E. R. G.: Surgery of the sympathetic for Meniere's disease, tinnitus and nerve deafness. Arch. Otolaryng., 57:257, 1953.

Strong, M. S.: Dorsal sympathectomy in labyrinthine disease. Arch. Otol., 65:342, 1957.

## Stacey Rufus Guild

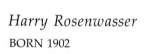

BORN 1890
DIED 1966

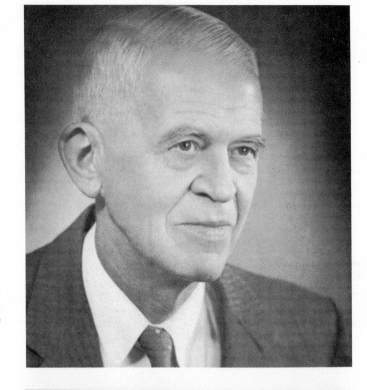

Discovered the glomus jugularis, source of the most common neoplasm of the middle
ear.

## Harry Rosenwasser

BORN 1902

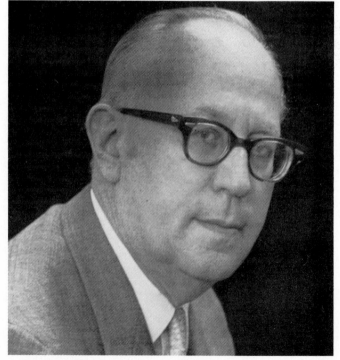

First described a vascular
tumor of the middle ear as
arising from the glomus jugularis.

Chapter 22

# Surgery of Tumors of the Ear

VARIETIES OF CYSTS AND TUMORS OF THE EAR AND
  TEMPORAL BONE
FIBROUS DYSPLASIA
HISTIOCYTOSIS
CARCINOMA OF THE OUTER AND MIDDLE EAR
    BASAL CELL CARCINOMA OF THE AURICLE
    SQUAMOUS CELL CARCINOMA OF THE MEATUS
      AND MIDDLE EAR
GLOMUS TUMORS OF THE MIDDLE EAR AND SKULL
  BASE
    HISTORICAL ASPECTS
    THE GLOMUS BODY OF GUILD
    PATHOLOGY OF GLOMUS TUMORS
    CLASSIFICATION OF GLOMUS TUMORS
    DIAGNOSIS
    TREATMENT
    COMPLICATIONS
    RESULTS

## VARIETIES OF CYSTS AND TUMORS OF THE EAR AND TEMPORAL BONE

For each of the three divisions of the organ of hearing, a particular neoplasm of serious import is characteristic. For the nerve of hearing, *acoustic neurinoma* is a fairly frequent tumor that begins most often within the internal acoustic meatus, producing at first tinnitus and sensorineural hearing loss. Only later does it protrude intracranially, producing Cushing's cerebellopontine angle syndrome. The early diagnosis and surgical removal of this tumor is considered in Chapter 23.

The labyrinth itself is not the site of primary neoplasia, and it is remarkably resistant to tumor invasion from without. This is because tumors spread through bone in vascular channels and the labyrinth is encased in its avascular endosteal bony capsule surrounded by the sparsely vascular endochondral capsule. Thus the entire petrous pyramid may be invaded and replaced by meningioma save for the labyrinth surrounded by a thin bony capsule.[1] Invasion of the labyrinth generally occurs only in metastatic carcinoma or brain tumor from the internal acoustic meatus via the cribriform areas, through which the eighth nerve fibers reach the labyrinth.[2]

**595**

In the middle ear, **glomus jugulare** tumors are the most frequent neoplasms. They present special surgical problems because of their extraordinary vascularity and bone-invading property.

For the external auditory meatus and middle ear, **squamous cell carcinoma,** though rare, is noteworthy because of the very poor prognosis unless it is discovered quite early and removed by wide-block excision.

Before discussing in greater detail these important tumors of the outer and middle ear, we should mention the wide variety of cysts and benign and malignant tumors that may occur in and around the ear and temporal bone, reflecting the complicated embryonic origin and resultant diversity of tissues found in this area. Noteworthy are branchial cysts and fistulas found in front of and sometimes beneath the auricle, as shown in Figures 14–2 and 14–5. Congenital epidermal rests occurring in the temporal bone produce the interesting congenital cholesteatomas, which are not the result of antecedent suppuration or attic retraction. These were considered in Chapter 7.

Sebaceous cysts are frequent in the outer ear, especially behind the lobule or in the floor of the external auditory meatus. Equally common, especially in swimmers, are exostoses of the inner end of the bony external auditory meatus. Among Negroes and persons with deeply pigmented skin keloid formations tend to follow surgical incisions or piercing for earrings. These common benign tumors were considered in Chapter 8. Metastatic malignant tumors sometimes occur in the temporal bone. Benign or malignant neoplasms of fat, cartilage, bone, connective tissue, smooth or striated muscle, blood vessels, lymphatics, nerves, ceruminous glands and salivary glands all may be found, though uncommonly, in and around the outer ear.

A tumor-like enlargement of the mastoid bone may be the result of histiocytosis (Hand-Schüller-Christian disease) or of fibrous dysplasia of bone; both of these are rare non-neoplastic diseases of bone of unknown etiology.


## FIBROUS DYSPLASIA

Fibrous dysplasia may involve a single bone (monostotic fibrous dysplasia) or, less often, several bones (polyostotic fibrous dysplasia).[3] When it occurs in the mastoid, a painless asymmetric swelling of the bone is noted, and conductive hearing loss due to bony occlusion of the external auditory meatus is the only complaint. Atypical radiographic loss of cellular structure and increased radiolucency due to replacement of osseous substance by fibrous tissue may give a clue to the diagnosis. As a rule the correct diagnosis is made only when the surgeon encounters a cyst-like mass of gritty fibrous tissue beneath a normal-appearing but thinned cortex and submits a specimen for pathologic study. This reveals a mass of fibrous tissue interspersed with sparse irregular bony spicules (Fig. 22–1).

The **treatment** of fibrous dysplasia is removal of sufficient diseased bone to re-establish a patent external auditory meatus. If there is insufficient meatal skin, split or full thickness skin grafts from behind the ear should be applied to the walls of the enlarged meatus. Since this is usually a disease of childhood, tending to become quiescent after puberty, there is probably no need to try to remove the entire lesion, as would be necessary for a true neoplasm.[4]


## HISTIOCYTOSIS

Histiocytosis, like fibrous dysplasia, is a disease of bone of unknown etiology occurring during childhood. It is characterized by replacement of normal osseous

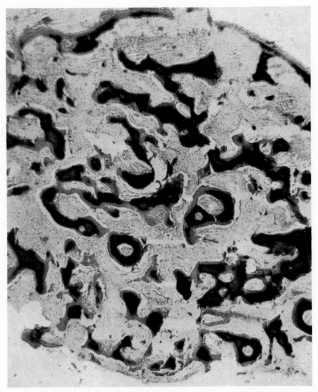

**Figure 22–1**   Fibrous dysplasia of mastoid. (Courtesy of Dr. Charles Vaughan.)

substance by tumor-like masses of foam-like reticuloendothelial cells containing lipoid droplets, with many eosinophiles and increased connective tissue. The bones of the skull are most often affected. When the bony enlargement produces exophthalmos and diabetes insipidus, the condition is known as the Hand-Schüller-Christian syndrome. Xanthomatosis, lipoid granulomatosis and eosinophilic granuloma are other names for this disease. Involvement of the temporal bone causes aural suppuration and granulations in the external auditory meatus in about half of all cases of histiocytosis. The diagnosis is made by pathologic study of granulations from the external meatus or tissue removed from the mastoid.

The **treatment** of histiocytosis is irradiation of the affected bone areas, with frequent checkup of the skeletal system by x-ray to detect any additional lesions. Some cases, after temporary radiation-induced remissions, proceed to a fatal outcome; when the temporal bone alone is involved, the prognosis is more favorable, and long-lasting remission may follow irradiation.[5]

## CARCINOMA OF THE OUTER AND MIDDLE EAR

### Basal Cell Carcinoma of the Auricle

Basal cell carcinoma of the auricle accounts for 5 to 8 per cent of all skin cancers, and occurs nearly always in males of advanced years who have been exposed to excessive sun. Blonde persons are more susceptible and Negroes are

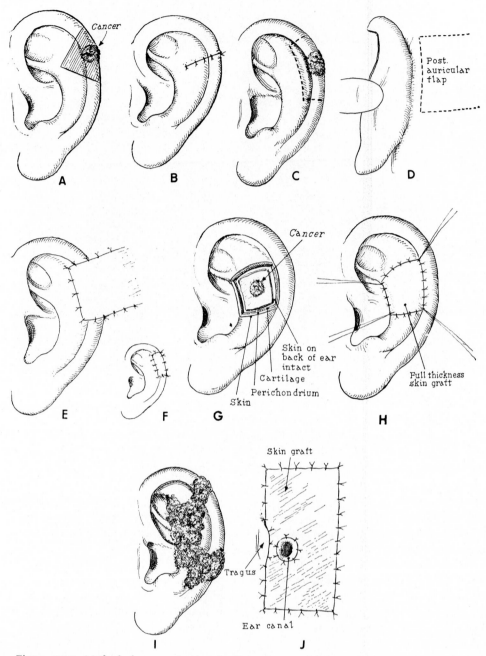

**Figure 22–2**   Methods for removing basal cell carcinoma of the auricle. *A* and *B*, Resection and approximation of wound. *C, D, E* and *F,* Resection and repair by postauricular pedicle released in 3 weeks. *G* and *H,* Excision of small cancer of prehelix, and repair by full thickness postauricular skin graft. *I* and *J,* Extensive carcinoma requiring excision of auricle and skin graft wound. (From Conley, J. J., and Novack, A. J.: The surgical removal of malignant tumors of the ear and temporal bone. Arch. Otol., 71:635, 1960.)

almost never afflicted, eloquent testimony of the protective effect of skin pigmentation against the harmful effects of actinic rays.[6]

The lesion begins in 50 per cent of cases on the most exposed upper edge of the helix as a small, painless, circumscribed, chronic ulcer, covered by a crust and with a slightly indurated and elevated border, which increases slowly in size. The correct diagnosis should be self-evident but may need to be confirmed by histologic examination. In the case of a small early ulceration, rather than cutting into it first for a biopsy, the surgeon should use a V-incision to remove the lesion with a zone of normal tissue and then examine it histologically.[7] Figure 22–2 shows various methods for removing such a lesion from the auricle.

An alternative piecemeal method of removing basal cell carcinoma of the auricle has been described by Mohs.[8] A special cauterizing solution is applied to the visible lesion, followed by excision and microscopic examination of the cauterized tissue. Wherever tumor tissue is found the cautery is repeated until a final layer of microscopically tumor-free tissue has been removed. Although in experienced hands this method results in 90 per cent cures, simple surgical excision at one time is the better method for most surgeons, with care to include an adequate zone of normal tissue. In the difficult case that recurs after surgical excision, referral to a physician experienced in chemosurgical removal should be considered.

## Squamous Cell Carcinoma of the Meatus and Middle Ear

Squamous cell carcinoma of the ear originates most often in the external auditory meatus, extending thence into the middle ear and mastoid, but the initial site of origin is difficult to determine in advanced cases.

A unique variety of epidermoid carcinoma **primary in the mastoid** occurs in radium-dial painters. The deposition of radium in bone results in a cumulative radiation effect on epithelium wherever it lies closely applied to bone, such as in the mastoid air cells. A similar mechanism may produce primary carcinoma of the mastoid in patients who received radium water or radium-containing salts three or four decades ago.[9]

The **earliest symptom** of carcinoma of the ear is bleeding or a **blood-tinged discharge. Pain** is the next symptom in point of time and frequency of occurrence, and **facial paralysis,** though not an early symptom, is highly suggestive of carcinoma. For the reasons noted before, the labyrinth is involved seldom and late in carcinoma of the ear.

The **diagnosis** of carcinoma of the ear requires histologic examination of tissue removed from the lesion. Because the prognosis is poor even in cases diagnosed reasonably early and subjected to radical excision, it is essential that the otologist possess a **high index of suspicion** and submit for **histologic examination every polyp or bit of granulation tissue** removed from the ear. Carelessly discarded tissue from the meatus or middle ear has cost many a life because of delayed diagnosis in carcinoma of the ear![7]

Primary carcinoma of the mastoid has an even poorer prognosis than that beginning in the outer meatus or middle ear, for there may be **no symptoms** until the tumor is so widespread that it is inoperable. For this reason radium-dial painters and others who received radium water or salts in the past should have **regular routine repeat mastoid x-ray examination,** with prompt surgical exploration of the mastoid if it begins to develop areas of bone destruction.[9] Except for these cases, x-ray is of little help in the early diagnosis of carcinoma of the ear. The demonstration of cancer cells in aural discharge by the Papanicolaou technique has been useful in establishing the early diagnosis in a few cases.[10]

The **treatment** of squamous cell carcinoma of the outer and middle ear is **surgical excision.** Irradiation by itself is not successful because of finger-like projections deep into bone along vascular channels, and for the same reason surgical removal must be far more radical than may seem necessary when the patient is first seen. Just as with cancer elsewhere, the patient's best and almost only hope of survival lies in a well planned and well executed **first operation.**

In the rare case of very early carcinoma confined to the **cartilaginous portion of the external auditory meatus,** a sleeve excision of the soft and cartilaginous tissues of the canal with a wide zone of normal tissue may suffice, as shown in Figure 22–3A. A primary split thickness skin graft is applied and held in place by a surgical rayon sleeve filled with cotton balls soaked in Gantrisin otic solution.

In early carcinoma of the skin of the **osseous meatus** it is necessary to excise the entire bony meatus and tympanic membrane in continuity (Fig. 22–3B). The outer meatal opening is widely outlined, as shown in Figure 22–4A and B, and incised to bone. A postauricular radical mastoidectomy is then performed, with exposure of the attic and removal of the malleus head and incus (Fig. 22–4 C). The fallopian canal is opened, exposing the facial nerve from the geniculate ganglion to the stylomastoid foramen (Fig. 22–4 D). With a small burr a new groove is made for the facial nerve from the horizontal semicircular canal to the digastric groove deep to the fallopian canal. The facial nerve, freed by blunt-scissor dissection well into the parotid gland to give it added length, is lifted from the fallopian canal and reset into the new deeper groove. With a fine cutting burr a series of perforations are made from the evacuated fallopian canal in a forward direction into the tympanic cavity,

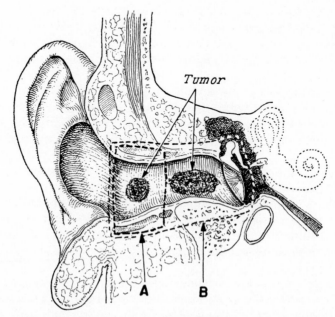

**Figure 22–3** Methods for removing squamous cell carcinoma of the external auditory meatus. *A,* Sleeve excision of skin and cartilaginous canal for small cancer of the outer meatus. *B,* Block excision of entire meatus and tympanic membrane for cancer of osseous meatus. (From Conley, J. J., and Novack, A. J.: The surgical removal of malignant tumors of the ear and temporal bone. Arch. Otol., 71:635, 1960.)

as shown in Figure 22–4 E. The roof of the temporomandibular fossa and the floor of the osseous meatus are then grooved deeply with a burr. A thin straight chisel is applied to the grooves, and with a few strokes of a mallet the residual bony attachment is fractured. The freed specimen includes the bony external auditory meatus with the sulcus tympanicus and tympanic membrane at the inner end (Fig. 22–4 G). The eustachian tube and middle ear are closed off with a full thickness graft from behind the ear, and the remainder of the cavity is dressed with a split thickness skin graft.[7]

When carcinoma of the external meatus involves the parotid gland, or a primary parotid carcinoma has become fixed to the mastoid tip or external auditory meatus,[11] a preliminary dissection of the anterior and posterior triangles of the neck is carried out as in Figure 22–5. The tissue dissection from the neck includes the sternocleidomastoid muscle still attached to the mastoid tip, the internal jugular vein still attached to the jugular bulb, the digastric muscle and glands from the neck. The curved vertical skin incision for the neck dissection is now continued upward postaurally and curved forward over the top of the auricle. The outer meatal opening is widely outlined as in Figure 22–4A, the meatal skin and tympanic membrane are lifted out like a sleeve and a postauricular mastoidectomy is performed, exposing the sigmoid sinus plate and digastric ridge (Fig. 22–5). The fallopian canal is opened from the posterior pyramidal bend at the horizontal semicircular canal to the stylomastoid foramen. Since the parotid gland is involved, the facial nerve cannot be preserved and is divided below the pyramidal segment. With straight chisels the mastoid tip and floor of the bony external auditory meatus are divided as indicated by the dotted lines in Figure 22–5. The mastoid tip is pushed downward, fracturing the bone through the hypotympanum (Fig. 22–5). This exposes the posterior aspect of the mandibular fossa and the deep lobe of the parotid gland. This gland is dissected from the masseter muscle, or the muscle may be removed. If necessary, the mandibular ramus can be disarticulated and removed. Branches of the facial nerve are identified and marked by 6–0 black silk ligatures and then divided, completing the freeing of the block dissection. A nerve graft taken from the cervical plexus is sutured to the stump of the vertical segment of the facial nerve and to the peripheral branches (Fig. 22–5). A pedicle temporal muscle flap may be turned down to fill the mastoid bowl and cover the nerve graft. The ear canal and tympanic membrane are replaced, and the wound is closed.

When extensive carcinoma involves the middle ear and mastoid, the only possibility of cure is by subtotal excision en masse of the temporal bone, including if necessary a portion of dura, sigmoid sinus, parotid gland and mandible, with no attempt to preserve the facial nerve, which generally is already involved. Any less radical piecemeal removal in the hope of sparing the facial nerve and labyrinth is doomed to failure.

The auricle, if it is not involved, is freed from the external auditory meatus and elevated upward with a flap of skin from the temporal region, as shown in Figure 22–6A and B. The deep vessels and nerves of the neck are exposed by transection of the zygoma and ascending ramus of the mandible, and most of the parotid gland, masseter muscle, posterior belly of the digastric, stylohyoid, external and internal pterygoid muscles and sternocleidomastoid muscle are removed (Fig. 22–7 A). The external carotid artery is ligated and sectioned close to the common carotid bifurcation, and the internal carotid, internal jugular vein, sympathetic chain and ninth, tenth, eleventh and twelfth cranial nerves are all exposed and followed to the base of the skull. The petrous bone is fractured by chisels and by a rocking maneuver

*Text continued on page 612.*

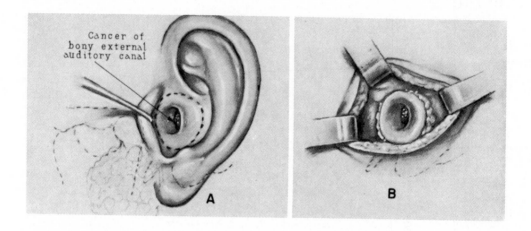

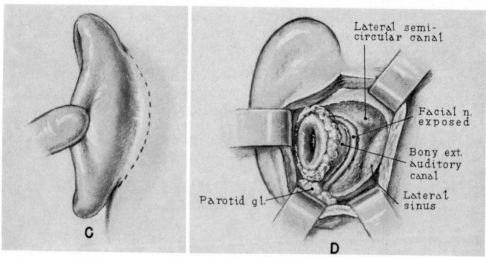

**Figure 22–4** Block excision of entire bony meatus and tympanic membrane for carcinoma of external auditory meatus. *A*, Wide meatal skin incision. *B*, Exposure of bone on all sides of the meatus. *C*, Postaural incision for simple mastoidectomy. *D*, Exposure of the facial nerve. (Continued on the opposite page.)

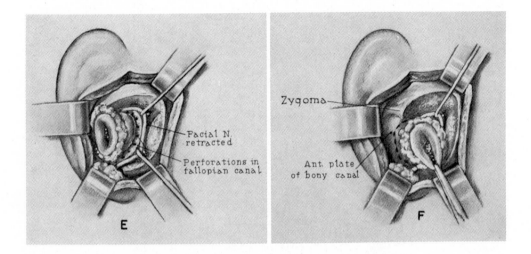

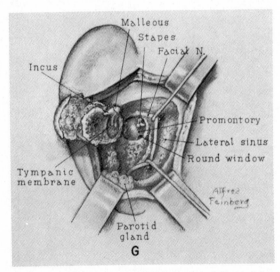

**Figure 22–4** (*Continued*)   E, Roof of the mandibular fossa and floor of the osseous meatus grooved deeply with burr. F, Dotted line indicates the site of fracture by chisel. G, Specimen freed by straight chisel. (From Conley, J. J., and Novack, A. J.: The surgical removal of malignant tumors of the ear and temporal bone. Arch. Otol., 71:635, 1960.)

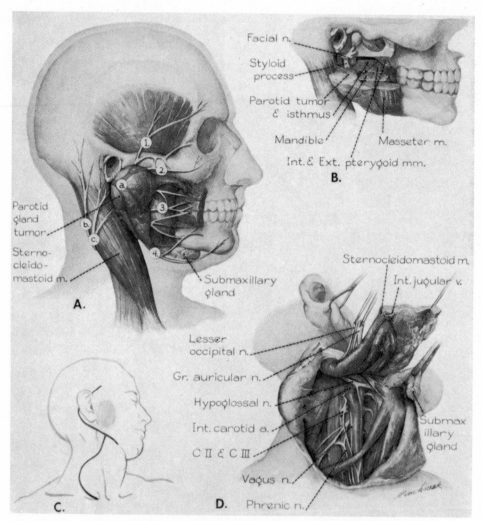

**Figure 22–5**  Method for removing carcinoma involving external meatus and parotid gland. *A*, Outer aspect of parotid tumor, anatomic relationships. *a*, Facial nerve. *1*, Temporal branch. *2*, Zygomatic branch. *3*, Buccal branch. *4*, Mandibular branch. *b*, Lesser occipital nerve. *c*, Greater auricular nerve. *B*, Inner portion of parotid tumor, anatomic aspects. *C*, Skin incision. *D*, Radical neck dissection up to the tumor (From Allen, G. W.: Total parotidectomy—technique in surgical removal of advanced cases. Laryngoscope, 74:1060, 1964.) (Continued on the opposite page.)

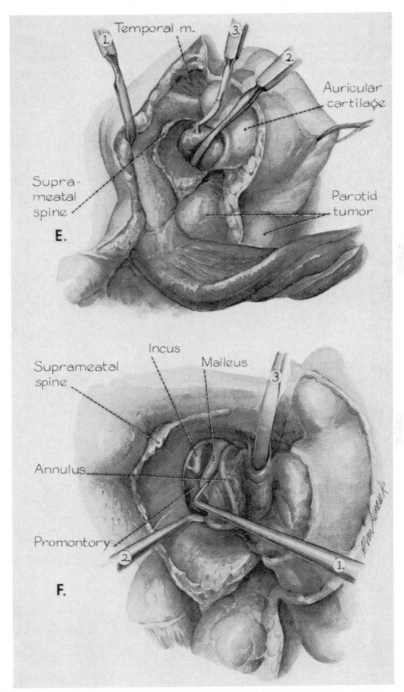

**Figure 22–5** *(Continued)* *E*, Removal of meatal skin. *F*, Removal of tympanic membrane from malleus. (Continued on page 606.)

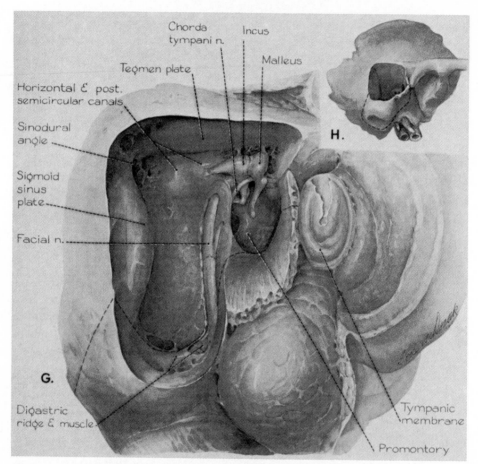

**Figure 22–5** (Continued)   G, Line of application of chisel to divide mastoid tip and floor of meatus.
*H,* Seen from below. (Continued on the opposite page.)

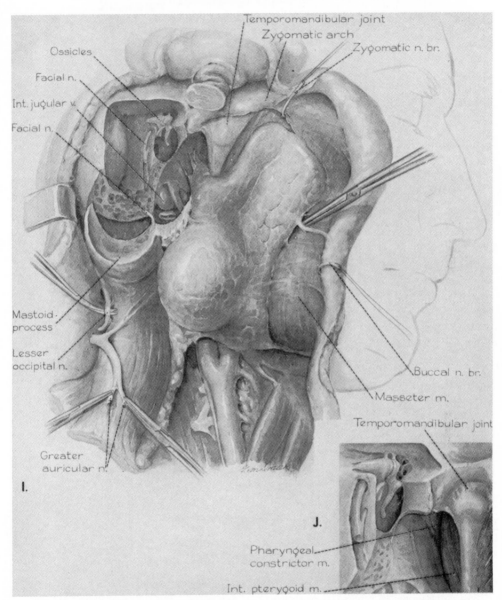

**Figure 22–5** *(Continued)*   *I*, Removal of tumor from retromandibular space. Branches of facial nerve identified and marked by 6–0 black silk sutures. *J*, Exposure of infratemporal fossa by tumor removal. (Continued on page 608.)

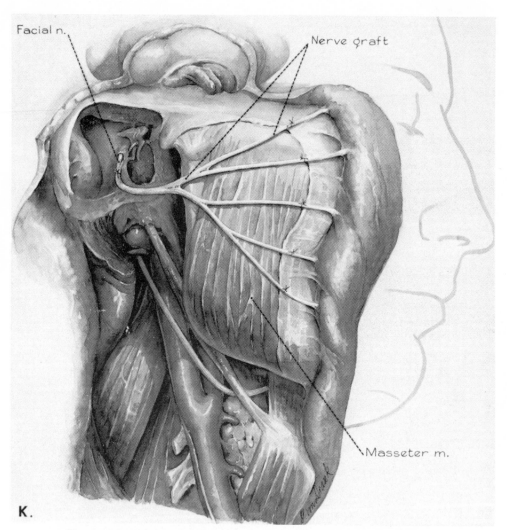

**Figure 22–5** (Continued)   K, Facial nerve continuity restored by nerve graft.

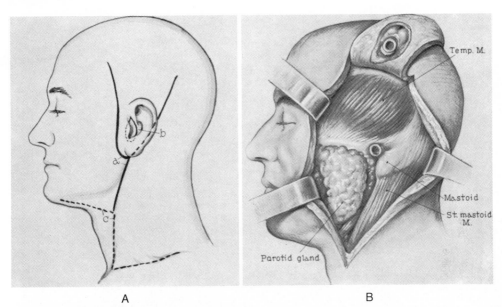

A           B

'**Figure 22–6** Method for block excision of temporal bone for carcinoma of the middle ear and mastoid. *A,* Skin incisions. *a,* Temporal skin flap. *b,* Meatal incision. *c,* Extension of skin incisions when radical neck dissection is indicated. *B,* Elevation of temporal skin flap and retraction of tissues. (Continued in Figure 22–7.) (Figures 22–6 and 22–7 from Conley, J. J., and Novack, A. J.: The surgical removal of malignant tumors of the ear and temporal bone. Arch. Otol., *71*:635, 1960.)

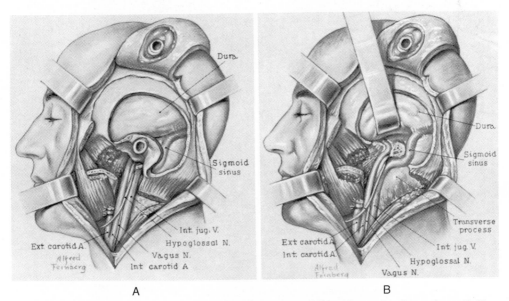

A           B

**Figure 22–7** *A,* Exposure of deep vessels and nerves, middle and posterior fossae durae. *B,* Temporal bone removed, leaving the petrous apex. (Continued from Figure 22–6.)

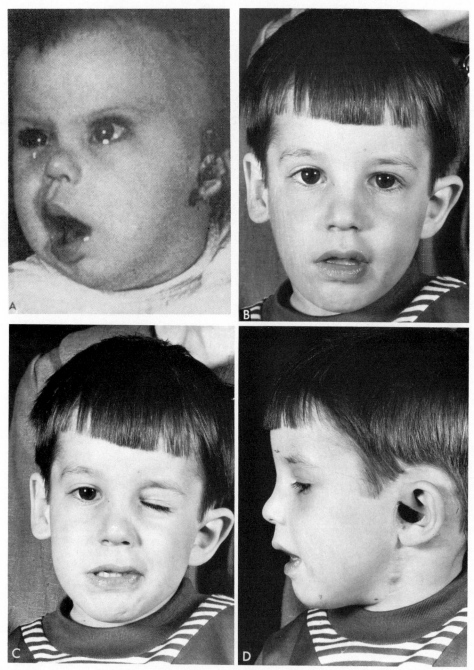

**Figure 22–8** *A,* Rapidly growing fungating malignant glomus tumor involving external ear with complete facial paralysis, child of 16 months. *B,* Result 2½ years after radical excision with immediate repair of the facial nerve by hypoglossal anastomosis; patient in repose. *C,* Voluntary contraction of face. *D,* Appearance of healed external ear. (Courtesy of Dr. John J. Conley.)

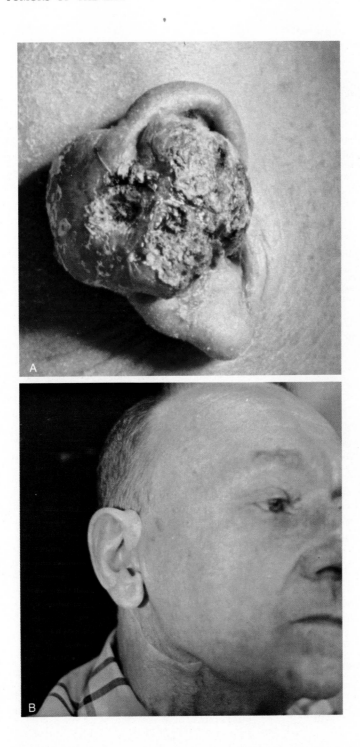

**Figure 22–9**  *A*, Fungating carcinoma of the auricle. *B*, Prosthetic ear after excision of entire auricle except for the tragus. (Courtesy of Dr. Robert Norman and Dr. Tawfic Girgis.)

just lateral to the internal carotid canal, and is removed after it is carefully separated from the carotid artery, the sigmoid sinus and jugular bulb and the inferior and superior petrosal sinuses. Any tears and bleeding from these structures is controlled by packing, transfixion and coagulation, with at least 3000 cc. of blood on hand for replacement transfusion. This final part of the operation is facilitated if spinal fluid from the lumbar spine is withdrawn through a previously implanted plastic catheter, allowing the temporal lobe and cerebellum beneath the middle and posterior fossae durae to be retracted. Spinal fluid leak from the internal acoustic meatus or any dural tear or defect is closed by a pedicle or free temporal muscle graft. The entire cavity, reduced by the muscle graft, is dressed with a split thickness skin graft. The skin flaps are repositioned and sutured.

**Results** of surgical removal of carcinoma of the middle ear and mastoid have been exceedingly poor except when radical block excision of the temporal bone was done. With this method Lewis[6] reports 13 cases with 4 successes but only one followed for more than 5 years. Conley and Novack[7] report 14 cases with 4 successes, 2 free from disease after 5 years, 2 followed for less than 5 years (Figs. 22–8 and 22–9).

## GLOMUS TUMORS OF THE MIDDLE EAR AND SKULL BASE

### Historical Aspects

Primary vascular tumors of the middle ear diagnosed as hemangio-endotheliomas or angio-endotheliomas began to be reported as early as 1906.[12] In 1941 Guild[13] discovered a tiny structure in the adventitia of the jugular bulb that he named the "glomus jugularis." In 1945 Rosenwasser[14] reported a primary vascular tumor, arising in the hypotympanum, that resembled in its histologic structure the carotid body, and suggested that it might have arisen from the glomus jugularis of Guild. Many series of cases of these tumors were reported in the following years under various names, including "glomus jugulare tumor" applied by Winship[15] in 1948 and "nonchromaffin paraganglioma of the middle ear" suggested by Lattes and Waltner in 1949;[16] "chemodectoma"[17] "receptoma,"[18] "glomerocytoma" and "tympanic body tumor" have also been used to refer to the same type of tumor.[19] Rosenwasser,[20] who first identified this neoplasm with the glomus jugularis of Guild, prefers the name "glomus jugulare tumor" rather than one of the names implying a function not yet proved.

### The Glomus Body of Guild

According to Guild,[13] the usual site for this tiny ovoid body, measuring scarcely 0.5 mm. broad by 0.25 mm. thick, is in the dome of the jugular bulb near the tympanic branch of the glossopharyngeal nerve (Jacobson's nerve). Additional glomus formations may occur along the course of Jacobson's nerve between the jugular fossa and the middle ear, or on the cochlear promontory, or along the auricular branch of the vagus nerve. In 88 temporal bones Guild[21] found a total of 248 glomus formations, half in the dome of the jugular bulb and half equally distributed along Jacobson's nerve and the auricular branch of the vagus.

Guild observed that the histologic structure of this body is a mass or glomus

(Latin for "ball") of vessels of capillary or precapillary size lined by uniform large epithelioid cells which fail to stain with chromium salts (non-chromaffin). This structure and the nerve and blood supply from the glossopharyngeal nerve and ascending pharyngeal artery are the same as for the carotid body.

The function of glomus bodies is believed to be similar to that of the carotid body: chemoreceptors sensitive to oxygen tension and possibly to $CO_2$ tension. Hormonal activity with production of epinephrine and norepinephrine has been demonstrated in carotid body tumors, and in one out of seven glomus jugulare tumors.[22]

## Pathology of Glomus Tumors

These tumors may begin wherever glomus jugularis tissue occurs, namely in the dome of the jugular bulb, in the bone between the bulb and hypotympanum, in the hypotympanum or on the promontory and along the auricular branch of the vagus. From the site of origin the tumor grows, usually very slowly, infiltrating and invading adjacent structures, including the bone of the jugular fossa, the jugular bulb, the tympanic membrane, the mastoid, the facial nerve, the nerves of the jugular foramen (ninth, tenth and eleventh), the labyrinth, and in some cases the petrous apex, fifth nerve, cranial cavity and even extending into the nasopharynx. It may compress the sigmoid sinus and jugular bulb from without, or protrude polyp-like into the bulb and internal jugular vein.[23] The rate of growth varies greatly among individual cases; some tumors change little in 15 to 20 years and others terminate fatally within a year of the first symptom, owing to intracranial extension.[20]

**Microscopically** glomus tumors resemble the glomus jugularis of Guild with a rich network of vascular spaces lined by large epithelioid cells. In the usual very slowly growing tumor (Fig. 22–10 A and B), these cells are uniform in size and appearance; tumors that grow rapidly and sometimes metastasize are more cellular and pleomorphic (Fig. 22–10 C).

The gross appearance of a glomus tumor resembles that of a vascular polyp of inflammatory origin with which it is often confused. In the tympanic cavity the tumor has a smooth, slightly lobulated appearance (Fig. 22–10 D), but as it grows into and infiltrates the tympanic membrane and adjacent bone there is no capsule or limiting membrane. The involved bone becomes soft and hemorrhagic, without a sharp line of demarcation from normal bone. The normal bone near the tumor develops an increased vascularity as it contributes to the nutrition of the adjacent tumor tissue. The tumor itself bleeds profusely at the slightest trauma, with very little tendency for the bleeding to stop by itself, since the vascular spaces have no contractile elements. However, the bleeding is readily controlled by a firm pack left in place for several minutes. If compressed Gelfoam is placed immediately against the bleeding surface, the gauze pack can be removed after several minutes, with the Gelfoam left in place.

## Classification of Glomus Tumors

Over the years there has been confusion concerning the terminology associated with glomus tumors. Alford and Guilford[24] were the first to clearly define a clinical classification of these neoplasms according to their point of origin and the extent of their involvement in the temporal bone: tumors limited to the middle ear and

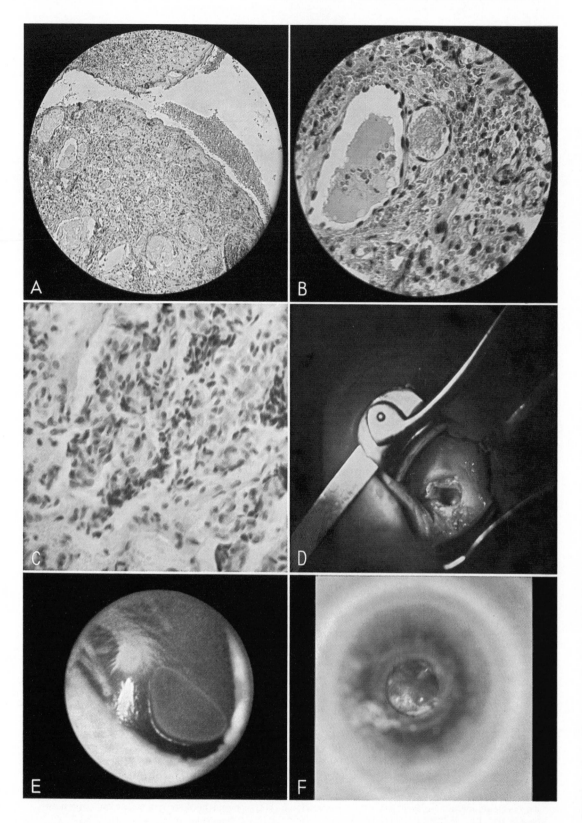

See legend on the opposite page.

mastoid were given the name **glomus tympanicum tumors**, while larger lesions involving the jugular bulb, middle ear and skull base were defined as **glomus jugulare tumors.**

This classification is important because it allows the surgeon to differentiate between small middle ear tumors and the larger, more treacherous and invasive skull base neoplasms. There are two distinct advantages to this differentiation. First, it makes a tremendous difference in the surgical preparations for removal of one of these tumors, the surgical approach, the allotted blood for replacement, ancillary assistance and so on, and secondly, it allows surgeons and radiologists to more accurately assess their therapeutic results. It is impossible to compare the removal of a 5 mm. tumor limited to the promontory to that of a lesion taking eight to ten hours to extract from the skull base. In like manner, the radiotherapist cannot make an accurate statement about cure rate without having some knowledge of the size and extent of the lesion prior to treatment.

Too often in the earlier literature, both of otolaryngology and radiology, broad statements were made concerning the surgical and radiation treatment of these tumors. By combining all glomus tumors under the general heading of "jugulare" it has been difficult to determine the true results obtained by either mode of therapy.

## Diagnosis of Glomus Tumors

The diagnosis of glomus tumors is a clinical one based upon a thorough history and physical and audiometric, vestibular and x-ray studies.

### History

The most characteristic symptom associated with glomus tumors is a pulsating tinnitus followed by a hearing loss. This loss is usually conductive; however, should the tumor invade the labyrinth or cochlea, it may be sensorineural.

As a general rule, glomus tympanicum tumors are diagnosed earlier than jugulare lesions. The reason is that the tumor, lying on the promontory, usually touches the underside of the umbo, producing the characteristic pulsating tinnitus and hearing loss. The jugulare tumors, on the other hand, may extend extensively into the base of the skull before they appear in the hypotympanum as a small red mass.

Many times glomus tumors of both types are found quite by accident during a

---

**Figure 22–10** *A*, Glomus jugulare tumor involving the middle ear and mastoid, showing a tremendous number of vascular spaces under low power. *B*, Same under high power, showing epithelioid cells. *C*, Glomus jugulare tumor that had destroyed the bone around the jugular bulb, carotid artery and hypotympanum and had begun to involve the nerves of the jugular foramen. Note the large number of epithelioid cells. *D*, Small glomus jugulare tumor, confined to the lower half of the tympanic cavity, removed by hypotympanotomy. *E*, Typical early glomus jugulare tumor resting against the lower half of the tympanic membrane. *F*, Otoscopic appearance of an early glomus jugulare tumor. The red color may be mistaken for a Schwartze's sign of otosclerosis and the pulsating bruit may be mistaken for carotid aneurysm.

routine physical examination by the family physician. Occasionally this will occur before any symptoms have manifested themselves.

Both types of tumor can attain great size (Fig. 22–19), completely blocking the middle ear and extending out into the external auditory canal. This situation is most often seen in the patient who fails to seek medical advice in the face of pulsating tinnitus and hearing loss.

Glomus tumors are commonly associated with carotid body tumors, tumors of the vagus nerve and carcinoma of the thyroid. In obtaining a history and in performing the physical examination, it is important to remember this as well as the fact that in some instances these lesions occur bilaterally.

### Physical Examination

The most important aspect of the physical examination is the otoscopic evaluation of the drum membrane because most glomus tumors can be seen behind an intact tympanic membrane. A hand-held otoscope may be sufficient for this purpose, but certainly the operating microscope is the instrument of choice.

If the examiner can see around the edges of the tumor (its border does not touch the annulus), the lesion is most likely a tympanicum and no further workup is necessary. Should the tumor extend past the annulus in any direction, it is impossible, by otoscopic examination, to determine whether the lesion is a tympanicum or jugulare. Unfortunately, many an unsuspecting surgeon has seen a small red mass lying in the hypotympanum and has mistakenly taken it for a glomus tympanicum tumor. Upon surgical exploration of the ear, this surgeon might find that he had only exposed the "tip of an iceberg," finding an extensive glomus jugulare tumor involving a large part of the skull base.

Brown[25] has described an interesting diagnostic test to demonstrate pulsations of the tumor. Using a pneumatic otoscope, pressure is exerted on the tympanic membrane which in turn brings the drum membrane into contact with the tumor. Pulsations are easily seen through the compressed membrane.

A permanent record of the pulsations can be obtained by performing a tympanogram with an impedance bridge. The tracing demonstrates the vascularity of the tumor by means of a series of sine waves traced out by the recorder.

### Myringotomy and Biopsy

Myringotomy and biopsy are mentioned to be avoided and to caution the inexperienced surgeon regarding the dangers associated with both of these procedures in the management of glomus tumors. It is most dangerous to perform a myringotomy when one sees a red mass behind an intact tympanic membrane. The mass might just as well be a misplaced and uncovered carotid artery. The literature is full of accounts relating instances where an unsuspecting physician performed a myringotomy in his office and had to deal with a profusely bleeding ear. Glomus tumors may bleed so briskly after a myringotomy that the entire external ear canal must be packed, and on occasion, blood replacement may be necessary.

Biopsy to establish the diagnosis should not be done through a myringotomy. There are several reasons for this. First, following such a procedure, there is a tendency for the tumor to grow into the tympanic membrane, necessitating the removal of the drum membrane at surgery.

Secondly, in most cases, the diagnosis can be made without biopsy based upon the characteristic x-ray examination. A pathologist with experience in reading frozen specimens of glomus tumors will hasten to make the diagnosis for the surgeon at the time of surgery. If the pathologist does not possess this skill, then perhaps a formal biopsy should be made before the definitive operative procedure is scheduled.

There is one other instance in which biopsy may be necessary, and that is if the lesion is not going to be treated surgically. In such a case, exposure of the middle ear should be done by lifting the tympanic membrane or through the mastoid approach. In either case, the biopsy should be performed under direct vision with ample supplies of Gelfoam, topical thrombin and iodoform gauze packing to control hemorrhage.

### Audiometric Studies

All otologic patients require a pure-tone air and bone conduction audiogram with speech discrimination scores. The hearing loss in glomus tumors is usually conductive but may be sensorineural. Occasionally, an individual will present with a "dead ear." It is important to establish this fact prior to the surgical removal.

### Vestibular Studies

Vestibular studies in the diagnosis of glomus tumors play a very small role. Due to the bulk of the tumor mass in the middle ear, one would expect the caloric response to be diminished. Should the caloric test response be absent, one might consider invasion of the labyrinth by tumor.

### X-ray Studies

Of all the lesions involving the temporal bone, glomus tumor diagnosis relies especially heavily upon x-ray examination, including polytome, arterial and venous studies, as well as posterior fossa myelograms and computerized axial tomography scan (CAT scan).

*Plane Films.* Routine x-ray examination of the temporal bone with special head units such as the Compere and Franklin is of little use in the diagnosis of glomus tumors. The base view is the only one of any real value because it demonstrates the jugular bulb. If one bulb is larger and appears on the same side as the hearing loss, this fact may be of clinical significance. It must be remembered that in most cases the right bulb is normally larger than the left.

*Polytome X-rays of the Temporal Bone.* The most valuable x-ray study for distinguishing between tympanicum and jugulare tumors is the polytome.

Anterior-posterior views are important in demonstrating enlargement of the jugular bulb and destruction of bone in the skull base. Figure 22–11 demonstrates a normal bulb, while Figure 22–12 shows the destruction by a jugulare tumor extending medially beneath the internal auditory canal (IAC).

Lateral views are invaluable in determining the extent of involvement in the carotid canal. Figure 22–13 clearly demonstrates the normal "V-shaped" piece of bone separating the jugular bulb posteriorly from the carotid canal. This "crotch" or

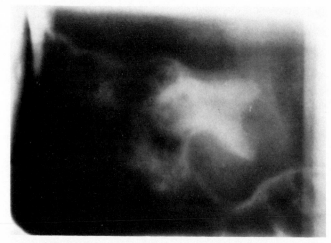

**Figure 22–11**   Polytome of normal jugular bulb.

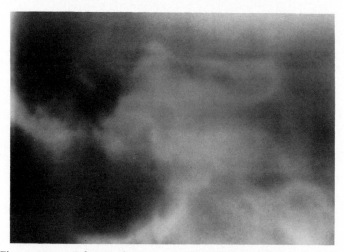

**Figure 22-12**   Polytome demonstrating destruction of the jugular bulb.

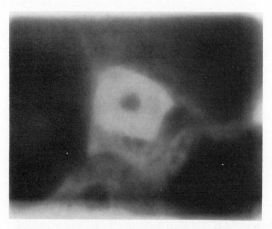

**Figure 22–13**   Lateral polytome demonstrates normal "V" shaped piece of bone separating jugular bulb from carotid canal.

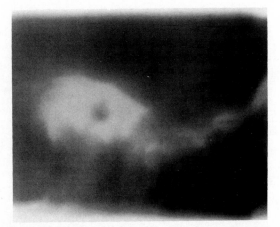

**Figure 22–14**  Lateral polytome shows destruction of normal "V" shaped piece of bone separating jugular bulb from carotid canal.

"vascular crest," as it has been termed, has been destroyed in Figure 22–14, indicating that the tumor has invaded the carotid canal.

Special base views will demonstrate extension of the disease into the clivus and occipital bone. While the polytome is accurate and is extremely helpful in determining the extension of the tumor, it does have limitations. Occasionally the surgeon will be amazed to find extensive invasion of the skull base when there has been no suggestion of the extent by polytome examination.

*Arteriogram.*   When the polytome x-rays are positive and one suspects that a jugulare tumor is present, a carotid arteriogram should be performed. In the past the junior author limited the use of this examination because of the risks involved.[26] However, after careful consideration and further clinical experience, this examination is being used more often as it gives a good estimate of the vascularity and origin of the blood supply (Fig. 22–15). In addition, it will demonstrate associated carotid

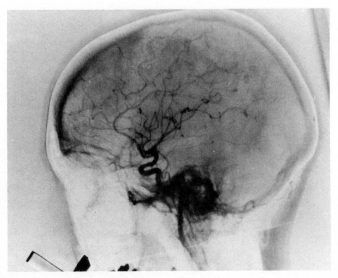

**Figure 22–15**  Carotid arteriogram demonstrating vascularity of glomus tumor.

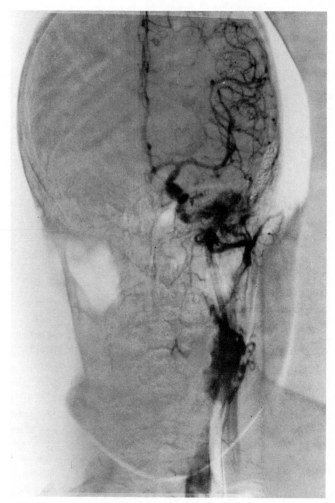

**Figure 22–16** Arteriogram demonstrating an associated carotid body tumor.

body tumors (Fig. 22–16). Bilateral studies are now performed routinely to demonstrate cross-flow collateral circulation from the opposite side. The arteriogram will also demonstrate vagal tumors (these lesions consist of glomus body type tumors occurring within the substance of the vagal nerve).

One further advantage of the carotid arteriogram is that the venous phase can be used to establish blockage of the jugular bulb, thus making a retrograde venogram unnecessary.

Vertebral artery studies are occasionally ordered to determine if there is intracranial extension of the tumor and to assess the extent of blood supply to the neoplasm from the vertebral artery.

*Retrograde Venogram.* When the polytome x-rays do not clearly delineate involvement of the jugular bulb, a retrograde venogram is helpful. However, this procedure is employed less frequently since bilateral carotid arteriograms are now performed on a more routine basis.

The venogram can be accomplished by a direct venopuncture in the neck or by means of a long catheter threaded up through the femoral vein. Figure 22–17 shows A-P and lateral views of a normal internal jugular vein and bulb. Figure 22–18

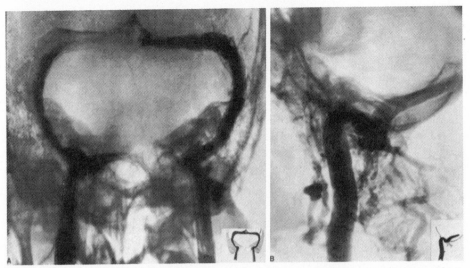

**Figure 22–17**  Jugularogram. *A*, Normal. Anteroposterior view. Both transverse sinuses and internal jugular veins are clearly shown. *B*, Same lateral view showing inferior petrosal sinuses. (from Gejrot, T., and Laurén, T.: Retrograde jugularography in diagnosis of glomus tumours in the jugular region. Acta oto-laryng., 58:191, 1964.)

demonstrates a lateral view of a filling defect most likely a glomus jugulare tumor.

These venograms make it quite evident that any surgical procedure for the removal of glomus jugulare tumors would be destined for failure if a resection of the internal jugulare vein was not a routine part of the operation.

*Posterior Fossa Myelogram.*  This dye study is reserved for those cases in

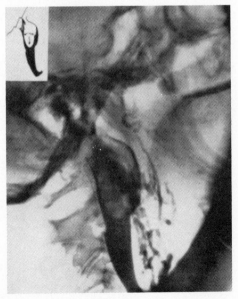

**Figure 22–18**  Jugularogram showing a large rounded mass filling expanded upper part of internal jugular vein in a patient with a glomus tumor. (From Gejrot, T., and Laurén, T.: Retrograde jugularography in diagnosis of glomus tumours in the jugular region. Acta oto-laryng., 58:191, 1964.)

which intracranial extension of the tumor is suspected. As a rule, only those individuals with cranial nerve deficits are considered as candidates for the myelogram and then only if a CAT scan is negative.

*Computerized Axial Tomography.*   This new x-ray examination is not only of value in determining intracranial extension into the posterior fossa, but new experience with coronal cuts of the temporal bone suggests that this procedure may allow the radiologist to determine the extent of bony involvement.

### Treatment of Glomus Tumors

Glomus tumors are managed by either radiation, surgical removal, embolization or a combination of these methods.

### *Radiation*

Considerable disagreement exists concerning the use of radiation as a mode of primary treatment for glomus tumors. The literature is full of papers claiming cures by radiation when no pretherapy evaluation was performed. The therapist, in these cases, did not know whether the involved tumor was either large or small or tympanicum or jugulare. This lack of information coupled with the fact that these lesions are sometimes extremely slow growing precludes a statement concerning x-ray cure rates over a five-year period. The same holds true for surgery. When a physician is dealing with a tumor that may remain relatively dormant for 15 to 20 years, it is difficult to assess any mode of therapy.

There is no question that some glomus tumors are more aggressive than others and that some are more vascular. There is good evidence that, to some extent, vascular tumors probably do respond to radiation therapy.[27] There is little evidence, however, that radiation cures the lesion;[28] rather it may arrest its growth and reduce it somewhat in size.

The junior author suspects that many times radiation is offered to the patient as an alternative to surgery because it is the easier route to take and surgical results in the past have not been satisfactory. Newer, more thorough operative procedures alter this argument. The senior author has observed recurrences years after apparently successful surgical removal, whereas radiation has arrested many, but not all glomus tumors.[37] With arrest the tumor may decrease in size and vascularity, and pulsating tinnitus subsides.

Irradiation has a place in therapy: it should be considered in those cases that are considered inoperable, or where mutilating and dangerous surgery is required in older individuals who are not candidates for extensive skull base surgery (Fig. 22–19).

In some instances a combination of surgery and radiation may be indicated,[27] using x-ray therapy as a means of decreasing vascularity prior to surgery. When a glomus tumor continues to increase in size after preliminary irradiation, surgery is required.

### *Embolization of Glomus Tumors*

At the time of surgery, embolization of a glomus jugulare tumor[29] will greatly lessen its vascularity and reduce the need for replacement blood. The ascending

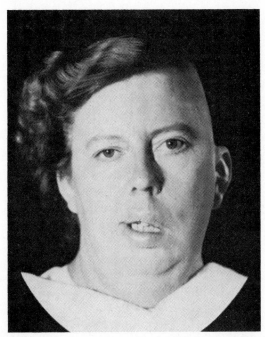

**Figure 22–19** Enormous glomus jugulare tumor producing a pulsating mass of the temporal and mastoid area with facial paralysis and dead labyrinth. The pulsations ceased the moment the external carotid artery was ligated below the markedly enlarged ascending pharyngeal artery. The main mass of tumor was the removed; a remnant left in the petrous apex was treated by postoperative irradiation. Death from cerebral extension occurred 3 years later.

pharyngeal artery, the initial and principal blood supply of these tumors, is embolized with small Teflon balls, Gelfoam, liquid Silastic or pieces of muscle. This procedure is not without danger, as the embolized particles can pass completely through the tumor and be picked up by the internal carotid artery, resulting in an embolus to the brain with subsequent stroke.

A second use for embolization is in inoperable patients who have reached the limit of radiation they can tolerate. In such an instance, repeated embolizations may be performed several months apart to periodically reduce the amount of vascularity of the lesion. Ligation of the ascending pharyngeal artery reduces the bleeding at surgery and will reduce annoying pulsating tinnitus in inoperable tumors.

### Surgical Removal of Glomus Tumors

Surgical excision of glomus tumors is the treatment of choice of some surgeons, including the junior author. There are, however, some very stringent guidelines that the surgeon must follow. Small tympanicum tumors can be removed with a minimum of morbidity and mortality; thus, if the patient's general health is good, age is not a limiting factor in the removal of these lesions. Such is not the case for larger tympanicum and jugulare tumors. In a 20- to 30-year-old individual, these lesions should be aggressively approached. However, the neoplasm in a 60- to 70-year-old might better be managed by radiation. The difficult age group is those individuals in their mid-fifties who are having very little difficulty or discomfort from a large, questionably resectable glomus jugulare tumor. Obviously, the decision for surgery or irradiation must be made on an individual basis and will

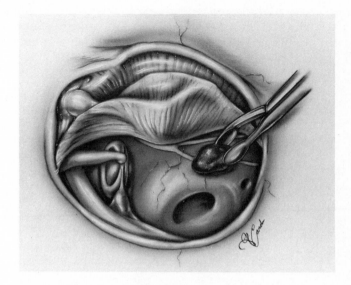

**Figure 22–20** Transcanal removal of a small glomus tympanicum tumor.

vary from patient to patient. Do the possible surgical benefits justify and outweigh the risks and mutilation of an operation of such magnitude? Or should palliative irradiation to arrest the tumor be given a trial?

### Transmeatal Surgical Removal

The authors reserve this procedure for very small glomus tympanicum tumors limited to the promontory. By otoscopic examination all borders of the lesion must be visible and cannot extend past the annulus of the drum membrane.

The procedure is as follows. Working through the ear canal under local anesthesia, a stapes type of endomeatal flap is created, elevating the tympanic membrane forward. The drum membrane is lifted off the malleus handle to expose the anterior portion of the middle ear. A cup forceps is used to grasp the tumor, which is then extracted in one piece, if possible, under direct vision (Fig. 22–20). Bleeding is controlled by placing Gelfoam soaked in 1:1,000,000 epinephrine into the middle ear and holding it in place with iodoform gauze packing. Once the hemorrhage is controlled, the Gelfoam is left in place, the tympanic membrane is placed into its original position and the external auditory canal is filled with an ointment.

The senior author[30] has described a transmeatal method for removing glomus tympanicum tumors that extend into the hypotympanum by "hypotympanotomy."

Under general or local anesthesia, the usual endaural incision is made, extending upward from the meatus. A supplementary incision is made from the lower end of the endaural incision along the lower two thirds of the anterior meatal wall at the level of the outer edge of the osseous meatus (Fig. 22–21A).

The skin and periosteum of the anterior-inferior and posterior osseous meatal walls are elevated and pushed upward, thus exposing almost the entire extent of the tympanic bone from the tympanomastoid suture behind nearly to the tympanosquamous suture in front (Fig. 22–21B).

The osseous meatus is enlarged by thinning down the anterior and inferior osseous meatal walls with a cutting burr (Fig. 22–21C). The position of the facial nerve at the stylomastoid foramen is kept in mind. The facial nerve is safely avoided if the removal of the floor of the osseous meatus is confined to the area in front of a vertical line through the tympanomastoid suture and posterior edge of the sulcus tympanicus.

The annulus tympanicus is elevated from its sulcus posteriorly, inferiorly, and anteriorly, similar to the exposure for stapes operations, but confined to the lower half of the tympanic cavity rather than the posterior-superior quadrant. As the tympanic membrane is folded upward upon itself, the tumor comes into view (Fig. 22–21D). Should the tumor be adherent to the tympanic membrane, that portion of the drum membrane should be removed with the tumor.

Resection of the bony sulcus tympanicus inferiorly without trauma to the tumor fully exposes the hypotympanum and the tumor within it (Fig. 22–21E). The extent of the tumor in all directions is determined, and any further bone that needs to be removed for full exposure of the tumor is taken down with a burr or curet (Fig. 22–21).

The tumor is rapidly dissected away from the promontory and floor of the hypotympanum with small periosteal elevators. The violent bleeding from the inferior tympanic artery is controlled with a Gelfoam or Surgicel pack.

After the field is dry, the tympanic membrane and skin of the meatus is replaced. Defects in the tympanic membrane are repaired by means of temporalis fascia. Removal of an extensive glomus tympanicum tumor by the endaural approach is shown in Figure 22–22.

### The Transmastoid Procedure of House

For large tympanicum tumors in which the border of the lesion extends beyond the annulus, the junior author prefers to use the transmastoid procedure described by House.[31] In most cases the anatomy and function of the ear can be maintained in that the posterior canal wall, tympanic membrane and ossicles are preserved.

A standard postauricular incision is made, and a simple mastoidectomy performed in the manner previously described. The facial nerve is identified, and the facial recess is opened in the routine manner.

The chorda tympani nerve is exposed and located just as it exits the facial nerve. It is sectioned at this point as well as in the middle ear and then discarded. A diamond burr is used to remove the bone between the vertical segment of the facial nerve and the fibrous annulus of the tympanic membrane. This annulus is used as the landmark for entering the hypotympanum. Referred to as the extended facial recess (Fig. 22–23), this allows the surgeon to completely expose the tumor in the middle ear and hypotympanum before any tumor removal is attempted. The horizontal segment of the facial nerve and the stapes can be inspected to make sure they are not involved with the tumor.

At this point a cup forceps is used to grasp the tumor and extract it from the middle ear. Occasionally tumor tissue will be found lying in the hypotympanic cell system, and these cells must be removed with a curet.

Similarly, the retrofacial cell tract is also involved with tumor, and this can be removed from beneath the facial nerve under direct vision. This is one of the advantages of this approach over one through the ear canal (Fig. 22–24).

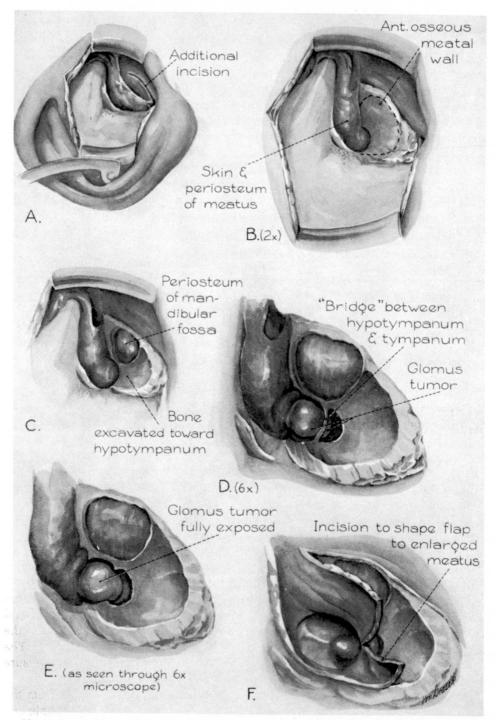

**Figure 22–21** Removal of a small glomus tympanicum tumor; hypotympanotomy approach. *A*, Skin incisions. *B*, Elevation of a flap to expose the floor of the osseous meatus (broken line showing area of bone to be removed). *C*, Bone removed to expose the hypotympanum. *D*, Hypotympanotomy with elevation of the lower half of the tympanic annulus from the sulcus. *E*, Tumor fully exposed. *F*, Incision of the skin flap preliminary to removal of the tumor. (Continued on the opposite page.)

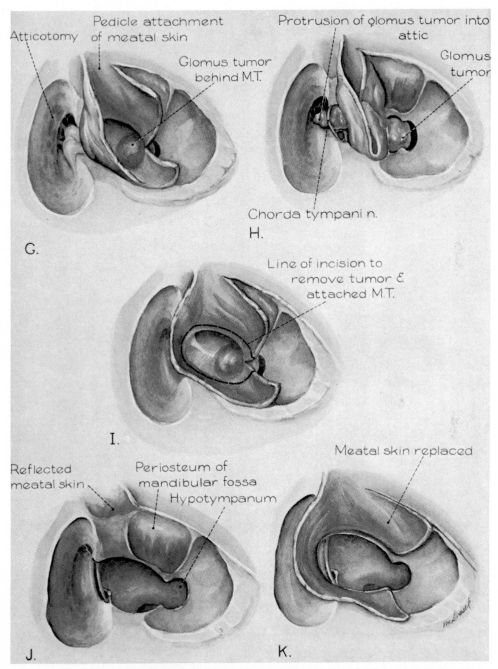

**Figure 22–21** *(Continued)* Supplementary atticotomy for extension of a glomus tympanicum tumor into the attic. *G,* Atticotomy; malleus and incus visualized. *H,* After removal of the incus and malleus, tumor seen protruding into the attic. *I,* Line of excision of the tympanic membrane with attached tumor. *J,* Appearance after removal of the tumor. *K,* Flap replaced. (From Shambaugh, G. E., Jr.: Surgical approach for so-called glomus jugulare tumors of the middle ear. Laryngoscope, 65:185, 1955.)

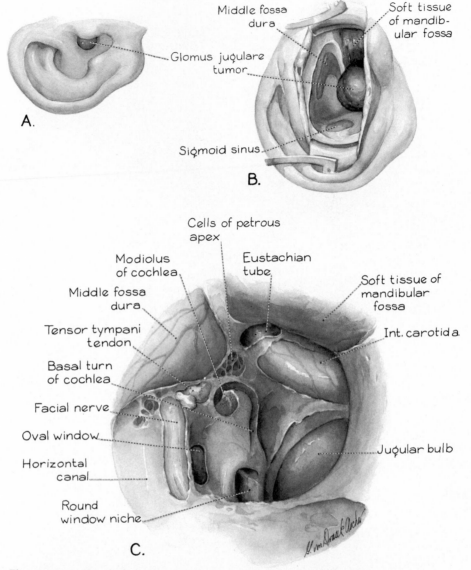

**Figure 22–22**  Removal of extensive glomus jugulare tumor in a child, age 9, with a 5 year history of earaches in the right ear, recent bleeding from the ear and vertigo. *A* and *B*, Initial exposure of tumor. *C*, After removal. The cochlea was eroded, the petrous apex excavated and the adjacent structures exposed as shown. Child died later of metastases.

Bleeding can be controlled with a Surgicel pack in the hypotympanum or with a piece of bone wax.

It is usually not possible to remove in this manner those tympanicum tumors that are extremely large, filling the external auditory canal and extending down the eustachian tube. In such a situation, the posterior canal wall must be removed and the ear converted to a radical cavity. Smith[32] has described a method of removing the posterior ear canal and wiring it back into place following removal of the tumor. This operation usually takes from one to two hours to complete, and the average blood loss is from one to three units.

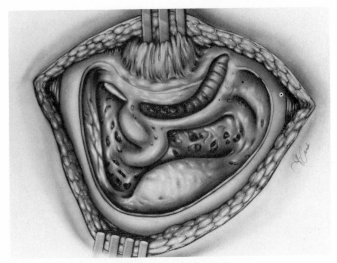

**Figure 22–23**  Extended facial recess.

## The Skull Base Approach

In order to completely remove glomus jugulare tumors, it is necessary to expose the great vessels and nerves of the neck and to resect the internal jugular vein and bulb as an *en bloc* specimen with the tumor.[33, 34, 37]

To accomplish this, a parotid type incision is made with the posterior arm extending into the postauricular area. The inferior portion runs along the anterior border of the sternocleidomastoid muscle (Fig. 22–25). A parotid flap is raised, exposing the superficial lobe. If the ear canal is to be preserved, the dissection stops here; otherwise, the superficial lobe is resected to expose the facial nerve overlying the deep lobe of the parotid.

Next, the facial nerve is identified in the usual manner and a plastic tape applied for later use. The dissection is carried into the neck where the common, external and

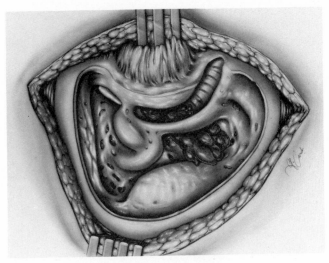

**Figure 22–24**  Retrofacial cell tract opened to gain better access to tumor.

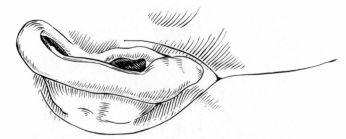

**Figure 22–25**   The post-auricular incision is carried into the neck along the anterior border of the sternocleidomastoid muscle.

internal carotid arteries are found and isolated with tapes. The spinal accessory, vagus and hypoglossal nerves are identified and tagged.

At this point, a simple mastoidectomy with exposure of the extended facial recess is carried out in the manner just described. It is possible to remove large glomus jugulare tumors with preservation of the posterior ear canal, tympanic membrane and ossicles if the tumor is not attached to the carotid artery and does not extend down the eustachian tube. Should this occur, a few alterations must be made in the surgical technique. These will be described after the standard method is set forth, as follows.

Once the extended facial recess has been exposed, the tip of the mastoid is removed (Fig. 22–26), and the facial nerve is taken out of the fallopian canal and draped along the posterior canal wall and out into the parotid. All of the bone and soft tissue are removed so that the jugular bulb is completely exposed, allowing the surgeon to follow it into the neck where it becomes the internal jugular vein.

At this point, the vein is ligated, severed and brought beneath the 11th nerve where it passes the lateral process of C2. Next the bone is removed from the sigmoid sinus; it is opened and packed with Surgicel. At this point the bulb is isolated except for the inferior petrosal sinus, which enters the bulb anteriorly.

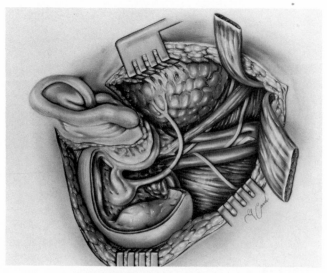

**Figure 22–26**   A simple mastoidectomy has been performed and the tip of the mastoid removed. The facial nerve has been exposed into the parotid.

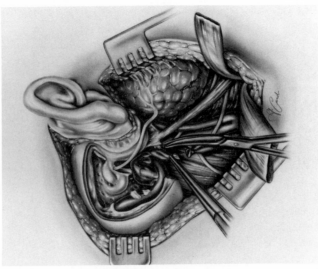

**Figure 22–27**   The jugular vein is grasped with a forceps, and the tumor is avulsed away from the carotid artery.

The jugular vein is grasped with a forceps, and under direct microscopic vision, the surgeon uses a pair of Metzenbaum scissors (Fig. 22–27) to dissect the vein and tumor away from the internal carotid artery. In most cases, it is possible to remain in the avascular areolar tissue plane that separates the artery and vein. When the tumor is free of the carotid, it is avulsed from the bulb, tearing the outer wall of the jugular vein away from the posterior fossa dura. At this point bleeding may be profuse from the inferior petrosal sinus. This is quickly and easily managed by placing a small plug of Surgicel directly into the orifice of the sinus as it enters the bulb. There may be other sinuses, such as the inferior petro-occipital sinus, draining into the bulb as well, and these will require similar treatment.

Most of the time the isolated and fully exposed tumor will avulse in one piece, but occasionally it will break in two. When this occurs, the second half is removed after the bleeding is under control. One can actually visualize the surgical defect quite well, and any bits of residual tumor are easily removed with forceps and curet (Fig. 22–28).

In removing tumor from the posterior aspect of the bulb, it is not unusual to obtain cerebrospinal fluid (CSF). Should this occur, the posterior belly of the digastric and sternocleidomastoid muscle are taken as free grafts and placed into the wound.

As the tumor is removed from the posterior fossa dura, it may become evident that the lesion actually invades the dura and has extended into the posterior fossa. There are two methods of dealing with this situation. One is to approach the posterior fossa through a separate incision, using the standard neurosurgical suboccipital exposure. This technique has been well demonstrated by Kinney.[29] The junior author prefers, when possible, a more direct route. In this method the dura is simply incised, and a neurosurgical cottonoid is placed into the posterior fossa to isolate the tumor from the brainstem. This cottonoid serves another purpose in that it protects the brainstem from instrumentation.Once the brain has been isolated, the dura is removed with a sharp pair of microscissors. In this manner, dura with the attached tumor is lifted away from the brainstem. Again, muscle is placed into the defect to prevent CSF leak, and the wound is closed in the usual manner.

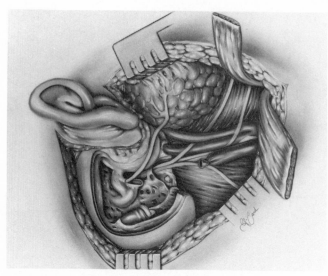

**Figure 22–28**   When the tumor has been removed the posterior canal wall, tympanic membrane and ossicles are still intact.

When the ear canal has been saved, the incision is closed in layers, and interrupted skin sutures are used. A hemovac is used under the parotid flap but not in the deep part of the wound because of the CSF.

When it is necessary to remove the ear canal wall, the procedure is somewhat more extensive.[34] All steps are the same, with the following exceptions. The superficial lobe of the parotid is removed and the branches of the facial nerve are dissected free of the deep lobes. (This is done in order to give maximal movement of the nerve for anterior displacement out of the fallopian canal.)

Before the anterior and posterior ear canal walls are removed, the skin of the ear canal and the tympanic membrane are dissected free and lifted out. Next, the root of the zygoma is drilled away, the incudostapedial joint separated and the malleus and incus removed. At this point the posterior canal wall is fractured free, and the anterior wall is removed with a cutting burr. It is taken down to the level of the eustachian tube. At this time a diamond burr is used to expose the internal carotid artery lying on the floor of the eustachian tube. The artery is then followed down to the entrance of the vessel into the carotid canal just anterior to the jugular bulb. In order to obtain enough exposure to accomplish this, it is necessary to displace the mandible forward out of the glenoid fossa for approximately 1 cm. Once the anterior and posterior canal walls have been removed and the carotid artery exposed, the facial nerve is displaced from the area of the geniculate ganglion, anteriorly to the artery (Fig. 22–29).

With this exposure, it is possible to remove a large tumor filling the middle ear and jugular bulb away from the internal carotid artery under direct vision from the most proximal portion of the artery to the most distal (Fig. 22–30). When the function of the ear has been compromised by removing the eardrum and ossicles, the external auditory canal is simply sutured closed to prevent the patient from having to care for a radical cavity.

The total operating time for this type of tumor is from eight to ten hours, with the average blood loss from six to ten units. Barring complications, the patient usually leaves the hospital seven to ten days following surgery.

In all surgical approaches to a glomus tumor, either of the tympanicum or the

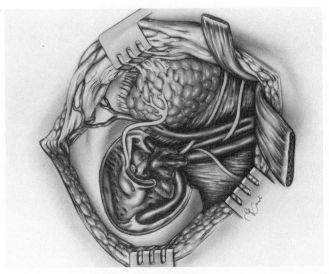

**Figure 22–29** Facial nerve laid forward after anterior and posterior ear canal walls have been taken down.

jugulare type, the problem of profuse bleeding flooding and obscuring the field each time the tumor is cut into is avoided by removal of bone around it before removal of tumor is attempted. Thus, "the patient is first removed from tumor, rather than the tumor from the patient," as so aptly stated by Weille.[34]

## Complications

There are numerous complications that can occur following the removal of glomus tumors. If the lesion has invaded the posterior semicircular canal or the basal coil of the cochlea, there is a very real possibility that postoperatively the individual will have a dead ear.

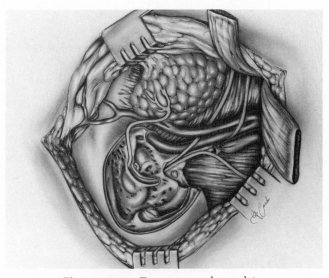

**Figure 22–30** Tumor removal complete.

Work on or near the internal carotid artery is fraught with danger, and if the artery is injured, there is a good chance the individual will suffer a stroke. If there is good collateral blood supply from the opposite side, the patient might survive without paralysis. Should there be no or poor collateral circulation, death may occur.

Facial weakness is a rare complication of glomus tympanicum removal, but it is common when the nerve must be rerouted out of the fallopian canal, as is the case with most large jugular tumors. All jugulare patients are warned that they most likely will experience a total facial paralysis for six to twelve months following surgery. In some cases, the nerve has been invaded by the tumor, and the individual may present with a facial paralysis. Whether the tumor has already destroyed the nerve function or has just invaded the nerve, it must be resected with the lesion. This requires a graft as described in Chapter 20 to rehabilitate the face.

If, for some reason, it is not feasible to use a graft, it is possible to perform a 7–12 anastomosis. However, this must be done as a separate procedure for the reason that the 12th nerve can be injured during tumor removal and the patient has to be awake to make sure the nerve is intact. The anastomosis is usually done several days after the initial operation.

When the subarachnoid space has been entered, persistent CSF leak is always a possibility. Most leaks require exploration of the wound for placement of more fat or muscle. Whenever CSF is present, the possibility of meningitis is a real threat. Fortunately, this is a rare complication.

In removing the tumor from the jugular bulb, it is possible to injure the 9th, 10th, 11th and 12th cranial nerves. Seldom are all these nerves lost, but it is not unusual to lose one or two. The loss of the vagus nerve presents the greatest problem because of its supply to the pharynx and larynx. These individuals have difficulty swallowing and have a tendency to aspirate. Thus a tracheotomy should be performed when this complication occurs. After a period of time, the patient will compensate and the tracheotomy can be removed. The other symptom associated with the loss of the 10th nerve is hoarseness due to the paralyzed vocal cord. If after one year the voice has not returned to normal, the cord can be injected with Teflon paste[35] with excellent results.

### Results of Surgery

Because of the slow growth rate of some glomus tumors, it is impossible to state that a patient is free of recurrent disease until at least a 10 to 15 year period has lapsed following surgery. Certainly, with the newer techniques now available for the complete removal of these lesions, it is the junior author's opinion that the problem of residual recurrent tumor will not be as great as in the past.

Spector et al.[36] recently reviewed a large series of tumors removed over a long time span and concluded that the best method of tumor eradication is by means of surgery. They quote a success rate for tympanicum and glomus jugulare tumors as 91 per cent and 78 per cent respectively. While irradiation has resulted in remission of symptoms and arrest of growth lasting more than 40 years,[37] destruction of tumor cells and disappearance of the growth cannot be expected. In cases of radiation failure to arrest the growth Spector et al. report a remarkable 80 per cent cure rate.

# REFERENCES

1. Nager, G. T.: Meningiomas Involving the Temporal Bone. Springfield, Ill., Charles C Thomas, 1964.
2. Oshiro, H., and Perlman, H. B.: Subarachnoid spread of tumor to the labyrinth. Arch. Otol., *81*:328, 1965.
3. Lichtenstein, L., and Jaffe, H. L.: Fibrous dysplasia of bone. Arch. Path., *33*:777, 1942.
4. Wong, A., Vaughan, C. W., and Strong, M. S.: Fibrous dysplasia of the temporal bone. Arch. Otol., *81*:13, 1965.
5. Kelemen, G.: Histiocytosis involving the temporal bone. Laryngoscope, *70*:1284, 1960.
6. Lewis, J. S.: Cancer of the ear. Laryngoscope, *70*:551, 1960.
7. Conley, J. J., and Novack, A. J.: The surgical removal of malignant tumors of the ear and temporal bone. Arch. Otol., *71*:635, 1960.
8. Mohs, F. E.: Chemosurgical treatment of cancer of the ear; microscopically controlled method of excision. Surgery, *21*:605, 1947.
9. Beal, D. D., Lindsay, J. R., and Ward, P. H.: Radiation-induced carcinoma of the mastoid. Arch. Otol., *81*:9, 1965.
10. House, H. P.: Early detection of middle ear malignancy. Ann. Otol. Rhin. & Laryng., *58*:789, 1949.
11. Allen, G. W.: Total parotidectomy-technique in surgical removal of advanced cases. Laryngoscope, *74*:1060, 1964.
12. Beck, J. C.: Angioendotheliomas of the middle ear, report of a case. Illinois M. J., *9*:137, 1906.
13. Guild, S. R.: A hitherto unrecognized structure, the glomus jugularis, in man. Anat. Rec., *79*:28, Suppl. 2, 1941.
14. Rosenwasser, H.: Carotid body tumor of the middle ear and mastoid. Arch. Otolaryng., *41*:64, 1945.
15. Winship, T., Klopp, C. T., and Jenkins, W. H.: Glomus jugularis tumors. Cancer, *1*:441, 1948.
16. Lattes, R., and Waltner, J. G.: Non-chromaffin paraganglioma of middle ear. Cancer, *2*:447, 1949.
17. Mulligan, R. M.: Chemodectoma in the dog. Am. J. Path., *26*:680, 1950.
18. Gaffney, J. C.: Carotid-body-like tumors of jugular bulb and middle ear. J. Path. & Bact., *66*:157, 1953.
19. Zettergren, L., and Lindstrom, J.: Glomus tympanicum. Acta Path. et Microbiol. Scandinav., *28*:157, 1951.
20. Rosenwasser, H.: Metastasis from glomus jugulare tumors. Arch Otolaryng., *67*:197, 1958.
21. Guild, S. R.: Glomus jugulare in man. Ann. Otol. Rhin & Laryng., *62*:1045, 1953.
22. Berdal, P., Braaten, M., Cappelen, C., Jr., and Mylius, E. A.: Glomus tumors or non-chromaffin paragangliomas of the head and neck. Acta oto-laryng., Suppl. 188, 1963.
23. Gejrot, T., and Laurén, T.: Retrograde jugularography in diagnosis of glomus tumours in the jugular region. Acta oto-laryng., *58*:191, 1964.
24. Alford, B. R., and Guilford, F. R.: A comprehensive study of the glomus jugulare. Laryngoscope, *72*: 765–805, 1962.
25. Brown, L. A.: Glomus jugulare tumors of the middle ear. Clinical Aspects. Laryngoscope, *63*:281, 1953.
26. Glasscock, M. E., Harris, P. F., and Newsome, G.: Glomus tumors: diagnosis and treatment. Laryngoscope, *84*:2006, 1974.
27. Gardner, G., et al.: Combined approach surgery for removal of glomus jugulare tumors. Laryngoscope, *87*:665, 1977.
28. Brackmann, D. E., et al.: Glomus jugulare tumors: effect of irradiation. Trans. Am. Acad. Ophthalmol. Otolaryngol., *76*:1423, 1972.
29. Kinney, S. E.: Glomus jugulare tumors with intracranial extension. Am. J. Otology, *1*:67, 1979.
30. Shambaugh, G. E., Jr.: Surgical approach for so-called glomus jugulare tumors of the middle ear. Laryngoscope, *65*:185, 1955.
31. House, W. F., and Glasscock, M. E.: Glomus tympanicum tumors. Arch. Otolaryngol., *97*:43, 1973.
32. Smith, M. F. W., and Shinn, J. B.: Glomus tympanicum—excision by radical mastoidectomy exposure with autograft reconstruction. Laryngoscope, *86*:431, 1976.
33. Fisch, U.: Infratemporal fossa approach for extensive tumors of the temporal bone and base of the skull. In H. Silverstein and H. Norrell (Eds.): Neurological Surgery of the Ear. Aesculapius Publishing Company, Birmingham, Ala., 1977.
34. Weille, F. L., and Lane, C. S., Jr.: Surgical problems involved in the removal of glomus jugulare tumors. Laryngoscope, *61*:448, 1951.
35. Arnold, G. E.: Vocal rehabilitation of paralytic dysphonia. Arch. Otol., *78*:179, 1963.
36. Spector, G. J., Fierstein, J., and Ogura, J. H.: A comparison of therapeutic modalities of glomus tumors in the temporal bone. Laryngoscope, *86*:690, 1976.
37. Silverstone, S.: Radiation therapy of glomus jugulare tumors. Arch. Otolaryngol., *97*:43, 1973.

*F. H. Quix*

BORN 1874
DIED 1946

Professor of otolaryngology
in Utrecht; first to remove an
acoustic neurinoma by the
translabyrinthine approach.

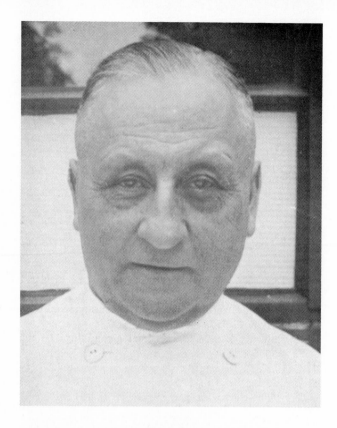

*William F. House*

BORN 1923

Developed and demonstrated
the advantages of transtemporal bone microsurgical removal of early acoustic
neurinomas.

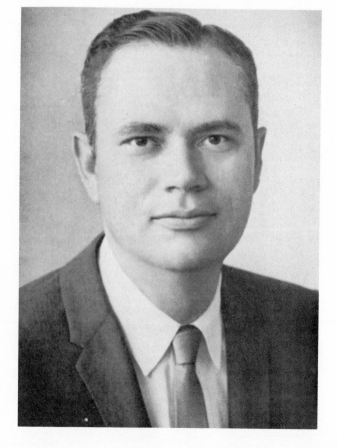

# Chapter 23

# *Acoustic Neuroma and Tumors of the Cerebellopontine Angle*

Tumors Producing the Angle Syndrome
Acoustic Neuroma
    Historical Aspects
    Pathology
    Diagnosis
    Surgical Removal
    Complications
    Results
Meningioma of the Temporal Bone
    Pathology
    Symptoms
    Diagnosis
    Treatment
Congenital Cholesteatoma of the Petrous
    Pyramid
    Pathology
    Symptoms
    Diagnosis
    Treatment

## TUMORS PRODUCING THE ANGLE SYNDROME

Harvey Cushing in his famous monograph "Tumors of the Nervous Acusticus and the Syndrome of the Cerebellopontine Angle"[1] defined the signs and symptoms of lesions of this area. By far, the most frequent lesion is acoustic neuroma. Eighth nerve symptoms appear first, followed by cerebellar, then fifth and seventh nerve involvement, and later the ninth and tenth nerves may be added. Headache, choked disc and diminished vision due to increased intracranial pressure complete the syndrome. Besides acoustic neuroma, the angle syndrome may be caused by meningioma or congenital cholesteatoma of the petrous pyramid, and by cystic arachnoiditis of the cerebellopontine angle.

## ACOUSTIC NEUROMA

### Historical Aspects

Acoustic neuroma (neurinoma, neurilemmoma, Schwannoma), first observed at autopsy in 1777,[2] was clearly described in 1830 in a patient by Charles Bell of Bell's palsy fame. The large tumor in the left cerebellopontine angle had caused total deafness on that side, facial paralysis, temporal and masseter muscle paralysis (fifth nerve), difficulty in speech and swallowing (tenth nerve), severe occipital pain, emaciation and difficulty in breathing (brainstem) leading to death.

At first deemed inoperable because of surgical inaccessibility, an acoustic neuroma was successfully removed for the first time in 1894 by the pioneer otologic and neurologic surgeon Sir Charles Ballance.[3] (The senior author heard a lecture on intracranial complications of cholesteatoma by this eminent neurologic and otologic surgeon in 1930.)

The occasional operations that followed in the next two decades carried an extremely high mortality of around 80 per cent. This was reduced dramatically in Cushing's first report[1] in 1917 to 30 per cent in his first thirty operations, and further to 4 per cent in his 1932 report.[4] Most of these were subtotal removals of tumor tissue from within the capsule, and many later required a second operation for recurrence of symptoms.

Early in the history of surgery for acoustic neuromas, an approach through the labyrinth had been proposed by Panse.[5] This was utilized in 1912 by Quix,[6] chiseling away with mallet and gouge the entire labyrinth through a radical mastoidectomy. Bleeding from the superior petrosal sinus necessitated termination of the operation with completion four days later when the walls of the internal acoustic canal were chiseled away, the carotid artery exposed and the tumor removed. Recurrence of headache after several months suggested regrowth of the tumor. Quix predicted that this translabyrinthine approach brings a small acoustic neuroma within the province of otology. Cushing's warning[4] that "while the otologist doubtless will be the first to recognize and diagnose these cases . . . there is no possible route more dangerous or difficult than this one . . . proposed by Panse" effectively dampened the otologic surgeon's interest in acoustic neuroma removals.

In 1961 William House,[7] using the middle fossa approach to the internal acoustic canal described seven years earlier by Clerc and Battise,[8] successfully removed a small acoustic neuroma. Soon House found the translabyrinthine approach best for all but very small early tumors with hearing worth preserving, and in 1964 he reported forty-seven consecutive translabyrinthine complete or subtotal microsurgical removals without a fatality, a record never before achieved for these common and eventually lethal tumors. The preservation of facial nerve function in the majority, the virtual absence of cerebellar trauma, and the amazingly brief convalescence compared with posterior fossa operations led to the remarkable series of more than a thousand operations for acoustic neuromas of all sizes by House and his associates with extremely low morbidity and mortality rates that have been duplicated by the junior author,[9] Maddox[10] and other followers of House.

House's great interest in acoustic tumors, coupled with his early diagnosis and techniques of surgical removal, has prompted other otologists and neurosurgeons to attempt new procedures. Smith[11] has advocated a microscopic suboccipital approach similar to that proposed by Rand and Kurze[12] for preservation of hearing in acoustic tumors. Several neurosurgeons have developed rather large series of cases using the suboccipital approach and the microscope. Among these are Mallis[13] and

MacCarty;[14] Rhoton[15] has also advocated this technique for preservation of hearing.

While the morbidity and mortality rates with the microsurgical suboccipital approach have improved greatly in the past 10 years, they still exceed those of the translabyrinthine and combined procedures.

If only one statement could be made about the progress made in the last 15 years in the removal of acoustic neuromas, it is that the operating microscope, first used by Nylén and introduced to America by the senior author, has revolutionized neurosurgical and neurotological surgical procedures.

## Pathology

Acoustic neuromas are benign, never malignant, encapsulated tumors that arise from the neurolemmal or Schwann cells of the eighth nerve, twice as often from the vestibular as from the cochlear division.[16] The great pathologist Rudolf Virchow called these neuromas, a name that persists despite agreement that neurilemmoma or Schwannoma is the more correct term. The usual site of origin within the internal auditory canal[17] is where the neurolemmal sheath terminates, the eighth nerve from there to the brainstem being clothed only in neuroglial fibers.

Acoustic neuromas account for 8 per cent of all intracranial tumors and are twice as frequent in women as in men. They are far more frequent than formerly appreciated; a rate as high as 2.4 per cent in the general population is suggested by the finding of six unsuspected small neuromas in the internal auditory canal in two hundred and fifty routine autopsies by Hardy and Crowe.[16]

Histologically, acoustic neuromas are composed of streams of elongated spindle cells with elongated nuclei often arranged in a palisade pattern (Fig. 23–1). Degenerative changes with cyst formation in the center often occur as the tumor

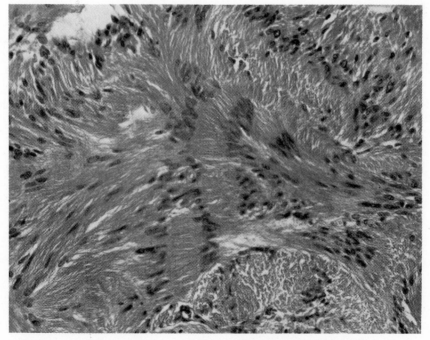

**Figure 23–1**  Typical acoustic neurinoma. (Courtesy of Dr. William House.)

slowly enlarges. For a while the tumor within the internal auditory canal is devoid of symptoms as it slowly fills the cerebrospinal space before it begins to press upon the nerves, artery and vein. Typical symptoms of endolymphatic hydrops can occur from the latter, while pressure on the eighth nerve begins to cause cochlear and vestibular nerve symptoms and impaired function. Slow growth of the tumor causes gradual enlargement of the internal auditory canal. Last of all, pressure on the more resistant motor facial nerve causes facial weakness, but this nerve may be stretched to a thin band on the surface of the tumor without impairment of function.

Protrusion of the slowly enlarging tumor into the cerebellopontine angle causes it to assume a pear shape, with pressure on the fifth nerve, later on the ninth, tenth, eleventh and twelfth nerves, and eventually, if the tumor is not recognized and removed, hydrocephalus, blindness and death due to herniation of the cerebellar tonsils into the foramen magnum.

### Diagnosis

The diagnosis of acoustic tumors is difficult in many cases simply because there is a lack of symptoms. If the tumor starts in the internal auditory canal and grows rapidly in diameter, it will produce tinnitus and hearing loss early in the course of its development. Should the lesion have its origin in the cerebellopontine angle or have an elongated shape, tinnitus and hearing loss might not become evident until the tumor has attained large size. This fact accounts for the continuing problem of large tumors in an era when diagnosis of small tumors has finally become a reality.

The differential diagnosis of an acoustic neuroma includes any peripheral entity that produces a unilateral sensorineural hearing loss with tinnitus, such as Meniere's disease. The next three most common lesions in the cerebellopontine angle are meningiomas, primary cholesteatomas and arachnoid cysts. Any of these lesions may mimic an acoustic tumor, and the true diagnosis may not be established until surgical exploration.

Early diagnosis depends upon a high index of suspicion on the part of the physician who sees any patient with unilateral tinnitus and unilateral hearing loss or both, as well as any form of spatial disorientation such as vertigo or imbalance. The patient presenting with these symptoms should have a basic neurotologic evaluation consisting of a thorough history and physical examination, screening neurological, routine audiometric and vestibular studies as well as plane x-rays of the petrous pyramid. Should the results of any of these studies be suspicious, further special audiometric testing should be performed, and, if indicated, more extensive x-ray studies should be made, such as polytomography, computerized axial tomography (CAT) scan and posterior fossa myelogram. However, no one test is always positive for an acoustic neuroma. The physician must take all the information available to him and put it together like a jigsaw puzzle. Only then will early diagnosis be possible.

### *History*

The typical patient with an acoustic neuroma will experience a unilateral tinnitus followed by hearing loss which progresses very slowly. Seldom does the patient complain of vertigo or imbalance because as the tumor grows it slowly destroys the vestibular function, and the individual has ample time to compensate for the loss of the labyrinth. Some patients complain of mild unsteadiness and a tendency to bump into doorways as they pass through.

## Physical

The routine head and neck physical examination is seldom abnormal, even in the presence of large cerebellopontine angle tumors.

## Neurological Screening

A neurological screening refers to a quick check of the cranial nerves while the examining physician is completing the routine head and neck physical. In tumors 2.5 cm. and larger the corneal reflex may be diminished and there may as well be a decrease in the sensation of touch on the involved side of the face. While the 5th nerve is frequently involved in larger tumors, the motor 7th is seldom weak or paralyzed by the tumor but the more vulnerable sensory fibers to the posterior meatal wall can be affected. It is unusual to have any cranial nerves involved other than the 5th or 7th; however, extremely large tumors extending deep in the posterior fossa may affect the 9th, 10th, 11th and 12th nerves.

## Audiometric Studies

Audiometric studies are the crux of early diagnosis because most often the initial audiogram is what catches the examining physician's attention and makes him suspicious of an acoustic tumor. All otologic patients receive a pure-tone air and bone conduction audiogram and speech audiometry. If the involved ear has a marked high-tone sensorineural hearing loss or if the speech discrimination score is out of proportion to the pure-tone level, then this patient is a prime suspect for having a tumor. It must be emphasized, however, that the authors have seen patients with low-tone and flat sensorineural losses who had tumors. An occasional patient will be seen who has normal hearing with a 100 per cent discrimination score but a 4 to 5 cm. cerebellopontine angle lesion.

When the patient with a suspicious audiogram is seen, there are numerous special audiometric tests to aid the audiologist and otologist in determining the presence of a tumor. One that was in vogue for several years was the Jerger classification[18] of the Békésy tracings. This test as traditionally administered has been replaced in recent years by more valuable audiometric studies.

One of the most practical and useful of these is the modified tone decay test of Carhart.[19] When there is decay in excess of 30 dB, one must suspect a retrocochlear lesion. The alternate binaural loudness balance (ABLB)[20] and small increment sensitivity index (SISI)[21] tests are useful in establishing that a hearing loss is cochlear rather than retrocochlear. These tests are helpful but cannot be relied upon as absolute proof of whether a tumor is present or not.

Brief-tone audiometry,[22] distorted speech, and other special tests have some usefulness in distinguishing cochlear from retrocochlear hearing loss but are probably more suited to a training situation than to a clinical practice.

One of the newer and extremely valuable audiometric studies is the stapedial reflex decay test. By means of an impedance bridge the stapedial reflex is elicited at suprathreshold level and a decay to half-amplitude in five seconds or less is suggestive of retrocochlear pathology. Current investigations indicate that this test is more sensitive than the preceding tests for retrocochlear pathology.

Of all the new audiometric evaluations that have become available to the audiologist in the last few years, one of the most sensitive is brainstem evoked response audiometry. This computerized hearing test has an accuracy rate of better than 90 per cent for the diagnosis of acoustic tumors. These results have been confirmed in at least two separate series of cases in different sections of the country.[23, 24]

This test is of such value that it deserves to be discussed in some detail. The study can be performed with the patient awake or asleep. It makes no difference, as this is a completely objective study of the 8th nerve and central auditory pathways and does not require patient cooperation. A vertex electrode picks up the averaged electrical response produced by a large series of clicks in the ear being tested as the response passes through the 8th nerve and the central pathways toward the auditory cortex. These responses are in microvolts and are numerous. The apparatus contains an averaging computer that looks at 1000 of these responses and then produces a characteristic wave form on an oscilloscope. These waves are labeled I through V and are believed to occur at different levels in the brainstem. In the diagnosis of acoustic neuromas, the important wave form to observe is number V and I to V conduction.

The main drawback of the test is that the patient must have no greater than a severe loss for the click else the test will be of limited value. Another interesting sidelight seems to be that this test is almost specific for acoustic tumors and may not be as accurate for meningioma and primary cholesteatoma of the cerebellopontine angle.[23]

Not only is brainstem evoked response audiometry of invaluable help in the diagnosis of acoustic tumors, but it appears that it is going to be very beneficial in determining other lesions involving the brainstem, such as multiple sclerosis, intrinsic brainstem tumors and vascular infarcts.

### Vestibular Studies

It is important to know if the vestibular nerve is functioning in an ear with a sensorineural hearing loss. The reason for this is that one is more suspicious of neuroma in a unilateral sensorineural loss if there is a markedly reduced vestibular response on the same side — particularly if the patient does not complain of vertigo, indicating a slowly progressive loss of vestibular function.

For practical purposes an ice-water caloric test will determine the presence or absence of vestibular function. This can be performed in a number of ways, the objective being to stimulate the semicircular canals. One method has been described by Linthicum[25] in which a small amount of ice-water is left in the external auditory canal for 20 seconds. The small amount of fluid (0.2 to 0.8 cc.) does not make the patient vertiginous or sick by too strong a stimulus to a normal ear.

A more sophisticated method of determining vestibular function and one that is more widely used is electronystagmography (ENG).[26] This method has many advantages over the standard caloric study. In the routine ENG a bithermal caloric response is obtained after the technique of Hallpike and Cairns.[27] In addition, optokinetic nystagmus, pendular tracking and gaze nystagmus are elicited and recorded. Spontaneous and positional nystagmus can be detected as well, and all the recorded information can be kept in the patient's chart for further comparison with subsequent tests. Many times in large tumors, central findings are picked up on eye tracking and there may be spontaneous nystagmus present by ENG that could not be elicited with Frenzel lenses or the naked eye.

### X-ray Studies

While audiometric and vestibular testing make the physician suspicious of an acoustic tumor, it is by x-ray that he makes the definitive diagnosis.

*Plane Films.*   To obtain adequate views of the internal auditory canal in the confines of the petrous pyramid, it is essential to have a special head unit such as the Compere[28] or Franklin. Several views should be made and should consist of a right and left stereoscopic Stenvers, a Chamberlain-Town, transorbital, base view and lateral view of the skull. Figure 23–2*A* and *B* demonstrates an enlargement of the right canal as compared with the left. The accuracy of well-made plane films of the internal auditory canal is approximately 90 per cent. These are of tremendous value as a

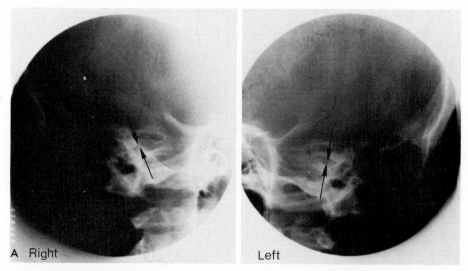

**Figure 23–2A**   Stenvers x-ray view showing right IAC markedly enlarged.

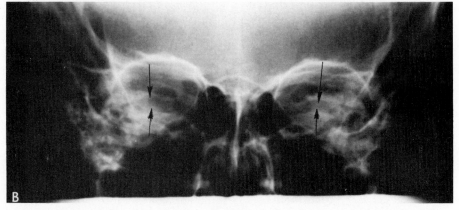

**Figure 23–2B**   Transorbital x-ray view showing right IAC to be enlarged.

screening device, and every otolaryngologist should have one of these head units in his office. There is no substitute for reading your own x-rays of the internal auditory canal.

What is considered a significant difference between sides? The junior author feels as little as 1 mm. difference in the two sides is important if the larger one is associated with a unilateral sensorineural hearing loss, tinnitus and a reduced vestibular response. In most instances of acoustic tumor there is definite enlargement of the canal.

*Polytome X-rays.*    The polytome x-ray plays a major role in the diagnosis of any lesion of the temporal bone. Because of the blurring effect of the planogram, polytome cuts of 1 mm. can be made through the temporal bone, demonstrating with extreme clarity all the structures hidden within. In most patients the plane views are adequate to visualize the internal auditory canal, and polytomes are simply not necessary. The one exception to this statement is the individual who has an extremely pneumatized petrous apex. In such a case, the internal auditory canal is lost in the complexity of the air cell system and cannot be well demonstrated with the best head unit available. Fortunately, the polytome will show the canal beautifully in this situation, as it can effectively block out the offending air cells.

The polytome has been used effectively with Pantopaque solution[29] to demonstrate filling defects at the porous acousticus. Known as the polytome Pantopaque study, this particular method has yet to gain widespread use outside of the Los Angeles area.

For this examination 2 cc. of Pantopaque are instilled by lumbar puncture into the subarachnoid space. The spinal needle is withdrawn and the patient positioned without the aid of a fluoroscope in such a manner that the dye gravitates toward and into the internal auditory canal. If a tumor is present, the dye does not enter the canal but outlines the filling defect caused by the tumor.

*Computerized Axial Tomography.*    The newest addition to the diagnostic armamentarium for acoustic tumors is the computerized axial tomography (CAT) scan.[30] This study is performed by placing the patient's head in a circular holder with a built-in waterbath to protect the patient from heat buildup. Multiple x-rays of the head are made, and a computer averages the responses. Extreme detail can be obtained, and it is almost as if the examiner were able to look through the top of the skull at the brain. Figure 23–3 delineates a 3 to 4 cm. cerebellopontine angle lesion. Particularly in posterior fossa studies, it is important that the lesion be enhanced with a bolus of intravenous iodine-based dye. In fact, many tumors will not be demonstrated on the CAT scan without enhancement. This does limit the usefulness of the study in those individuals who are allergic to iodine.

Tumors under 2 cm. are not well shown by CAT scan, and if the physician is suspicious that a tumor is present, a posterior fossa myelogram must be performed. If the CAT scan is positive, it is not necessary to order a myelogram. If both studies are to be requested at the same time, it is important to perform the scan prior to the myelogram, as the Pantopaque creates "hot spots" on the scan, making it impossible to read accurately.

New generation scanners are being produced on a regular basis, and as the neuroradiologists gain more experience with them, we will be able to learn a great deal more from them. One example is the recent use of coronal sections through the petrous pyramid bone itself. These views very clearly demonstrate an enlargement of the internal auditory canal.

*Posterior Fossa Myelogram.*    This is the standard method of determining the

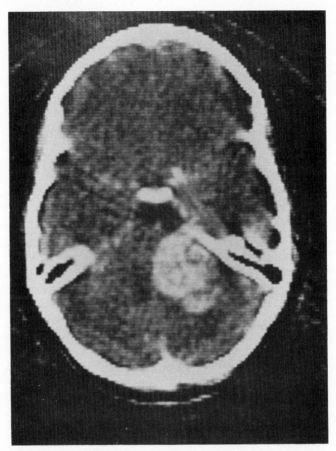

**Figure 23–3**  Abnormal CAT scan.

presence of a small acoustic neuroma and has stood the test of time. Most radiologists perform this study in the hospital under fluoroscopic guidance.[31] Gardner[32] has devised a method of performing this study in his office using a standard Compere unit. The individual is managed as an out-patient and is not admitted to the hospital.

As an in-patient test, the patient is placed on a tilting x-ray table and a lumbar puncture is performed. CSF is withdrawn and sent to the laboratory for the determination of spinal fluid protein. Large tumors usually increase the protein content of the CSF, but small and medium-sized lesions have little effect. Once the Pantopaque has been instilled into the subarachnoid space (2–6 cc.), the patient is tilted head down, and the dye is followed into the posterior fossa under fluoroscopic guidance. By shaking the head vigorously and positioning the ear under test in a dependent attitude, dye enters the normal internal auditory canal (Fig. 23–4) but creates a filling defect on the side with the tumor (Figs. 23–5 and 23–6). The dye is removed and the patient kept at bed rest for eight hours.

Most individuals can go home the following morning, but about 5 per cent complain of headache or a sore back and are kept in the hospital for a few days. On rare occasions (less than 1 per cent) an individual may develop a chemical meningitis due to the Pantopaque that requires the use of steroids.

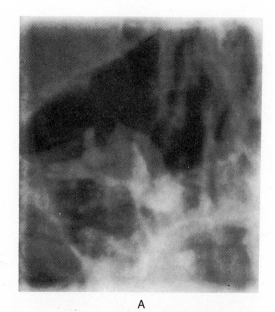

**Figure 23–4**  *A* and *B*, Normal opaque cerebellopontine cisternogram showing complete filling of the internal auditory canal. Note the well defined crista separating the superior and inferior compartments of the fundus of the canal. (Courtesy of Dr. G. Valvassori.)

### Surgical Removal

There are four popular microsurgical approaches for the removal of acoustic tumors. These are the middle fossa, translabyrinthine, combined one-stage translabyrinthine–suboccipital, and the suboccipital. Most neurosurgeons utilize the suboccipital route for all lesions, while neurotologists tend to pick a procedure based upon the size of the tumor. Thus, in the junior author's series of well over 200 cases, small tumors (up to 1.5 cm.) have been removed through the middle fossa if

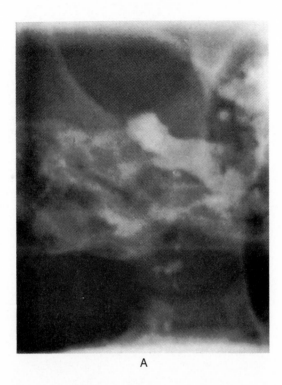

A

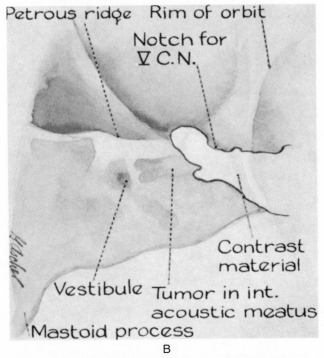

B

**Figure 23–5** *A* and *B*, Opaque cisternogram showing a small tumor filling the internal auditory canal to the porus. The neurinoma was removed by the translabyrinthine approach without neurologic defect. (Courtesy of Dr. J. Clemis.)

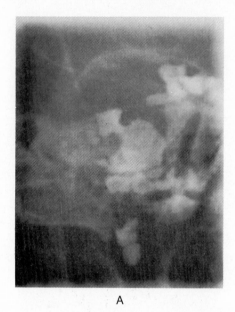

A

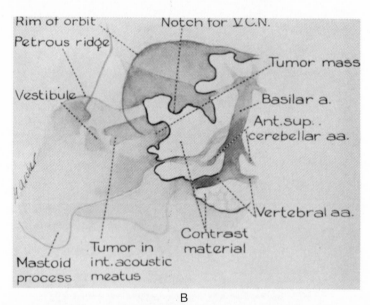

B

**Figure 23–6** *A* and *B*, Opaque cisternogram of a larger but still small tumor filling the internal auditory canal and protruding 1 cm. into the cerebellopontine cistern. Translabyrinthine removal resulted in immediate facial paresis, with recovery beginning after 2 months. (Courtesy of Dr. J. Clemis.)

the hearing was normal; medium-sized lesions (1.5 cm. to 4 cm.) through the translabyrinthine approach; and large tumors (over 4 cm.) through a combined approach.

### Middle Fossa Approach

This procedure is employed when there is normal or near normal hearing in the involved ear and the tumor is confined to the internal auditory canal or just protruding from it. In bilateral cases with von Recklinghausen's disease the indications will be stretched to include those tumors measuring 1.5 cm. outside the internal auditory canal.

The initial surgical technique is the same as described in Chapters 20 and 21. There are some major differences once the internal auditory canal has been exposed. After the superior semicircular canal blue line has been obtained and the facial nerve followed into the canal, all of the bone overlying the canal must be removed with a diamond burr. This exposes the underlying tumor. At this point, Mannitol (500 cc. of 20 per cent) is given intravenously to shrink the brain. The superior petrosal sinus is identified and opened. Surgical packing is rapidly placed in the proximal and distal segments of the sinus to control hemorrhage. Next, the blade of the self-retaining House-Urban retractor is pushed down into the posterior fossa. Care must be taken to locate the petrosal vein as it enters the superior sinus so that it can be cauterized with the bipolar tips. Pressure is exerted on the temporal lobe by the retractor to obtain more working room. Cottonoids are used to isolate the tumor and then the dura of the internal auditory canal is incised along its posterior border (Fig. 23–7). The facial nerve, Bill's bar and the superior vestibular nerve are identified, and the superior vestibular nerve is avulsed just as one would do in a middle fossa section. The tumor is carefully dissected free of the facial and cochlear nerves. Usually the inferior vestibular nerve is involved with the tumor and comes out automatically. Once out of the internal auditory canal, the stalk of the vestibular nerve is located and sectioned with a pair of sharp microscissors. This leaves the cochlear and facial nerves exposed and intact. A muscle plug is placed over the internal auditory canal,

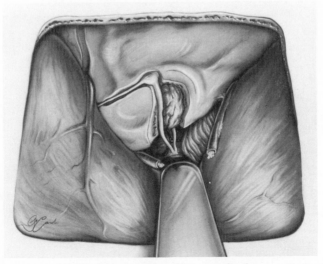

**Figure 23–7**   Middle fossa exposure of intracanalicular acoustic tumor.

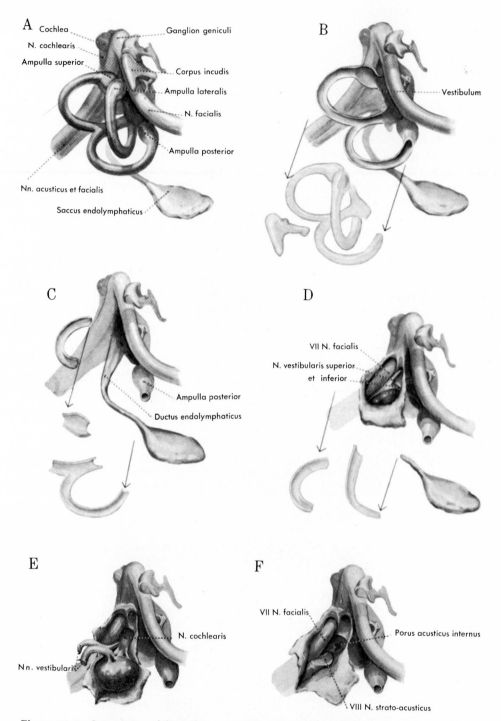

**Figure 23–8**   Steps in translabyrinthine exposure of internal acoustic meatus for a small tumor, showing structures that need to be removed. *A*, Anatomic relationships. *B*, Removal of the incus and semicircular canals. *C*, Exposure of the endolymphatic sac and duct. *D*, Dura of the internal acoustic meatus opened. *E*, Exposed tumor partially removed. *F*, After removal.

and the temporal lobe is allowed to expand. The patient is observed overnight in the recovery room and undergoes routine craniotomy checks.

### Translabyrinthine Approach

This procedure can be used for all tumors of the cerebellopontine angle, but the junior author prefers to limit it to tumors under 3 to 4 cm. (Figs. 23–8 and 23–9).

A standard postauricular incision is used (Fig. 23–10A). The edges of the wound are held open by a retractor, and a simple mastoidectomy is performed, exposing the middle and posterior fossa dural plates, the sinodural angle, sigmoid sinus, antrum and digastric ridge (Fig. 23–10B). Next, the vertical course of the facial nerve is identified and the facial recess opened (Fig. 23–10C and D). The incudo-stapedial joint is separated and the incus removed and placed in the bone bank. The anterior attic is opened and the head of the malleus removed. This is pushed into the

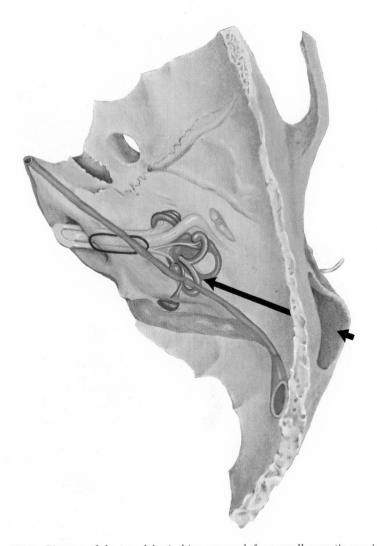

**Figure 23–9** Diagram of the translabyrinthine approach for a small acoustic neurinoma.

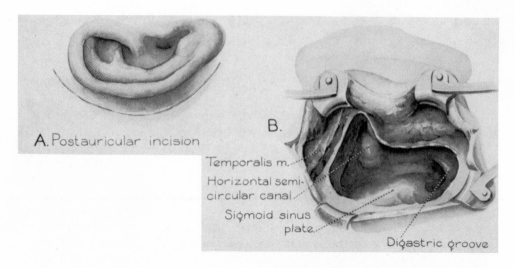

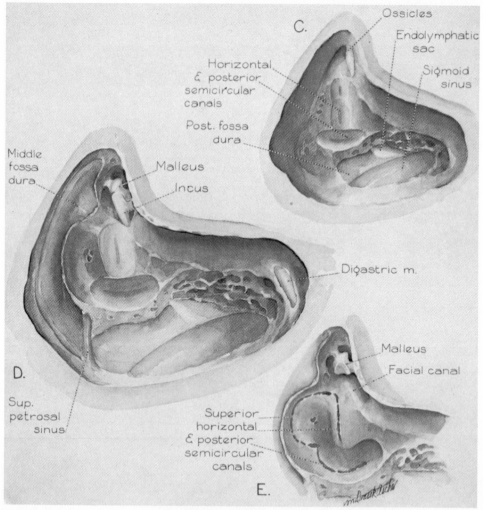

**Figure 23–10**   Translabyrinthine removal of acoustic neurinoma. *A*, Postauricular incision. *B*, Mastoidectomy. *C*, Gray lines of horizontal and posterior semicircular canals; endolymphatic sac and dura exposed. *D*, Further definition of semicircular canals and dural exposure. *E*, Semicircular canals partly opened. (Continued on the opposite page.)

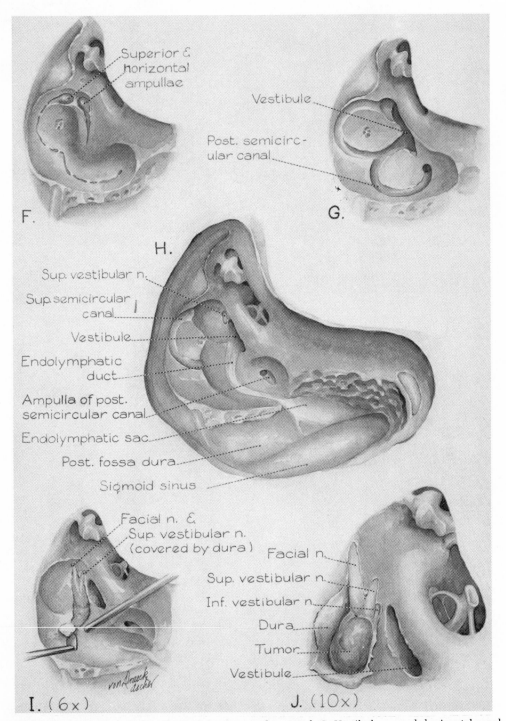

**Figure 23–10** *(Continued)*  F, Semicircular canals opened. G, Vestibule opened; horizontal canal removed. H, Posterior canal removed; endolymphatic sac and duct exposed; superior vestibular nerve uncovered. I, Exposure of the petrous portion of the facial nerve. J, Internal acoustic meatus opened. (Continued on page 654.)

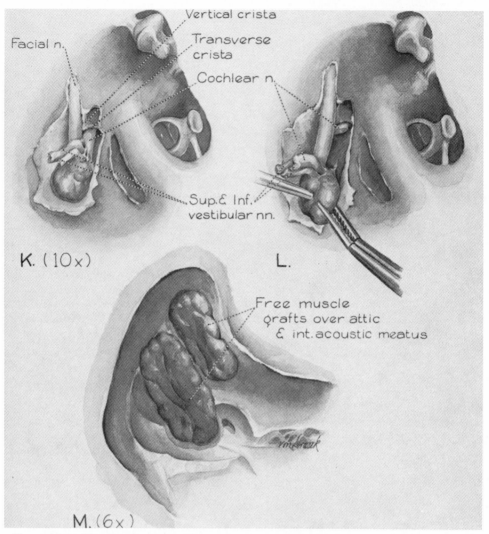

**Figure 23–10** *(Continued)*   *K,* Vestibular nerves sectioned; cochlear nerve exposed. *L,* Cochlear nerve sectioned; removal of tumor. *M,* Attic and internal acoustic meatus sealed by free muscle grafts.

eustachian tube orifice, and the middle ear is filled with small pieces of temporalis muscle.

Using a cutting burr and irrigation suction, the three semicircular canals are systematically removed, starting with the horizontal, moving to the posterior, and following that, to the common crus and then to the superior (Fig. 23–10E). Once the canals have been drilled away, the bone from the superior, inferior and posterior aspects of the internal auditory canal is removed, exposing its dura (fig. 23–10I). Bone is now removed from the middle and posterior fossa dura and sigmoid sinus. It is important to carry this bone removal back behind the sinus in order that it may be retracted for better exposure. A bipolar cautery is used to coagulate and shrink the sinus. This improves the view and gives better access to the cerebellopontine angle.

An incision is made in the posterior fossa dura with a No. 11 Bard Parker knife blade, and a cottonoid strip is placed against the cerebellum. Microscissors are used to cut away the dura, exposing the cerebellum and the angle. Telfa strips are placed over the cerebellum to protect it, and the tumor is isolated by cottonoids. Small tumors are removed at this point without reducing them in size (Fig. 23–10L). Lesions over 1.5 cm. require reduction before they can be extracted. To do this, the capsule is incised, and a cup forceps is used to gut the interior. The capsule is gently pulled toward the center of the field, being careful to cauterize (bipolar) all blood vessels that are attached to it. Cottonoids are used to protect the brainstem as the capsule is carefully dissected free. Once the tumor mass has been reduced to approximately 1 to 1.5 cm., the tumor is removed *in toto*. To accomplish this, the surgeon directs his attention to the most lateral extent of the internal auditory canal where he identifies Bill's bar and avulses the superior vestibular nerve with the tumor (Fig. 23–10K). This exposes the facial nerve anteriorly. A right-angle hook is placed into the inferior quadrant of the canal, and the inferior vestibular and cochlear nerves are avulsed.

The tumor is removed from the canal, dissecting it away from the facial nerve. The facial nerve is followed to the brainstem where the 8th nerve is located and severed. The tumor mass is extracted in one piece at this time. Copious amounts of irrigating solution (Tis-U-Sol) are used to wash clean the cerebellopontine angle and to determine if there is any bleeding. All cottonoids and Telfa are removed from the wound. Once the hemorrhage has been controlled with a bipolar cautery, a large piece of Gelfoam is placed over the cerebellum, and fascia lata is draped over the dural defect. (The fascia lata along with the adipose tissue was taken at the beginning of the operation from the lateral aspect of the thigh.) The wound is filled with fat or muscle and then closed in layers; the skin is approximated with a

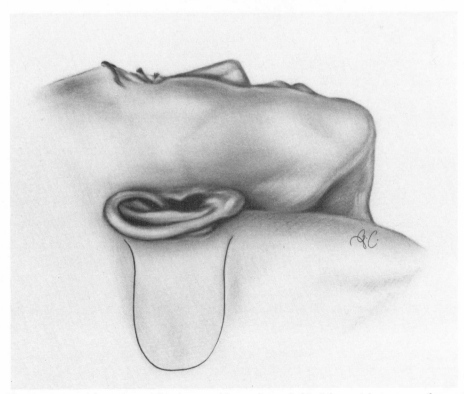

**Figure 23–11**   A large (6 cm.) flap is created in two layers behind the auricle to expose the mastoid and suboccipital area.

running, interlocking, subcutaneous suture, employing Dixon R #3. A bulky dressing is applied, and the patient is observed in the recovery room overnight and undergoes routine craniotomy checks.

### One-Stage Combined Translabyrinthine-Suboccipital Approach

This procedure is used by the junior author for tumors over 3 to 4 cm. A larger postauricular flap is created (Fig. 23–11) in order to expose the occipital bone. This flap is retracted forward and held in place by dural hooks. A complete translabyrinthine dissection is carried out as described previously (Fig. 23–12). Next, bone is removed from behind the sigmoid sinus for approximately 4 cm. (Fig. 23–13) as 500 cc. of 20 per cent Mannitol is given intravenously. At this point the dura over the cerebellum is incised and retracted with stay sutures. Telfa strips are placed over the cerebellum and a Janetta posterior fossa retractor is inserted to gently retract the cerebellum. Once this has been accomplished and the tumor isolated with cotton-oids, the mass is gutted (Fig. 23–14). The capsule is cut away as the size decreases. All blood vessels entering the tumor are cauterized with the bipolar cautery. At the

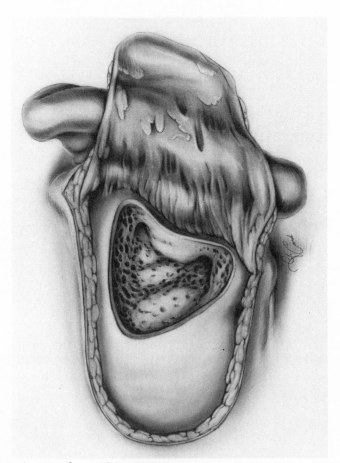

**Figure 23–12**  A cutting burr and irrigation/suction are used to perform a simple mastoidectomy, exposing the middle and posterior fossa dura, labyrinth, and sinodural angle.

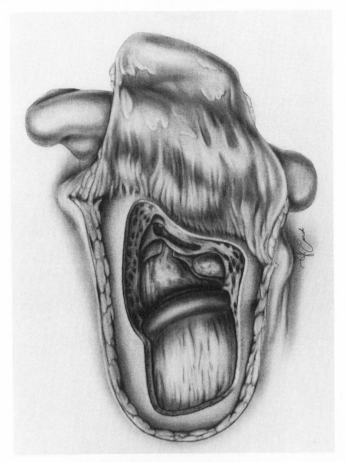

**Figure 23–13** Bone is removed from the suboccipital area for approximately 4 cm. posterior to the sigmoid sinus, allowing the surgeon access to the posterior portion of the tumor.

brainstem the capsule is carefully dissected free and cottonoids are placed on the stem to protect it. The tumor is reduced in size to approximately 2 cm. At this point the remainder of the surgery is performed through the translabyrinthine route as just described (Figs. 23–15, 23–16, 23–17, 23–18 and 23–19). Fascia lata and fat are used in the mastoid cavity, and the dura over the cerebellum is closed with 3–0 silk. The flap is approximated in a routine manner, and the patient is observed in the recovery room overnight.

### Suboccipital Approach

The unilateral suboccipital approach to the cerebellopontine angle was first advocated by Dandy[33] and has been the standard neurosurgical procedure since. In recent years, the microscope has been incorporated on a routine basis and the technique improved upon by removal of the posterior lip of the internal auditory canal for identification and preservation of the facial and occasionally cochlear nerves (Fig. 23–20).

This procedure is performed with the patient supine, prone or seated. There are

*Text continued on page 666.*

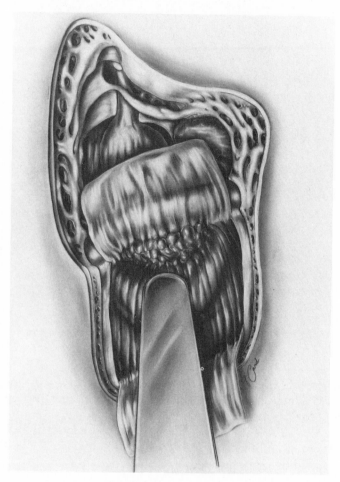

**Figure 23–14**  Note that the Heifetz retractor exposes the tumor without excessive tension on the cerebellum.

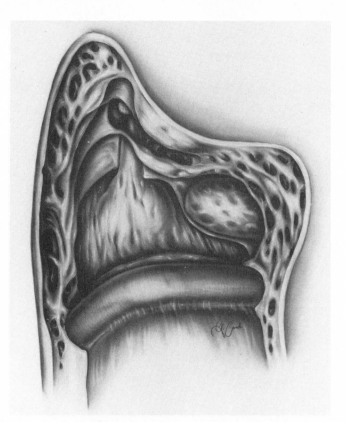

**Figure 23–15** Once the tumor has been reduced in size the table is rotated back toward the surgeon and the posterior fossa dura is opened. In this illustration the dura has not yet been excised.

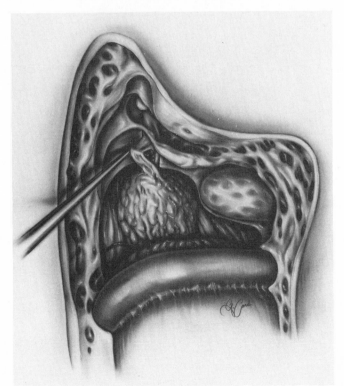

**Figure 23–16** The superior vestibular nerve is avulsed from its canal, exposing the facial nerve anterior to Bill's bar.

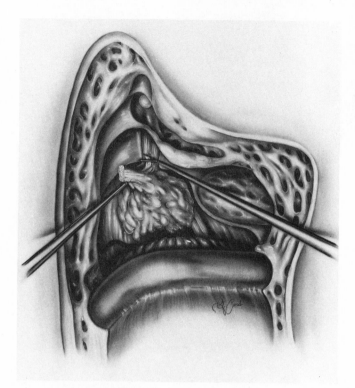

**Figure 23–17**   The tumor is removed from the facial nerve by blunt dissection.

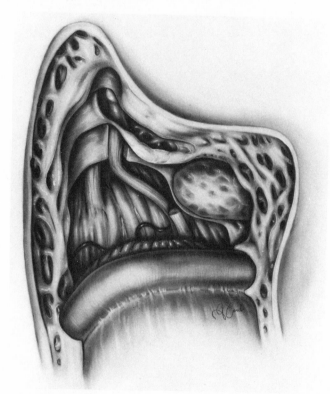

**Figure 23–18**   Note the excellent view of the CPA (cerebello-pontine angle) obtained through the translabyrinthine route. The facial and trigeminal nerves can be seen lying in the angle.

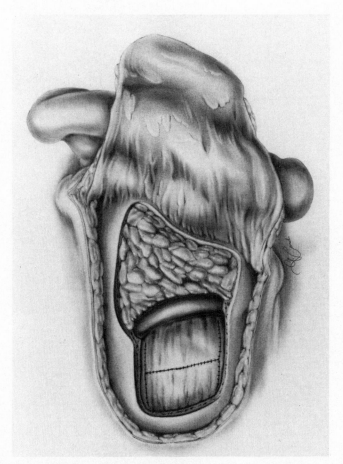

**Figure 23–19**  Fat is placed in the mastoid cavity, and the dura is closed with interrupted sutures.

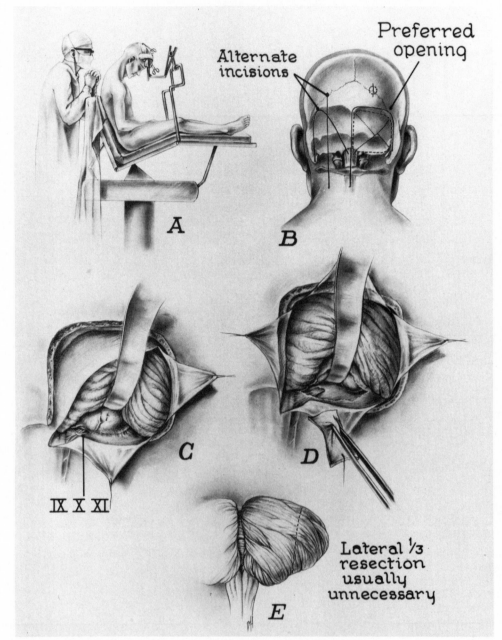

**Figure 23–20**   Suboccipital approach for a large acoustic neuroma. *A*, The patient is operated upon in the seated position. *B*, The incision may be midline or midway between the midline and the auricle. *C*, By lifting the cerebellum the surgeon can identify cranial nerves IX, X and XI. *D* and *E*, The cerebellum is retracted, or one-third of its lateral aspect is removed to expose the tumor lying in the cerebellopontine angle. (Continued on the opposite page.)

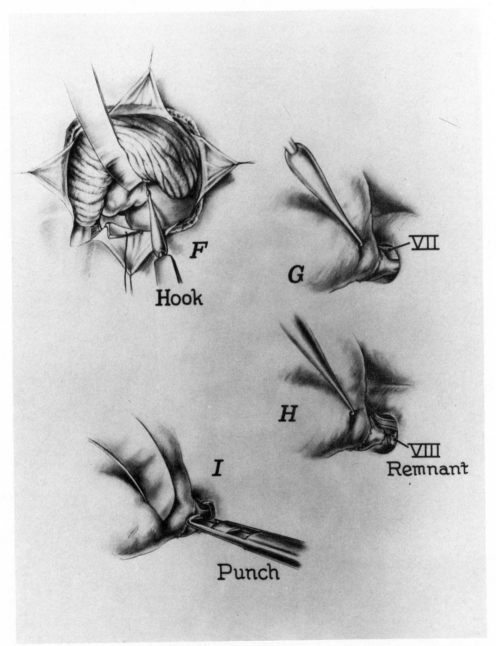

**Figure 23–20** *(Continued)*    *F,* A hook is used to rotate the tumor away from the petrous apex to expose the internal auditory canal from behind. *G,* Note the VII nerve lying anterior to stattico-acoustic nerve. *H,* The VIII nerve is identified leaving the tumor. *I,* With a punch the posterior lip of the internal auditory canal is removed to further identify the VII cranial nerve. (Continued on page 664.)

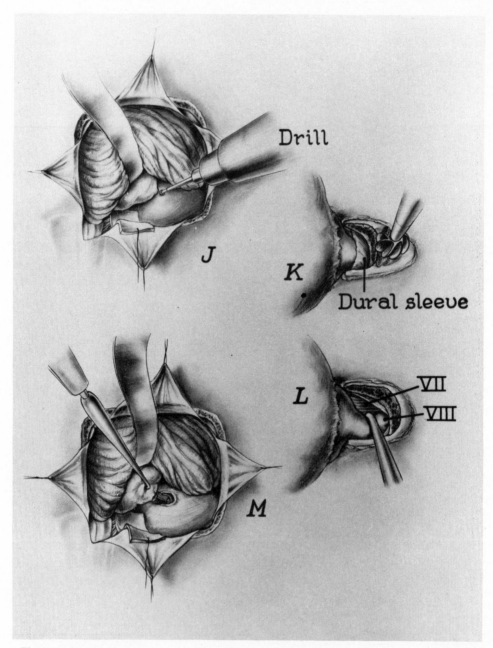

**Figure 23–20** *(Continued)*   *J,* A rotating drill is employed to carry the dissection more laterally to identify the VII nerve in the lateral aspect of the IAC. *K, L,* and *M,* Once the lateral aspect of the IAC has been uncovered, the tumor is carefully stripped away from the VII nerve until it is free of the temporal bone. (Continued on opposite page.)

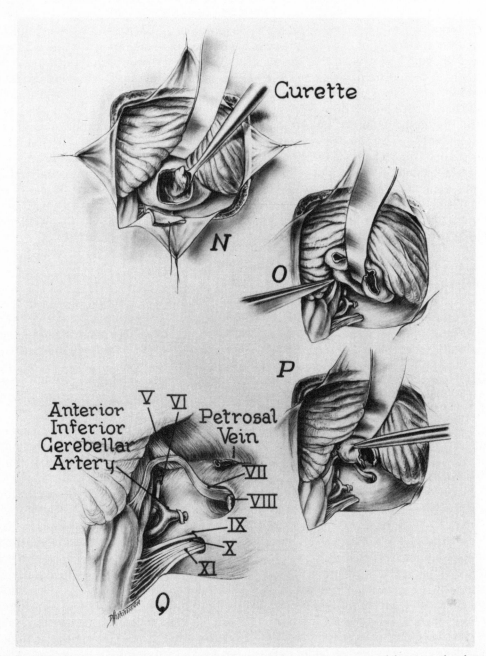

**Figure 23–20** *(Continued)*   N, A curet or forceps is used to gut the contents of the tumor thereby reducing it in size. O and P, The capsule is dissected away from the brainstem and VII nerve. Q, Note the exposed cerebellopontine angle with a complete removal of the neuroma. The VII nerve can be seen lying intact across the angle and entering the IAC. The VIII nerve has been removed with the tumor. Cranial nerves IX, X, XI and XII are intact and uninjured.

numerous disadvantages to the seated position (air embolism, lumbar disc rupture and so on), and most neurosurgeons are using it less often.

A large suboccipital flap is created, and the occipital bone overlying the cerebellum is removed, exposing the underlying dura. This is incised and held back by stay sutures. The cerebellum is retracted to expose the cerebellopontine angle. The tumor capsule is opened and the mass gutted as in the previous descriptions if the lesion is large. If it is small, the tumor is simply dissected free of the facial nerve and removed. The exposure of the facial nerve from this approach requires that the dura over the posterior portion of the petrous apex be removed. A diamond burr is used to remove the posterior lip of the canal. This dissection must be taken as far laterally as possible. At this point the tumor is pulled away from the facial nerve and carefully dissected free of this structure. The nerve is followed into the angle much as one would using the translabyrinthine route at this point in the operation. The major disadvanatage of this approach to the facial nerve is that the surgeon does not have the benefit of the bony landmark of Bill's bar and the dissection is very deep, requiring extra-long instruments.

Once the tumor has been removed and the cerebellopontine angle is free of bleeding, the dura is closed and the flap is approximated in layers. The patient is observed in the recovery room overnight in the usual manner.


## Complications

Complications in acoustic neuroma surgery depend upon the size of the tumor and the approach used. Obviously, large lesions carry a higher incidence of morbidity and mortality than smaller ones (a good argument for early diagnosis).

In the immediate postoperative period, hemorrhage is a serious complication that must be immediately controlled. This may require opening the wound and evacuating the blood clot in the recovery room. Such a patient must be returned to the operating suite for definitive management of the bleeding.

A second emergency complication is cerebral edema in the immediate postoperative period. These individuals must be returned to surgery as well, and an attempt made to bring the situation under control. Removal of infarcted cerebellar brain tissue is often required.

Loss of facial nerve function is considered a complication and occurs most often with large tumors. The junior author feels that the surgical approach has a lot to do with preservation of the facial nerve. The literature would tend to support this contention, as the suboccipital advocates cannot preserve the nerve as often as those using the translabyrinthine approaches. There are certain cases, of course, when it is simply impossible to preserve the nerve by any approach. Often it will literally be incorporated into the capsule so firmly that it cannot be separated. One must remember that the prime goal of acoustic tumor surgery is to remove the tumor totally and save the patient's life. While an attempt should be made to save the facial nerve, prolonged surgery should not be carried out, endangering the patient's well-being just to save the facial nerve.

Cerebrospinal fluid leak has been a particular problem with the translabyrinthine procedures, but in recent years the overall incidence has decreased. Packing the middle ear with muscle and the use of adipose tissue to fill the mastoid have improved this problem considerably.

Though not as frequent, leaks can occur with the suboccipital route as well, particularly in an individual who has a well pneumatized petrous apex.

These operative procedures can be quite lengthy, exposing the wound to air for long periods of time. This, coupled with spinal fluid leaks, accounts for the incidence of meningitis associated with this type of surgery.

Prolonged retraction or removal of the lateral hemisphere of the cerebellum (more common with the suboccipital approach) or both result in postoperative ataxia and other cerebellar signs such as tremors and dysmetria.

The ultimate complication is death. Mortality rates are much higher in large tumors and have to do mostly with their blood supply, which they share with the brainstem. The anterior cerebellar artery has been shown to be the key to survival. If this artery can be avoided, most likely the patient will survive. On occasion, just touching the vessel will put it into spasm resulting in brainstem infarction.

Hemiparesis, while rare, is a possible complication of this surgery. Subtotal removal in a young individual must be regarded as a complication, as recurrence is certain to occur requiring future further surgery or causing death, or both. All tumor removals should be total if at all possible. The exception, of course, is the older patient in poor health who is undergoing tumor removal for prolongation of life.

When attempting to preserve hearing through the middle fossa or suboccipital approaches, failure to do so should be considered a complication of that particular operation.

## Results

From the days of Sir Charles Ballance to the present time, the mortality rate for acoustic tumor surgery has been lowered from 80 per cent to less than 5 per cent. Several factors are responsible for this. The general supportive care of the patient in the operating suite, improved general anesthesia, antibiotics and so on have obviously been important. Improved instrumentation and particularly microsurgical technique have proved invaluable. And finally, the one single factor that has been most influential is the dedicated work of William House in the development of early detection and a general awareness of the problem as well as his contributions of new and improved surgical techniques. When future historians review the twentieth century, they will note that the three giants of acoustic neuroma diagnosis and surgery were Harvey Cushing, Walter Dandy and William House.

While the overall results of the suboccipital and translabyrinthine procedures have improved in the last 15 years, the temporal bone approaches would appear to have an edge according to the literature.

House's most recent reports[34] indicate that he has been able to reduce his subtotal removals to less than 10 per cent. He has always been able to preserve the facial nerve better than 90 per cent of the time. Morbidity and mortality by the translabyrinthine technique have been lowered to about 2 per cent for small tumors and less than 10 per cent for large ones.

In reviewing the work of others who use the translabyrinthine approaches,[9, 10] these results have been equaled. This confirms the fact that the procedure can be standardized.

By the use of microsurgical technique the neurosurgeons have improved their results. Thomsen[35] in 125 tumors was able to obtain total removal in 75 per cent and preserved the facial nerve in 35 per cent. His overall mortality was 22 per cent until he adopted the microscope, which allowed him to drop the rate to 13 per cent.

Rand[12] reported 31 cases with 93 per cent total removal and a 2 per cent mortality rate. McCarty[14] reviewed 132 cases and reported 82 per cent total removal with 5 per cent mortality. He preserved the facial nerve 53 per cent of the time. Rhoton[15] reported 24 tumors with preservation of the facial nerve in 83 per cent of the cases. No mention was made of total removals or mortality rate. Smith et al.[11] probably have the best suboccipital results in that out of 15 tumors they were able to remove 93 per cent totally and preserve the facial nerve in 80 per cent. Their mortality rate was 6 per cent.

Based upon the literature and the junior author's experience in well over 200 acoustic tumors, the translabyrinthine and combined approaches should be considered the standard by which all others are judged.

For results to be improved and complications reduced, a concerted effort must be made to diagnose these lesions early in their development when they are small.

## MENINGIOMA OF THE TEMPORAL BONE

Meningioma is a non-metastasizing but often locally invasive tumor that arises from the endothelial lining cells of the arachnoid villi found in the walls of the cranial venous sinuses and their tributary veins. Although meningiomas comprise 19 per cent of all brain tumors, only about 7 per cent of meningiomas arise from the petrous pyramid, about equally from its middle fossa surface and its posterior surface.[35] Occasionally a meningioma begins within the internal acoustic meatus, and rarely it arises in the middle ear, where arachnoid villi cells can be demonstrated at the geniculate ganglion and in the roof of the eustachian tube.[35]

### Pathology

Meningiomas arising from the internal surface of the temporal bone are generally of the ovoid, well circumscribed type, appearing as a firm dense tumor in the dura without a capsule. Less common is the flat plaque-like variety that grows carpet-like with little elevation above the dural surface, enveloping and infiltrating nerves and underlying bone.

Histologically meningiomas consist of masses of endothelial cells with large uniform nuclei occurring in whorls. Typical of these tumors are circular psammoma bodies consisting of concentric layers of hyalinization and calcification (Fig. 23–21). As a rule these tumors are quite vascular, and the histologic structure may be fibromatous or angiomatous.

### Symptoms

Meningiomas produce symptoms by involvement of adjacent nerves and by pressure on brain tissue. Those tumors that arise from the middle fossa surface of the petrous pyramid cause fifth nerve symptoms with facial or eye pain and sensory and motor changes of fifth nerve distribution, with convulsions, uncinate attacks and sensory or motor aphasia. These patients rarely consult the otolaryngologist.

Meningiomas arising from the posterior surface of the petrous pyramid produce the cerebellopontine angle syndrome resembling the clinical picture of acoustic neurinoma. When the tumor arises within the internal acoustic meatus, the symptoms are indistinguishable from acoustic neurinoma, but more often it begins outside the meatus and involves other adjacent cranial nerves and the cerebellum earlier than the eighth nerve. The greater tendency of meningioma to infiltrate bone causes invasion of the middle ear, and when they are first seen half the patients with meningioma of petrous origin have chronic otorrhea in addition to cranial involve-

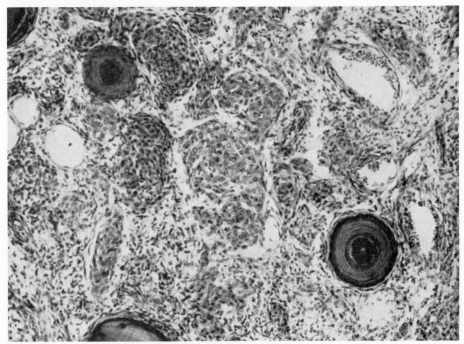

**Figure 23–21**   Typical meningioma showing psammoma body (lower right). (From Nager, G. T.: Meningiomas Involving the Temporal Bone. Springfield, Ill., Charles C Thomas, 1964.)

ment (Fig. 23–22).[35] The rare primary meningioma in the middle ear produces a conductive hearing loss, often with chronic otorrhea with polyps and granulations.[37]

## Diagnosis

Meningioma involving the temporal bone should be suspected in a patient with the cerebellopontine angle syndrome who has chronic otorrhea and extensive x-ray evidence of destruction of bone. Histologic examination of tissue showing the typical cellular whorls with psammoma bodies is required for conclusive diagnosis.

## Treatment

Meningiomas do not respond to radiation therapy; surgical removal is the only available treatment. The tendency of the tumor to infiltrate underlying bone renders complete surgical removal difficult when the temporal bone has been invaded, and the only chance for a permanent cure is early diagnosis combined with extensive resection of tumor and involved bone. Since these are very slowly growing tumors as a rule, with displacement rather than invasion of brain tissues, extensive surgical removal may relieve symptoms for a period of years, even when total eradication is not accomplished.

Meningiomas that arise from the middle fossa or posterior fossa surface of the petrous pyramid are neurosurgical problems; those that begin on the surface and deeply invade the temporal bone are combined otoneurosurgical problems; those that are confined to the internal acoustic meatus or that begin in the middle ear are otosurgical problems.

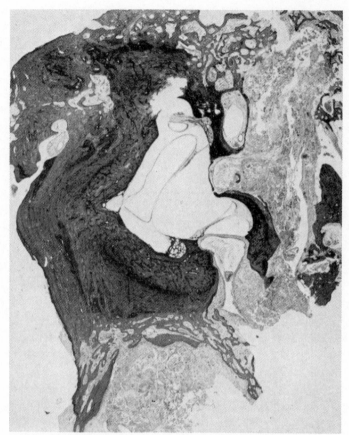

**Figure 23–22**  Meningioma invading the entire petrous pyramid and middle ear, sparing the round window membrane, stapes footplate and labyrinth. Same patient as in Figure 23–21. (From Nager, G. T.: Meningiomas Involving the Temporal Bone. Springfield, Ill., Charles C Thomas, 1964.)

## CONGENITAL CHOLESTEATOMA OF THE PETROUS PYRAMID

Cholesteatomas that originate within the temporal bone with no initial connection with the external auditory canal are believed to be the result of an embryonic epidermal rest, and are known as primary or congenital cholesteatomas. When they arise in the middle ear, attic or mastoid, they produce a conductive hearing loss without otorrhea until they rupture into the external auditory canal. When they arise deep within the petrous pyramid, they produce early labyrinthine and facial nerve involvement and sometimes the picture of the cerebellopontine angle syndrome.[38]

### Pathology

Like cholesteatomas acquired by the ingrowth of epidermis through a tympanic membrane perforation or by invagination of Shrapnell's membrane, primary congenital cholesteatomas have a lining of keratinizing stratified squamous epithelium, sometimes termed the matrix. Unlike acquired cholesteatomas, which as a rule are secondarily infected by putrefactive organisms from the external meatus, the primary congenital type consists of flaky, dry, odorless masses of desquamated

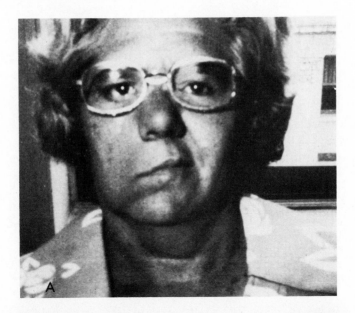

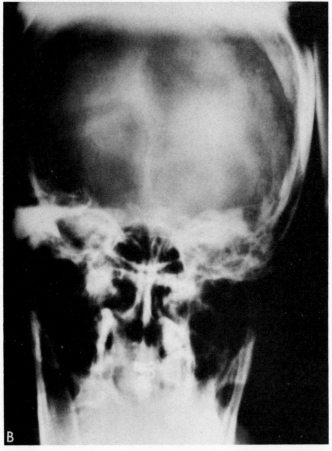

**Figure 23–23**   Case of congenital petrous cholesteatoma. Cawthorne type. *A*, Mrs. R. B., chronic foul discharge of the right ear for 22 years, preceded 3 years before by facial paralysis on the same side. At operation an enormous cholesteatoma was found, reaching the petrous apex with exposure of the carotid artery and middle fossa dura and erosion of horizontal semicircular canal and cochlea. Exteriorized cavity symptom free for 11 years. *B*, Pantopaque placed in cavity of right ear extends to the apex.

keratinized epithelium, which have a pearly sheen when first exposed to air.[39] The bone-eroding property of acquired cholesteatomas is shared by the primary congenital variety, the epidermal cyst slowly enlarging as the contained desquamated material continues to accumulate.

## Symptoms

Of nine patients with primary congenital cholesteatoma arising in the petrous pyramid, seven sought treatment because of progressive facial paresis occurring on the same side as a long-standing profound sensorineural deafness.[39] Vestibular symptoms of intermittent unsteadiness had been present in four of the seven. In two, meningitis occurred secondary to otitis media, owing to rupture of the cholesteatoma into the external auditory canal, and one of these had facial palsy and complete loss of cochlear and vestibular function.

## Diagnosis

The occurrence of facial paralysis in a patient with long-standing severe deafness in the same ear suggests the probability of a primary cholesteatoma of the petrosa. X-ray studies, including tomographic views, are often characteristic; finding the typical epidermal cyst at operation establishes the diagnosis.

## Treatment

The usual treatment for a primary congenital cholesteatoma should be surgical exteriorization by means of a radical mastoidectomy (Fig. 23–23). If there is good residual hearing, and if the surgeon is confident that he has removed every microscopic remnant of epidermal matrix with the operating microscope, a radical mastoidectomy with exteriorization might be omitted. However, complete removal of every vestige of epidermal lining may be difficult to attain in extensive invasive or deep-seated petrosal lesions. In removing the cholesteatoma material and the epidermal lining particular care must be taken to identify and avoid injury to the facial nerve. When the cholesteatoma has eroded into the posterior or middle cranial fossa, it tends to creep between the dura and the bone, in which case dura must be exposed by removal of overlying bone to the farthest extent of the epidermal cyst.

Finally, mention should be made of intracranial primary cholesteatomas that do not arise within bone, a third of which occur in the cerebellopontine angle.[40] These affect the fifth nerve earlier than the seventh, they are primarily neurosurgical problems and only rarely will be encountered by the otologic surgeon.[41] For these intracranial epidermoid cysts, removal of the entire matrix is difficult and probably not necessary since, in the absence of infection, reaccumulation of epidermal debris occurs very slowly.[41]

## REFERENCES

1. Cushing, H.: Tumors of the Nervus Acusticus and the Syndrome of the Cerebellopontine Angle. Philadelphia, W. B. Saunders Co., 1917.
2. Bell, C.: The Nervous System of the Human Body. Washington, Green, 1833.
3. Ballance, C.: Some Points in the Surgery of the Brain and Its Membranes. London, Macmillan & Co., 1907.

4. Cushing, H.: Intracranial Tumors. Springfield, Ill., Charles C Thomas, 1932.
5. Panse, R.: Clinical and pathological observations. IV. A glioma of the akusticus. Arch. Ohrenh., 61:251, 1904.
6. Quix, F. H.: Case of acoustic tumor with translabyrinthine removal. Verhandl. Deutsch. Otol. Gesellsch., 1912.
7. House, W.: Surgical exposure of the internal auditory canal and its contents through the middle cranial fossa. Laryngoscope, 71:1363, 1961.
8. Clerc, P., and Batisse, R.: Access to the intrapetrous structures from the intracranial aspect. Ann. oto-laryng., 71:20, 1954.
9. Glasscock, M. E., and Hays, J. W.: The translabyrinthine removal of acoustic and other cerebellopontine angle tumors. Ann. Otol. Rhinol. Laryngol., 82:415, 1973.
10. Maddox, H. E.: Experiences in acoustic tumor surgery. Laryngoscope, 79:652, 1969.
11. Smith, M. F. W., Miller, R. N., and Cox, D. J.: Suboccipital microsurgical removal of acoustic neurinomas of all sizes. Ann. Otol. Rhinol. Laryngol., 82:407, 1973.
12. Rand, R. W., and Kurze, T. L.: Micro-neurosurgery in acoustic tumors (suboccipital transmeatal approach. Trans. Am. Acad. Ophthal. Otolaryngol., 71:682, 1967.
13. Mallis, L.: Personal communication, 1979.
14. MacCarty, C. S.: Acoustic neuroma and the suboccipital approach (1967–1972). Mayo Clin. Proc., 50:15, 1975.
15. Rhoton, A. L.: Microsurgical removal of acoustic neuromas. Surg. Neurol., 6:211, 1976.
16. Hardy, M., and Crowe, S. J.: Early asymptomatic acoustic tumor: report of 6 cases. Arch. Surg., 32:292, 1936.
17. Henschen, F.: Concerning the history and pathogenesis of cerebellopontine angle tumors. Arch. Psychiat., 56:21, 1915.
18. Jerger, J.: Bekesy audiometry in analysis of auditory disorders. J. Speech & Hearing Res., 3:275, 1960.
19. Carhart, R.: Clinical determination of abnormal auditory adaptation. Arch. Otolaryngol., 65:32, 1957.
20. Fowler, E. P.: The recruitment of loudness phenomenon. Laryngoscope, 60:680, 1950.
21. Jerger, J.: The SISI test. Int. Audiol., 1:246, 1962.
22. Sanders, J. W., Kemker, F. J., and Josey, A. F.: Brief tone audiometry in patients with VIIIth nerve tumor. J. Speech Hear. Res., 14:172, 1971.
23. Selters, W. A., and Brackmann, D. E.: Acoustic tumor detection with brain stem electric response audiometry. Arch. Otolaryngol., 103:181, 1977.
24. Glasscock, M. E., Jackson, C. J., and Josey, A. F., et al.: Brainstem evoked response audiometry in a clinical practice. Layngoscope, 89:1021, 1979.
25. Linthicum, F. H., and Churchill, D.: Vestibular test results in acoustic tumor cases. Arch. Otolaryngol., 88:56, 1968.
26. Rubin, W.: Electronystagmograph. Arch. Otolaryngol., 89:19, 1966.
27. Hallpike, C. S., and Cairns, H.: Observations on pathology of Meniere's syndrome. J. Laryngol., 53:625, 1938.
28. Compere, W. E.: Radiographic Examination of the Petrous Portion of the Temporal Bone. Book I of Radiographic Atlas of the Temporal Bone. St. Paul, Minnesota, American Academy of Ophthalmology and Otolaryngology, 1964.
29. Glasscock, M. E., Overfield, R. E., and Miller, G. W.: Polytomography in an otologic practice. Southern Med. J., 69:1433, 1976.
30. Scott, W. R., et al.: Computerized tomography of the cerebellopontine angle. In Silverstein, H., and Norrell, H. (Eds): Neurological Surgery of the Ear. Birmingham, Alabama, Aesculapius Publishing Co., 1977, pp. 206–215.
31. Scanlan, R. L.: Positive contrast medium (Iophendylate) in diagnosis of acoustic neuroma. Arch Otolaryngol., 80:698, 1964.
32. Gardner, G.: Personal communication, 1978.
33. Dandy, W. E.: An operation for the total removal of cerebellopontine (acoustic) tumors. Surg. Gyn. & Obst., 41:129, 1925.
34. House, W. F.: Personal communication, 1979.
35. Thomsen, J.: Suboccipital removal of acoustic neuromas: results of 125 operations. Acta Otolaryngol., 81:406, 1976.
36. Nager, G. T.: Meningiomas Involving the Temporal Bone. Springfield, Ill., Charles C Thomas, 1964.
37. Bucy, P. C., and Isamot, F.: Tumors of the cerebellopontine angle. Arch. Otol., 73:29, 1961.
38. Cawthorne, T., and Griffith, A.: Primary cholesteatoma of the temporal bone. Arch. Otol., 73:252, 1961.
39. Olivecrona, H.: Cholesteatomas of the cerebellopontine angle. Acta Psychiat. et Neurol., 24:639, 1949.
40. Mahoney, M.: Epidermoids of the central nervous system. Ztschr. Neurol. u. Psychiat., 155:463, 1936.
41. House, W., and Doyle, J. B., Jr.: Early diagnosis and removal of primary cholesteatoma causing pressure to the VIII nerve. Laryngoscope, 73:1053, 1962.

# Surgical Anatomy of the Temporal Bone Through Dissection

RICHARD J. WIET, M.D.

Assistant Professor of Clinical Otolaryngology and Maxillofacial Surgery
Department of Otolaryngology and Maxillofacial Surgery
Northwestern University
Chicago, Illinois

MICHAEL E. GLASSCOCK, III, M.D.

Associate Clinical Professor of Surgery (Otology and Neurotology)
Vanderbilt University School of Medicine
Nashville, Tennessee

GEORGE E. SHAMBAUGH, Jr., M.D.

Professor (Emeritus) of Otolaryngology and Maxillofacial Surgery
Department of Otolaryngology and Maxillofacial Surgery
Northwestern University
Chicago, Illinois

**1980**
W. B. SAUNDERS COMPANY
Philadelphia London Toronto

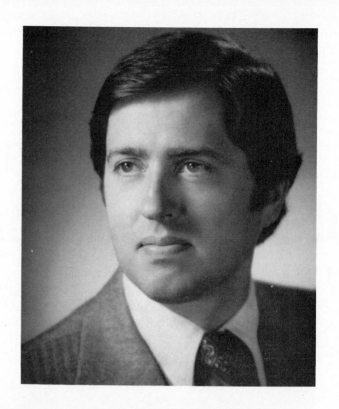

*Richard J. Wiet,*
*M.D.*

Assistant Professor of Clinical Otolaryngology and Maxillofacial Surgery, Northwestern University of Chicago; Staff, Hinsdale Sanitarium and Hospital, Shambaugh Ear Institute, Hinsdale, Illinois.

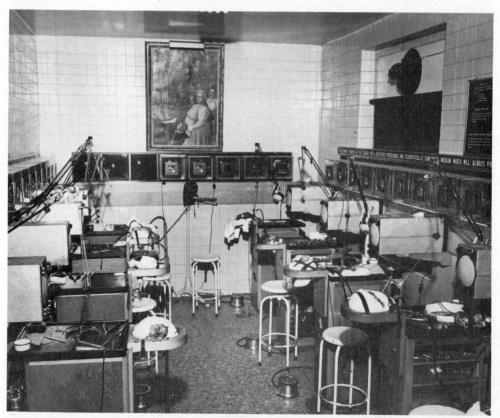

Julius Lempert, a European immigrant to the United States, was well known for his ability as a teacher of temporal bone anatomy. Shown here is his famous laboratory in New York, where students would dissect under the direction of his otologic genius.

**676**

# Foreword

Three quarters of a century ago the great pioneer otologist Friedrich Bezold, in his *Textbook of Otology,* warned that "the danger to the patient of an incompetent operator, who does not know the many anatomical details crowded together in the narrow space of the temporal bone and their extreme variability, is much greater here than in any other region of the body." Only by cadaver dissections can the aspiring ear surgeon learn to safely traverse the perilous anatomy of the temporal bone so as to avoid injury to the many vital structures concealed in an area no larger than an olive. Postoperative facial nerve paralysis continues to be a frequent source for malpractice suits in our specialty.

Otologic surgery has changed remarkably since Lempert introduced the first consistently successful operation to restore hearing in 1938. Before that date, otologic surgeons were preoccupied almost exclusively with the relief of middle ear suppuration and its complications. Bezold observed that around 5 per cent of all deaths occurring between ages 10 and 30, the healthiest and strongest years of life, were due to suppurations of the ears. Thrombophlebitis of the sigmoid sinus, brain abscess and uncomplicated meningitis each accounted for a third of these fatalities.

The observation by Alexander Fleming in 1928 of lysis of staphylococcus colonies by penicillium mold, and the discovery in 1932 by Gerhard Domagk of the antistreptococcal effect of sulfanilamide, progressively and dramatically reduced the mortality and the indications for surgical intervention in acute ear infections. By the time that Lempert introduced the one-stage fenestration operation for otosclerosis, chemotherapy and antibiotic therapy of acute otitis media were well accepted.

Operations to improve hearing were not new; stapes mobilization and stapedectomy for otosclerosis, operations for congenital meatal atresia and for repair of tympanic membrane perforations had begun more than a century ago, only to come to an abrupt halt at the 1900 International Congress of Otology, where the leaders in the specialty united in condemning surgery for deafness as "not only useless, but dangerous to life." So complete was the rejection of operations to improve hearing that during the residency of the senior author (George E. Shambaugh, Jr., M.D.) the 1930 standard text on otology disposed of surgical measures for the relief of deafness in half a page, concluding that "these operations mentioned for their place in otologic history are quite obsolete today."

With considerable courage in the face of this concerted opposition, Bárány in 1911, Jenkins in 1912 and Holmgren in 1914 began to operate to try to improve hearing in otosclerosis. In 1921, Nylén, a young assistant in Holmgren's clinic, first employed a monocular operating microscope to assist in a radical mastoidectomy. Holmgren immediately recognized the advantage of magnification and began to use a binocular operating microscope for his operations on otosclerosis. He demonstrat-

677

ed that by careful aseptic technique, a semicircular canal could be opened safely and a temporary hearing improvement achieved.

In 1924 Sourdille observed Holmgren's operations and returned to France to devise his two- or three-stage "tympanolabyrinthinopexy." With this, he created a fistula in the horizontal semicircular canal and covered it with a skin flap from the meatus. For the first time, permanent hearing improvements in otosclerosis were achieved. In 1947 the senior author observed and tested the hearing of two patients operated by Sourdille more than ten years earlier. In both, the fistula (fenestra) in the horizontal semicircular canal was clearly visible through the thin covering of skin, and the operated ear had a maintained improvement of hearing to "the serviceable practical level."

Sourdille's 1937 lecture before the New York Academy of Medicine prompted Julius Lempert to apply the technique, using the endaural (rather than postaural) approach and a surgical-dental drill, with the surgery being completed in a single-stage operation. In 1938 the senior author became Lempert's first pupil and began a series of more than 5000 fenestration operations. When the operating microscope was first applied by the senior author to Lempert's fenestration operation in 1940 (Sourdille and Lempert relied upon the loupe for magnification), with the subsequent addition by the senior author of continuous irrigation, enchondraliza- tion, and a diamond drill for construction of the fenestra, the lasting hearing improve- ments reached 80 per cent of fenestrations.*

The success of Lempert's fenestration (essentially Sourdille's operation with improvements) led to the revival of operations for congenital meatal atresia and then in 1950 to the techniques of tympanoplasty to rebuild a sound-conducting system in the ear damaged by previous infection or trauma. The operating microscope, pioneered by the senior author for Lempert's fenestrations in America, was applied to tympanoplasty by Zöllner and Wullstein. Their work encouraged the Zeiss optical company to construct the first otomicroscope, an instrument specifically designed for ear surgery.

Meanwhile, Lempert, a great surgeon, a great teacher and a great innovator, continued to use the loupe, insisting that the microscope "made things look bigger, but no clearer."

When Rosen revived stapes mobilization in 1952 and Shea revived stapedec- tomy in 1958, the use of the operating microscope spread until it became the indispensable tool of all modern temporal bone surgery.

In 1958 William House applied the method of Clerc and Batisse of approaching the internal meatus and the geniculate ganglion from the middle cranial fossa. This led three years later to his first operation to remove an acoustic neuroma by this approach. Soon House reported an impressive series of 47 acoustic neuroma operations without a fatality and with preservation of facial nerve function in the majority. Previous neurosurgical removals of similar tumors had carried a mortality of around 20 per cent, and permanent facial nerve paralysis in nearly all. House, a brilliant innovator and skilled otologic surgeon, became a devoted enthusiast of the operating microscope for all types of temporal bone surgery. In addition to his magnificent contributions to surgery for acoustic neuromas, he revived Portmann's operations for Meniere's disease and with James Sheehy modified Claus Jansen's operation for cholesteatoma without creating a radical cavity. House utilized the

---

*Shambaugh, G. E., Jr., and Juers, A. L: Surgical treatment of otosclerosis, a preliminary report on an improved fenestration technique. Arch Otolaryngol., 43:549, 1946.

postaural approach to the temporal bone, whereas Lempert had taught that the endaural operation was best for nearly all ear surgery.

The dissection manual in this last part, by Dr. Richard J. Wiet, is meant to emphasize the anatomy of the two most common approaches to the temporal bone: the lateral and superior approaches. It is not meant to teach surgery but rather should be used as a supplement by the otolaryngologist in the dissection laboratory. The manual makes no attempt at histology but emphasizes normal gross anatomy. All sketches and photographs in the manual are done in the surgical position on a right temporal bone.

RICHARD J.WIET, M.D.

MICHAEL E. GLASSCOCK, III, M.D.

GEORGE E. SHAMBAUGH, JR., M.D.

*Hinsdale, Illinois*
*Nashville, Tennessee*

## PROCEDURE FOR REMOVAL OF TEMPORAL
## BONES

Partly because of the recent sharp decline in the rate of hospital autopsies and partly because of physician apathy, there has been a steady decrease in the supply of temporal bones available for dissection. Otolaryngologists should encourage the practice of autopsy because of its crucial role as a source of temporal bones for continuing medical education. The removal of temporal bones is implied in most "complete" autopsies, but it is wise to check local laws and practices within the Pathology Department at each hospital.

Temporal bones may be removed by either the core or block method. At the time of autopsy, it is of value to study related neuroanatomy, especially the brainstem, cranial nerves and skull base.

The authors prefer the "block method" over the "plug method" for several reasons: (1) more structural features are retained in a larger sample, (2) the eustachian tube can be removed, (3) related cranial nerves can be viewed, and (4) it is easier to teach on a larger sample. At autopsy, care is taken to remove only the skull cap in such a way as to leave two pyramidal eminences anteriorly and posteriorly to avoid slipping of the cap over the skull base later on (Fig. 1). The brain is then removed.

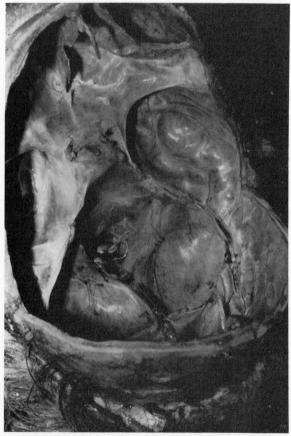

**Figure 1**  Preparing the head for temporal bone removal. Here the brain has been removed. The seventh and eighth cranial nerves are sectioned at the level of the internal auditory canal.

To remove the temporal bone four saw cuts are made. The first cut and the second are at a right angle to the superior angle of the petrous bone. Cut one is made near the apex of the bone as the size and shape of the posterior cranial fossa permits. In any case, it is well anteromedial to the cochlea. The farther forward this cut is made, the larger is the portion of the eustachian tube obtained. Cut two is made roughly parallel to cut one and through the middle mastoid region as near to its lateral wall as the saw can be held.

Cut three is made vertically in the floor of the middle cranial fossa about one inch in front of the petrous ridge and laterally as close to the cranial wall as possible. This cut should join the forward ends of cuts one and two. If this is correctly done, cut three is about 3/8 inch lateral to and in front of the tympanic membrane. The block tissue removed includes the deeper part of the osseous external auditory canal.

Cut four is an undercut of the block of tissue outlined by the preceding three cuts. It is made as nearly as possible in the anatomically horizontal plane and as near to the floor of the posterior cranial fossa as the saw can be placed. Usually it is possible to make the cut pass through or below the dual exit of the vagus nerve. The posterolateral end of cut four should be made first; thus it is possible to carry the cut nearer to the apex of the petrous portion of the bone than in the case when the cut is started at the narrow anterior part of the posterior cranial fossa.

Removal of the block outlined by the four cuts is often the most difficult part of the entire procedure. If the cuts have not overlapped at the deep corners (often they do not), the block of tissue is held in place not only by some remaining bony connections, but also by the dense fibrous tissue of and near the medial side of mandibular articulation. If any attempt is made to remove the block forcibly by the use of ordinary large forceps, it usually results in crushing of the pneumatized areas or making of a crack along the plane of the middle ear. It is best to use the lion-jawed forceps. The block is grasped by placing the two prongs of the jaw of the forceps in cut four and closing down the other jaw in such a manner that its prongs grasp the superior angle of the petrous bone pyramid, because this region of the superior surface is usually more free of underlying pneumatized or marrow spaces than are the more lateral portions of the superior surface. With the block grasped as described, gentle back and forth movement of the handle of the forceps causes the unsevered bony connections at the deep corners to break without damage to important structures. After the bone becomes completely loose, it is elevated with the forceps to allow insertion of a knife along cuts three and four to sever the dense fibrous connections remaining. A wide sharp chisel is useful, especially at the styloid process.

After removal of the bone two important things have to be done for the undertaker: The internal carotid artery is grasped and ligated, and the external auditory canal is sutured with silk with a piece of muscle plugged between the suture. This is done to avoid leakage of fluids from the cranial cavity to the outside through the external auditory canal.

## THE OPERATING MICROSCOPE AND TEMPORAL BONE DISSECTION LABORATORY

The difficult anatomy of the temporal bone and techniques of otologic surgery obviously cannot be mastered by simply reading about them. Actual dissection is imperative for the development and maintenance of a "three-dimensional concept" of the temporal bone. Furthermore, rapid advancements in our field make continuing study of this structure necessary. Courses on the surgical anatomy of the temporal bone are offered in universities and otologic foundations throughout the United States and Europe. Such programs are unsurpassed for concise, concentrated study of the anatomy under the guidance of experienced otologists and are strongly recommended.

This section is devoted to the otolaryngologist who wishes to set up his own dissection "laboratory" at his home or office so he may review anatomy and technique at his convenience.

### The Operating Microscope

Since the introduction of the operating microscope for ear surgery to the United States 40 years ago, it has been used increasingly by a growing number of medical disciplines. Shambaugh was most influential in the popularization of magnification for ear surgery by means of the binocular microscope.

Some of the most commonly used microscopes are those made by the Carl Zeiss Company (Fig. 2). At the front of the Zeiss Operating Microscope is an objective lens of large diameter which focuses the image towards infinity. The distance between

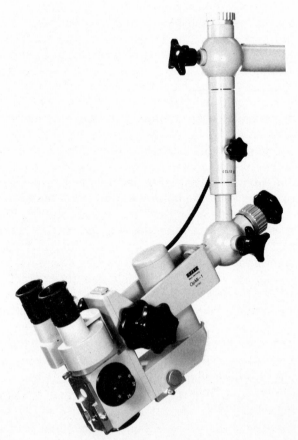

**Figure 2**   The Zeiss Operation Microscope (OpMi-1). Straight oculars and 200 mm lens are recommended for ear surgery.

the lens and the object in focus is the **focal length.** Side-by-side behind the objective lens, two magnification changer systems increase or decrease the initial magnification of the front lens system. Behind this, a binocular tube serves to further magnify and invert the image. The two eyepieces in the binocular tube permit highly magnified stereoscopic vision. The higher the magnification, the shorter is the depth of the focused field.

### Obtaining Par Focal Vision*

One of the most common problems experienced by surgeons using the operating microscope is eye strain. Most often this seems to be due to a misunderstanding of how to obtain par focal vision. Continued eyestrain may mean the optics are not optimally adjusted to the operator's eyes or that there is a refractive error.

For surgeons with normal vision, comfortable binocular vision can be achieved by setting the diopter adjustment to "0" and moving the eyepiece assembly either apart or together to adjust for interpupillary distance. Wearers of eyeglasses can use the 'scope without them by setting the diopter adjustment to their lens correction. Astigmatics may be forced to wear their eyeglasses while using the microscope or to modify the eyepiece assembly with an astigmatic correction lens.

For the majority of surgeons, however, par focal vision can be achieved by following these simple steps:

1. Position microscope over steady flat area.
2. Make a small crosshatch (#) mark on white paper for use as a focusing target.
3. Make sure eyepieces are fully inserted into binocular eyepiece tubes, and set diopter corrector ring to "0."
4. Focus microscope on crosshatch target and set magnification changer to 40×. Critically focus microscope (using focusing knobs) at this 40× setting and carefully lock all arm tension knobs to prevent any movement of the microscope or change in focus setting.
5. Carefully, so as not to disturb focus setting, revolve magnification changer to 6× (opposite 40×).
6. Carefully, again so as not to disturb focus setting, while closing the opposite eye adjust each individual eyepiece to produce the sharpest image and note reading of diopter scale.
7. Adjust binocular eyepiece interpupillary distance for good convergence.
8. Microscope is now par focal and the magnification changer can be rotated to all positions and the image will remain in focus.

### The Dissection Laboratory

A temporal bone dissection "laboratory" can be easily established in a small room with adequate electrical outlets, ventilation and lighting. For clean-up, access to a sink with a trap for pieces of bone and tissue is necessary.

A dissection bench (24″ deep × 22″ long × 30″ high) with drawers for instruments is most convenient (Fig. 3), though a simple desk can be adequately converted for this purpose.

---

*Courtesy of Mr. Jack Urban, Los Angeles.

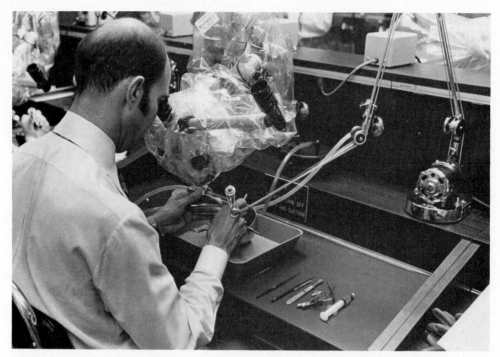

**Figure 3**   Temporal bone dissection bench at Sam Sanders' Temporal Bone Laboratory, Nashville, Tennessee (Courtesy of the E.A.R. Foundation).

Drilling should be done with a desk-mounted, electric bone engine with a foot switch, using a surgical handpiece of your choice. A House-Urban temporal bone holder (Figs. 4 and 5) allows movement of the specimen in many planes, for simulation of surgical positioning of the patient, and is, therefore, preferable to stationary temporal bone holders. This holder should be set within an 8″ × 10″

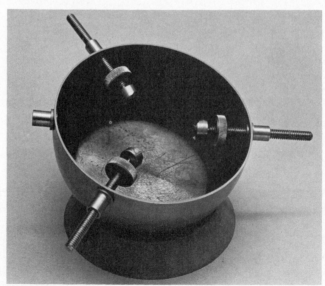

**Figure 4**   The House-Urban temporal bone holder positioned on the neoprene ring allows surgical positioning.

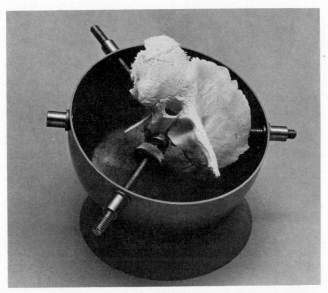

**Figure 5**  The House-Urban temporal bone holder with specimen mounted.

plastic tray (such as that used for photographic developing) to catch water and debris. Gloves and gown should be worn during dissection, especially when working with unpreserved bones.

It is recommended that a separate set of instruments be kept for dissecting in the laboratory (Fig. 6). An assortment of diamond and cutting burrs is necessary for mastoid work. A Lempert periosteal elevator will be necessary for stripping periosteum and temporalis muscle prior to dissection. Canal elevators, picks, sickle

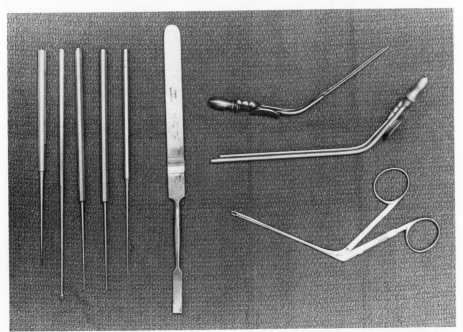

**Figure 6**  A minimum number of instruments are necessary. These include heavy scissors, suction irrigation, cup forceps, periosteal elevators and an assortment of canal skin elevators and picks.

knives, cup forceps and microscissors are also needed. A knife handle and blades will also be necessary, for dissecting soft tissue from the bone. A light lubricating oil is needed for the drill and handpiece.

There is no substitute for suction-irrigation in modern ear surgery. Various sizes of suction-irrigators are needed: smaller sizes for tight areas such as the facial recess and larger sizes for removing large amounts of bone dust on the mastoid cortex. If built-in suction is not available, an ordinary Gomco or SMR suction unit may be used. Gravity-flow irrigation can be provided by genitourinary irrigation bags with regular IV hookups. Silastic tubing is recommended for the water, while PVC plastic tubing of 1/4 inch diameter is preferred for the suction because it is stiffer and less likely to collapse.

## EXTERNAL TEMPORAL BONE ANATOMY

### Lateral Surface

The external anatomy of the lateral surface of the temporal bone is best visualized by studying the surface of a dry bone.

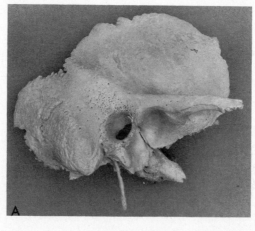

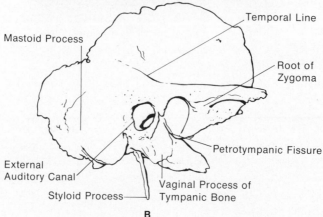

**Figure 7** Lateral surface of temporal bone. Note the petrous, squamous zygomatic, mastoid and tympanic segments of the bone.

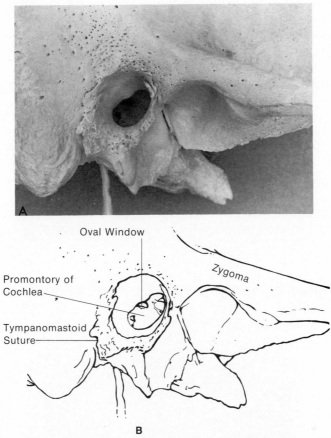

**Figure 8**  Lateral surface of external auditory canal. Note the promontory, suprameatal spine, zygoma and tympanomastoid suture — a good external landmark to the facial nerve below.

The lateral surface of the temporal bone demonstrates the mastoid, styloid, zygomatic and petrous portions of the temporal bone (Figs. 7 and 8). Planning postauricular incisions in adults requires palpation of the mastoid tip. Anterior to the tip, the facial nerve lies between the styloid process and anterior surface of the mastoid. The temporal line serves as an attachment for the temporal fascia and limits the origin of the temporalis muscle. MacEwen's triangle (suprameatal triangle) is a standard landmark to the mastoid antrum. Its borders are the external canal itself, inferior temporal line and the spine of Henle (a variably sized eminence on the superior wall of the external acoustic meatus).

The zygomatic process has two roots. The anterior root, continuous with the lower border of the zygomatic process, is marked by the articular tubercle (this tubercle demarcates the anterior boundary of the mandibular fossa and thus is covered with cartilage [see Fig. 12]). Posterior to the articular tubercle, the mandibular fossa is bounded medially by a fissure, part of which is formed by the narrow petrotympanic fissure, which serves as passage for the chorda tympani. The posterior root, continuous with the upper border of the zygomatic process, is marked anteriorly by the postglenoid tubercle, then extends posteriorly over the external auditory meatus and terminates as the supramastoid crest.

Posteriorly the tympanomastoid suture is a fairly reliable external landmark to the exit of the facial nerve.

**Superior Surface** (Fig. 9)

An accurate knowledge of the anatomy of the superior surface of the temporal bone is mandatory in planning middle fossa surgery.

The superior surface of the temporal bone forms the floor of the middle cranial fossa. Just medial to the squamous portion is the tegmen. The petrous portion of the temporal bone is marked by depressions and eminences for the convolutions of the brain. The arcuate eminence indicates the landmark of the superior semicircular canal. A shallow groove, the hiatus of the facial canal, marks the passage of the greater superficial petrosal nerve. Just anterior to the facial hiatus is the foramen lacerum for the carotid canal. Parallel and lateral to the facial hiatus is the semicanal of the tensor tympani muscle.

Near the apex of the petrous bone and medial to the carotid is the trigeminal impression for the reception of the semilunar ganglion. Proximal to the semicanal for the tensor tympani is the tympanic canaliculus for passage of the lesser superficial

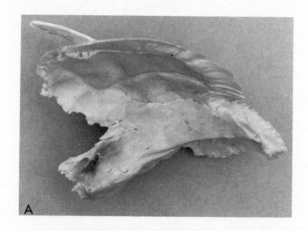

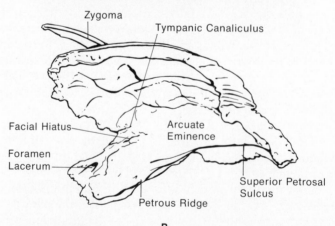

**Figure 9**  Superior surface of temporal bone. Important to the middle fossa surgeon is a knowledge of the facial hiatus, arcuate eminence and superior petrosal sulcus. Note also the location of the foramen lacerum and the tympanic canaliculus.

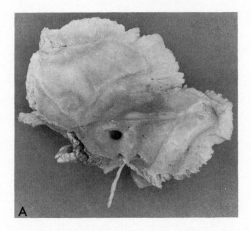

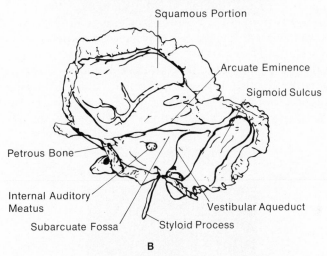

**Figure 10**   Posterior surface of the temporal bone. The sigmoid sulcus forms a large part of the posterior surface of the temporal bone, but more important are the relationships at the internal auditory canal. Note also the vestibular aqueduct, the subarcuate fossa and the arcuate eminence.

petrosal nerve (a branch of the glossopharyngeal nerve which eventually supplies secretory fibers to the parotid).

**Posterior View** (Fig. 10)

The posterior surface of the temporal bone forms the anterior aspect of the posterior cranial fossa. Its intracranial surface, the sigmoid sulcus, forms the medial aspect of the mastoid. The subarcuate fossa is located anteromedial to the sigmoid sulcus and just behind the internal auditory canal. The canal itself opens its meatus toward the occiput and houses the vestibular nerves, facial and acoustic nerves and blood vessels. Further lateral is the vestibular aqueduct for transmission of the endolymphatic duct and sac. The cochlear canaliculus (not shown on Fig. 10) transmits the perilymphatic duct. At the juncture of the middle and posterior fossae lies the sulcus for the superior petrosal sinus.

## Internal Auditory Canal (Fig. 11)

The internal auditory canal opens on the posterior surface of the temporal bone. There is a short posterior lip to the canal. The acoustic meatus is about 1 cm. in length and transmits the facial and acoustic nerves, the nervus intermedius and the internal auditory artery. The transverse (horizontal) crest, called the crista falciformis, separates the canal into two portions. A vertical crest of bone (Bill's bar) separates the facial nerve from the superior vestibular nerve. Below the crista falciformis lie multiperforate areas of bone that transmit the singular, the inferior vestibular and cochlear nerves.

## Inferior Surface of the Temporal Bone (Fig. 12)

A much neglected aspect of temporal bone anatomy is the inferior surface. On first examination, one is immediately struck by the jugular fossa, which houses the jugular bulb. Just anterior to it lies the carotid canal. Immediately behind the styloid process is the stylomastoid foramen for transmission of the facial nerve. Posterior to this foramen are the mastoid tip and the mastoid notch (digastric groove). Medial to the jugular fossa is the cochlear aqueduct or canaliculus. In the ridge between the carotid and the jugular fossa is the small inferior tympanic canaliculus for passage of the glossopharyngeal nerve. This canaliculus is traversed by the inferior tympanic

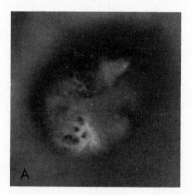

A

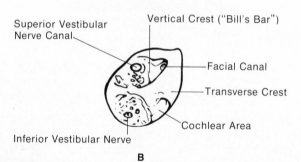

B

**Figure 11** Internal auditory canal. Note Bill's bar and the transverse crest. Also note the areas of the vestibular, cochlear and facial nerves.

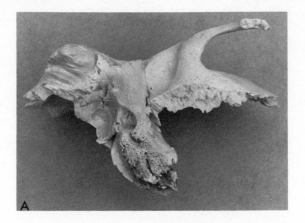

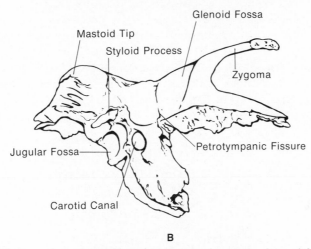

**Figure 12**   Inferior surface of the temporal bone. Note the relationships of the carotid canal to the jugular bulb. In glomus tumor surgery the facial nerve is intimately related to the jugular bulb; note the stylomastoid foramen.

artery (a branch of the ascending pharyngeal artery) and the tympanic branch of the glossopharyngeal nerve (Jacobson's nerve).

**Petrous Apex (Medial Portion)** (Fig. 13)

The petrous apex is that pyramid-shaped section of the temporal bone wedged between the sphenoid and occipital bones. It is directed medially and anteriorly in the cranial cavity. The superior surface of the bone (over the middle ear) is called the tegmen tympani. Looking straight down the carotid canal as a reference, one can locate the hiatus for the facial nerve (greater superficial petrosal), the arcuate eminence (superior semicircular canal), the trigeminal impression and the semicanal for the tensor tympani. The eustachian tube is located parallel to the carotid canal. Its medial wall is at times dehiscent, leaving the carotid vulnerable to trauma during middle ear surgery.

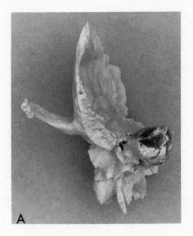

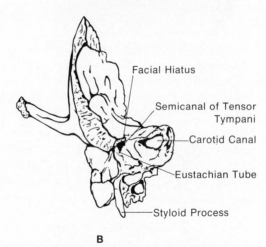

**Figure 13** The petrous apex. Important in this figure is the relationship of the carotid artery to the Eustachian tube.

## MAJOR VESSELS AND RELATED CRANIAL NERVE ANATOMY

### Major Vessels

For the purposes of the otologist we will discuss only those venous sinuses in immediate contact with the temporal bone, mainly the sinuses of the dura mater, the emissary veins to the mastoid and the sigmoid sinus.

The transverse (lateral) sinuses begin at the internal occipital protuberance, one (generally the right transverse sinus) being the continuation of the superior sagittal sinus and the other of the straight sinus. The transverse sinus leaves the tentorium, curves downward behind the mastoid as the sigmoid sinus and turns medially to terminate as the internal jugular vein.

The superior petrosal sinus connects the cavernous sinus with the sigmoid sinus and runs in the superior petrosal sulcus of the temporal bone. The inferior petrosal sinus is formed by the junction of the inferior part of the cavernous sinus and passes directly into the jugular foramen, ending in the superior bulb of the internal jugular vein. Though not commonly described by anatomists, a confluence of sinuses is often seen here.

The principal emissary vein of concern to the otologist is the mastoid emissary vein. It runs through the mastoid foramen close to the juncture of the temporal and occipital bones from the post-auricular or occipital vein to the transverse sinus.

The carotid artery enters the inferior surface of the temporal bone through its own canal (Fig. 12) and exits the temporal bone (Fig. 13) after taking an anterior, almost right-angle bend. It may be encountered through the middle ear or tympanic approach on the medial wall of the eustachian tube; here it is occasionally dehiscent and at times may be present in the middle ear as a mass.

To expose the carotid clearly from the lateral approach one must drill away the cochlea because its bend in the temporal bone is medial to this structure. Additionally, inferiorly the carotid is separated from the jugular bulb by a thin plate of pneumatic bone known as the "vascular crest" by radiologists.

### Related Peripheral Cranial Nerve Anatomy

Knowledge of the cranial nerves as they relate to the temporal bone is becoming more essential to the otologist as infra-temporal surgery progresses.

*Third Nerve (Oculomotor).*   The third nerve supplies motor fibers for innervation of the levator palpebrae and all the extraocular muscles except the superior oblique and lateral rectus. The oculomotor nucleus is located ventral to the aqueduct in the upper midbrain. The oculomotor nerve contains autonomic fibers for the ciliaris muscle and the sphincter pupillae. The oculomotor nucleus is intimately related to the medial longitudinal fasciculus, which lies on its ventral aspect.

*Fourth Nerve (Trochlear).*   The fourth cranial nerve contains the motor fibers for the superior oblique muscle of the eye. The nucleus for the trochlear nerve is located beneath the cerebral aqueduct at the level of the inferior colliculus. The nucleus receives terminals from the medial longitudinal fasciculus and contains proprioceptive connections similar to those of the oculomotor nucleus.

*Fifth Nerve (Trigeminal).*   The large Gasserian ganglion (semilunar) lies on the apex of the petrous portion of the temporal bone, indenting its bony surface. The trigeminal supplies both motor and sensory components to the face. The trigeminal has two roots: The main root is the sensory, which enters the lateral surface of the pons at the superior aspect of the cerebellopontine angle; the motor root is more medial, leaving with the sensory trunk and joining the mandibular division to supply the muscles of mastication.

*Sixth Nerve (Abducent).*   The nucleus of the abducent nerve is located close to the fourth ventricle. The nerve trunk lies in a furrow between the inferior border of the pons and the superior end of the medulla oblongata. Apical lesions can compress the sixth nerve by edema as it passes through Dorello's canal beneath the petrosphenoid ligament at the tip of the petrous apex (Gradenigo's syndrome). The abducent supplies motor fibers to the ipsilateral lateral rectus muscle.

It should be noted that the nuclei of the third, fourth and sixth cranial nerves are adjacent to or interconnected with the medial longitudinal fasciculus. Cells in the vestibular nuclei send their axons to the cerebellum, to the lateral vestibulospinal tract and to the medial longitudinal bundle. Thus, the vestibular organ may influence eye movements (nystagmus).

*Seventh Nerve (Facial).*    Secretomotor fibers of the lacrimal, submandibular and sublingual glands begin in the cell bodies of the superior salivary nucleus and lacrimal palatal nasal nuclei. These fibers are preganglionic parasympathetic nerves that are joined by special sensory fibers for taste and form what is known as the *nervus intermedius.* This sensory root joins the larger motor root to form the main trunk of the facial nerve. The nervus intermedius lies more laterally between the motor root of the facial and the auditory nerve. The nerve enters the temporal bone through the internal auditory canal. At the geniculate ganglion, the greater superficial petrosal nerve branches off the facial and runs anteriorly, passing through the facial hiatus onto the petrous apex. The greater superficial petrosal nerve carries secreto-motor fibers to the lacrimal gland by way of the pterygo-palatine ganglion. The remainder of the facial nerve runs posteriorly through the superior border of the middle ear. At the lateral semicircular canal the nerve turns inferiorly and runs toward the stylomastoid foramen. The chorda tympani nerve diverges from this vertical portion and crosses the middle ear, exiting through the petrotympanic fissure. Motor fibers from the facial nuclei supply the stapedius muscle and muscles of facial expression as well as the posterior belly of the digastric and stylohyoid muscles.

Axons from the facial nerve nucleus in the pons leave its dorsal surface, run along the medial side of the abducent nucleus in what is called the internal genu of the facial nerve, then emerge between the olive and inferior cerebellar peduncle at the caudal border of the pons. Neurons that innervate the lower part of the face are entirely crossed, while those to the upper part of the face are both crossed and uncrossed.

*Eighth Nerve (Cochlear Division).*    The cochlear nerve arises from the bipolar cells of the spiral ganglion, and its peripheral fibers pass to the organ of Corti. Central fibers pass through the modiolus, through the foramen of the tractus spiralis foraminosus, and thence into the fundus of the internal auditory canal. The cochlear nerve is inferior to the facial in the internal canal.

*Eighth Nerve (Vestibular Division).*    Cell bodies of the vestibular division (Scarpa's ganglion) are located within the internal auditory canal. The vestibular nerve enters the medulla oblongata pons between the inferior cerebellar peduncle and the spinal tract of the trigeminal nerve. There are two rami of the vestibular nerve: (1) the upper ramus goes from the superior vestibular area in Scarpa's ganglion to the superior cribrose macula and divides into the following: the utricular to the acoustic macula of the utricle; the superior ampullary to the superior membranous ampulla; and the lateral ampullary to the lateral membranous ampulla. (2) The lower ramus divides into the saccular nerve to the acoustic macula of the saccule; and the posterior ampullary, which passes through the singular foramen to the membranous ampulla of the posterior canal.

*Ninth Nerve (Glossopharyngeal).*    The ninth cranial nerve leaves the medulla at its upper lateral portion along with the vagus and accessory nerves to pass through the jugular foramen. It is distributed to the tongue and pharynx, as its name implies. After it exits from the skull in a separate sheath of dura mater, it runs anteriorly between the internal jugular vein and internal carotid artery posterior to the styloid process and its muscles. While the ninth nerve has multiple branches, including those supplying taste to the posterior one third of the tongue and sensation to the adjacent pharyngeal mucosal, the one of greatest importance to the otologist is the branch that forms the tympanic nerve. The tympanic nerve supplies parasympathetic fibers to the parotid gland and receives sensory fibers from the middle ear. It enters the temporal bone through its own canaliculus on the inferior surface and continues upward on the promontory. At the level of the processus cochleariformis it passes internal to the semicanal for the tensor tympani and continues as the lesser superficial petrosal nerve.

*Tenth Nerve (Vagus).*   The longest of cranial nerves, the vagus begins with 8 to 10 rootlets that emerge from the medulla oblongata in a groove between the olive and the fasciculus cuneatus. The roots unite into a main trunk that passes beneath the flocculus of the cerebellum to the jugular foramen. The vagus and accessory nerves lie in the same dural sheath. After passing through the jugular and nodose ganglia, the vagus passes vertically down the neck into the carotid sheath deep to and between the internal jugular and common carotid arteries, passing through the thorax and into the abdomen.

*Eleventh Nerve (Spinal accessory).*   This nerve emerges from the medulla inferior to the ninth and tenth nerves. It consists of a cranial and spinal motor part. The otologist is more concerned with the spinal part. These fibers originate from a cell column in the anterior horn, which extends from C5 or C6 to the level of the pyramidal decussation. The nerve then passes proximal to the foramen magnum into the cranial cavity, and there it crosses the occipital bone to the jugular notch and passes through the jugular foramen. It passes posterior to the digastric muscle to pierce the sternocleidomastoid muscle and supply it and the trapezius muscle.

*Twelfth Nerve (Hypoglossal).*   The hypoglossal has its origins in the medulla and emerges by means of a series of rootlets located in the sulcus between the pyramid and olive. It pierces the dura and exits in the hypoglossal canal of the occipital bone. As the nerve emerges from the skull it lies deep to and runs between the internal carotid and internal jugular vein, and becomes superficial near the angle of the mandible. It passes over the external carotid below the digastric tendon, curving upward at the lateral aspect of the hyoid bone before it innervates the musculature of the tongue.

## ANATOMY OF THE MIDDLE EAR OR TYMPANIC CAVITY

The tympanic cavity is divided into three portions: the attic, or epitympanum; the tympanum proper, or mesotympanum; and the hypotympanum below the level of the tympanic membrane.

Superiorly, the middle ear cavity is separated from the brain by a thin plate of bone known as the tegmen. Inferiorly, a thin bony floor separates the cavity from the jugular bulb. Laterally lies the tympanic membrane and medially lies the labyrinth.

In adults the tympanic membrane lies at a 45 degree angle from the long axis of the petrous pyramid. The ring of bone into which the membrane fits, the tympanic sulcus, is deficient superiorly. Here it is called the notch of Rivinus. From the ends of this notch two bands (anterior and posterior malleolar folds) extend down and attach to the lateral process of the malleus. This part of the drum is known as the pars flaccida or Shrapnell's membrane. The most depressed portion of the drum, called the umbo (Fig. 14), lies at the tip of the malleus manubrium. In the region of the notch of Rivinus, the chorda tympani branches off the facial nerve, enters the tympanic cavity beneath the tympanic membrane and exits the tympanic cavity through the petrotympanic fissure (Fig. 8).

The medial wall of the tympanic cavity contains numerous structures in a width of scarcely 15 mm. A mound of bone on this medial wall is termed the promontory (basilar turn of the cochlea, on end). On the promontory are branches of the tympanic plexus. Above the promontory is the oval window (fenestra vestibuli) in which the footplate of the stapes is inserted. Just inferiorly is the round window

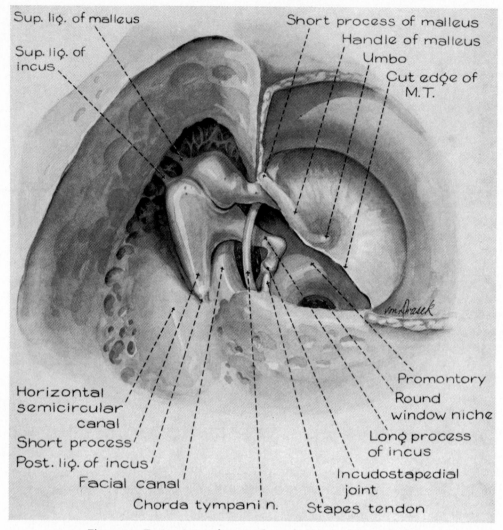

**Figure 14**  Tympanic membrane and ossicles (surgeon's eye view).

(fenestra cochleae), which leads into the scala tympani of the cochlea and is closed by the secondary tympanic membrane.

The tensor tympani tendon (Fig. 15) comes out of its semicanal at the bony eminence known as the cochleariformis process (Fig. 16) and inserts onto the malleus. The facial canal lies just above the oval window and runs in an anteroposterior direction known as the tympanic segment. At the cochleariformis the facial nerve takes a sharp bend toward the internal auditory canal. It marks the approximate level of the geniculate ganglion on the superior aspect of the temporal bone.

A fairly standard landmark on the promontory of the cochlea is Jacobson's nerve, or the tympanic branch of the glossopharyngeal. It enters the tympanic cavity through a canaliculus between the internal jugular and carotid arteries and divides into branches that ramify on the promontory, pointing to the cochleariformis process. The terminal branch of the tympanic nerve, the lesser superficial petrosal, runs on the

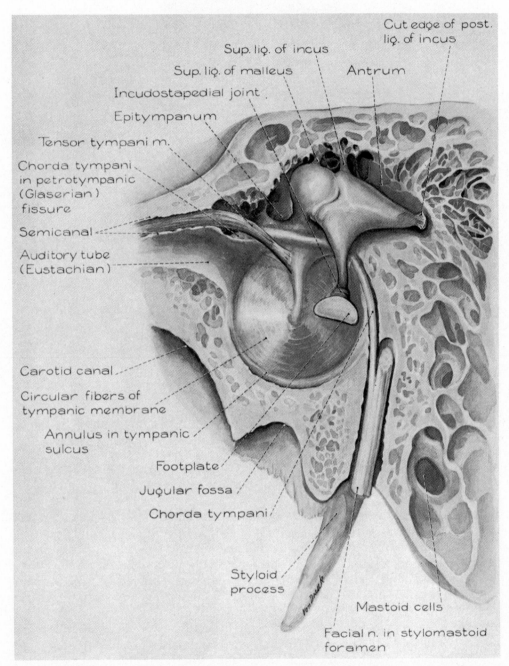

**Figure 15** Tympanic membrane and ossicles as viewed from within looking outward.

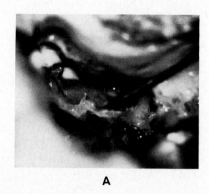

**A**

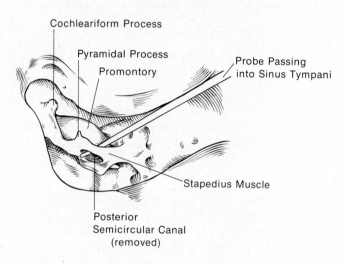

**B**

**Figure 16**   In this figure, the facial nerve has been intentionally sectioned and removed to show the stapedius, muscle which runs below and parallel to it. Also surgically created is a potential space where the posterior canal and the sinus tympani come in close contact. Note the cochleariformis process.

superior surface of the temporal bone lateral to the facial hiatus. It sends preganglionic fibers to the parotid gland.

The posterior wall (attic) of the middle ear leads to the antrum, the primitive first air cell that communicates to the other cells of the mastoid process. Below this is the pyramidal eminence containing the tendon to the stapedius (Fig. 16). The sinus tympani, which is not visible from a posterior dissection, lies in the posterior tympanum between the labyrinthine capsule and the styloid complex. Above this area and the facial nerve is an area known as the facial recess (see below). The fossa incudis is a small depression that is an important landmark for facial nerve surgery.

On the anterior wall of the middle ear is the semicanal of the tensor tympani muscle. It runs almost parallel to the eustachian tube. The tensor tympani originates on the cartilaginous portion of the eustachian tube, passes across the cochleariforme process as a tendon and inserts on the manubrium of the malleus. The eustachian tube connects the tympanum with the nasopharynx, allowing passage of air between the two. In the adult it consists of an upper bony one third and lower cartilaginous two thirds.

*The Auditory Ossicles.* The auditory ossicular chain consists of three bones held together by delicate articulations and ligaments (Figs. 17 and 18). The malleus has a head, neck and three processes. The head articulates with the incus in the epitympanum. The manubrium is attached to the medial surface of the tympanic membrane.

The incus consists of a body and two process, known as the short and long crus. On the anterior surface there is a facet which articulates with the malleus. The short crus is attached into the fossa incudis by the posterior ligament of the incus. The long crus articulates with the stapes at its lenticular process.

The stapes has a footplate, anterior and posterior crus and a capitulum. The neck is constricted for attachment of the stapedius tendon.

*Sinus Tympani.* The medial wall of the posterior mesotympanum is divided into discrete bony pockets by the ponticulus (Fig. 19) and the subiculum. Below the ponticulus on the posterior aspect of the tympanum is the sinus tympani. The depth of the sinus tympani is not directly visible from the posterior approach.

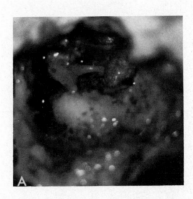

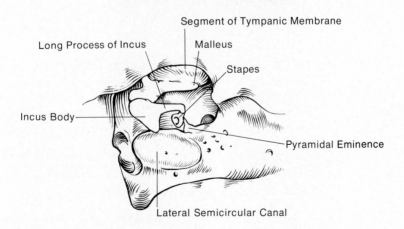

**Figure 17** The auditory ossicles. Here the bony canal wall was removed and the posterior one-half of the tympanic membrane removed to show structures in the middle ear. Note the auditory ossicles and their articular relationships.

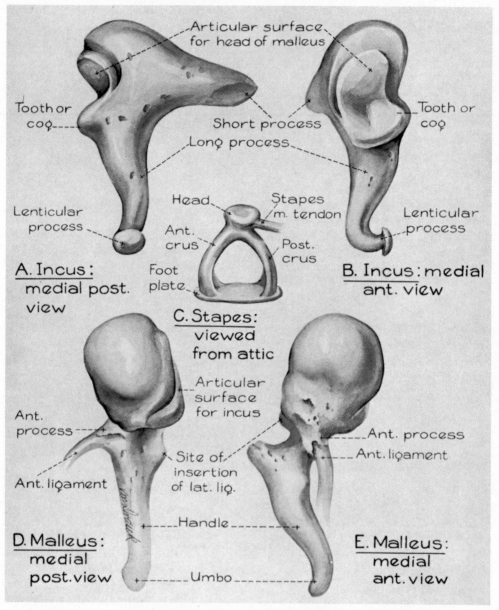

**Figure 18**  Ossicles under high magnification.

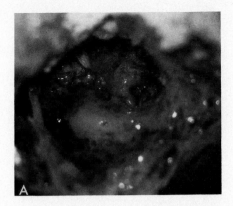

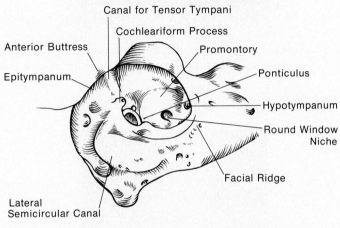

**Figure 19**   Here the tympanic membrane and auditory ossicles as well as the posterior bony canal wall have been removed. Otologic terminology applicable here is the facial ridge, infra-annular mass of bone, and the anterior buttress areas. This is a radical cavity.

## Eustachian Tube and Tensor Tympani

The osseus portion of the eustachian tube begins in the carotid wall of the tympanic cavity below the semicanal of the tensor tympani muscle. At the isthmus this tube becomes cartilaginous and travels for a length of another 24 mm.

The tensor tympani muscle is contained in its own bony canal above the osseus portion of the auditory tube and the adjoining part of the greater wing of the sphenoid. It ends in a slender tendon, makes a sharp bend at the processus cochleariformis and inserts into the manubrium of the malleus.

## ANATOMY OF THE MASTOID CAVITY

The goal of a "complete" mastoidectomy is never truly attained, owing to the extent of pneumatization of the air-cell system. Nevertheless, during mastoid surgery one can identify critical structures that help to develop a thorough mastoidectomy.

Prior to beginning mastoid surgery one must be familiar with external landmarks.

After examining the surface of the temporal bone to locate the inferior temporal line, the spine of Henle (suprameatal spine), the external canal and MacEwen's triangle, an initial cut is made with the rotating cutting burr parallel to the inferior temporal line (Fig. 20).

### Widening the Mastoid Antrum (Fig. 21)

The antrum of the mastoid lies just superior, lateral and posterior to the posterior and superior semicircular canal walls, within a few millimeters lateral to the annulus and sulcus tympanicus. After the antrum is widened, the lateral semicircular canal becomes apparent. Visualization is increased by working su-

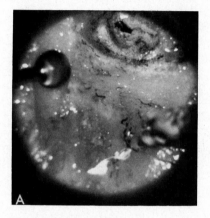

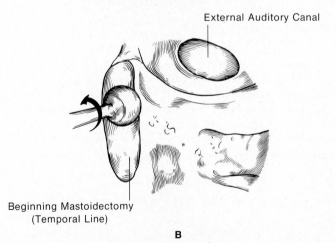

External Auditory Canal

Beginning Mastoidectomy
(Temporal Line)

B

**Figure 20**   The initial cut prior to mastoidectomy should parallel the *linea temporalis*.

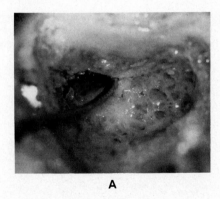

**A**

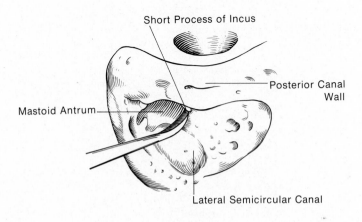

**B**

**Figure 21**  Having entered the antrum, identify immediately the lateral semicircular canal. The instrument points to the short process of the incus, giving these two key points for identification of the facial nerve.

periorly toward the tegmen, anteriorly toward the zygoma, posteriorly to the sigmoid sinus and inferiorly to the mastoid tip.

### Fossa Incudis and Facial Nerve (Mastoid Segment)
(Figs. 21 and 22)

Important relationships for the otologic surgeon exist at the fossa incudis with regard to the facial nerve. From the tip of the short process of the incus, the mean distance to the facial nerve is 1.7 mm. to 0.92 mm.* By lowering the pneumatic cells over the facial nerve with the cutting burr, one carefully approaches the facial nerve. The facial nerve lies on the infero-medial side of the lateral semicircular canal. Using

---

*Anson, B., and Donaldson, J.: Surgical Anatomy of the Temporal Bone and Ear, 2nd ed. Philadelphia, W. B. Saunders, 1973.

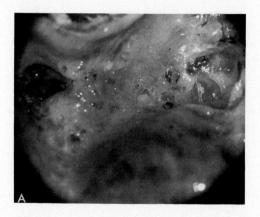

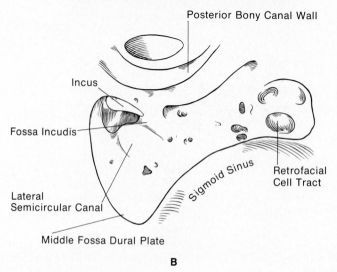

**B**

**Figure 22**    The mastoid cells over the facial nerve may be lowered after establishing a sense of depth of the facial nerve using the digastric ridge.

the fossa incudis, the lateral canal and the digastric ridge inferiorly, the surgeon can outline the periosteal sheath that covers the facial nerve. One must recall that in the descending portion of the facial nerve below the level of the lateral canal, there is some variation in its medial to lateral slant. Additionally, the facial nerve lies 2 to 3 mm. anterior to the posterior semicircular canal. Here endochondral bone can be observed as the nerve approaches the stylomastoid foramen.

## Facial Recess (Figs. 23 and 24)

By cutting a trough just below the tip of the short process of the incus inferiorly toward the mastoid tip, the facial recess may be opened, exposing the mesotympanum. The surgically created limits of the facial recess are (1) the facial nerve inferiorly, (2) the chorda tympani superiorly and (3) bone adjacent to the incus superiorly. The facial recess has been known by such alternative names as "lateral facial recess," "posterior tympanotomy" and "lateral tympanic sinus." The facial recess gives visualization of the superior and posterior mesotympanum.

Through the facial recess one can observe the pyramidal process and stapes superstructure. The oval and round windows, incus and malleus, as well as the eustachian tube, may be identified. After removal of the bar of bone protecting the incus, the horizontal course of the facial nerve comes into clear view, as do the tensor tympani and cochleariformis process (Fig. 25). While not easily seen, the ponticulus is a ridge of bone separating the oval window inferiorly from the sinus tympani. The subiculum is that eminence which persists from the pyramidal eminence to the posterior lip of the round window niche, separating the tympanic sinus from the round window.

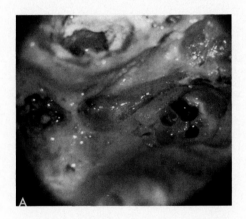

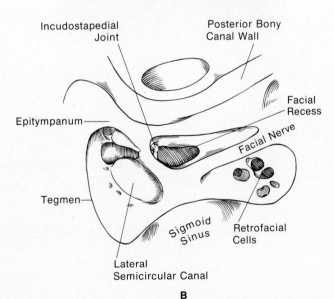

**Figure 23**   A trough of bone is opened just over the facial nerve to gain access to the middle ear.

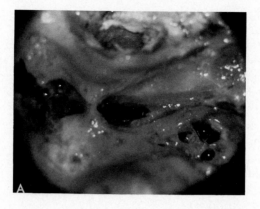

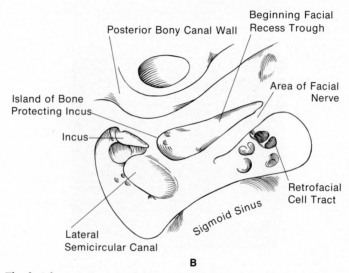

**Figure 24**   The facial recess is opened. Note the incudo-stapedial joint, the Eustachian tube, the malleus, the promontory, and the hypotympanum.

### Extended Facial Recess (Fig. 26)

By extending the facial recess inferiorly until its floor is flush with the hypotympanum, one gains better visualization of the mesotympanum and hypotympanic cells. This necessitates section of the chorda tympani nerve. By enlarging the aperture to the limit of the sulcus tympanicus and the facial nerve, one improves visualization. This procedure is useful in removal of glomus tympanicum tumors.

### Jugular Bulb

The area of pneumatized mastoid cells below or medial to the facial nerve is termed the "retrofacial cell tract" (Fig. 24). This area is inferior to the labyrinth and

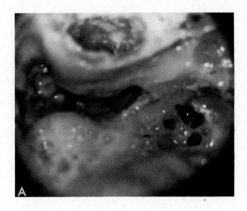

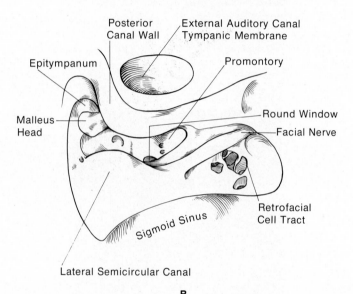

**Figure 25** The bar of bone protecting the incus is now removed, exposing better the view of the tympanic segment of the facial nerve. Note also the cochleariform process, the canal for the tensor tympani, the malleus head in the epitympanum.

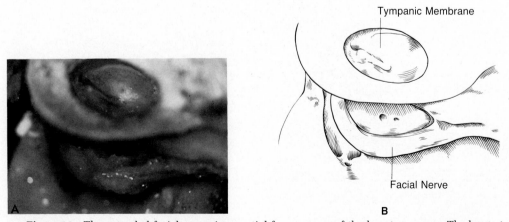

**Figure 26** The extended facial recess is essential for exposure of the hypotympanum. The bone at the area of the styloid eminence is removed; this necessitates sectioning of the chorda tympani nerve.

extends toward the inferior surface of the temporal bone and anteriorly toward the cochlea. Because it is pneumatized bone, cholesteatoma can occasionally invade this area, avoiding the dense endochondral bone of the labyrinth. Graham* has pointed out that the jugular bulb can be variably positioned in the mastoid and hypotympanum. The bulb lies in a fossa on the inferior surface of the temporal bone. The top of the bulb may in some cases lie 20 mm. above the horizontal limb of the sigmoid sinus. The bulb usually lies on the floor of the middle ear which in some cases is dehiscent. The inferior petrosal sinus (which may be a system of sinuses) empties into the inferior aspect of the jugular bulb.

### Area of Endolymphatic Sac (Fig. 27)

The superior limit of the endolymphatic sac is located by drawing an imaginary line (Donaldson's line) from the lateral semicircular canal, bisecting the perpendicu-

*Graham, M.: The jugular bulb: Its anatomic and clinical considerations in contemporary otology. Laryngoscope, 87:105, 1977.

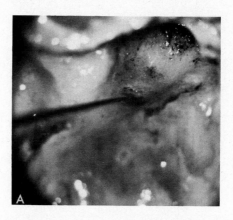

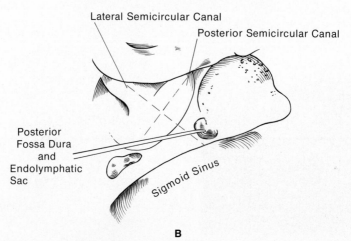

**Figure 27**   An imaginary line (Donaldson's line) delimits the top of the endolymphatic sac. Note the posterior and lateral semicircular canals.

lar formed by the posterior semicircular canal. The top of the sac is located here in the posterior fossa dura.

While Arenberg* has shown that the location of the endolymphatic sac varies with the amount of periaqueductal pneumatization, it is typically located in the dura of the posterior fossa medial to the sigmoid sinus. There is a wide variation in size, shape and location of the endolymphatic sac. The duct takes its characteristic "J" shape while approaching the operculum from the vestibule. The endolymphatic sac is pear shaped, the bottom being the endolymphatic duct.

## ANATOMY OF THE EPITYMPANUM

By superior dissection along the zygomatic root and preservation by thinning of the superior osseous canal wall, one explores an area known as the attic, or epitympanum. Here one can visualize initially the short process of the incus, the ossicular ligaments, the head of the malleus and the horizontal (tympanic) course of the facial nerve.

The attic lies in the potential space above the tensor tympani fold, but some authors describe a definite bony plate between the attic and mesotympanum. It is essential to know exactly where the geniculate ganglion is located in the anterior epitympanum. It can be found slightly superior-anterior to the cochleariforme process as the nerve turns inward toward the internal auditory canal, bending around the cochlea. The geniculate ganglion sits like a cap over the anterior portion of the external genu of the facial nerve. Sheehy makes note of a spine of bone ("the cog") that hangs inferiorly from the tegmen. The facial nerve lies anterior to the cog just before it turns into its first genu. The cog extends inferiorly just above the cochleariformis process.

Anterior to the head of the malleus is a large cell separating the main epitympanic space by an incomplete or membranous bony wall. This is called the anterior epitympanic recess. It is a common place for recurrent disease (i.e., cholesteatoma).

## ANATOMY OF THE RADICAL CAVITY

The radical cavity will always remain to be dealt with in modern otolaryngology (see Fig. 19). The objective of the surgical creation of the radical cavity is to exteriorize all areas of the temporal bone. Incomplete surgery may modify the author's concept of what a radical cavity truly is. After the osseous canal wall is removed, those areas in which the canal is attached to the tympanic ring are called the anterior and posterior buttresses. The canal is taken down to the level of the facial nerve, and the tympanic membrane and all ossicles are removed. The plate of bone just covering the facial nerve is called the "facial ridge." The bone just anterior to the facial nerve in its descending course is called the "infra-annular mass of bone" and separates the mastoid from the middle ear. The epitympanum is flush with the mesotympanum and hypotympanum, so one large cavity is created. Ideally, the floor of the mastoid cavity is level with the floor of the osseous meatus.

---

*Arenberg, I. K., Anderson, H. R., Wilbrand, H., and Stahle, J.: The surgical anatomy of the endolymphatic sac. Arch. of Otolaryngol., *103*:1, 1977.

## LABYRINTHINE AND TRANSLABYRINTHINE ANATOMY

The osseous (bony) labyrinth consists of three parts: the cochlea, the vestibule and the semicircular canals. On lateral dissection the three semicircular canals can be skeletonized more or less easily, depending on the amount of pneumatization of the temporal bone (Fig. 28).

The membranous labyrinth is contained within the bony labyrinth. The cochlea contains the cochlear duct, and the three semicircular canals each contain a semicircular duct. The vestibule contains the utricle, saccule and endolymphatic duct leading to the endolymphatic sac.

On opening the bony labyrinth (Fig. 29) at the lateral semicircular canal, one next proceeds toward the posterior canal. The non-ampullated ends of the posterior and superior canals form the common crus (Fig. 30). The ampulla of the posterior canal lies under the facial nerve (Figs. 31 and 34), adjacent to the sinus tympani, and opens

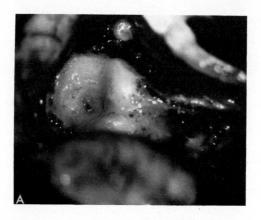

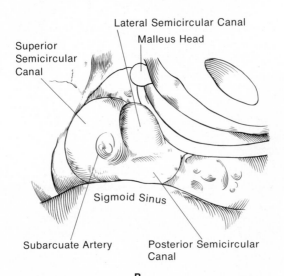

**B**

**Figure 28**   The semicircular canals skeletonized to show right angle relationships. Note the subarcuate artery in the center of the superior canal.

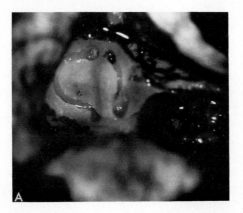

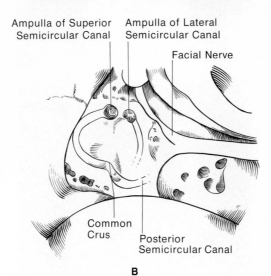

Ampulla of Superior
Semicircular Canal

Ampulla of Lateral
Semicircular Canal

Facial Nerve

Common
Crus

Posterior
Semicircular Canal

B

**Figure 29**   The bony labyrinth opened to show the ampullae and the canals of the membranous labyrinth.

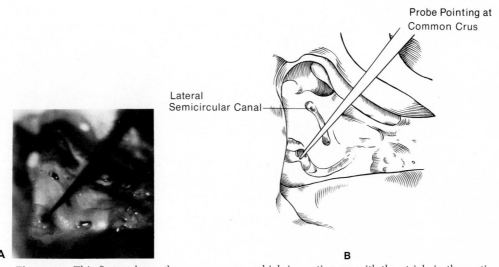

Probe Pointing at
Common Crus

Lateral
Semicircular Canal

A                                                                              B

**Figure 30**   This figure shows the common crus, which is continuous with the utricle in the vestibule.

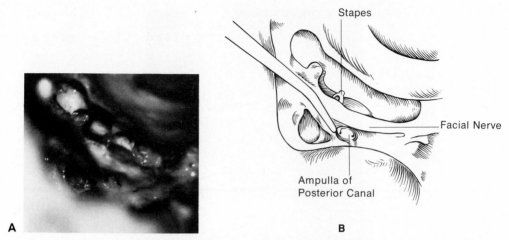

A

B

**Figure 31** Note that the posterior ampulla lies under the facial nerve adjacent to the sinus tympani.

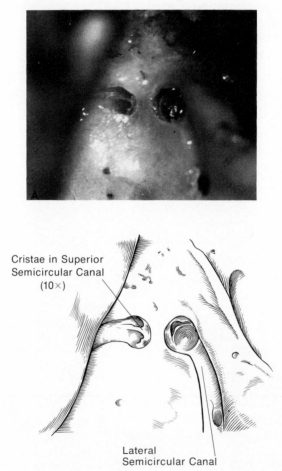

B

**Figure 32** The ampullae of the lateral and superior semicircular canals at 16×. Note the crista inside the ampulla. These ampullae are adjacent to each other. Inferior to the lateral ampulla is the facial nerve.

in the floor of the vestibule, while the ampullae of the lateral and superior canals are next to each other. The canals lie at right angles to each other.

The ampulla of the lateral semicircular canal is just above the fenestra vestibulae (oral window). Within the ampullated end of each semicircular canal is the crista, the end organ of the vestibular nerve (Fig. 32).

The bony cochlea is conical in form and has its apex directed laterally, downward and forward. From apex to base it measures 5 mm., and the diameter of the base is about 10 mm. The cochlea has two and three-fourths turns.

Between the cochlea and the semicircular canals lies the vestibule (Fig. 33). Its lateral wall contains the oval and round windows. The medial wall of the vestibule

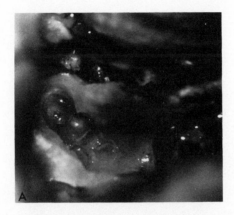

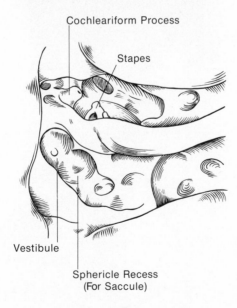

**Figure 33** The anatomy of the vestibule is rather complex. The bony anatomy in the vestibule corresponds rather well to the membranous labyrinth. The saccule lodged in the spherical recess of the vestibule receives fibers of the vestibular nerve through foramina that pass from the inferior vestibular area of the fundus of the IAC and cribrose macula of the vestibule. The utricle that lies in the elliptical recess is adjacent to the superior cribrose macula of the vestibule that conducts branches of the upper terminal ramus of the vestibular nerve.

presents an anterior area known as the recessus sphericus, which lodges the saccule, and a posterior area known as the recessus ellipticus, in which the utricle is attached. These two recesses are separated by a vertical crest (the crista vestibuli) which bifurcates inferiorly to form the recessus cochlearis in which are found some perforations through which pass a few fibers of the vestibulocochlear nerve that are delivered to the lower vestibular portion of the cochlear duct.

In the spherical recess are perforations (the macula cribrosa media) for passage of nerve fibers to the macula of the saccule. In the elliptical recess are perforations (the macula cribrosa superior) through which nerve fibers pass to the ampullae of the superior and horizontal semicircular ducts. This area in the elliptical recess has been nicknamed "Mike's dot" by Michael Glasscock's associates (Fig. 34) and is a useful landmark to the lateral end of the internal auditory canal.

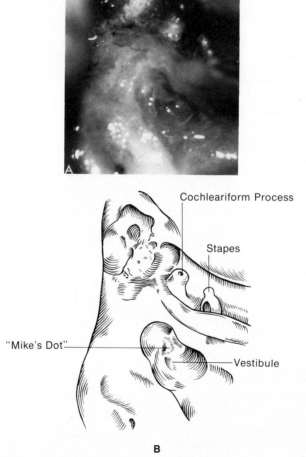

**B**

**Figure 34** "Mike's dot," a cribriform area of bone (macula cribrosa superior) that transmits the vestibular nerve to the ampulla of the lateral and superior semicircular canals. It is a useful landmark to the lateral end of the internal auditory canal located in the vestibule.

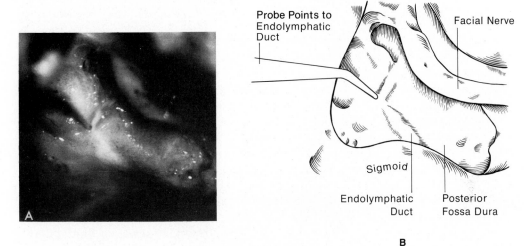

**Figure 35**   This light "J" shaped structure is the endolymphatic duct seen only after labyrinthec-tomy.

The membranous components of the vestibule are the utricle and saccule. The utricle, in the elliptical recess, is about 5 mm. in length and communicates with the three semicircular ducts. The macula of the utricle lies on the roof of the elliptical recess. It is oval in shape and composed of sustenticular cells and sensory epithelium.

The saccule that lies in the spherical recess of the vestibule is slightly more anterior. It communicates with both the endolymphatic duct via the saccular duct and the cochlear duct via the ductus reuniens. The saccule has its own macula.

In the inferior portion of the recessus ellipticus is found the orifice of the aqueductus vestibuli which contains the endolymphatic duct proceeding to the posterior surface of the mastoid (Fig. 35).

Posterior to this orifice is an area of perforation (foramen singulare) for nerve fibers going to the ampulla of the posterior semicircular duct.

The subarcuate artery (Fig. 28) is a vessel forming a connection between meningeal vessels and those of the inner ear. The contained vessel usually becomes atrophic by the fifth year of life, but occasionally does contain an active blood supply in the adult.

## THE INTERNAL AUDITORY CANAL

The vestibular portion of the eighth nerve is divided into two branches before it is distributed to the membranous labyrinth. The superior ramus sends branches to the utricle and to ampullae of the lateral and superior semicircular ducts, and a small branch to the saccule. The inferior ramus sends branches to the saccule and to the ampulla of the posterior semicircular duct, and a small branch to the most proximal portion of the cochlear duct.

Besides the vestibular nerves, the facial and cochlear nerves (with the nervus intermedius) are located in the internal auditory canal. The singular nerve to the posterior canal is also observed.

After removing all the bone between the labyrinth and the jugular bulb, the internal auditory canal is skeletonized by removing bone above (the roof) and below (the floor) as well as in the area near the posterior lip (Fig. 36). One must recall the plane of the internal canal and remember that the vestibule is the most lateral neighboring structure to the canal itself, while the medial end is lower or more medial in the lateral approach. Bone is thus removed so as to approach the posterior wall of the internal auditory canal; all dura is exposed first. A horizontal crest, the falciformis crest (Fig. 37), separates the fibers of the superior vestibular nerve (Fig. 37) from the thin filaments of nerve to the saccule (inferior vestibular nerve) (Fig. 38). There is a further vertical bony bar on the medial side of the superior vestibular nerve (Bill's bar) (Fig. 39) which is seen more clearly when the meatus is opened from the middle fossa side.

It is important to conceptualize the relationships of the nerves inside the canal prior to opening into the internal auditory meatus. The meatus should not be opened until all the preliminary bone work of the exposure has been completed. The facial nerve (Fig. 39) is situated above and in front; indeed, it may not be seen until the superior vestibular nerve is divided. It enters the canal above the falciform crest and in front of the vertical crest (Bill's bar). The superior vestibular nerve, which covers the facial nerve, is situated more superficially than the inferior vestibular nerve. Further inside the canal, the two vestibular nerves may intertwine. The cochlear nerve can only be seen after resection of the inferior vestibular nerve.

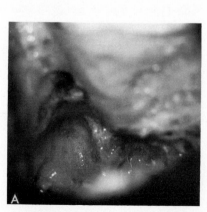

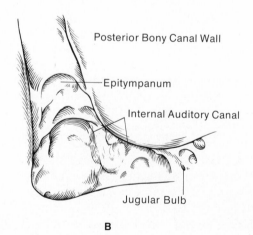

Posterior Bony Canal Wall

Epitympanum

Internal Auditory Canal

Jugular Bulb

**A**                                                                      **B**

**Figure 36**  This depicts the internal auditory canal still covered by a thin layer of bone. Bone has been removed from the roof of the canal, near the posterior lip and at the floor.

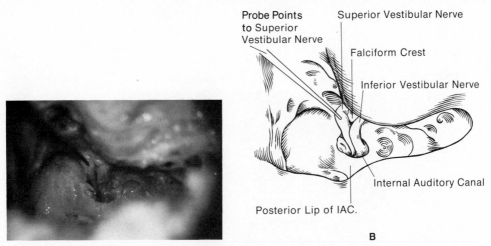

**Figure 37** The superior vestibular nerve supplies fibers to the utricle and ampullae of the lateral and superior semicircular canals. The inferior vestibular nerve gives fibers to the posterior ampulla and the saccule.

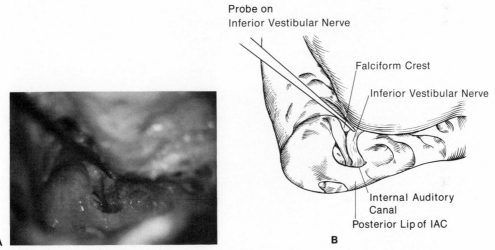

**Figure 38** From the lateral approach, the superior vestibular nerve is the most dominant, and is cephalad, often covering the facial nerve. The probe points to the inferior vestibular nerve.

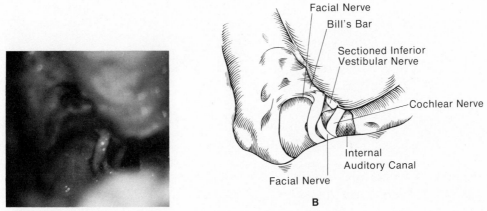

**Figure 39** After sectioning the inferior vestibular nerve, one can observe the cochlear nerve more easily. Also note that the superior vestibular nerve covers the facial nerve.

717

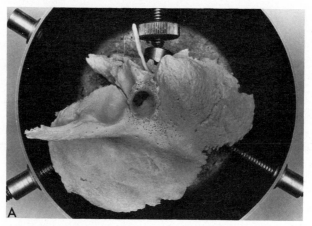

**Figure 40**  Orientation to the student of middle fossa surgery must be obtained in the surgical position shown on a dry temporal bone here.

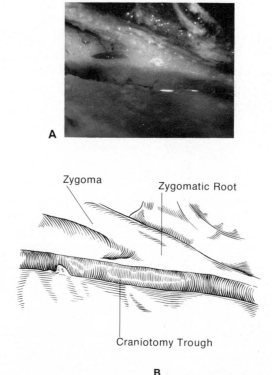

**Figure 41**  It is useful to remember that the external acoustic meatus and the most posterior edge of the posterior root of the zygoma are in the same axis as the internal auditory canal.

## SUPERIOR (MIDDLE FOSSA) APPROACH TO THE TEMPORAL BONE

### Positioning of the Bone

Most confusing to students of temporal bone anatomy is the correct position for superior anatomical exposure of the temporal bone. All dissection should be done in the surgical position as if the operator were sitting at the head of the patient and looking toward the feet. The bone then simply has the mastoid tip pointing away from the dissector (Fig. 40). A preliminary craniotomy flap is done above the zygoma as shown to expose the superior surface of the temporal bone (Fig. 41). If the bone still has dry dura, this is carefully removed so as not to avulse the greater superficial petrosal nerve or geniculate ganglion, which are at times dehiscent.

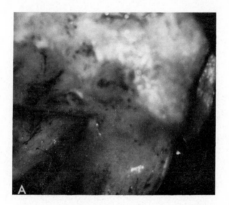

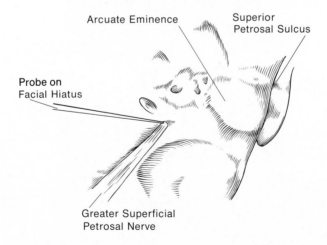

**B**

**Figure 42**    The greater superficial petrosal nerve is a flat thin structure on the superior surface of the temporal bone. Its identification is essential in middle fossa surgery. This nerve exits the facial hiatus just medial to the foramen spinosum for the middle meningeal artery and nearly on the same plane.

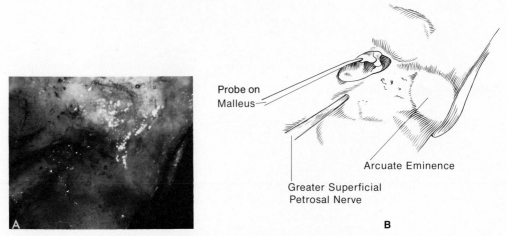

**Figure 43** The malleus is shown with the pointer. On a plane slightly anterior to it, but located considerably more medially, is the internal auditory canal.

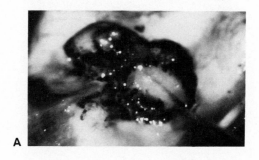

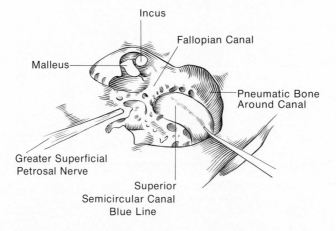

**Figure 44** Professor U. Fisch has found the superior semicircular canal also to be a useful landmark to the internal auditory canal. After it has been "blue lined," the semicircular canal is on a 60° angle with the internal auditory canal.

## Orientation

Identification of the greater superficial petrosal nerve is essential, as it acts as a guide to the internal auditory canal. By careful dissection the nerve is isolated and, using a diamond burr, its origin is traced back posteriorly to the geniculate ganglion beyond the facial hiatus (Fig. 42). In some bones the foramen spinosum for the middle meningeal artery can be observed. The lesser superficial petrosal nerve runs parallel to the greater.

By removing the tegmen covering the malleus and incus (Fig. 43), further identification of the canal is insured as the internal auditory canal is on a plane just anterior with this ossicular juncture. Care must be used here so as not to disrupt the tympanic segment of the facial nerve.

Lastly, by cautiously thinning the bone over the arcuate eminence one can identify the superior semicircular canal. It is skeletonized until a "blue line" appears (Fig. 44). The segment between the blue line and the internal auditory canal is an angle of about 60 degrees and facilitates exposure of the posterior aspect of the internal canal. The fundus of the internal auditory canal is bordered by the basal

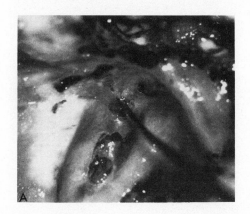

A

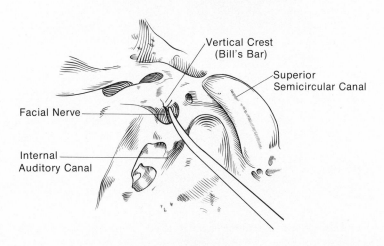

B

**Figure 45** The vertical crest ("Bill's bar") is a useful landmark to the facial nerve. It separates the facial nerve from the superior vestibular nerve at the most lateral extent of the IAC.

turn of the cochlea anteriorly and by the superior semicircular canal posteriorly. The area medial to the geniculate ganglion is the narrowest portion in the dissection of the internal auditory canal.

### Fundus of Canal

The internal auditory canal is lined by an extension of dura. The dura surrounds the seventh nerve and becomes neurolemma of the nerve. The facial and superior vestibular nerves pass through the fundal portion of the canal to enter distinct bony channels. They are separated by a distinct bony crest (Bill's bar) (Fig. 45).

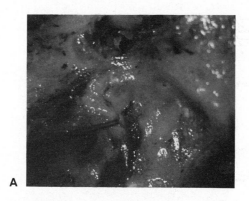

A

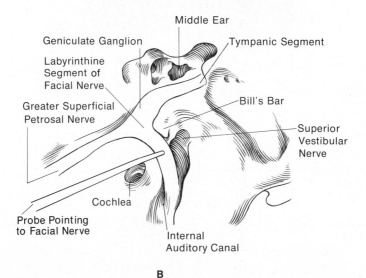

B

**Figure 46**  This figure shows how the facial nerve descends into the internal auditory canal and its relationship to the geniculate ganglion and the greater superficial petrosal nerve. The cochlea is intentionally fenestrated to demonstrate its proximity to the facial nerve and its vulnerability in middle fossa surgery.

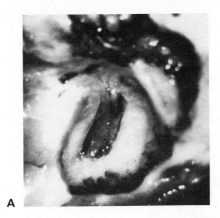

**A**

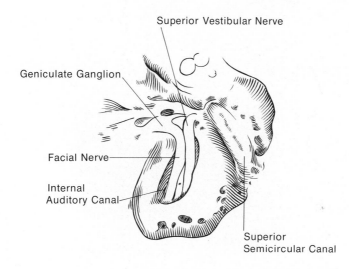

**B**

**Figure 47**  Nicely demonstrated in this specimen is the facial nerve as it relates to the superior vestibular nerve. Note that the posterior semicircular canal makes a 60° angle with the internal auditory canal. The facial nerve is higher at the lateral aspect of the internal auditory canal and descends into the internal canal.

The fundus of the internal auditory canal is divided into two parts by a falciform crest which is on a horizontal plane (Figs. 11 and 45) and a vertical crest, Bill's bar, that separates the facial from the superior vestibular nerves.

The facial nerve (Fig. 46) is the most superiorly placed of the nerves. It enters the internal acoustic meatus at the lateral rim, then curves downward into the fundus of the canal. It is anterior and superior in position in the canal. Immediately beneath and behind the facial nerve is the nervus intermedius of Wrisberg, which proceeds toward the brainstem in its own trunk.

The superior vestibular nerve (Fig. 47) is observed passing through the fundus of the internal acoustic meatus and there presents with a swelling, Scarpa's ganglion. It receives fibers from the utricular macula and ampullae of the lateral and

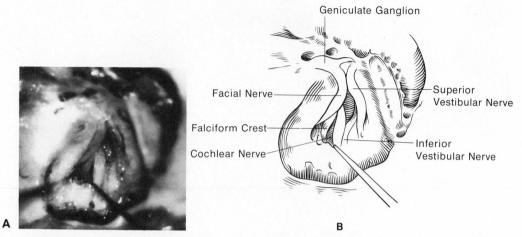

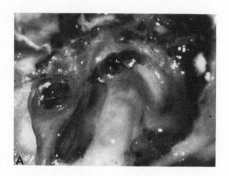

**Figure 48**   Here the facial nerve has been moved aside to demonstrate the falciform crest and the cochlear nerve.

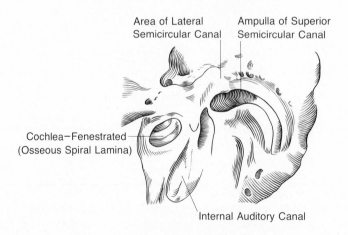

**Figure 49**   The labyrinth has been drilled open to demonstrate the ampulla of the superior semicircular canal, the semicircular canal itself and the cochlea. Note that there is more bone between the semicircular canal and the internal auditory canal than between the cochlea and the internal auditory canal.

superior semicircular ducts that pass through the minute foramina of the macula cribrosa superior.

The inferior vestibular nerve (Fig. 48) receives fibers from the ampulla of the posterior duct by way of the foramen singulare as well as the macula of the saccule.

The cochlear nerve (Fig. 48) travels from the osseous spiral lamina (Fig. 49), passing through foramina in the cochlear recess inferior to the facial and slightly below the level of the inferior vestibular nerve, and proceeds toward the brainstem.

*Acknowledgment:*

The author wishes to express his gratitude to J. Michael Barret, Ph.D., and Willis K. Paull, Ph.D., Department of Anatomy, The Medical College of Georgia, for their editorial comments.

# Index of Names

Page numbers in *italics* indicate bibliographic citations.

Adams, W. S., 281, *287*
Adamson, M., *367*, *468*
Adelman, N., *265*, *314*
Adour, K. K., 533, *557*
Aenaldi, M., *152*
Agazzi, C., *152*
Alberti, P. W. R. M., *314*
Alexander, G., 381, *406*
Allen, G. W., *29*, *635*
Almour, R., *264*, *290*, *314*, 345, 347
Alt, F., *556*
Altmann, F., *406*, *474*, *591*
Amjad, A. H., *495*, *499*
Anderson, J. R., *592*
Anjou, A., *152*
Anson, B. J., 4, 5, *29*, *406*, *460*, *461*, *475*, *568*, *591*
Arenberg, I. K., 585, *592*, *709*
Arnold, G. E., *635*
Arslan, M., *461*, *475*, 584, *592*
Aschoff, L., 215, *220*
Austin, D., 432, 433, 437, *453*
Avicenna, 289

Babbit, J. A., *182*
Badger, G. F., *220*
Bagby, R. A., *220*
Baker, H. L., *475*
Ballance, C. A., *264*, *290*, *314*, 426, 452, 516, 520, 521, 522, *556*, 638, 667, *672*
Banzer, M., 408, *422*
Bárány, R., 502, *515*
Baron, S., 268, *286*
Barrois, J. J., *152*
Barsky, A. J., *407*
Basek, M., *499*
Bast, T. H., 4, 5, *29*, *406*, *460*, *461*, *475*, *568*, *591*
Batisse, R., 587, *592*, *593*, 638, *673*, *678*
Beal, D. D., *635*
Beck, J. C., *313*, *635*
Becker, O. J., *230*, *249*
Békésy, G. von, 352, 357, 359, 372, *379*, *422*, *427*
Bel, J., *475*
Bell, C., 520, 522, 638, *672*
Bell, H. L., *422*
Berdal, P., *635*
Bergès, J., *460*, *469*, *474*
Bergmann, E. von, *286*
Bernstein, P., *592*
Berthold, E., 409, *422*, 425, *452*

Bezold, F., 2, 3, *202*, 214, *220*, 255, *264*, 353, *379*, 456, *677*
Blake, C. J., 408, *422*, *478*, *498*, 502, *515*
Blatt, I. M., 313, *314*, 532, *556*
Bloch, W., *152*
Bondy, G., 268, *286*
Boucheron, E., 425, *452*, *478*, *498*
Bourjat, P., *152*
Boyd, L. J., *249*
Boyle, W. F., *83*
Braaten, M., *635*
Brackmann, D. E., *635*, *673*
Braun, A., *314*, 347
Bret, P., *152*
Bretlau, P., *475*
Brown, L. A., 616, *635*
Brown, M. R., *592*
Brownrigg, G. M., *249*
Brünner, S., *152*
Bryan, M. P., *592*
Bryan, W. T. K., *592*
Buckingham, R. A., *152*
Bucy, P. C., *315*, *673*
Bunnell, S., 518, 520, *556*

Cairns, H., 560, 565, *591*, *673*
Campbell, E. C. R., *557*
Campbell, P. A., 353, *379*
Cappelen, C., Jr., *635*
Carhart, R., 366, *379*, 504, *673*
Cauldwell, E. W., *461*
Causse, J., *460*, *461*, *469*, *473*, *474*, *475*, *496*, *498*
Cawthorne, T., 180, 184, *219*, *220*, 313, 345, *347*, 522, *556*, *557*, 560, 576, *591*, *592*, *673*
Celsus, 289
Chailkin, J. B., *83*
Chandler, J. R., *249*, *556*
Chevance, L. G., *460*, *461*, *469*, *474*, *475*, *498*
Churchill, D., *673*
Clemis, J. D., *83*, *152*, 153, *453*
Clerc, P., 587, *592*, 638, *673*, *678*
Cody, D. T. R., 281, *287*, 473, *475*, 583, 590, *592*
Coiter, V., 352, *378*
Colman, B. H., *315*
Compere, W. E., *111*, *152*, *673*
Conley, J. J., *557*, 612, *635*
Corti, A., 352, *378*, 568
Costen, J. B., *83*
Cotugno, D., 352, *378*

Courville, C. B., 265, *314*
Cova, P. L., *152*
Cox, D. J., *673*
Crabtree, J. A., 397, *407*
Crowe, S. J., 560, *591*, 639, *673*
Cushing, H., 637, 638, 667, *672, 673*
Cutt, R. A., *592*

Dahmann, H., 352, 357, *379*
Dandy, W. E., *592*, 657, 667, *673*
Danforth, H. B., *557*
Davis, G. S., *249*
Davis, H., 352, 353, 378, *379*, 426, *452*, 504, *515*
Davison, R. C., *83*
Dawes, J. D. K., *314*
Day, K. M., 213, 214, *220*, *593*
Day, L. A., *592*
de Kleijn, A., 461, *475*
Dean, L. W., 381, *406*
Dearmin, R. M., 340, *347*
Dederding, D., 560, 576, *591*
Deka, R. C., *475*
der Hoeve, J. van, 461, *475*
Derlacki, E. L., *83*, 220, 287, *407*, 409, 415, 422, 437, *453*, 478, 499, 507, 565, *591*
Diamant, M., 29, 214, 220
Dietzel, K., *556*
Dix, M. R., 560, *591*
Doefler, L., *83*
Domagk, G., 252, 288, 677
Donaldson, J. A., *591*
Dott, N. M., 521, *556*
Dowling, H. F., *314*
Doyle, J. B., Jr., *673*
Doyle-Kelly, W., *453*
Dra, F. W., *453*
Drobnick, T., 520
Druss, J. G., *314*
Dubs, R., *407*
Duel, A. B., 467, 520, 521, *556*
Duke, W. W., 565, *591*
Dunlap, A. M., 411, *422*
Duquesnel, J., *152*
Duverney, J. G., *378*

Eagleton, W. P., *264*, 290, *314*, 340, *347*
Eby, L. G., *347*
Echols, D. F., *249*
Empedocles, 351
English, O. S., *83*
Engström, H., 502, *515*, *591*
Eustachius, B., 352, *378*
Eysell, C. G., *264*, *452*

Fallopio, G., 352, *378*, 518
Faraci, G., 478, *498*
Farrior, J. B., 220, 290, *314*, 340, *347*
Faunce, C. B., *220*, *314*
Feller, A. E., *220*
Fick, I. A., 583, 590, *592*
Fisch, U., 533, 548, 556, *556, 557*, 587, *592*, 635, *720*

Fischgold, H., *152*
Fish, W., *249*
Fleming, A., 252, 288, 677
Fowler, E. P., 467, 560, 579, 591, *673*
Fowler, E. P., Jr., 238, *249*, 499, *556, 592*
Franceschetti, A., *406*
Francois, J., *152*
Frank, O., 352, *379*
Fraser, J. S., *83*, *406*
Frenckner, P., 290, *314*, 340, *347*
Frey, K., *152*
Friesner, I., *314, 347*
Furstenberg, A. C., 576, *592*

Gaffney, J. C., *635*
Galen, C., 351, *378*
Gandhi, K., *422*
Garcia-Ibánez, L., *453*
Gardner, G., *635*
Gardner, W. J., 555, *557*, 645
Gejrot, T., *635*
Gianturco, C., *111*
Gillies, H., *407*
Gilse, P. H. G. von, 238, *249*
Giraud, M., *152*
Githler, F. J., 372, *379*, *422*
Gittins, T. R., *406*
Glasscock, M. E., 51, *407, 422, 453*, 556, *557*, 587, *592*, 635, *673*, 714
Glorig, A., *83*, *314*
Goldman, J. L., *314*
Goodhill, V., *315, 347*
Gowers, W., 520
Gradenigo, G., 290, *314*, 316, *347*
Graham, M., *422*, 708
Griffith, A., *220, 673*
Groen, J. J., *379*
Gross, J. P., *152*
Grunert, K., 307, *314*
Guild, S. R., 458, 465, 474, 568, 594, 612, *635*
Guilford, F. R., 281, *286, 287*, 437, 439, *453, 635*
Guillen, G., *152*

Habermann, J., 213, *220*
Hagen, W. E., *592*
Hall, A., 427, *453*
Hallberg, G. E., *592*
Hallpike, C. S., 560, 565, *591*, *673*
Hamrick, P. E., *592*
Hansel, F. K., *220*
Hanson, D. G., *592*
Hardin, W. B., Jr., 556, *557*
Hardy, M., 639, *673*
Harpman, J. A., *314*
Harris, P. F., *635*
Harrison, W. H., *379, 422, 453*
Harvey, T., *557*
Heerman, H., 167, 182, *422*, 427, 478, *499*
Heimendinger, E., *152*
Heine, B., *313*
Hellmann, K., 214, *220*
Helmholtz, H. L. F. von, 350, 352, 353, 357, 359, 364, *378*, 425, 426, *452*
Helsper, J. T., 522, *556*

Henschen, F., *673*
Herzog, H., 352, *379*
Hickey, R. P., *557*
Hilding, A. C., *219*
Hildyard, V. H., *407*
Hilger, J. A., *557*, *592*
Hinsberg, V., 335, *347*
Hippocrates, 1, 251, 289
Hodges, R. G., *220*
Holderman, J. W., 469, *475*
Holmgren, G., 177, 353, 426, *452*, 502, 515, 677
Homsy, C. A., *453*
Hood, J. D., 560, *591*
Hoogland, G. A., *379*
Horton, B. T., *592*
Hough, J. V. D., *407*
House, H. P., 51, 381, *406*, 407, 409, 422, 473, *475*, *635*
House, W. F., 29, 83, 407, 422, *453*, 584, 587, 590, *592*, *635*, 636, 638, 667, *673*, 678
Hoyne, A. L., *314*
Hughes, R. L., *83*
Huizing, E. H., *379*
Hunt, J. R., *557*

Ingrassia, G. F., 352, *378*
Isamot, F., *673*
Ishiyama, E., *592*

Jack, F. L., 478, *498*, 502, *515*
Jackson, C. J., *673*
Jannetta, P. J., 555, *557*
Jansen, A., 290, *314*, 335, *347*
Jansen, C. L., 437, *453*
Jansen, V., *678*
Jasser, 251
Jeanes, A., *346*
Jenkins, G. J., 502, *515*, 677
Jenkins, W. H., *635*
Jensen, A. M., *314*
Jepson, O., *557*
Jerger, J., 475, 560, *591*, *673*
Johansen, H., 353, 366, *379*
Jones, I. H., *379*
Jongkees, L. B. W., 503, 533, *557*, *592*
Jordan, R. E., *83*, *220*
Jordan, W. S., Jr., *220*
Jørgensen, M. B., 461, *475*
Joseph, R. B., *453*
Josey, A. F., *673*
Joynt, J. A., 409, *422*
Juers, A. L., *183*, 213, 353, 360, *379*, 414, 422, 426, *452*, 503, 504, 507
Juster, M., *152*

Kacker, S. K., *475*
Kakizaki, I., 460, *474*
Kaplan, J., *422*
Katz, J., *83*
Kelemen, G., 461, *635*
Kemble, J., *264*
Kemker, F. J., *673*
Kerrison, P. D., 425, *452*

Kerth, J. D., *183*
Kessel, J., 154, 167, 269, 425, 426, *452*, 477, *498*, 502, 504, 515
Kettel, K., *347*, 521, 533, *556*
Kimura, R. S., 570, *591*
Kinney, S. E., 631, *635*
Kirikae, I., *591*
Kisch, J., *286*
Kisselbach, W., *406*, 425, *452*
Kitlowski, E. A., *249*
Kley, W., *423*, *453*
Kline, O. R., *249*
Klopp, C. T., *635*
Klotz, G., *152*
Knapp, H., 560, *591*
Knudsen, V. O., *379*, 560, *591*
Kobrak, H. G., 352, 364, *379*
Koch, H., *422*
Konishi, T., *592*
Kopetsky, S. J., *220*, *264*, 265, *286*, 290, *314*, 345, *347*, 381, *406*
Körner, O., 268, *286*, 289, 293, *314*, *591*
Kornfeld, M., *591*
Kranz, F. W., 366, *379*
Kurze, T. L., 638, *673*
Küster, E., 426, *452*

Lake, R., 560, *591*
Lane, C. S., *635*
Lane, W. A., *314*
Lang, E. R., *315*
Lange, K., *249*
Lange, W., 214, *220*
Langfeldt, B., *152*
Lashment, F. H., *592*
Lattes, R., *635*
Laumans, E. P., Jr., *557*
Lauren, T., *635*
Law, F., *111*
Lawrence, M., 352, *356*, 357, 362, *378*, *379*
Lebert, 289, *314*
Leicher, H., *406*
Lele, D. N., *249*
Lempert, J., 167, 177, *182*, *264*, 268, 269, 273, *286*, 290, *314*, 344, *347*, 349, 426, *452*, 478, 500, 502, 503, *515*, 676, 677
Lenz, W., *406*
Lepper, M. H., *314*
Lermoyez, M., 565, *591*
Levine, R., *557*
Lewis, J. S., 612, *635*
Lichtenstein, L., *635*
Lindsay, J. R., *153*, *347*, *361*, 460, 474, 560, *591*, *635*
Lindstrom, J., *635*
Linn, E. G., 409, *422*
Linser, P., *314*
Linthicum, F. H., *453*, 461, 473, *673*
Lund, W. S., *314*
Lundquist, P., *591*
Lüscher, E., 352, 364, *379*

MacCarty, C. S., 639, 667, *673*
Macewen, W., 289, *314*
Maddox, H. E., 638, *673*

Mahoney, M., *673*
Mallis, L., 638
Manasse, P., *83, 474*
Marovitz, W. F., *557*
Martin, H., 522, *556*
Maxwell, J. H., *557*
May, M., 532, 533, *556, 557*
Mayer, E. G., *111*
Mayer, O., *83*
McCabe, B. F., 555, *556, 557, 592*
McGee, T. M., *315*
McKenzie, D., 214, *220*
McLaughlin, C. R., *423*
McMinn, R. M. H., *422*
McNally, W. J., *346*
Meckel, P. F., *352, 378*
Melkersson, E., 554, *557*
Mendoza, D., 461, *475*
Meniere, P., 558, 559, 560, *591*
Meryman, H. T., 223, *249*
Meurman, Y., 281, *286, 381, 387, 406*
Michaux, P., *475*
Millard, D. R., Jr., *407*
Miller, G. W., *453, 592, 673*
Miller, R. N., *673*
Milligan, W., 560, *591*
Mills, W. J., 223, *249*
Miot, C., 425, *452, 478, 498, 502, 515*
Mogan, R. F., *593*
Mohs, F. E., 599, *635*
Mounier-Kuhn, P. L., *152*
Morand, S. F., 289, *314*
Morgagni, G. B., 289
Moritz, W., *426, 452*
Morrison, A. W., 585, *592*
Müller, J., 352, 364, *378*
Mulligan, R. M., *635*
Mündnich, K., *152, 396, 406*
Myers, D., *592*
Myerson, M. C., *347*
Mygind, S. H., 560, 576, *591*
Mylius, E. A., *635*

Nager, F. R., 214, *220, 502, 515, 591*
Nager, G. T., *635, 669, 673*
Nash, C. S., *83*
Newsome, G., *635*
Nilsson, G., 353, *378, 379*
Nixon, K. H., *557*
Norris, C. H., *83, 249, 592*
Novack, A. J., 612, *635*
Nylén, C. O., 348, *426, 502, 639, 677*

O'Brien, F. H., *346*
Ochsner, A., *183*
Ogier, M., *152*
Ogilvie, R. L., 461, *475*
Ojala, L., 214, *220*
Okuneff, W. N., 409, *422*
Olivecrona, H., *673*
Ombrédanne, M., *152, 381, 406, 426, 427, 452*
Oppenheimer, P., 413, *422*
Orr, M. F., *557*
Oshiro, H., *635*

Osmun, P. M., 238, *249*
Overfield, R. E., *673*
Owen, G. R., *111*

Page, J. R., 381, *406*
Palva, T., 281, *287, 437, 453*
Panse, R., 638, *673*
Paparella, M. M., 585, *592*
Paré, A., 251
Parry, R. H., 560, *591*
Passe, E. R. G., *593*
Passow, K. A., 281, *286, 502, 503, 515*
Pattee, G. L., 381, *406, 426, 427, 452*
Patterson, M. E., *51, 407, 453*
Payne, M. C., 372, *379, 422*
Peacock, R., *592*
Peer, L. A., *407*
Pennington, C. L., *407, 432, 453, 584, 590, 592*
Perlee, J. H., *249*
Perlman, H. B., *635*
Perozzi, L., 460
Petersen, O., *152*
Petit, J., 251, 264
Petrovic, A., *472, 475*
Petti, G. H., *347*
Pierce, R., *153*
Piffl, O., 307, *314*
Plester, D., *422, 453*
Podesta, R., *347*
Pohlman, A. C., 352, *378, 379*
Pohlman, M. E., 408, *422*
Politzer, A., 52, *381, 406, 456, 474, 478, 502*
Portmann, G., 558, 584, *591*
Portmann, M., *152*
Pulec, J. L., *83, 347*

Quix, F. H., 636, 638, *673*

Raber, R., *152*
Rainer, A., *347*
Ramadier, J., *264, 290, 314, 344, 347*
Rambo, J. H. T., *347, 453*
Rammelkamp, C. H., Jr., *220*
Rand, R. W., 638, 667, *673*
Rask-Andersen, H., *592*
Reger, S., *379*
Retzius, G., 352, *378*
Rhoton, A. L., 639, *673*
Ricci, V., 461, *475*
Richards, C. S., *406*
Richards, J. D., 335, *347*
Richardson, A. T., *557*
Riff, E. R., *314*
Rinne, H. A., 52
Rius, M., 461, *475*
Rohrbach, R., *314*
Roosa, D. B. St. J., 409, 410, *422*
Rosen, S., *426, 452, 476, 478, 499, 678*
Rosenblith, Q. A., *379*
Rosenthal, C., 554, *557*
Rosenwasser, H., *265, 314, 594, 612, 635*
Roux, J., *314*

Rubin, W., 83, 592, 673
Rüedi, L., 220, 381, 406, 454, 458, 460, 461, 463, 469, 474, 475, 479, 499
Ruggles, R. L., 453
Rius, M., 475
Rumstrom, G., 111
Ruttin, E., 334, 347
Rytzner, C., 427, 453

Sanders, J. W., 673
Sava, G., 557
Sawicki, B., 556
Saxen, A., 214, 220
Scanlan, R. L., 673
Scaramella, L. F., 557
Scheer, A. A., 490, 499
Scheibe, A., 196, 220, 381, 406
Schmitt, H., 453
Schuknecht, H. F., 83, 313, 315, 411, 422, 459, 474, 492, 570, 579, 591, 592
Schulhof, E., 409, 422
Schuster, A., 83
Schwabach, D., 366, 379
Schwartze, H. H., 83, 250, 252, 264, 381, 406, 426, 452
Scott, A., 475
Scott, W. R., 673
Seifi, A. E., 315
Selters, W. A., 673
Senaldi, M., 152
Sercer, A., 461, 475
Shambaugh, G. E., Sr., 467, 469, 475, 560, 568
Shambaugh, G. E., Jr., 83, 183, 220, 265, 287, 314, 347, 367, 378, 379, 381, 406, 407, 422, 468, 475, 499, 515, 557, 568, 570, 591, 592, 635, 677
Shea, J. J., 409, 422, 427, 453, 476, 478, 499, 584, 592, 678
Sheehy, J. L., 51, 402, 407, 422, 423, 437, 453, 494, 678
Sheer, A. A., 494, 495, 499
Shinn, J. B., 635
Shuster, A., 83
Shuster, B., 83
Siebenmann, F., 264, 287, 456, 459, 474, 478, 498, 502, 515
Siirala, U., 381, 406
Silverstone, S., 635
Simpson-Hall, L., 180, 461, 475
Skoog, T., 353, 378, 379
Smith, K. P., 453
Smith, K. R., 379
Smith, M. F. W., 635, 638, 673
Smythe, G. D. L., 287, 437, 453
Sooy, F. A., 422
Sourdille, M., 177, 353, 426, 452, 500, 502, 503, 506, 515, 678
Spalteholz, W., 556
Spector, G. J., 634, 635
Spoendlin, H., 458, 474, 499
Stacke, L., 268, 286, 426, 452, 520, 556
Stahle, J., 592
Stenvers, H. W., 111
Stevens, E. L., 592
Stevenson, E. W., 249, 453
Stewart, K., 83
Stoksted, P., 152

Storrs, L. A., 249
Strong, M. S., 593, 635
Stroud, M., 557
Stuart, E. A., 346
Sullivan, J., 556, 557
Symonds, C. P., 309, 314

Tabb, H. G., 249, 409, 422, 584, 592
Tabor, J. R., 423
Talbot, F., 592
Talbott, J. H., 592
Tardy, M. E., 232, 249
Tarf, O., 152
Tarkkanen, J. V., 347
Tato, J. M., 347
Taverner, D., 533, 557
Taylor, H. K., 111
Taylor, M., 422
Teed, R. W., 214, 220
Thies, F., 266
Thies, F., Jr., 167, 182, 286
Thomsen, J., 667, 673
Tody, T., 437
Tonndorf, J., 379
Towne, E. D., 111
Toynbee, J., 408, 413, 422, 454, 455, 474
Trautmann, F., 381, 406
Tresley, I. J., 231
Tröltsch, A. F. von, 268, 286, 456, 474
Tucker, H., 553, 557
Tumarkin, A., 214, 220

Valdez, G., 409, 422
Valsalva, A. M., 30, 152, 153, 455, 461, 469, 474, 570
Vaughan, C. W., 635
Ventry, I. M., 83
Vernon, J. A., 379
Vesalius, A., 352, 378
Virchow, R., 639
Voss, O., 307, 314

Wallner, L. J., 220
Walsh, P. J., 592
Walsh, T. E., 353, 378, 379, 426, 452, 504, 515, 556
Waltner, J. G., 612, 635
Ward, P. H., 313, 315, 635
Warpeha, R. L., 591
Weber, E. H., 366, 379
Weille, F. L., 633, 635
Weiss, E., 83
Weiss, P., 556
Wette, R., 556, 557
Wever, E. G., 352, 356, 357, 362, 364, 378, 379
Whaley, R., 249
Whitaker, C. F., 183
White, L. E., 314
Whiting, F., 307, 314
Whiting, T., 252, 264
Wiet, R. J., 676, 679

Wilbrand, H., *592*
Wilde, W., 154, 252, *264*
Williams, H. L., *346, 347, 591, 592*
Wilson, J. G., 467
Winch, T. R., *591*
Winship, T., 612, *635*
Wittmaack, K., *29*, 214, 215, *220*, 461, *475*
Wolfson, R. J., 590, *592*
Wong, A., *635*
Wright, A. J., 329, *347*, 565, *591, 593*
Wright, J. W., III, *453*
Wright, J. W., Jr., *453*
Wright, W. K., 167, *183*, 281, *287*, 409, 415, *422, 423*, 437, *453*

Wullstein, H., 269, *286*, 353, 376, *379*, 409, *422, 424, 425, 427, 452, 453*, 503, 504, 678
Wullstein, S. R., 437, 439, 448, *453*

Yearsley, J., 408, *422*

Zaufal, E., 266, 268, *286, 290, 314*, 426, *452*
Zechner, G., *474*
Zettergren, L., *635*
Zöllner, F., 269, *286*, 353, 376, *379*, 409, *422, 424, 427, 452, 453*, 503, 504, 678
Zwahlen, P., *406*

# Index of Subjects

Page numbers in *italics* indicate illustrations. A (t) following a number indicates a table.

Abducens nerve, 44, 693

ABLB test. See *Alternate binaural loudness balance test.*

Abscess. See specific type.

Accessory nerve, 54, 695

Acid cautery, for closure of tympanic membrane perforation, 414

Acoustic meatus. See *Auditory meatus.*

Acoustic nerve, 45

Acoustic neurilemmoma. See *Acoustic neuroma.*

Acoustic neurinoma. See *Acoustic neuroma.*

Acoustic neuroma, 80, 530, 639–668
  and tumors of the cerebellopontine angle, 637–673
  diagnosis of, 139–147, *140–145*, 640
  graft after removal of, 521, *521*
  hearing loss in, 640
  pathology of, 639–640, *639*
  radiologic appearance of, *108, 109, 109, 110, 643–646, 643, 645, 646*
  screening tests for, 138–139, *138*
  surgical removal of, 646–666
    complications of, 666–667
    middle fossa approach for, 649–651, *649*
    results of, 667–668
    suboccipital approach for, 657, *662–665*, 666
    translabyrinthine approach for, 651–656, *651–654*
    translabyrinthine-suboccipital approach for, *655, 656–657, 656–661*
  tomography in, 137–147, *138, 140–145*
  vs. endolymphatic hydrops, 574–575

Adenocarcinoma, 530

Air cells, of temporal bone, embryologic development of, 24–25, *24*

Air conduction, in diseased ear, mechanics of, 366–378

Air-water sound barrier, 18, *19*

Allergic otitis media, 207–208

Allergy, endolymphatic hydrops and, 578

Alternate binaural loudness balance test (ABLB), 64, *66*
  in hearing loss, 66

Anastomosis, facial nerve, for facial nerve repair, 550, 552–553, *553*

Anatomy of the ear, developmental, 5–29

Anatomy of the temporal bone, 31–51
  through dissection, 675–725

Anemia, progressive, in lateral sinus thrombophlebitis, 302
  secondary, in coalescent mastoiditis, 199, 256

Anesthesia, for ear surgery, 163–166, *164, 166*
  for fenestration operation, 506–507, *506*
  for myringotomy, 247, *248*
  for radical and Bondy modified mastoidectomy, 273
  for stapes operations, 166
  for tympanoplasty, 532
  local, points of injection in ear operations, 34–35, *35*

Angiography, intracranial, in diagnosis of brain abscess, 324

Angle syndrome. See *Cerebellopontine angle syndrome.*

Anterior curotomy mobilization, 484–486
  instruments for, *486*

Anthelix, *32*
  creation of, in lop ears, *230, 231, 232*

Antibiotic therapy, after simple mastoid operation, 263
  and incidence of meningeal complications of otitis media, 290–291
  for temporal bone surgery, 160–163
  in generalized meningitis, 300, 301

Antitragus, *32*

Antrum, 45
  cholesteatoma of, 102, *102*
  embryologic development of, 382(t)
  location of, in mastoid operation, 261

Aphasia, in left temporal lobe abscess, 322

Arcuate eminence, *38, 39*

Arteriogram, in facial paralysis, 535
  in glomus tumor, 619–620, *619, 620*

Artery. See specific artery.

Aseptic technique, in temporal bone surgery, 155–161, *157–159, 161*

Ataxia, in cerebellar abscess, 323
  in endolymphatic hydrops, 614

Atresia, congenital, radiologic appearance of, *104, 105*
  meatal. See *Auditory meatus, external, atresia of.*

Attic, 45. See also *Epitympanum.*
  dry perforation, *206*
  extension of glomus jugulare tumor to, atticotomy for, *627*

**733**

Attic (*Continued*)
  retraction cholesteatoma of, 213–216
Attico-antrotomy, in construction of osseous
    meatus, 395
  in horizontal canal labyrinthotomy, 581, *582*
Atticotomy, for exposure of facial nerve, *548, 549*
  for extension of glomus jugulare tumor to
    attic, *627*
  in fenestration operation, *508*
  in radical and Bondy modified mastoidectomy,
    273, *274, 277*
  in radical mastoid operation, 282
Audiogram. See *Audiometry.*
Audiometry, Békésy, 64, *65*, 66(t)
    in acoustic neuroma, 641
    in cochlear hearing loss, 66(t)
    in conductive hearing loss, 66(t)
    in endolymphatic hydrops, 573
    in retrocochlear hearing loss, 66(t)
  brainstem evoked response, in acoustic
    neuroma, 642
  Carhart notch. See *Carhart notch.*
  mass tilt in, cerumen as cause of, *372*
    fluid in tympanic cavity as cause of, *369*
  in acoustic neuroma, 641–642
  in facial paralysis, 534
  in glomus tumors, 617
  pure tone, 57–58, *58*
    in endolymphatic hydrops, *563*
    in stapedial and cochlear otosclerosis, *466*
    in stapedial otosclerosis, *467*
  speech, 58–59
Auditory canal, internal, anatomy of, 690, *690,
    716–718, 716–718*
  fundus of, 722, *723*
Auditory meatus, external, atresia of, acquired,
    240–242, *242*
    congenital, surgery for, 393–397, *394, 396*
      hearing result in, 400–401, *400, 401*
      skin-lined opening to antrum, 390, *391*
      substitute tympanic membrane in, 398,
        *399*
    tomography of, 123, *125*
    with exostoses, 240
    with osteoma, 240, *240*
  carcinoma of, squamous cell, 599–612
    removal of, 600–601, *600, 602–604*
    tomography of, 131, *133*
  cartilage of, 32, *32*
  cholesteatoma of, 244
  cicatricial stenosis of, 240–242, *242*
  embryologic development of, 20, *21*
  foreign body in, 243
  furuncle of, 241, 243
  increased air pressure in, effect of, *369*
  infections of, 244–245
    varieties of, *370*
  occlusion of, hearing loss in, 371–372
  polyp of, 243–244
  sensory nerve supply to, 33–35, *33, 34*
  skin grafts from, for myringoplasty, 415,
    *416, 417*
  skin of, 222
  surgical conditions of, 238–245, *239, 240, 242*
  internal, anatomy of, 49–50, *50*, 522–523, *523*
  osseous, and mandibular joint, *40*
    carcinoma of, removal of, 600–601, *602–603*
    caries of, 244

Auditory meatus, osseous (*Continued*)
    construction of, 393–395, *394*
    embryologic development of, 382(t)
    exostosis of, 238–240, *239*
    in coalescent mastoiditis, sagging of posterior
      wall, 198, *255*
    necrosis of, 244
    osteoma of, 238–240, *239*
    skin grafting of, 398, *399*
    wall of, plastic flap from. See *Meatal plastic
      flap.*
    removal of, in fenestration operation, *506*
Auditory tests, diagnostic significance of, 66
Aural discharge. See *Otorrhea.*
Auricle, absent, reconstruction of, 391–393
  attachment to head, 43
  carcinoma of, 601, *611, 612*
    basal cell, 597–599, *598*
  cartilage of, 32, *32*
  congenital absence of, *20*
  development of, 21–22, *21*, 382(t), *384*
  displacement of, by subperiosteal abscess, 255,
    *255*
  erysipelas of. See *Erysipelas.*
  frostbite of. See *Frostbite.*
  Hansen's disease of, 225, *225*
  hematoma of. See *Hematoma.*
  keloid of. See *Keloid.*
  leprosy of, 225, *225*
  malformation of, with atresia, *384*
  microtic, reconstruction of, 391–393, *392*
  perichondritis of. See *Perichondritis.*
  sebaceous cyst of. See *Sebaceous cyst.*
  sensory nerve supply to, 33–35, *33, 34*
  skin of, 32–33, 222
  surgical conditions of, 222–237
Auricular artery, posterior, 35
Auricular branch of the vagus, 34–35, *34*
Auricular nerve, great, 33–34, *33, 34*
    anesthesia for, 165, *166*
  posterior, 33, *33*
Auriculotemporal nerve, *33*, 34–35
    anesthesia for, 165, *166*
Autophonia, in patent eustachian tube, 73
Axial projection, in tomography, 121, *122*
Axon, degeneration of, 525–526
Axonotmesis, 525

Babinski test, in otitic meningitis, 297
Basal cell carcinoma, of auricle, 601, *611, 612*
Békésy audiometry. See under *Audiometry.*
Bell's palsy, 532–533
  after fenestration, 513
  decompression of facial nerve for, 521, *521*
Bezold's abscess, in coalescent mastoiditis, 255
"Bill's bar," *721*
"Biscuit footplate," in otospongiosis, 490, *491*
Bleeding, after removal of acoustic neuroma, 666
  from bone, control of, *176, 177*
  in carcinoma of ear, 599
  in glomus tumors, 616
  venous, in simple mastoid operation, 264
Blood culture, in lateral sinus thrombophlebitis,
    304
Bondy modified radical mastoid operation. See
    *Mastoid operation, radical, Bondy modified.*

Bone(s), bleeding, control of, *176, 177*
   ear surgery on, techniques for, 171–177, *174,*
     *175, 176*
   endochondral, in otic capsule, 15–18, *16, 17*
   endosteal, in otic capsule, 15–18, *17*
   erosion, extension of infection by, 196
     in otitis media, 293, 294
   intrachondral, in otic capsule, 15, *16*
   periosteal, of labyrinthine capsule, 18
   removal of, in fenestration, 509–510, *510, 511*
     instruments for, 172–173, *174*
   surgery on, techniques for, 171–177, *174, 175,*
     *176*
   temporal. See *Temporal bone.*
Bone conduction, compressional, 363–364
     movement of skull in, *363*
   hearing by, 363–364, *363*
   in diseased ear, 365–366
   occlusion of external auditory meatus and, 366,
     *366*
   translatory, 363–364
     movement of skull in, *363*
   transmitted, 364
Bone dust, removal of, in fenestration, 509–510,
   *510, 511*
Brain, abscess of, 317–326
     diagnosis of, 323–324, 323(t)
     differential diagnosis of, 323
     drainage of, technique for, 325
     pathology of, 318–321, *318, 319, 320*
     prognosis for, 326
     residual neurologic defects in, 326
     stages of, 318–319, *320*
     surgery for, 289–290
     symptoms and signs of, 321–323
     treatment of, 324–326
     vs. suppurative labyrinthitis, 323(t)
   dehydration of, for brain abscess, 326
   scanning of, in diagnosis of brain abscess, 324
Branchial apparatus, development of sound-
   conducting system from, 381, 382(t)
Bridge, bony, from malleus to stapes, congenital
   malformation in, *402*
Brudzinski sign, in otitic meningitis, 297
Burr(s), for bone cutting, *175*
     technique of using, 173–175, *175*

Caloric test, cold water, 67–68, *67*
     in acoustic neuroma, 642
   in endolymphatic hydrops, 572
Carcinoma, basal cell, 530
     of auricle, 597–599, *598*
   squamous cell, 530
     of auditory meatus, 599–612
Carhart notch, of audiogram, after stapes surgery,
   *367*
   elimination by surgery, *468*
   in stapedial otospongiosis, 366, *366, 467, 467*
Carhart tone decay test, in acoustic neuroma,
   641
Caries, of osseous meatus, 244
Carotid artery, 44
CAT scan. See *Computerized axial tomography.*
Catheter inflation of eustachian tube, 75–77, *77*
"Cauliflower ear," 32, 226
Cautery, acid, for closure of tympanic membrane
   perforation, 414–415

Cawthorne's head exercises, after labyrinthectomy
   surgery, 588–589
Cawthorne's labyrinthotomy, for endolymphatic
   hydrops, technique, *582, 583*
Central auditory tests, 64–65
Cerebellar abscess, 321
   symptoms of, 323
   vs. suppurative labyrinthitis, 323(t)
Cerebellopontine angle, opaque cisternogram of,
     in acoustic tumors, 644–645, *647, 648*
   normal, *646*
   tumors of, 637–673
     vs. endolymphatic hydrops, 574
Cerebellopontine angle syndrome, meningioma
   producing, 669
   tumors producing, 637
Cerebral ischemia, vs. endolymphatic hydrops, 574
Cerebrospinal fluid, hydrostatic function of, 8
   leak of, after acoustic neuroma removal, 666
     after glomus tumor removal, 634
     with fracture, 126, *127*
Cerumen, against tympanic membrane, mass tilt
   of audiogram in, *372*
   occlusion of auditory meatus by, hearing loss
     in, *370*
Chamberlain-Towne position, in otologic x-ray,
   89, *93*
Chausse III position, in otologic x-ray, 89, *92, 95*
Chemotherapy, prophylactic, for temporal bone
   surgery, 160–163
Chocolate cyst, after radical mastoid operation,
   285–286
Cholesteatoma, attic retraction, 213–216
     appearance of, *206*
     Bondy modified radical mastoid operation
       for, 270–271
     conservative management of, 271
     diagnosis of, 270–271
     etiology of, 213–216
     myringostapediopexy for, 282
     radical and Bondy modified radical mas-
       toidectomy for, 272–284, *274–276, 279–281*
     tympanoplasty for, 437–439, *438*
   congenital, 216–217, *217, 218*
     of petrous pyramid, 670–672, *671*
     radiologic appearance of, 104, *104*
     tomography in, 132–134, *133, 134*
   exposure of facial nerve by, without paralysis,
     346, *346*
   extension into mesotympanum, pars tensa
     excision in, 282
   facial paralysis and, 530, 531
   fistula of labyrinth from, 327
   in the attic and antrum, 101–102, *101, 102*
   of external auditory meatus, 244
   osteoplastic epitympanotomy for, 448–450,
     *448–450*
   radiologic appearance of, 101–102, *101, 102*
   recurrence after radical mastoid operation, 286
   secondary acquired, 212–213
     radical mastoid operation for, 270
     therapy for, 213
   tympanoplasty for, 437–439, *438*
     canal wall down, 441–442, *440–441*
     intact canal wall, 442–450, *443–450*
   vs. acoustic tumor, 640
   vs. chronic suppurative otitis media, 73
   with chronic otorrhea, Bondy modified radical
     mastoidectomy for, 270

Cholesteatoma (*Continued*)
  with otitis media, tomography in, 128–129,
    *129, 130*
  with otitis media and fistula of lateral semi-
    circular canal, tomography in, *131*
Chorda tympani nerve, test of, 536
  trauma to, in stapedectomy, 493
Cigarette smoking, in endolymphatic hydrops,
  578–579
Cisternogram, opaque cerebellopontine, in
    acoustic neuroma, 645, *646–648*
  in neoplastic conditions, 139–145, *140–145*
  normal, *646*
Coalescent mastoiditis. See under *Mastoiditis.*
Cochlea, embryologic development of, 6, *7*, 382(t)
  frequency analysis by, 364–365
  in endolymphatic hydrops, 561, *562, 564*
  otosclerosis of. See *Otosclerosis, cochlear.*
  protection of, by ossicles, 365
  response of, to sound, 364–365
  spiral ganglion cells, in endolymphatic
    hydrops, 561, *563*
  loss of, in presbycusis, *564*
Cochlear aqueduct. See *Perilymphatic duct.*
Cochlear duct, dilatation of, after obliteration of
    endolymphatic duct in guinea pig, *570*
  embryologic development of, 10, *10*
Cochlear nerve, anatomy of, *694, 717, 724, 725*
  section of, for endolymphatic hydrops, 583
Cochlear otospongiosis. See *Otospongiosis.*
Cochlear reaction, in serous labyrinthitis after
  fenestration, 513
Cold water caloric test. See *Caloric test, cold
  water.*
Columella effect, 375
Common cold virus, otitis media from, 188–189
Common crus, anatomy of, *711*
Computerized axial tomography (CAT), in
    acoustic neuroma, 644, *645*
  in facial paralysis, 535
  in glomus tumors, 622
  in neoplastic conditions, 146–147, *146, 147*
Concha, *32*
Concussion, hearing loss in, 79
Conductive hearing loss, air-bone gap as measure
  of, 365–366. See also *Hearing loss,
  conductive.*
Congenital malformations, of sound-conducting
    system, case reports of, 403–406, *405, 406*
  surgical correction of, 380–407
  tomography of, 122–126, *124, 125*
Congenital nerve deafness, 78
Convulsions, in brain abscess, in children, 321
  in meningismus in infants, 297
  Jacksonian, in brain abscess, 322
Cortilymph, 568
Costen syndrome, 74
Cranial nerves, in temporal bone, 44–45, 693–695
Cribriform area, 36, *36*
Cryosurgery, for endolymphatic hydrops, 584
CT. See *Computerized axial tomography.*
Cupola technique, for fenestration operation, *512*
Curet, technique of using, 175, *176*
Cyst(s), "epidermoid," of tympanum, *218*
  of ear, varieties of, 595–596
  of radical mastoid cavity, 285
  preauricular, congenital, 235, *385*
  sebaceous, of auricle, 228

Dandy's syndrome, 589
Deafness. See also *Hearing loss.*
  labyrinthine, sudden, unilateral, 80
    vs. endolymphatic hydrops, 575
  nerve, congenital, 80
  progressive hereditary, 79
    syphilitic, acquired, 79
      congenital, 79
      toxic, 79
  psychogenic, 80–81
  sensorineural, in acute necrotic otitis media,
    205
Decompression, and repair of facial nerve, 519–557
  of endolymphatic sac, 584–586, *585, 586*
  subtemporal, in temporal lobe abscess, 325
Dehydration, after labyrinthine operations, treat-
    ment of, 180
  in brain abscess, 326
Diet, in endolymphatic hydrops, 576
Digastric groove, 36
Digastric muscle, 35–36
Diplacusis, in endolymphatic hydrops, 560, 573
  in serous inflammatory labyrinthitis, 332
  test for, 60–61, *61*
Diplopia, in petrositis, 339
Disorientation, in brain abscess, 322
Diuretics, in endolymphatic hydrops, 576–577
Doerfler-Stewart test, in psychogenic deafness, 81
Dorello's canal, 45
Drainage, in endolymphatic sac operations,
  procedure for, 584, *585, 586*
Drapes, sterile, in temporal bone surgery, *159,
  160, 161, 162*
Dressing(s), after ear surgery, 180–182, *181*
  mastoid, *181*
Drills, surgical, for bone removal, 172–173, *174*
Drowsiness, in brain abscess, 321
  in localized otitic meningitis, 297
Dura, incision of, in brain abscess, 325
  injury of, in simple mastoid operation, 264
  laceration of, in fenestration operation, 511
Dysplasia, fibrous, of mastoid, 596, *597*


Ear, carcinoma of, 597–612
  "cauliflower," 32
  congenital malformations of, causes of, 386–387
    diagnosis of, 388–389, *389*
    surgical correction of, age of patient for, 390
      cases of, 403–406, *405, 406*
      hearing results of, 400–403, *400–403*
      postoperative care for, 400
      techniques for, 390–399, *391, 392, 394–397,
        399*
  cysts of, varieties of, 595–596
  disease of, air conduction in, 366–378
    bone conduction in, 365–366, *366, 367*
    diagnosis of, 53–83
      differential, 78
      equipment, 54–55, *55, 56*
      eustachian tube examination in, 73–78
      hearing tests in, 57–66
      otoscopy in, 71–73
      procedure for, 54
      vestibular tests in, 66–71
    psychosomatic, 53

Ear (*Continued*)
  embryologic development of, 5–29, 382(t),
    *383, 384*
  external. See *External ear.*
  fenestrated, mechanics of, *377, 378, 378*
  internal. See *Internal ear.*
  lop. See *Lop ears.*
  middle. See *Middle ear.*
  outer. See *External ear.*
  sound sensitivity of, 353–355, *354*
  speculum, technique of holding, *71*
  surgery of. See also *Temporal bone, surgery of;*
      and specific operations.
    anesthesia for, 163–166, *164, 166*
    magnification in, 177–180, *178, 179*
    postoperative care in, 180–182, *181*
    postoperative dressings for, 181–182, *181*
    preoperative sedation for, 163–165
  surgery on bone of, techniques for, 171–177,
      *174, 175, 176*
  threshold of feeling of, 353–355
  threshold of hearing of, 353–355, *354*
  tumors of, surgery of, 595–635
    varieties of, 595–596
Earache, in acute suppurative otitis media,
    hyperemia stage, 191
Eggshell technique, for fenestration operation, *512*
Eighth cranial nerve, 45, 694
  hearing disorders of, Békésy audiogram of, *65*
Electrodiagnosis, in facial paralysis, 538–539
Electroencephalography, in diagnosis of brain
    abscess, 324
Electromyography (EMG), in facial paralysis, 539
Electronystagmography (ENG), 68–71, *70*
  in acoustic neuroma, 642–643
Eleventh nerve, 45, 695
Emaciation, in cerebellar abscess, 323
  in lateral sinus thrombophlebitis, 303
Embolization, for glomus tumors, 622–623
Embryology, of ear, 5–29, 382(t), *383, 384*
EMG. See *Electromyography.*
Enchondralization, in fenestration operation, *509*
Endaural incision, in fenestration operation, *506*
  in horizontal canal labyrinthotomy, *582*
  in radical mastoid operation, 269
  in simple mastoid operation, 258
  local anesthesia for, 165, *166*
  technique of, 168–170, *169*
Endolymph, and perilymph, pressure equilibra-
    tion between, 569–572, *570, 571*
  hydrostatic function of, *8, 9*
  production and resorption of, 568–569, *569*
    and endolymphatic hydrops, 570
Endolymphatic duct, *567, 569*
  anatomy of, *715*
  dilatation of, 560, *561*
  embryologic development of, 6, *7*
Endolymphatic hydrops (Meniere's disease), 80,
    559–593
  after fenestration, 514
  atypical, 575
  audiogram in, *563*
  caloric tests in, 572
  cochlear changes in, *562*
  diagnosis of, 572–573
  differential diagnosis of, 573–576
  etiology of, 565
  hearing loss in, 573

Endolymphatic hydrops (Meniere's disease)
    (*Continued*)
  medical treatment of, 576–579
  pathology of, 561–565, *562–564*
  secondary, 575–576
  surgical treatment of, 579–593
    exercises after, 588–589
    indications for, 579–580
    postoperative course of, 587–589
    results of, 590–591
    risks and complications of, 589–590
  symptoms and signs of, 572–573
  tinnitus in, 573
  vertigo in, 572
  vs. cerebellopontine angle tumor, 574–575
  with presbycusis audiogram in, *563*
Endolymphatic (otic) labyrinth, embryologic
    development of, 6–10
  extraction of, in horizontal canal labyrin-
    thotomy, *582*
  perforation of, in fenestration operation, 511
Endolymphatic sac, anatomy of, 708–709, *708*
  decompression of, 584–586, *585, 586*
  embryologic development of, 8–9, *8*
  surgery of, for endolymphatic hydrops, 584–
    586, *585, 586*
Endolymphatic-subarachnoid shunt, for endo-
    lymphatic hydrops, 584, *586*
Endomeatal incision, in tympanoplasty, 437, *438*
  technique of, 170–171, *170, 171*
ENG. See *Electronystagmography.*
Eosinophilic granuloma, 596–597
Epidermoid tumor, primary, in mastoid, 599
  tomography in, 132–134, *133, 134*
"Epidermoid cyst," of tympanum, *218*
Epidural abscess. See *Extradural abscess.*
Epitympanotomy, osteoplastic, for cholesteatoma,
    448–450, *448–450*
Epitympanum, 45. See also *Attic.*
  anatomy of, *709*
  embryologic development of, 24, 382(t)
  normal pneumatic pattern in, *96*
ERA. See *Evoked Response Audiometry.*
Erysipelas, of auricle, 227–228
Eustachian tube, catheter inflation of, 75–77, *77*
  closure of, in radical mastoid operation, *279,*
    280
  embryologic development of, 23, 382(t)
  examination of, 73–78, *76, 77*
  inflation of, 73–77, *76, 77*
    interpretation, 77–78
  occlusion of, audiogram in, *369*
    causes of, 73–75
    effect on hearing, *369*
    hearing loss in, 374–375
    vs. endolymphatic hydrops, 574
  Politzer inflation of, 75–76, *76*
  Wright prosthesis for, 436, *436*
Evoked Response Audiometry (ERA), 65–66
Exostosis, of auditory meatus, 238–240, *239*
External ear, anatomy of, 32–35, *32, 33, 34*
  blood supply to, 35
  carcinoma of, 597–599, *598*
  embryologic development of, 18–24, *19, 20, 21*
  glomus tumor of, *610*
  innervation of, 33–35, *33, 34*
  malformation of, 381, *383, 384*
  muscles of, 35–36

External ear (*Continued*)
    nerve supply of, *164*
    resonance and efficiency of, 362–363
    skin of, 222
    surgery of, 221–249
Extradural abscess, 295–296
    etiology of, 295
    pathology of, 295–296
    symptoms of, 296
    treatment of, 296
Eye, care of, in facial paralysis, 539–540
Eyeground changes, in brain abscess, 322
    in right lateral sinus thrombophlebitis, 303

Facial nerve, 46–49, *47, 48, 49*
    anastomosis of, 550, 552–553, *553*
    anatomy of, 522–525, *523, 524,* 694, 703–704,
        *703, 704, 722, 723*
    atticotomy exposure of, *548, 549*
    cholesteatoma exposing, without paralysis, 346,
        *346*
    decompression of, and repair of, 519–557
        technique for, 540–547, *541–543, 545–549*
    edema of. See *Bell's palsy.*
    graft of, 547–553, *550–553*
    iatrogenic injury to, 528–529
    in malformations of external and middle ear, 386
    injury to, in simple mastoid operation, 263–264
        in stapedectomy, 490–491
    mastoid exposure of, 540–544, *541–543*
    mastoid portion of, *47, 48,* 524, 525
    middle fossa exposure of, 540–544, *541–543*
    neuromuscular transfer for repair of, 553
    paralysis of. See *Facial paralysis.*
    paresis of. See *Facial paresis.*
    pyramidal turn of, *47, 48,* 524, *525*
    repair of, by anastomosis, 550–553, *553*
        by nerve graft, 547–550, *548–552*
        by neuromuscular transfers, 553–554
        by rerouting and approximation, 544, *547*
    section of, in fenestration operation, 511
    surgery of, complications of, 555–556
        results of, *555,* 556
    tympanic portion of, *47,* 47, 524, 525, *707*
        exposure of, in fenestration operation, 511
    vertical segment of, *47, 48,* 524, *525*
Facial paralysis, 345–346, *346*
    after fenestration, 513
    after glomus tumor removal, 634
    after iatrogenic injury, 528–529
    after radical mastoid operation, 285
    after simple mastoid operation, 263–264
    after stapes operation, 493
    after temporal bone fracture, 527–528, *527, 528*
    diagnosis of, 533–537, *536*
    electrodiagnosis in, 538–539
    electromyography in, 539
    eye in, care of, 539–540
    facelifts for, 554
    fascia lata sling for, 554
    flaccid, etiology of, 526–533
    idiopathic, 532–533
    in congenital cholesteatoma, 672
    in diabetics, 531
    infection as a cause of, 530–532, *532*
    postoperative, care of, 180

Facial paralysis (*Continued*)
    prognostic studies in, 537–539
    radiologic examination in, 534–535
    surgical rehabilitation following, 540–554
    topographic studies in, 535–537
    traumatic, tomography in, 128, *129*
    tumor as cause of, 529–530
Facial paresis, after radical mastoid operation, 285
    in left temporal lobe abscess, 322
    in petrositis, 339
"Facial recess," 48
    anatomy of, 704–706, *705, 706, 707*
Falciform crest, *724*
Fallopian canal, anomalies, 525
    petrous segment of, 522
    pyramidal segment of, 523
    tympanic segment of, 523
Fascial grafts, for myringoplasty, 415–422
Femoral cutaneous nerve, graft from, for facial
    nerve repair, 549–550, *551*
Femoral thrombophlebitis, postoperative, care of,
    180
Fenestration operation, 501–515
    anesthesia for, 506–507, *506*
    after radical mastoid operation, 284
    atticotomy in, *508*
    closure of fenestra after, 514–515
    complications of, early, 513
        late, 514–515
    creation of fenestra, *512*
    cupola technique for, *512*
    development of, 502–503
    eggshell technique for, *512*
    enchondralization in, *509,* 510
    endaural incision for, *506*
    for otospongiosis, 501–515
    hearing results in, *377, 378, 378*
    indications for, 504–505, *505*
    infection after, secondary, 514
    mechanics of, 503–504, *504*
    ossiculectomy in, partial, *510*
    postoperative care in, 512–513
    removal of osseous meatal wall, *508*
    results of, Shambaugh formula for, 504–505,
        *505*
    selection of cases for, 504–505, *505*
    stapedectomy after, 494–496, *495*
    surgical accidents during, 511
    technique for, 505–510, *506–510*
    tympanomeatal skin flap for, construction of,
        *507*
Fibrosis, ossicular fixation by, 398–399
Fibrous dysplasia, of mastoid, 596, *597*
Fifth cranial nerve, 44, 693
    involvement in acoustic neuroma, 641
Fissula ante fenestram, and otospongiosis, 459,
    *460, 462*
    embryologic development of, 11–14, *12, 13, 14*
    new bone formation in, 11, *13, 14*
    normal connective tissue of, replaced by car-
        tilage, 11, 13, *13*
Fistula, of labyrinth. See under *Labyrinth.*
    second branchial, in congenital absence of
        auricle and deformed meatus, *20*
Fluoride. See *Sodium fluoride.*
Footplate, floating, in stapedectomy, 490
Foreign body, in external auditory meatus, 243
Fork 64 by air test, 60

Fossa mastoidea, 36, *36*
Fossula post fenestram, 14
Fourth cranial nerve, 693
Fowler test, for recruitment. See *Alternate binaural loudness balance test.*
Franceschetti-Zwahlen syndrome, 385
Frequency, of tone, 353
Frequency analysis, by cochlea, 364–365
Frontal projection, in tomography, 114–116, *114, 115*
Frostbite, of auricle, 222–224, *223*
    etiology and pathology of, 222–223
    treatment of, 223–224
Furstenberg diet, for endolymphatic hydrops, 576
Furuncle, of external auditory meatus, 241, 243
    vs. coalescent mastoiditis, 256

Ganglion cells, of cochlea, loss of, in presbycusis, *564*
Gill apparatus, development of sound-conducting system from, 381, 382(t)
Glasscock air drill, 173, *174*
Glomus tumor, and facial paralysis, 530
    classification of, 613, 615
    diagnosis of, 615–622
    endaural approach for, 625, *628*
    jugulare, radiologic appearance of, 109, *110*
        tomography in, 136–137, *136, 137*
        venography in, *137*
    location of, 612–613
    of external ear, *610*
    of middle ear and skull base, 612–634
    pathology of, 613, *614*
    radiologic examination of, 109, *110*, 617–622, *618–621*
    skull base approach to, 629–633, *630–633*
    surgery of, complications of, 633–634
        results of, 634
    surgical removal of, 623–633, *624, 626–633*
        hypotympanotomy for, 624–625, *626–627*
        transmastoid procedure of House for, 625, *628, 629*
        transmeatal surgical method for, 624–625, *624, 626, 627*
    treatment of, 622–633
        embolization for, 622–623
        radiation for, 622, *623*
        surgery for, 623–633
    tympanicum, tomography in, 135–136, *136*
Glossopharyngeal nerve, 45, 694
Gradenigo's syndrome, 45, 339
Graft. See specific type, e.g., *Nerve graft; Skin graft; Vein graft.*
Granuloma, eosinophilic, 596–597
Granulomatosis, lipoid, 596–597
Greater auricular nerve, graft from, for facial nerve repair, 549, *549, 550*
Greisinger's sign, in lateral sinus thrombophlebitis, 303
Grommet tubes, 247–248, *248*
Gustometer, electronic, in diagnosis of flaccid facial paralysis, 537

Hand-Schüller-Christian syndrome, 597
Hansen's disease, of auricle, 225, *225*

Head exercises, Cawthorne's after labyrinthectomy surgery, 588–589
Head holder, Juers, for temporal bone surgery, *159, 160*
Headache, in brain abscess, 322
    in initial encephalitis stage, 321
    in otitic hydrocephalus, 309
    in otitic meningitis, generalized, 300
        localized, 297
    in right lateral sinus thrombophlebitis, 303
Healing, promotion of, for closure of tympanic membrane perforation, 413–415
Hearing, binaural, 355
    bone conduction, 363–364, *363*
    in acute suppurative otitis media, hyperemia stage, 191
    in attic retraction cholesteatoma, 216
    mechanics of, 351–379
    tests of, 57–66. See also specific tests.
        before tympanoplasty, 431
    threshold of, 353–355, *354*
Hearing aid, for otospongiosis, 505
Hearing loss. See also *Deafness.*
    cochlear, after fenestration, 513
        test results in, 66(t)
    conductive, after radical mastoid operation, 284
        audiograms in, *61*
        in coalescent mastoiditis, 256
        in interruption of ossicular chain, 428
        pure, high frequency, audiogram of, 58
        test results in, *66*
        types of, 81–83
    differential diagnosis of, 78
    etiologic types of, 78–83
    fluid in tympanic cavity as cause, audiogram in, *369*
    in absence of ossicles, 374, *374*
    in acoustic neurinoma, 80, 640
    in atresia of external auditory meatus, *370, 371*
    in attic retraction cholesteatoma, 216, 270
    in concussion, 79
    in eighth nerve lesions, test results, 65
    in endolymphatic hydrops, 80, 560, 573
    in eustachian tube occlusion, 73, 74, 81, *369*, 374–375, *375*
    in glomus tumor, 615
    in labyrinthitis, serous, 79
        after fenestration, 513
        suppurative, 80
    in mumps, 80
    in occlusion of external auditory meatus, 81, *369, 370, 371–372, 372*
    in otitis media, 82
    in otospongiosis, cochlear, 81
        stapedial, 82, 377, *369, 377*
    in pars tensa perforation, 81
    in round window closure, 376–377
    in serous labyrinthitis, 79
    in skull fracture, 79
    in tubercular otitis media, 210
    in tympanic membrane perforation, 372–373, *372–373*
    increased air pressure in external auditory meatus as cause, audiogram in, *369*
    labyrinthine, sudden, unilateral, 80
    moist cotton on tympanic membrane as cause, audiogram in, *369*
    noise and, 80

Hearing loss (*Continued*)
  sensorineural, after fenestration, 465–466
    after stapes surgery, 496–498
    in endolymphatic hydrops, 573
    low frequency, audiogram in, *58*
    of central origin, 80
    otospongiotic origin of, 470–471, *471*
    types of, 78–81
Helix, *32*
Hemangioma, 530
Hematoma, of auricle, 224, *224*
Hemifacial spasm, clonic, 554–555
Hemorrhage. See *Bleeding.*
Hereditary nerve deafness, 79
Heredity, and congenital malformations, 387
Herpes zoster oticus, 531, *532*
Histamine, in endolymphatic hydrops, 577–578
Histiocytosis, 596–597
History, patient, in otologic diagnosis, 56
Horizontal projection, in tomography, 121–122, *123*
House suction irrigator, *176*
House-Urban temporal bone holder, *684, 685*
Hydraulic ratio, of middle ear, 359, 365
Hydrocephalus, otitic, 309, 312
Hydrops, endolymphatic. See *Endolymphatic hydrops.*
Hyperostosis, of osseous meatus, 238
Hypoglossal nerve, 695
Hypotympanotomy, for removal of glomus tumor, 624–625, *626–627*
Hypotympanum, 45

Imbalance, in acoustic tumors, 640
Impedance, formula for acoustic system, 368, *368*
  measurements of, 61–63, *62, 63*
Incisura terminalis, 32, *32*
Impressio trigemini, 45
Incus, *50*. See also *Ossicle(s)*.
  anatomy of, *699, 700*
  dislocation of, in simple mastoid operation, 264
    traumatic, tomography in, 126, *127, 128*
  embryologic development of, 23, 385
  fitted, in tympanoplasty, 432–433, *434*
  fixation of, management of, 435
  fused with malleus, *396*
  lenticular process of, congenital absence of, *402*
    hearing tests in, *406*
    myringostapediopexy for, *405*
  long process of, fracture of, in stapedectomy, 492
  mobilization of, by amputation of head of malleus, *396*
  ossification of, 23
  removal of, in simple mastoid operation, 264
    in translabyrinthine labyrinthectomy, 582
  sculptured, in tympanoplasty, 432–433, *433, 434*
  transposition of, in tympanoplasty, 432
Incus replacement prosthesis (I.R.P.), for stapedectomy after fenestration, 494–496, *495*
Infant, temporal bone of, compared with adult, *25, 26, 27, 28*
Inner ear. See *Internal ear.*
Intensity, of tone, 353–354, *354*

Internal ear, abnormalities of, tomography in, *125*
  embryologic development of, *19*
  normal, tomographic section of, *41*
Intratympanic muscles, function of, 364
I. R. P. See *Incus replacement prosthesis.*
Irrigation, House apparatus, *176*
  Shambaugh apparatus, *176*

Jaw joint, 39, *40*
Juers head holder, for temporal bone surgery, *159, 160*
Jugular bulb, anatomy of, 42, 706, 708, *706*
  polytome of, in glomus tumor, *618, 619*
  thrombosis of. See under *Thrombosis.*
Jugular vein, internal, 42
  ligation, in lateral sinus thrombophlebitis, 308–309, *310, 311*
    in sigmoid sinus thrombus, 306
Jugularogram, in glomus tumor, *621*

Keloid, of auricle, 228–229, *228*
Kernig sign, in otitic meningitis, 297, 300, 301
Kerr electric drill, 173, *174*
Körner's septum, 27, *28*
Korogel insert, for closure of tympanic membrane perforation, 408, 413

Labyrinth, anatomy of, 49–51, *50, 51,* 710–715, *710–715*
  bony, development of, 15–18
  dead, 337
  drainage of, technique for, 335–337, *336*
  endolymphatic, development of, 6–10
  fistula of, 326–329
    creation and filling of, in horizontal canal labyrinthotomy, 581
    diagnosis of, 327–328, *327*
    pathology of, 326–327
    surgically produced, 327
    symptoms of, 327–328, *328*
    test for, 327–328, *328*
    treatment of, 328–329
  membranous, canal of, *711*
    embryologic development of, *7*
    lumen of, *7*
  otic. See *Labyrinth, endolymphatic.*
  perilymphatic, embryologic development of, 10–14
  periotic. See *Labyrinth, perilymphatic.*
  pressure equilibration in, 569–572, *570, 571*
  sequestrum of, 337
  skull fracture involving, 126, *127*
Labyrinthectomy, technique for, *336*
  translabyrinthine, for endolymphatic hydrops, 581, 583
Labyrinthine capsule, embryologic development of, 382(t)
  enchondral layer, exposure of, in fenestration, 510
  ossification stages, *17*
  otosclerosis focus in, 458, *458*
Labyrinthine deafness, sudden, unilateral, 80
  vs. endolymphatic hydrops, 575

Labyrinthine fluids, hydrodynamics of, 565–572
Labyrinthine hydrops. See *Endolymphatic hydrops.*
Labyrinthitis, 326–337
  latent, 337
  purulent, treatment, development of, 290
  serous inflammatory, 329–332
    after fenestration, 513
    etiology of, 329
    hearing loss in, 79–80
    pathology of, *330, 331, 331*
    symptoms and diagnosis of, 331–332
    treatment of, 332
    vs. endolymphatic hydrops, 574
    vs. suppurative, 332
  suppurative inflammatory, 332–337
    drainage for, 335–337, *336*
    etiology and pathology of, 332–333, *333*
    hearing loss in, 80
    prognosis for, 334–335, *335*
    symptoms of, 333–334
    treatment of, 334
    vs. cerebellar abscess, 323, 323(t)
    vs. endolymphatic hydrops, 574
Labyrinthotomy, horizontal canal, for endolymphatic hydrops, 581, *582*
  oval window, for endolymphatic hydrops, 580, *581*
Lacrimation, test for, in flaccid facial paralysis, 535–536, *536*
Lateral femoral cutaneous nerve, graft from, for facial nerve repair, 549–550, *551*
Lateral projection, in tomography, 116–118, *117, 118*
Lateral semicircular canal, fistula of, and cholesteatoma and otitis media, tomography of, *131*
Lateral sinus(es), 42, *43*
  sigmoid portion. See *Sigmoid sinus.*
  thrombophlebitis of. See under *Thrombophlebitis.*
Law position, in otologic x-ray, 84, *85*
Lempert-Ramadier petrosectomy, 340, *342, 343,* 344–345
Leprosy, of auricle, 225, *225*
Leucocytosis, in coalescent mastoiditis, 198, 256
Lever factor, of middle ear, 365
Lipoid granulomatosis, 596–597
Longitudinal sinus, superior, 42, *43*
Lop ear, 229–238
  surgical correction of, 229–238, *230, 231, 233–238*
Lymph node, mastoid, suppuration of, vs. coalescent mastoiditis, 256


Malleus. See also *Ossicle(s).*
  anatomy of, *696, 699, 700, 720*
  ankylosis of, in stapedectomy, 491–492
    lysis of, 491–492
    management of, 435
  embryologic development of, 23, 385
  fused with incus, *396*
  head of, ankylosis of, tympanoplasty for, 435
  mobility of, test for, in stapes operation, 487
  ossification of, 23
Mandibular-facial dysostosis, 385, *386*
Mandibular joint, 39, *40*

Mass tilt, in audiogram. See under *Audiometry.*
Mastoid, air cells of, embryologic development of, 24, *24*
  exenteration of, in simple mastoid operation, 259–261
  carcinoma of, 601, *609*
    removal, *609*
    results of, 612
  cortex of, removal of, in simple mastoid operation, 258
  dressing for, 180, *181*
  embryologic development, 382(t)
  fibrous dysplasia of, 596, *597*
  glomus jugulare tumor of, *614*
  in infant, 27
    and line for incision, *166*
  lymph node, suppuration of, vs. coalescent mastoiditis, 256
  pneumatization of, 24
    Mayer position x-ray, *98*
    Owen position x-ray, *96, 97*
    Stenvers position x-ray, *98, 99*
  tenderness of, in acute suppurative otitis media, exudative stage, 193
  in coalescent mastoiditis, 197, 254
Mastoid cavity, anatomy of, 701–709, *702–708*
Mastoid emissary vein, 37
Mastoid operation(s), in fistula of labyrinth, 328–329
  in lateral sinus thrombophlebitis, 304, 306
  radical, and Bondy modified, 267–287
    anesthesia for, 273
    atticotomy in, 273, *274, 277*
    cavity of, inspection of, 280–281
      obliteration of, 280, *280, 281*
      radiologic appearance of, 103, *103*
    complications of, 285–286
    contraindications for, 272
    development of, 268–269
    endaural approach for, vs. postaural approach, 269
    facial ridge removal in, *275, 277–278*
    pedicle graft for, *280, 281, 281*
    postoperative care of, 284–285, *286*
    problems following, 284
    skin flap for, *276, 278*
    skin grafting of cavity in, 282–284, *283*
    technique for, 272–284
  Bondy modified, indications for, 270–271
    contraindications for, 272
    for atypical chronic otorrhea, 272
    for chronic osteitis, 271–272
    for osteomyelitis, 271–272
    indications for, 269–270
  simple, 251–265
    accidents during, 263–264
    after-care of, 263
    anesthesia for, 258
    cortex removal in, 258
    development of, 251–252
    dressing for, *262*
    exenteration of cells in, 259–262, *260*
    for exposure of facial nerve, 544, *545*
    for petrositis, 339
    incision for, 258, *259*
    indications for, 252–257
    suture of wound in, 262–263
    technique of, 257–263, *259, 260, 262*

Mastoidectomy. See *Mastoid operation(s)*.
Mastoiditis, acute, radiologic appearance of, 97–100
    Law position, *100*
    Owen position, *99*
    "acute hemorrhagic," 199
    atypical, 257
    chronic, radiologic appearance of, 100–103, *101–103*
        Mayer position, *101, 102, 103*
        Owen position, *101, 102, 103*
        with cholesteatoma, 100–101, *101, 102*
    coalescent, 195–198, *196, 197*
        acute, *196, 197*
        atypical, 257
        differential diagnosis of, 256
        latent, 257
        masked, 257
        radiographic changes of, 256
        silent, 257
        simple mastoid operation for, 252–253
        symptoms and signs of, 253–256
    facial paralysis and, 531
Mayer position, in otologic x-ray, 85, 87, *87, 88, 89*
    technique for filming, 95
Meatal plastic flap, in radical and Bondy modified radical mastoid operation, placement of, *276, 282*
    preparation of, *275, 276, 278*
Meatus, auditory. See *Auditory meatus*.
Meckel's cartilage, of first branchial arch, development of malleus and incus from, 385
Melkersson's syndrome, 554
Meniere's disease. See *Endolymphatic hydrops*.
Meningeal artery, middle, *38, 39*
Meninges, temporal bone and, 39–41, *41*
Meningioma, of temporal bone, 668–670
    diagnosis of, 669
    pathology of, 668, *669*
    symptoms of, 668–669, *670*
    treatment of, 669
    vs. acoustic tumor, 640
    tomography in, 134–135, *135*
Meningitis, otitic, generalized, 299–302
        diagnosis of, 300
        pathology of, 299–300
        suppurative labyrinthitis from, 335, *335*
        symptoms of, 300
        treatment of, 300–302
    localized, 297–299, 298(t), *299*
        diagnosis of, 298, 298(t)
        pathology of, 297
        signs of, 297–298
        symptoms of, 297
        treatment of, 298–299, *299*
    purulent, in otitis media, 290
    spinal fluid findings in, 298(t)
Microscope, operating, *158, 177, 178,* 180, 682–683, *682*
    par focal vision for, 683
Microtia, surgical reconstruction in, 391–393, *392*
Middle cranial fossa, dura of, exposure of, in ear surgery, 40
    injury of, in simple mastoid operation, 264
Middle ear, anatomy of 695–701, *696–701*
    carcinoma of, 597–612
        surgical excision of, 600–601, *609*
            results of, 612

Middle ear (*Continued*)
    dimensions of, comparison with wavelength of 1000 cycles, *361*
    embryologic development of, 18–24, *20, 22,* 285
    glomus tumor of, 612–634. See also *Glomus tumor*.
    hydraulic ratio of, 365
    lever factor of, 365
    infection of, facial paralysis and, 531
    inflammatory diseases of, classification of, 188
        pathology and course of, 186–220
    mucoperiosteum of, structure and defense mechanisms of, 187–188
    position in skull, *41*
    pressure transformation in, 355–357
        hydraulic effect in, 359
        lever effect of ossicular chain in, 357–359, *358*
        phylogenetic evolution of, 355–357, *356, 357*
    resonance and efficiency of, 362–363
    transformer ratio of, 365
Middle ear spaces, 45–46
Middle fossa exposure of facial nerve, 540–544, *541–543*
Middle fossa incision, technique of, 171, *172*
Middle fossa removal of acoustic tumor, 649–651, *649*
"Mike's dot," *714*
Mollusc, otolithic organ of, 356, *356*
Mucoperiosteum, of middle ear, structure and defense mechanisms of, 187–188
Mucopus, formation of, 187
Mucous cyst, after radical mastoid operation, 285–286
Multiple sclerosis, hearing loss in, 80
    vs. endolymphatic hydrops, 574
Mumps, hearing loss in, 80
Muscle. See specific muscles.
Muscle graft, pedicle, in radical and Bondy modified mastoid operation, *280, 281, 281*
Myelogram, posterior fossa, 621–622
    in acoustic neuroma, 644–645, *646–648*
Myringitis, chronic, of tympanic membrane, 249
Myringitis bullosa, of tympanic membrane, 245–246
Myringoplasty, 415–422
    overlay technique of, 415–418, *416, 417*
        complications of, 418
    undersurface technique of, 418–422, *420, 421*
Myringostapediopexy, in attic retraction cholesteatoma, 282
    in congenital absence of lenticular process of incus, 404–405, *405, 406*
    in meatal atresia, 401, *401*
    in radical and Bondy modified radical mastoid operation, 282
    "nature's," 282, 375, *376*
Myringotomy, in acute suppurative otitis media, 246, *247*
    in serous otitis media, 246–248, *248*


Nausea, in brain abscess, initial encephalitis stage, 321
    in endolymphatic hydrops, 572
Neck, retraction of, in generalized otitic meningitis, 300
    rigidity of, in localized otitic meningitis, 297

Necrosis, localized, of osseous meatus, 244
Neoplastic disease, tomography of, 130–147, *133–138, 140–147*
Nerve(s). See also specific nerves.
  and temporal bone anatomy, 44–45
  cranial, anatomy of, 693–695
  physiologic block of, pathology of, 525–526
Nerve excitability studies, in facial paralysis, 538–539
Nerve graft, for facial nerve, 547–553, *550–553*
  in removal of carcinoma of external auditory meatus and parotid gland, 601, *608*
Neurapraxia, 525
Neurilemmoma. See *Acoustic neuroma.*
Neurinoma, acoustic. See *Acoustic neuroma.*
Neurofibroma, 530
Neuroma, acoustic. See *Acoustic neuroma.*
Neuromuscular transfer, for facial nerve repair, 553
Neurotmesis, 525
Ninth cranial nerve, 44, 694
Noise, excessive, hearing loss in, 80
Nystagmus, in cerebellar abscess, 323
  in endolymphatic hydrops, 572
  in labyrinthine fistula test, 327
  in serous inflammatory labyrinthitis, 331


Occipital sinus, 42, *43*
Ocular paralysis, in brain abscess, 322
Oculomotor nerve, 693
Opisthotonos, in infants with meningismus, 297
Osseous meatus. See *Auditory meatus, osseous.*
Ossicle(s). See also *Incus; Malleus; Stapes.*
  absence of, hearing loss in, 375–376
  anatomy of, *696, 697, 699, 699, 700*
  axis of rotation of, *358*
  chain of, and tympanic membrane, sound-pressure transformer ratio of, 359
    interruption of, hearing loss in, 374
      tympanoplasty for, 432–436, *433–436*
    lever effect of, in pressure transformation of middle ear, 357
    restoration of continuity of, in tympanoplasty, 451–452
  congenital malformation of, 395–398, *396, 397, 399*
    cases of, 403–406
    hearing loss in, 82
    hearing results in, 401–406, *402*
    management of, 395–398, *396, 397, 399*
    vs. otosclerosis, 388–389
  embryologic development of, 22–24, *22,* 382(t)
  fixation of, by fibrosis, postoperative, 398–399
    by tympanosclerosis, 435
  fractures and dislocation of, 126, *127, 128*
  homograft, in tympanoplasty, 435–436
  in tympanoplasty, 432–436
  interruption of, types of, 432–435, *433, 434, 435*
  malformed, correction by substitute tympanic membrane against stapes, 395, *396*
  ossification of, 23
  protection of cochlea by, 365
Ossiculectomy, partial, in fenestration operation, *510*
Osteitis, and otitis, vs. osteitis and cholesteatoma, 129

Osteitis (*Continued*)
  chronic, radical mastoidectomy for, 271–272
    suppurative otitis media from, 217–218
Osteocytes, death of, and otospongiosis, 460
Osteogenesis imperfecta, and otospongiosis, 461
Osteoma, of osseous meatus, *206,* 238–240, *239*
  audiogram in, *370*
  of temporal bone, radiologic appearance of, 106, *107*
Osteomyelitis, suppurative otitis media from, 217–218
  radical mastoidectomy for, 271–272
Osteoplastic epitympanotomy, for cholesteatoma, 448–450, *448–450*
Osteothrombophlebitis, extension of infection in otitis media by, 293
Otic capsule, ossification of, 14–18, *16, 17*
  in pig embryo, *16, 17*
  intermediate stage of, *566*
Otic labyrinth. See *Endolymphatic labyrinth.*
Otic pit, 6, *6*
Otic placode, 6
  in embryologic development of ear, 382(t)
Otitis externa, malignant, 245
  facial paralysis and, 531
Otitis media, acute, facial paralysis and, 531
  adhesive, chronic, hearing loss in, 82
  allergic, 207–208
    contraindication to radical mastoid operation, 272
  bacterial, acute, complicating viral head cold or influenza, 189
  brain abscess from, 317–326
  catarrhal, chronic, 82
  complications of, meningeal, 289–315
    non-meningeal, 317–347
  differential diagnosis of, 218–219
  hearing loss from, 82
  labyrinthitis following, 326–337
  meningeal complications of, 289–315
    pathways of spread of, 292–295
  necrotic, acute, 200–207, *204*
    findings, 205
    in scarlet fever, *204*
    pathology, 203–205, *204*
    results, *206, 207*
    symptoms, 205
    therapy, 205–207
  non-meningeal complications of, 317–347
  petrositis following, 337–345
  purulent, acute. See *Otitis media, suppurative, acute.*
  secretory, myringotomy in, 246–248, *248*
    radiologic appearance of, 105–106, *105, 106*
    with fluid in middle ear, audiogram in, *56*
  suppurative, acute, 188, 189–200
    characteristics of, 191
    coalescent mastoiditis in, 195–198, *196, 197*
    complication stage, 198–200
    etiology of, 190
    exudation stage, 193–194
    frequency of, 190
    hyperemia stage, 191–193, *192*
    myringotomy for, 246, *247*
    resolution stage, 202
    stages of, 191–200
    suppuration stage, 194–195
    tympanic membrane perforation from, 410

Otitis media, suppurative (*Continued*)
    chronic, 210–218
        atypical, radical mastoid operation for, 272
        benign, 210–212
        cholesteatoma in, 212–217, *217*
        osteitis or osteomyelitis as cause, 217–218
        facial paralysis from, 345, 530–531
        hearing loss in, 82
    tomography in, 128–130, *130, 131, 132*
    tubercular, 208–210, *209*
    viral, 188–189
    with cholesteatoma, tomography in, 128–129,
        *129, 130*
    with cholesteatoma and fistula of lateral
        semicircular canal, tomography in, *131*
Otocyst, 6
    development of sensory labyrinth from, 381
    embryologic development of, 382(t)
Otodystrophies, tomography in, 147–152
Otolithic organ, of mollusc, 356, *356*
Otorrhea, after simple mastoid operation, causes,
        263
    cerebrospinal, 312–313
    chronic, atypical, mastoidectomy for, 272
    in cholesteatoma, secondary acquired, 270
    in coalescent mastoiditis, 198, 253
    in otitis media, necrotic, acute, 205
        suppurative, benign chronic, 211
        tubercular, 210
    in petrositis, 339
    radical mastoidectomy for, 270
Otosclerosis. See *Otospongiosis.*
Otosclerotic notch. See *Carhart notch.*
Otoscopic inspection, 71–73, *71*
Otoscopy, 71–73, *71*
Otospongiosis (otosclerosis), 455–475
    cochlear, diagnosis of, 469–470
        criteria for, 470
        hearing loss in, 81
        sodium fluoride for, 470, 472–474
        tomography in, 148, *149, 150,* 470
    diagnosis of, 466–471, *466, 467, 468, 470*
    etiology of, 459–465, *460, 462–464*
    familial predisposition in, 465
    fenestration operation for, 501–515. See also
        *Fenestration operation.*
        selection of cases for, 471–472
    histologic, lesion of, *457*
        silent, *457,* 465
    medical treatment for, 472–474, *472, 473*
    natural history of, 465–466
    new bone formation and, in fissula ante
        fenestram, 11, 13, *14, 15*
        in fossula post fenestram, 14
    of oval window, 490
    pathology of, gross, 456–457
        microscopic, 457–459, *457, 458*
    sensorineural hearing loss due to, criteria for,
        470–471, *471*
    sex incidence of, 458
    sodium fluroide for, *463, 464,* 470, 472–474,
        *472, 473*
    stapedial, 13, 14, *15,* 456, *458*
        and cochlear otospongiosis, audiogram in,
            *466*
        ankylosis in, of anterior end of stapes
            footplate, *458*

Otospongiosis (otosclerosis), stapedial (*Continued*)
        audiogram air curve in, *369*
        bone conduction curve in, *366, 367*
        diagnosis of, 466–468, *467, 468*
        hearing loss in, 81, 82, *473,* 480
    stapes operation for, 477–499. See also
        *Stapes operations.*
    surgery for, 471–472
    tomography in, 148–152, *148–151*
    vs. ossicular malformations without atresia,
        388–389
    vs. Paget's disease, 461, *464, 465*
Outer ear. See *External ear.*
Oval window, and round window, phase
        difference between, 360–362, *360, 361*
    congenital absence of, tomographic appearance
        of, *125*
    in tympanoplasty, sound-pressure transforma-
        tion for, 428
    otospongiosis of, 490
Overlay technique, of myringoplasty, 415–418,
        *416, 417*
Owen position, in otologic x-ray, 88–89, *90,* 95


Paget's disease, of temporal bone, 461
    radiologic appearance of, 106, *107*
    vs. otospongiosis, 461, *464, 465*
Pain, in coalescent mastoiditis, 254
    in petrositis, 339
Palsy, Bell's. See *Bell's palsy.*
Papilledema, in otitic hydrocephalus, 309
Parotid gland, carcinoma of, from external
        auditory meatus, removal of, 601, *604–608*
Pars flaccida, of tympanic membrane, retraction
        of, in attic retraction cholesteatoma, 213–216
Pars tensa, in cholesteatoma, excision of, 282
    in suppurative otitis media, acute, 246, *247*
    layers of, 413–414
    perforation of, hearing loss in, 81
    tear of, traumatic, 248–249
Partial ossicular replacement prosthesis
        (P.O.R.P.), 427, *433, 435*
P.B. score, 63–64, *66*
Pedicle muscle graft, in radical and Bondy modi-
        fied mastoid operation, 280, 281, *281,* 282
Performance-intensity function, 63–64, *66*
Perichondritis, after radical mastoid operation,
        285
    of auricle, 226, *227*
Perilymph, and endolymph, pressure equilibra-
        tion between, 569–572, *570, 571*
    flow of, in stapedectomy, 492
    formation and resorption of, 566–568, *567*
Perilymph fistula, after stapes operation, 493–494
Perilymphatic duct, 11, *567*
    embryologic development of, 11, 12
Perilymphatic labyrinth, embryologic develop-
        ment of, 10–14
Periosteum, retraction of, in radical and Bondy
        modified radical mastoid operation, 273, *274*
    thickening of, in coalescent mastoiditis, 198,
        254
Periotic duct. See *Perilymphatic duct.*
Periotic labyrinth. See *Perilymphatic labyrinth.*
Perisinus abscess, 295–296

Petro-occipital sinus of Englisch, inferior, 42
Petrosal nerve, greater superficial, 719
Petrosal sinus, inferior, 42, 43
  superior, 38, 39, 42, 43
Petrosectomy, Lempert-Ramadier, 340, 342, 343, 344–345
Petrositis, 337–345
  definition and pathology of, 337–338
  diagnosis of, 339
  etiology of, 338
  radiologic appearance of, 100
  symptoms of, 338–339
  treatment of, 339–345, 341–343
    development of, 290
    surgical, 340, 341–343, 344–345
Petrosquamous suture, 28, 37
Petrosquamous suture line, 27, 28
Petrous apex, anatomy of, 691, 692
Petrous pyramid, congenital cholesteatoma of, 670–672, 671
  meningioma of, 670
  semiaxial projection of, in tomography, 120–121, 120
Phlebitis, femoral, after fenestration, 513
Pneumatic cell(s), temporal bone, 50–51
  embryologic development of, 24–25, 25
Pneumatization, of mastoid. See under Mastoid.
  of temporal bone, 24–25, 24, 386
Pneumococcus, in petrositis, 338
Pneumoventriculography, in diagnosis of brain abscess, 324
Politzer inflation of eustachian tube, 75–76, 76
Polyp(s), of ear canal, removal of, 436
  of external auditory meatus, 243–244
Polytome x-ray, in acoustic neuroma, 644
  in facial paralysis, 535
  in glomus tumors, 617–619, 618, 619
P.O.R.P. See Partial ossicular replacement prosthesis.
Portmann's endolymphatic sac operation. See Endolymphatic sac, surgery of.
Postaural incision. See Postauricular incision.
Postauricular incision, in simple mastoid operation, 258, 259
  in tympanoplasty, 440, 443
  local anesthesia for, 165, 166
  technique of, 166, 167–168
  Wilde incision, in simple mastoid operation, 258, 259
Posterior cranial fossa, dura of, in ear surgery, 41
  injury of, in simple mastoid operation, 264
Preauricular cyst and fistula, congenital, 235, 385
Preformed pathway, extension of infection in otitis media by, 294–295
Pregnancy, and otosclerosis, 461
Preoperative sedation, for ear surgery, 163–165
Presbycusis, 81
  loss of ganglion cells of cochlea in, 564
  with endolymphatic hydrops, audiogram in, 563
  horizontal semicircular canal in, 564
Pressure transformation. See Sound-pressure transformation in middle ear.
Prosthesis, for closure of tympanic membrane perforation, 413
  in tympanoplasty, 432–435, 435

Prosthesis (Continued)
  partial ossicular replacement (P.O.R.P.), 433, 435
  total ossicular replacement (T.O.R.P.), 434, 435
Psammoma body, in meningioma of temporal bone, 668, 669
Pseudomonas aeruginosa, and perichondritis of auricle, 226
Pseudomonas infection, in diabetics, 531
Psychogenic deafness, 80–81
Psychosomatic ear disease, 53

Queckenstedt test, for lateral sinus thrombophlebitis, 304

Radiation therapy, for glomus tumors, 622, 623
Radical cavity, anatomy of, 709
Radical mastoid operation. See Mastoid operation, radical.
Radiologic examination, in acoustic neuroma, 108, 109, 109, 110, 643–646, 643, 645, 646
  in acute mastoiditis, 97–99, 99, 100
  in acute suppurative otitis media, exudative stage, 193
  in benign tumor, 106, 107
  in chronic mastoiditis, 100–103, 101–103
  in coalescent mastoiditis, 198, 256
  in congenital atresia, 104, 105
  in congenital cholesteatoma, 104, 104
  in facial paralysis, 534–535
  in fractures, 106, 107
  in glomus tumors, 109, 110, 617–622, 618–621
  in otospongiosis, 109
  in Paget's disease, 106, 107
  in petrositis, 100
  in secretory otitis media, 105–106, 105, 106
  of temporal bone, 84–111
    interpretation of, 96–110
    positions for, 84–96
    technique of filming, 94–95, 94
Ramsay Hunt syndrome, 531, 532
Recruitment of loudness, in endolymphatic hydrops, 560, 573
  test for. See Alternate binaural loudness balance test.
Rectus sinus. See Straight sinus.
Rinne tuning fork test, 59
  in endolymphatic hydrops, 573
  in stapes fixation, 472
Rongeur, technique of using, 175, 177
Round window, and oval window, phase difference between, 360–362, 360, 361
  border of, otospongiosis focus in, 457
  closure of, hearing loss in, 376–377
    in otospongiosis, 492
  function of, 359–360
  in diseased ear, 428
  in normal ear, 428
  in tympanoplasty, sound protection for, 427, 428
Rubella, and congenital malformations of ear, 387

Saccular duct, embryologic development of, 6, 7
Saccule, 356
  dilatation of, in endolymphatic hydrops, 571
Sacculotomy, for endolymphatic hydrops, 583
Sagittal sinus, superior. See Longitudinal sinus, superior.
Salivary flow studies, in facial paralysis, 537–538, 538
Salt, restriction of, in endolymphatic hydrops, 576
Scala tympani, embryologic development of, 11
Scala vestibuli, embryologic development of, 11
Scapha, 32
Schirmer test, in facial paralysis, 535–536, 536
Schuknecht's transtympanic labyrinthotomy for endolymphatic hydrops, 580, 581
Schüller position, in otologic x-ray, 85, 86, 95
Schwabach tuning fork test, 59
Schwannoma. See Acoustic neuroma.
Schwartze sign, in otospongiosis, 456, 458, 470
Sebaceous cyst, of auricle, 228
Sedation, in endolymphatic hydrops, 577
  preoperative, for ear surgery, 163–165
Sedimentation rate, in coalescent mastoiditis, 198, 256
Semiaxial projection of the petrous pyramid, in tomography, 120–121, 121
Semicircular canal(s), anatomy of, 51, 708, 710
  embryologic development of, 6, 382(t)
  horizontal, fistualization of, in Cawthorne's labyrinthotomy, 581, 582
    identification of, in endolymphatic sac surgery, 584, 585
    in endolymphatic hydrops with presbycusis, 564
    osseous, enchondralization of, in fenestration, 509
  lateral, anatomy of, 703
  superior, 720, 721
    ampulla of, 712, 724
Sensorineural function, bone-conducted hearing as measure of, 365–366
Sensorineural hearing loss, etiologic types of, 78–81
Sensory end-organs, embryologic development of, 10
Seventh cranial nerve, 44, 45, 694
Shambaugh continuous irrigator-suction, 176
Shambaugh formula for prediction of results of fenestration, 505, 505
Shambaugh operating microscope, 178
"Shambaugh's gland," 568
Shea electric drill, 173, 174
Shea technique of stapedectomy, vein graft for, 488, 489
Short increment sensitivity index (SISI), 64. 66
  in endolymphatic hydrops, 573
  in hearing loss, 66
Sigmoid sinus, 42–44, 43
  perforation of, in fenestration operation, 511
  thrombus of, jugular vein ligation for, 306, 310, 311
Sigmoid sinus plate, 44, 44
Sinodural angle, 44, 46
Sinus. See specific sinuses.
Sinus tympani, anatomy of, 699, 701
SISI. See Short increment sensitivity index.

Sixth cranial nerve, 44, 693
  paralysis of, in otitic hydrocephalus, 309
Skin, sterilization of, in temporal bone surgery, 158–159
Skin grafts, in osseous meatus, 398, 399
  in radical mastoid cavity, 282–284, 283
  meatal, in myringoplasty, incision for, 416
    placement of, 417
Skull base, glomus tumor of, 612–634
  surgical approach to, 629–634, 630–633
Skull fracture, extralabyrinthine, tomography in, 126, 127
  facial paralysis in, 526–529, 527, 528
    facial nerve decompression in, 540–547, 541–547
  hearing loss in, 79
Smoking, tobacco, in endolymphatic hydrops, 578–579
Sodium fluoride, for otospongiosis, 463, 464, 469–470, 470, 472–474, 472, 473
  tomographic follow-up for, 151, 151
Sodium restriction, in endolymphatic hydrops, 576
Solid angle, 46, 46
Sound, nature of, 353–355, 354
Sound-conducting system, congenital malformations of, diagnosis of, 388–389, 389
  indications for surgery of, 389–390
  surgical correction of, 380–407
  surgical technique for, 390–399
  embryologic development of, 381–388, 382(t)
  evolutionary development of, 18
Sound conduction, mechanics of, 355–370
Sound-pressure transformation in middle ear, 355–357
  hydraulic effect in, 359
  lever effect of ossicular chain in, 357, 358, 359
Sound-pressure transformer ratio of middle ear, 359, 365, 428
Speculum, ear, technique of holding, 71
Speech discrimination tests, 58–59
Speech reception threshold (SRT), 58
Spina helicis, 32
Spinal fluid, drainage from ear, 312–313
  examination of, in suppurative inflammatory labyrinthitis, 334
  findings in meningitis, 298(t)
  in brain abscess, 322
  leak of, after translabyrinthine removal of acoustic neuroma, 666
    surgical, 40–41
  pressure of, in lateral sinus thrombophebitis, 302
    in otitic hydrocephalus, 309
Spiral ganglion cells of cochlea. See under Cochlea.
Splinting, for closure of tympanic membrane perforation, 413
Squamous cell carcinoma, of ear, 596, 599–612
  removal of, 600, 602–611
  tomography in, 131–132, 133
SRT. See Speech reception threshold.
Stapedectomy, 486–498
  after fenestration, 494–496, 495
  "biscuit footplate" in, 490, 491
  complications of, 493–494
  facial nerve in, 481, 490
  fixed malleus in, 491–492

Stapedectomy (Continued)
  floating footplate problem in, 490
  fracture of incus in, 492
  indications for, 480
  instruments for, 488
  obliterative otospongiosis problem in, 490
  perilymph fistula after, 493–494
  perilymph leak in, 492
  postoperative care in, 492–493
  problems during, 490–492, 491
  procedure for, 486–489, 487, 488, 489
  revision of, 496, 497
  round window closure in, 492
  sensorineural hearing loss after, 496–498
  Shea technique for, 488, 489, 489
    vein graft for, 488, 489
Stapedial otospongiosis (otosclerosis), 82–83
Stapedial reflex, absence of, in facial paralysis,
    537
Stapedius muscle, anatomy of, 698
  function of, 364
Stapes. See also Ossicle(s).
  anatomy of, 699, 700
  ankylosis of, congenital, 386
  congenital absence of crural arch and tendon,
    402
  congenital fixation of, 402
  emaciation of, after ossification, 386
  embryologic development of, 22–23, 22
  exposure of, instruments for, 484
  fixation of, by fibrosis, 398–399
    congenital, 402
    hearing loss in, 377
    otospongiotic. See Otospongiosis, stapedial.
    surgical correction of, 397
  footplate, embryologic development of, 23
    otospongiotic focus in, 490, 491
  malformation of, 386
  mobilization of, by anterior crurotomy, 484–486,
    485, 486
    instruments for, 486
    technique for, 485
  development of, 477–479
Stapes operations, anesthesia for, 166, 482
  for otospongiosis, 477–499
    exposure of oval window in, 482, 483, 484,
      484
    indications for, 480
    postoperative care in, 492–493
    principles underlying, 479–480
    revisions of, 496, 497
    sensorineural loss after, 496–498
    technique for, 481–489, 481, 483–489
      anesthesia in, 482
      oval window exposure in, 482–484, 483,
        484, 485
      preoperative preparation for, 481–482, 481
      tissue graft for, 482
  secondary, after radical mastoid operation, 284
  selection of cases for, 471–472
Stenosis, cicatricial, of auditory meatus, 240–241
Stenvers position, in otologic x-ray, 89, 91, 94–95
  in tomography, 118–120, 119, 120
Sternocleidomastoid muscle, 35
Steroids, for brain abscess, 326
Stiffness tilt, in stapedial otospongiosis audio-
  gram, 467, 467

Straight sinus, 42, 43
Streptococcus, beta hemolytic, in petrositis, 338
Streptomycin, for endolymphatic hydrops, 579
Stress, endolymphatic hydrops and, 578–579
Submento-vertex position, in otologic x-ray, 89,
    93
Subperiosteal abscess, in coalescent mastoiditis,
    254–255, 255
  postaural, in infant, incision for, 27, 166
Suction, House apparatus, 176
  Shambaugh apparatus, 176
Sulfonamides, and incidence of meningeal
    complications of otitis media, 290–291
Suprameatal spine of Henle, 36
Sural nerve, graft from, for facial nerve repair,
    550, 552
Syphilitic nerve deafness, 79


Taste test, in facial paralysis, 536–537, 536
Tear test. See Schirmer test.
Tegmen, of attic and antrum, 45
Television, for viewing surgery, 179
Temporal artery, superficial, 35
Temporal bone, 36, 38
  air cells, development of, 24–25, 24
  anatomy of, surgical, 31–51, 675–725
  cysts of, varieties of, 596
  development of, from birth to adulthood, 26
  dissection of, 675–725
    House-Urban bone holder for, 684
    instruments for, 685
    laboratory for, 683–686, 684, 685
    microscope for, 681–683, 682
      par focal vision for, 683
    removal of bone for, 680–681, 680
  external, anatomy of, 686–692, 686–692
  facial nerve in, 524
  fracture of, and facial paralysis, 527–528,
    527, 528
    radiologic appearance of, 106, 107
  in infant, 25
    landmarks on, 37, 37
    vs. adult, 26–29, 26
  incisions for exposure of, 167–172,
    169–172
  inferior surface of, anatomy of, 690–691, 691
  lateral surface of, anatomy of, 686–687
    surgical landmarks of, 36–37, 36, 37
  meninges and, 39–41, 41
  meningioma of, 668–670, 669, 670
  nerves with, 44–45
    anatomy of, 693–695
  pneumatic cells of, 50–51
    development of, 24–25, 25
  posterior surface of, anatomy of, 689
  radiologic examination of. See Radiologic
    examination.
  removal of, procedure for, 680–681, 680
  stages of development of, 26
  superior approach to, anatomy of, 719–725
  superior surface of, anatomy of, 688–689
    surgical landmarks of, 38–39, 38
  surgery of, 155–183. See also Ear, surgery of;
      and specific operations.
    anesthetic for, 34–35, 35

Temporal bone, surgery of, (*Continued*)
    antibiotic therapy for, 160–163
    aseptic technique for, 155–160
    postoperative care in, 180–182, *181*
    postoperative dressings for, 181–182, *181*
    principles of, 155–183. See also specific
        operations.
    surgical anatomy of, 31–51
        through dissection, 675–725
    surgical landmarks of, 36–39, *36, 37, 38*
    tomographic anatomy of, 113–122
    tomography of, 112–153
    tumors of, benign, radiologic appearance of,
        106, *107*
        varieties of, 596
    vessels with, anatomy of, 692–693
Temporal bone dissection, 675–725
Temporal fascia grafts, in myringoplasty, 415, 419
    incision for, *416*
        placement of, *417, 421*
    in tympanoplasty, *438, 441*
Temporal line, 36–37, *36*
Temporal lobe abscess, 319, 321
    symptoms of, 322
Temporal muscle, 36
Tensor tympani muscle, function of, 364
Tenth cranial nerve, 44, 45, 695
Thalidomide, and congenital malformations of
    ear, 387–388, *387*
Third cranial nerve, 693
Thrombophlebitis, extension of ear infection by,
    199
    femoral, after surgery, prevention of, 180
    lateral sinus, 302–309
        diagnosis of, 303–304
        jugular vein ligation for, 308–309, *310, 311*
        mastoidectomy for, 304, 306
        pathology of, 302–303
        symptoms of, 303
        treatment of, 304–309, *305*
Thrombosis, of jugular bulb, surgery for, 307
    of lateral sinus, in otitis media, 290
    of sigmoid sinus, jugular vein ligation for, 306,
        *310, 311*
Tinnitus, in acoustic neuroma, 640
    in endolymphatic hydrops, 573
    in glomus tumors, 615
    in labyrinthine deafness, sudden, 575
Tissue grafts, in tympanoplasty, 444, *444*
    complications of, 451
Tobacco smoking, in endolymphatic hydrops,
    578–579
Tobey-Ayer-Queckenstedt test, for lateral sinus
    thrombophlebitis, 304
Tomography, in acoustic neuroma, 146–147, *146,*
    *147*
    in pathologic ear conditions, 122–152
    of temporal bone, 112–153
    projections in, 114–122
Tone decay tests, 63, 66
Topographic studies, in facial paralysis, 535–537,
    *536*
Torcular Herophili, 42, *43*
Total ossicular replacement prosthesis (T.O.R.P.),
    427, 434, *435*
Toxic nerve deafness, 79
Toynbee's artificial tympanic membrane, 408,
    *409*
Tragus, *32*

Transformer ratio. *See Sound-pressure*
    *transformer ratio of middle ear.*
Translabyrinthine anatomy, 710–715, *710–715*
Translabyrinthine labyrinthectomy, for
    endolymphatic hydrops, 581, 583
Translabyrinthine removal of acoustic neuroma,
    650, 651–656, *651–654*
Translabyrinthine-suboccipital removal of
    acoustic neuroma, *655*, 656–657, *656–661*
Transverse sinus(es). See *Lateral sinus(es).*
Trauma, acoustic, hearing loss in, 79
    to skull, tomography in, 126–128, *127, 128, 129*
    tympanic membrane perforation from, 410
Trautmann's triangle, 46, *46*
Treacher-Collins syndrome, 385, *386*
Trigeminal ganglion, 45, 693
Trochlear nerve, 693
Tullio phenomenon, in labyrinthine fistula, 328
Tumor(s), acoustic. See *Acoustic neuroma.*
    facial paralysis from, 529–530
    glomus, 612–634. See also *Glomus tumor.*
    of cerebellopontine angle, 637–673
    of ear, surgery of, 595–635
    tomographic appearance of, 130–147
    vs. endolymphatic hydrops, 574
Tuning fork tests, 59–61, *61*
Twelfth nerve, 695
Tympanic cavity, anatomy of, 695–701, *696–701.*
    See also *Tympanum.*
Tympanic membrane, absence of, hearing loss in,
    375–376
    anatomy of, *696, 697, 707*
    and ossicular chain, sound-pressure transformer
        of, 359
    artificial, Toynbee's, *409*
    axis of rotation of, *358*
    embryologic development of, 21
    in acute suppurative otitis media, 191, *192*
    in coalescent mastoiditis, 256
    in tuberculosis of middle ear, *209*
    incision of. See *Myringotomy.*
    movements of, for 2000 cycle tone, *356*
    myringitis bullosa of, 245–246
    myringitis of, 249
    pars flaccida, attic retraction cholesteatoma of,
        213–216
        therapy for, 216
    pars tensa. See *Pars tensa.*
    perforation of, *206*
        closure of, 408–423
            contraindications to, 412–413
            development of, 408–410, *409*
            indications for, 412
            myringoplasty for, 415–422
            promotion of healing for, 413–415
            prosthetic, 413
            splinting for, 413
        etiology and pathology of, 410–411, *411*
        hearing loss in, 372–373, 411–412
        in coalescent mastoiditis, 198
        in fenestration operation, 511
        in otitis media, chronic suppurative, 211
            necrotic, *206, 207*
        otoscopic examination of, 72
        spontaneous healing of, 410–411
        stratified squamous epithelium in, 411, *411*
        traumatic, 248–249
            splinting of, 413
            treatment of, 249

Tympanic membrane (*Continued*)
  position in skull, *41*
  substitute, against mobile stapes, *396*
    construction of, *398*
  surgical conditions of, 245–249
Tympanic sulcus, embryologic development of, 21
Tympanogram, types of, *62*
Tympanomastoid suture, *36, 37*
Tympanomeatal plastic flap, in fenestration operation, construction of, *507*
    placement of, *510*
    tear of, *511*
Tympanometry, 61–63, *62, 63*
Tympanoplasty, 425–453
  after radical mastoid operation, 284
  anesthesia for, 432
  canal wall down, *440–441, 441–442*
  complications of, 450–451
  contraindications to, 430–431
  definition of, 429–430, *429*
  development of, 425–427
  dressing for, *181*
  fitted incus in, 432–433, *433–435*
  for cholesteatoma, 437–439, *438*
  incus transposition in, 432
  indications for, 430–431
  intact canal wall, 442–450, *443–450*
  partial ossicular replacement prosthesis in, *433, 435*
  physiologic principles of, 427–429
  postauricular incision for, *440, 443*
  preoperative evaluation for, 431
  results of, 451–452
  staging of disease in, 439
  techniques of, 432–450
  total ossicular replacement prosthesis in, *434, 435*
  type II, *438*
  type III, *440, 441*
  types of, *429*
  with intact tympanic membrane, 432–436
  Wright eustachian tube prosthesis for, *436, 436*
Tympanosclerosis, vs. stapes ankylosis, 469
Tympanosquamous suture, *36, 37*
Tympanum, 45
  air-containing space in, at birth, 24
  embryologic development of, 23, 24, 382(t)
  "epidermoid cyst" of, *218*
  inspection of, in radical mastoid operation, 278–280, *279*
  promontory, 49

Undersurface technique, of myringoplasty, 418–422, *420, 421*
Ultrasound, for endolymphatic hydrops, 583–584
Utricle, dilatation of, in endolymphatic hydrops, 561, *562*
Utricular duct, embryologic development of, 6, 7
Utriculoendolymphatic fold (valve of Bast), 9–10, *9*

Vagus nerve, 45, 695
  auricular branch of, anesthesia for, 165, *166*
van der Hoeve's syndrome, *462*
Vein. See specific veins.
Vein graft, for Shea technique of stapedectomy, 488, *489*
Venogram, retrograde, in glomus tumor, 620–621, *621*
Venous sinuses, cranial, 41–44, *43, 44*
Vertigo, in endolymphatic hydrops, 572
  in labyrinthine deafness, sudden, 575
  in labyrinthine fistula test, 328
  in petrositis, 339
  postural, vs. endolymphatic hydrops, 574
Vestibular aqueduct, 566, *567*
Vestibular lesion, central, vs. endolymphatic hydrops, 574
Vestibular nerve, 694
  section of, for endolymphatic hydrops, 587, *588*
  superior, *717, 723*
Vestibular sterile labyrinthitis, after fenestration, 513
Vestibular tests, 66–71
  in acoustic neuroma, 642–643
  in facial paralysis, 534
  in glomus tumors, 617
Vestibule, anatomy of, *713*
Visual field defects, in left temporal lobe abscess, 322
Vomiting, in brain abscess, 321, 322
  in endolymphatic hydrops, 572
  in localized otitic meningitis, 300
von Recklinghausen's disease, 80, 649

Water, cold, and exostoses of external auditory meatus, 238, 240
  caloric response to. See *Caloric test, cold water.*
Weber test, 60
Wright eustachian tube prosthesis, for tympanoplasty, 436, *436*

Xanthomatosis, 596–597
X-ray. See *Radiologic examination.*

Zeiss magnifying loupe, *178*
Zeiss operating microscope, *682*
Zeiss otomicroscope, 180
Z-plasty, for reconstruction of microtic auricle, 392, *392*
Zygomatic abscess, in coalescent mastoiditis, 255